Cranial
Osteopathy

Torsten Liem DO is registered with the General Osteopathic Council (GB), and Principal of Osteopathie Schule Deutschland (Germany) and of an MSc program in Pediatric Osteopathy. He is a member of the Research Committee of the Akademie der Osteopathie (AFO), and is author of *Praktisches Lehrbuch der Kraniosakralen Osteopathie, Praxis der Kraniosakralen Osteopathie, Osteopathie – Die sanfte Lösung von Blockaden,* Coeditor of the *Lietfaden Osteopathie* and Cofounder and former Chief Editor of the journal *Osteopathische Medezin*.

All photography © **Karsten Franke**, Hamburg, Germany.

For Elsevier

Senior Commissioning Editor: Sarena Wolfaard
Project Development Manager: Claire Wilson
Project Manager: Ailsa Laing
Designer: Keith Kail

Cranial Osteopathy
Principles and Practice

SECOND EDITION

Torsten Liem DO Osteopath GOsC (GB)
Principal, Osteopathie Schule Deutschland, Hamburg, Germany

With a contribution by
Professor John M McPartland DO MSc
Associate Professor, School of Osteopathy, UNITEC, Auckland, New Zealand
Assistant Professor, Department of Family Practice, College of Medicine, University of Vermont, Burlington, USA

Evelyn Skinner BA DO
Lecturer, School of Osteopathy, UNITEC, Auckland, New Zealand
Clinical Director, The Twig Centre, Wellington, New Zealand

Forewords by
Jean Pierre Barral DO
Academic Principal of the Collège International d'Osteopathie in St. Etienne, Lecturer in the Faculty of Medicine in Paris Nord, the European School of Osteopathy in Maidstone and the Osteopathie Schule Deutschland

Fred L Mitchell jnr DO FAAO FCA
Professor Emeritus of the College of Osteopathic Medicine of Michigan State University, USA

Richard A Feely DO FAAO FCA FAAMA
Past President of the Cranial Academy, Associate Professor of the Chicago College of Osteopathic Medicine, Midwestern University, USA

Translated by
Elaine Richards, David Beattie and Mary Alexander

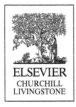

ELSEVIER
CHURCHILL
LIVINGSTONE

Edinburgh   London   New York   Oxford   Philadelphia   St Louis   Sydney   Toronto   2004

ELSEVIER
CHURCHILL
LIVINGSTONE

First and Second Editions published in German under the title
Praxis der Kraniosakralen Osteopathie
© 2000, 2003 Hippokrates Verlag in MVS Medizinverlage Stuttgart Gmb & Co. KG

Second edition published in English
© 2004, Elsevier Limited. All rights reserved.

First edition 2000
Second edition 2003
English edition 2004

ISBN 0 443 07499 2

British Library Cataloguing in Publication Data
A catalogue record for this book is available from the British Library

Library of Congress Cataloging in Publication Data
A catalog record for this book is available from the Library of Congress

Note

Every effort has been made by the Author and the Publishers to ensure that the descriptions of the techniques included in this book are accurate and in conformity with the descriptions published by their developers. The Publishers and the Authors do not assume any responsibility for any injury and/or damage to persons or property arising out of or related to any use of the material contained in this book. It is the responsibility of the treating practitioner, relying on independent experience and knowledge of the patient, to determine the best treatment and method of application for the patient, to make their own evaluation of their effectiveness and to check with the developers or teachers of the techniques they wish to use that they have understood them correctly.

The Publisher

ELSEVIER your source for books, journals and multimedia in the health sciences

www.elsevierhealth.com

Transferred to Digital Printing in 2009

The publisher's policy is to use paper manufactured from sustainable forests

Contents

Contents

Forewords

Life is motion. This principle applies just as surely to osteopathy and its subdivisions; as a science, as an art and as a philosophy, osteopathy is not static, but continually in motion. The great challenge before us is to remain firmly rooted in the principles of osteopathy as we simultaneously open ourselves to the dynamics of life, allowing ourselves to be affected by our daily contact with patients, by new scientific insights, by the exchange of ideas among colleagues, and by the demands of the time in which we live.

Torsten Liem's previous volume in German impressed me at first sight on account of its instructional layout and uniquely comprehensive and lively presentation of craniosacral osteopathy.

The present work continues that tradition. The anatomical and physiological aspects of the visceral structures of the cranium and their associated dysfunctions and methods of treatment are presented with the utmost detail and clarity. This work serves at the same time as a speedy reference manual in the course of practice, providing a description of the techniques relating to each cranial bone and the diagnosis and treatment of the facial organs, and systematically setting out their possible dysfunctions. The author meanwhile does not lose sight of the essential: that capacity to be inwardly touched by the uniqueness of each contact and of osteopathy itself.

I am convinced that students of osteopathy and practicing osteopaths will agree in welcoming this book.

France, 2004   Jean Pierre Barral

I have for some years been aware of the need for a comprehensive textbook of craniosacral work. For many years *The Cranial Bowl* (1939) by Sutherland and Magoun's *Osteopathy in the Cranial Field* (1951) were the sole works in this field, although neither had been conceived or written as a textbook. Each of these books focused in the first instance on the clinical relevance of investigating and treating the phenomenon that Sutherland called the primary respiratory mechanism, and providing a theoretical basis for craniosacral osteopathy.

Howard and Rebecca Lippincott compiled their first handbook of craniosacral techniques from the notes they made during their period of study under William G. Sutherland and published it in

1943 through the auspices of the Academy of Applied Osteopathy. A second revised edition was published in 1946 by the Osteopathic Cranial Association. This describes about 60 techniques, many of which were later exchanged or replaced by the authors or by other students of the cranial concept. Many of these changes, however, still remain to be written down.

Since the 1930s/1940s, cranial techniques have multiplied in the minds and hearts of creative students. Many of these students, such as Charlotte Weaver, Beryl Arbuckle and Viola Frymann, have emphasized the importance of embryology and the use of craniosacral osteopathy in practical pediatrics. Special techniques were developed for use in this field. Will Sutherland's courses must have attracted especially creative minds. Paul Kimberly, Alan R. Becker, Rollin Becker, Robert Fulford, Kenneth Little, J. Gordon Zink, Olive Stretch, Tom Schooley, Howard Lippincott, Rebecca Lippincott, Anne Wales and Harold Magoun Sr. were some of the students of Sutherland whose ideas formed my own craniosacral concept. Each of these made their own unique contributions as to methods.

Torsten Liem has produced outstanding work in research, and presents in this edition, an excellent selection of beautifully illustrated craniosacral techniques, which will provide the reader with well balanced instruction in the basics of craniosacral work. The section on temporomandibular dysfunctions will be an inspiration to many readers with its depth and detail.

A *word of caution*: gentleness is the first essential to master in any course of training in craniosacral osteopathy. Clinically effective craniosacral manipulation demands gentleness and patience. Craniosacral work is often described as 'non-invasive', but that is too simplistic. The art is to learn to reach down through the tissue with sympathetically attuned understanding and not just with the hands. The treatment route to be followed is decided on the basis of the clinical assessment, founded on scientific anatomical and physiological knowledge, which indicates whether particular techniques of manual medicine can helpfully be employed.

USA, 2004   Fred L. Mitchell Jnr

Torsten Liem's stimulating work on cranial osteopathy is designed for the osteopathic physician/student as well as the craniosacral therapist/student. In his German edition, he gave the historical background of the discoverer, William Garner Sutherland DO DSc(Hon). In this complete textbook, he provides a glossary in which he explains the most important concepts of cranial osteopathy, with extensive references.

Dr WG Sutherland was a student of Andrew Taylor Still MD, the founder of osteopathy. Late in his life, Dr Sutherland had this to say: 'In 75 years, in the crucible of time, not one statement made by Dr AT Still has needed revising'.

The beginning of this unique, truly American school of medicine dates back to 22 June, 1874, when after years of personal research and discovery, Dr Still on the wheat fields of Kansas, 'flung the banner to the breeze – Osteopathy'. The first school was founded in 1892 in Kirksville, Missouri. With the success of patient care and cures, osteopathy's fame spread and caught the attention of a young newspaper reporter from Minnesota, WG Sutherland. Sutherland entered the original American School of Osteopathy in Kirksville, Missouri in 1898 where Dr AT Still was to have said, 'There's a few right thinking people here'. Dr AT Still taught his students to think osteopathically; that is, that the Creator designed the human body perfectly and there is a reason and purpose for each and every structure, design, relationship and function. Reasoning from anatomy and physiology, the osteopath designs a treatment that restores the body to its maximum efficiency, wholeness and health. In 1899, while examining an open, disarticulated cranium at the American School of Osteopathy, WG Sutherland was struck by the observation of how closely the squama of the temporal bones resembled the gills of a fish. The next stage in his train of thought followed logically, that the structure of the skull must be designed for some sort of motion, gills – respiration – motion. This outrageous (for the time, 1899) thought, that the skull had motion, because of its anatomical design and the laws of physics, continued to plague Dr WG Sutherland for the rest of his life. Until at last, in 1938, he was able to prove to himself that the cranium does have an inherent capacity for motion, the Primary Rhythmic Impulse. He recognized the existence of the motility of the central nervous system; fluctuation in the cerebrospinal fluid; the mobility of the dura mater acts, in this respect, as a reciprocal tension membrane; articular mobility of the cranial bones, backed by the mobility of the sacrum between the alae of the ilium.

Dr AT Still gave the profession its concepts: the rule of the artery is supreme, the body has the inherent capacity to heal itself; and structure and function are reciprocally interrelated. Dr WG Sutherland added: The rule of the artery is supreme, but the cerebrospinal fluid is in command and its fluctuation can be observed by palpation with cranial technique. In 1950, Robert E Truhlar, DO neatly summed it all up, 'Osteopathy is divine geometry, physics, and chemistry'.

The author, Torsten Liem, brings to the profession a fresh, new and improved presentation of both well-known and recent advancements in the field of cranial osteopathy and craniosacral therapy. The author directs your attention to the intricate anatomical and physiological function that make up the dynamic cranial sacral mechanism. His direct and easy-to-read palpatory procedures for diagnosis and treatment are refreshing. Torsten Liem deals with each cranial bone in turn, describing its physiological mobility and restrictions to motion, as well as diagnostic and therapeutic methods and procedures. The reader is assisted in visualizing these methods and procedures by the magnificent photographs and illustrations that accompany the text.

The section dealing with the treatment of the bones and organs of the face is most interesting with a thorough treatment of the diagnostic and treatment procedures of the cranial structures. A selection of well-known pathologies is used to illustrate the osteopathic approach, providing guidance to the reader new to osteopathy. In this connection, the book follows the original theme in relation to diagnosis and treatment utilizing cranial osteopathy. Throughout, excellent references to the literature complete this work.

American osteopathic physicians and surgeons have long been aware of the healing and life-giving effect of the physiological phenomenon known as the Primary Rhythmic Impulse. Torsten Liem presents this effectively, while making no secret of the difficulties of the diagnostic and therapeutic methods needed to bring a favorable influence to bear on the life and health of patients. If the life and the condition of humanity are to be improved, precise understanding and correct application in the cause of restoration and wholeness of the entire person are indispensable. This art is a powerful psychomotor skill, and it is essential to use the knowledge contained in this book only in combination with personal instruction from competent masters of this skill. Personal training with validation of the development of your osteopathic skills is the only way to become sure and trustworthy practitioners, confident in diagnosis and treatment, able to rely on the desired outcome of your work.

Chicago, USA, 2004   Richard A. Feely

Preface to
the second edition

The original plan had envisaged a brief revision of *Praxis der Kraniosakralen Osteopathie*. This has now given way to a substantial reworking, and the chapter on the temporomandibular joint in particular has been considerably expanded. The results of new research and understanding of the anatomical structures and their physiological significance as well as additional diagnostic and therapeutic procedures are presented. Osteopathic approaches to the temporomandibular joint are increasingly being used in place of orthopedic treatments of the jaw. In the light of this it becomes essential for the osteopath to possess a sound body of knowledge.

All other chapters have also been updated to reflect the present state of knowledge. The instructional layout, which follows the treatment of each cranial bone and orofacial structure, of the organs of sight, hearing and balance and the upper respiratory tract, and in the case of headache, has proved helpful and has been retained in its existing form. It would give me great pleasure if the present manual and reference work is able in any degree to contribute to the further recognition of osteopathic treatment in the cranial field.

Hamburg, 2005   Torsten Liem

Preface to
the first edition

This book focuses primarily on those mechanisms of dysfunction and treatment techniques that belong to the more narrowly defined field of cranial and craniomandibular osteopathy. It also includes some material beyond this immediate field.

The reason for the somewhat mechanical presentation of the structures in this book is entirely didactic. It is by no means the intention to imply that therapeutic intervention is merely a matter of finely executed manual techniques. Intuition, caring attention and empathy on the part of the therapist, and the sensitivity of the practitioner's hands are just as important for the success of treatment. Listening, non-invasive attentiveness and consciousness in palpation activates the body's inherent healing powers. It is a great gift when hands begin to see, hear and know, and a still greater gift that this remains a constant adventure.

Practicing therapists know that each touch conveys new insights into the integrated working together of the body as a whole. Only an open spirit that has emptied itself is capable of receiving these insights. Just as much weight should therefore be placed on the approach, which must focus on the entirety, and on an open and listening touch, as on the learning and absorbing of the specific structures and their functional and anatomical relationships. It is less a question of 'doing' than the capacity of 'being' with the other person, and permitting the closeness and intimacy that open doors in the therapeutic encounter.

The repetition of material from the first book was inevitable; it is also practical from the instructional point of view, since it would otherwise have been necessary to make reference to the relevant parts of the first. That would make the text difficult to use, especially for quick reference.

The account of the localization, origin and treatment of dysfunctions of the various bones has been limited to the structures directly involved.

The format of the present work is to present techniques in relation to each cranial bone and the organ systems of the viscerocranium. A large number of additional variations and possible methods of performing them do in fact exist, and can be employed with at least as much success. During the course of a career, every therapist will to some extent develop individual approaches. These stem not only from experiences during that practice and from individual characteristics, but also from the fact that every patient, every treatment and each one of the body's structures is unique.

The basis of osteopathy according to Andrew Taylor Still was not in the first instance the teaching of particular techniques, but insight into particular principles that might give individual osteopaths the capacity to develop techniques of their own. The more a therapist internalizes the differentiation between the living tissues, their reciprocal anatomical and physiological relationships, and the osteopathic principles of diagnosis and treatment and develops manual sensitivity, the greater that capacity will be. In addition, the therapist has to expand his awareness to the reciprocal relationship of the patient to his cultural, social, emotional and natural surroundings.

The intuitive, 'living' and spiritual content of Sutherland's work and his concept of the 'Breath of Life' were to some degree deleted from the revised standard work by Harold Ives Magoun: *Osteopathy in the Cranial Field*, 3rd edition of 1976, published after Sutherland's death. The intention was to achieve greater political acceptance among the osteopaths living at that time and to make the cranial approach accessible to further research. In today's climate there is more readiness to consider these ideas too. An accompanying understanding of the historical associations and roots, as well as a common language, are important for the practice of cranial osteopathy, its further development and its transmission. For this reason the Glossary explains the fundamental principles using primarily the original Sutherland sources.

It simply remains for me to thank most sincerely all those who have written or sent ideas in response to the first book.

I wish you as much pleasure in reading this book, in palpation and in applying the techniques described, as I have had in writing it and experience day by day in my contact with patients.

In particular I wish you the same courageous spirit and devotion in your search and application of this living osteopathy as the founders of this unique discipline themselves possessed.

Hamburg, 2000   Torsten Liem

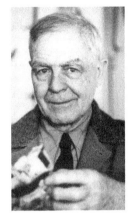

William G. Sutherland

Acknowledgments

I am greatly inspired by the teaching of Jean Pierre Barral DO MRO. This inspiration derives not only from his unique experience, the silent accompaniment to all his lectures, but especially from the effortless manner in which he helps both me and others, encouraging me to have confidence and find enjoyment in my palpation. He can make me believe almost anything; even that he could identify the color of the patients' underwear by palpation through their outer clothing.

I owe a great deal to Franz Buzet MREO MSBO. It feels so good to have someone believe in you.

The genius and intuition of Patrick van den Heede DO is a source of constant astonishment and a great inspiration to me.

I should also like to thank Beatrice Macazaga, who inspired me many years ago as a friend and involuntary mother-substitute.

Fred L Mitchell Jnr DO FAAO FCA is a teacher who combines empathy, clarity and comprehensibility, modesty and sheer competence, making him able to answer even stupid questions with the same constant concern and attentiveness!

I should like to thank Alan R Becker DO FAAO FCA, who took me into his heart as his pupil and taught me how simple it is to touch.

I am especially grateful for my contact with Renzo Molinari DO MRO, not only for his magnificent help and support, but because I could not imagine a more able, involved and empathic President of the European School of Osteopathy.

I cannot be thankful enough to Jim Jealous DO. He had a major influence in osteopathy and in osteopathic thought. He developed the biodynamic model from the pioneering work done by Sutherland, Becker, Schooley and Fulford. His support, appreciation and guidance are appreciated.

Robert Fulford DO FAAO FCA is a great figure, who has shown me that in osteopathy too it is important to follow one's heart and one's inner voice with conviction, even if it sometimes leads to conflict.

To Viola Frymann DO FAAO FCA, the 'grande dame' of cranial osteopathy, I express my gratitude for sharing with me her experience, and for her sensitive and knowledgeable hands. Her continuing dedication to the treatment of children is outstanding and exemplary.

When I remember Anne Wales DO FAAO FCA, I feel quite at ease about growing old as an osteopath (though I am still quite young). Even in later years she held her entire audience spellbound by her intellectual and spiritual perception. More than that, it is such a delight to see a person whose life is so imbued with uprightness, modesty and devotion that they are surrounded, even in old age, by a seemingly timeless youth, beauty and unique radiance.

I wish very much to thank Thomas Schooley DO FAAO FCA for the conversations in which he told me much about the original spirit of osteopathy.

I should like to thank John Upledger DO for the creativity and inspiration I found in his courses.

My thanks go too to John Wernham DO, now 97 years old; personally and in treatment sessions he passed on a wealth of information about classical European osteopathy and about his own experience with the principles of Littlejohn.

Artho Wittemann is both a therapist and a friend to me. I am especially grateful to him for supporting and helping me to make contact with many facets of myself. I am constantly surprised to discover what souls co-exist or alternate in my inner self.

If I ever believed that osteopathy had anything to do with strength, then it was Lawrence H Jones DO FAAO who convinced me of the opposite. I was impressed at the lightness and grace – like that of a dancer – of Dr Jones (himself advanced in age) as he touched, moved and treated me. It was through him and through John C Glover DO FAAO that I first understood that strain/counterstrain has nothing to do with rote-learned points.

I am very grateful to Guy Claude Burger. I discovered and learned through him that nutrition has a more profound effect on my body, spirit and emotional life that I would ever have dreamt, and that the body knows best what it needs.

A big thank you to Paul Chauffour DO. His original and global approach enlightened my hands in the palpation of every existing tissue in the body. Big thanks also to Bruno Chikly MD DO(Hons) for his friendship and inspiration in treating the lymph system. Above all, I owe Anthony G Chila DO FAAO FCA thanks for teaching me the importance of being empty oneself before beginning treatment of the patient, and of letting technique take a back seat.

I cannot thank Dr Frank Willard enough for his brilliant lectures on the interrelationships of anatomy and physiology. They were deeply impressing for me and offer ever-new perspectives or points of view of the osteopathic concept.

Thank you to Sat Hari and Robert, who inspired me in the midst of the great confusion of youth to turn to yoga. It is good to sense this gradual increase of confidence in 'self-regulation'.

I should also especially like to thank my friends Alain Abehsera, Celine Siewert, Christian Fossum, Michael Puylaert, Professor Dr Paul Klein, Peter Sommerfeld, Serge Paoletti, Jenny Parkinson, Peter Blagrave, Sabine Hansen, Uwe Senger and Zachary Commeaux, among other things for the many hours of osteopathic exchange, the interesting and inspiring discussions and the right to indulge in fruitful craziness and ask awkward questions. When I close my eyes, it is the closeness, openness and mutual caring, and the trust I have for my friends, that enable me to feel at home and grow, just as in one osteopathic family.

I also thank all my patients, who give me the opportunity to learn, to mature, and to pass on what I have learned. Thank you too to all those unnamed teachers and others who have assisted in the production of this book and my own growth process, and continue to do so.

I express special thanks to Sandra Bierkemeyer for her care and creative ideas in the production of the graphics for this book, and to Karsten D Franke for producing the photography.

Many thanks to Nathalie Trottier, whose diploma thesis helped me in producing the Glossary. I should also like to thank very much Dr Walter Schöttl (author of the excellent and very inspiring book, *Die craniomandibuläre Regulation*, Hüthig Verlag), Dr Carola Pfeiffer, Dr Michael Jaehne, Rainer Quast, Dr Stefan Schlickewei, Uwe Senger, Irene Özbay, Michael Kaufmann and Katja Hinz for their great help with proofreading.

I should like to give special thanks to the German publishers, Hippokrates Verlag, and to Frau D Seiz and Frau Horbatsch for their incredible patience, support and flexibility right through to the later stages of the publishing process.

Hamburg, 2005   Torsten Liem

Publisher's Acknowledgments

Figure 11.33 is reproduced from Arbuckle BE (1994) The Selected writings of Beryl E Arbuckle with the kind permission of American Academy of Osteopathy.

Figures 11.15, 11.20 and 14.23 are reproduced from Perlemuter L, Waligora J (1980) Cahiers d'anatomie 1, systeme nerveux central with the kind permission of Masson, Paris.

The publishers wish to express thanks to THIEME and HIPPOKRATES for their kind permission to reproduce the following Figures:

Figures 11.2, 11.10, 11.17, 11.18, 11.19, 12.1, 12.3, 12.8, 12.9, 12.11, 12.13, 12.14, 12.31, 12.35, 13.4, 13.13–2, 13.13–3, 14.8, 14.9, 14.10, 17.1 are from Tillmann B (1997) Farbatlas der Anatomie. Zahnmedizin-Humanmedizin. THIEME

Figures 12.2, 12.33, 12.34, 12.37 and 13.13 are from Feneis H (1988) Anatomisches Bildworterbuch 6E. THIEME

Figure 11.96 is from Upledger JE and Vreedevoogd JD (1994) Lehrbuch der Kraniosakrale Therapie 2E. Haug Verlag

Figure 12.32 is from Leonhardt H et al. (1987) Rauber/Kopsch: Anatomie des Menschen. Vol 1. Nervensystem. THIEME

Figure 14.3 is from Drews U (1993) Taschenatlas der Embryologie. THIEME

Figures 14.6, 14.7 are from Langmann J (1989) Medizinische Embryologie: die normale menschliche Entwicklung und ihre Fehlbildungen 8E. THIEME

Figure 14.11 is from Kahle W (1986) Taschenatlas der Anatomie: fur Studium und praxis. Vol 3. Nervensystem und Sinnesorgane 5E. THIEME

Figure 14.20 is from Liebmann M (1993) Basiswissen Neuroanatomie. THIEME

Figure 12.7 is from Pothmann VR (Eds) (1996) Systematik der Schmerzakupunktur. HIPPOKRATES

Quotations

... Everybody assumes consciousness is the exclusive province of the Brain. What a mistake! I've got my share of it, to be sure, but hardly enough to claim special privileges. The Knee has consciousness, and the Thigh has consciousness. Consciousness is in the Liver, in the Tongue ... It's coursing through you, too, and you're acting it out. You're each a part of it. In addition, there is consciousness in butterflies and plants and winds and waters. There is no Central Control! It's everywhere. So if Consciousness is what is required ...

Tom Robbins,
Even Cowgirls get the Blues

The truth is the I AM. The flower is my body. The song of the bird is my body. I encompass everything. In the stillness, when there are no ideas and no thoughts, there is room for knowledge. The wholeness of the whole becomes visible ... to be still simply means to live outside concepts.

Christin Lore Weber,
A Cry in the Desert. The Awakening of Byron Katie

An osteopath is taught that Nature is to be trusted to the end.

Andrew Taylor Still

Introduction

Osteopathy, developed at the end of the 19th century by AT Still, is a system of healing that professes to focus on wholeness and is characterized by its use of the hands to heal disease. The principles of osteopathy are based on the unity of the body, its self-regulating and healing powers, the interaction between structure and function, the great importance of perfusion, and the application of these principles in treatment.

The world of phenomena that surrounds us, including the tissues of the body that we touch in our work as osteopaths, is not rigidly set but temporary, the expression of interacting circumstances and forces. All depends on an infinity of other factors and contingencies.

The ability to recognize patterns of interacting contingencies and motion and interpret them diagnostically, and the ability to synchronize oneself with homeodynamic forces, play a decisive role in successful therapeutic work.

Technical skill is important, but limits should not be imposed on the potential for healing by excessive focus on technical performance. Healing is not just a one-way process from therapist to patient. The conscious participation of all those involved in the healing process and empathetic insight into the way that the signs and symptoms of disease relate and into the interrelationship of all the mutually linked phenomena of life are apparently of great importance.

PRINCIPLES AND METHODS OF PALPATORY DIAGNOSIS

Osteopathic diagnosis consists of more than just history-taking, visual assessment, tests and palpation; it may also include further specialized investigations. Every diagnosis in osteopathy must always consider the body as a whole. Examination as described below is limited to the palpation of the cranial system; this is for clarity of teaching. Most of the diagnostic procedures given here can also be used as appropriate in the rest of the body.

Barral's method of thermodiagnosis

This examination is carried out with the palm of the dominant hand. The area of the palm that is most sensitive to heat is also the area that responds most strongly to a gentle mechanical stimulus, and can be found by stroking a finger across the palm (Table 0.1).

Table 0.1 Areas of heat

Point-like, clearly defined	Structural changes: tumors, calcifications
Linear, clearly defined	Sutures, blood vessels, visceral channels
Large, circular, clearly defined	Part of an organ, e.g. lobe of brain
Large, linear, clearly defined	Elongated structures, e.g. esophagus
Large, circular, not clearly defined	Visceral or emotional disorders

Procedure:

➤ Place the hand, slightly cupped and relaxed, almost in contact with the skin at an area of heat and raise it gradually until you reach the level where the heat radiation can be felt most strongly. Then lower the hand again to the point where a slight resistance can be felt, usually about 10 cm above the skin.

➤ During thermodiagnosis the hand should always follow the contours of the body.

➤ Swing the hand gently from side to side. When performing this diagnosis it is important not to let the hand remain for too long in any one position so as not to influence the result. Examine the overall cranial contour to find the areas of greatest heat, which indicate possible dysfunctions.

Palpation of shape

The shape of the cranium can be used to help differentiate pathological or functional disorders. It also provides an initial indication of the severity of a dysfunction. 'Dysmorphism can be one of the first signs of cranial synostosis,[1] although it does not provide any indications as to the cause. There is still disagreement about whether pathological cranial shapes develop as a result of synostoses of the base or vault of the cranium. In young children, it is possible to assess the course of therapy by means of the cranial shape.' Particular attention should be paid to the ossification centers of the bones and asymmetries due to craniocervical rotation restrictions in young children.

Palpation of density[1]

Evaluation of the density and hardness of the tissue can be an indication of the severity of a dysfunction or can be used to assess the course of treatment.

➤ The density of the bone may be palpated through soft pressure with the hands.

Palpation of tissue elasticity

Tissue elasticity helps to evaluate bones, sutures, membranes, visceral structures and vessels.

> Spread your hands and place them swiftly on the various areas of the head. The hands exert brief light pressure on the particular region, which is then suddenly released, like a gentle recoil. The therapist notes the resistance of the tissue to gentle pressure (pliancy/hardness) and the reaction of the tissue when the pressure is released (resilience).

This is followed by local testing, e.g. of a suture or intraosseous structure.

Local tenderness

Tenderness to pressure is a sign of possible sutural dysfunctions.

Palpation of variation in rhythmic tension

A number of rhythms of varying clinical significance have been described after the manner of primary respiration (Table 0.2). These rhythms are claimed to be present in the entire body.

Various values exist for the frequency of primary respiration, also called the craniosacral rhythm. It may be that these are simultaneously present in a multi-layered complex, e.g.:

- 10–14 cycles per min: 4–6 s cycle (Magoun, Traube-Hering wave)[2-8]
- 6 or 8–12 cycles per min: 5–10 s cycle (Becker, Upledger)[9,10]
- 2.5 cycles per min: 24 s cycle (Jealous)[11]
- 6–10 cycles per 10 min: 60–100 s cycle (Becker's 'slow tide', Mayer wave)[8,12]
- 1 cycle per 5 min: 300 s cycle (Liem et al.)[13,14]
- Using CT scans, Lewer-Allen et al. also recorded phasic motion patterns of brain density and ventricular shape with a 33-min cycle (2000 s cycle).[14]

There are as yet no written details on the palpation of this last type of rhythmic pattern. Some personal findings from palpation do also seem to indicate very slow expansion and retraction impulses, but these results lack regularity or unity.

These and similar rhythmic values have been defined on the basis of: palpation findings by individual osteopaths; average values for palpation studies of the cranium (10–14 cycles per min); average values obtained in intra-rater and inter-rater reliability studies; the rhythmic motions of brain and cranial structures as measured in studies using a variety of instruments (ultrasound, CT, MRI); electromechanical measurements, sometimes carried out in combination with simultaneous palpation (e.g. the rhythm of 6–12 cycles per min).

The genesis of the rhythmic alternation of the inspiration and expiration phases, linked as it is with a tendency to oscillating

Table 0.2 Frequency of primary respiration

Investigator	Rhythm (cycles/min)	Method
Woods, Woods (1961)[2]	12.47 cycles/min	Palpation (1961)
Wallace, Avant, McKinney, Thurstone (1966)[15]	9 cycles/min	Ultrasound study of intracranial motion (1966)
Allen, Goldmann (1967)[16]	2–9 cycles/min	Ultrasound (1967)
Baker (1970)[17]	9 cycles/min	Measured at the molars
White, Jenkins, Campbell (1970)[18]; Jenkins, Campbell, White (1971)[19]	7 cycles/min	Ultrasound study of brain
Frymann (1971)[20]	12.8 cycles/min	Measured at the cranium
Michael, Retzlaff (1975)[12]	5–7 cycles/min	Measured using anesthetized apes (1975)
Becker (1977)[21]	0.6 cycles/min	Palpation of 'long tide'
Lay, Cicorda, Tettambel (1978)[6]	8 cycles/min	Motion detectors on frontal and temporal bones
Upledger (1979)[22]	6–12 cycles/min	Palpation (1979)
Brookes (1981)[23]	12–14 cycles/min in adults; 14–16 cycles/min in children	Palpation (1981)
Upledger et al. (1983)[24]	4.5 cycles/min	Palpation in coma patients (1983)
Podlas, Allen, Bunt (1984)[25]; Allen, Bunt (1989)[26]	2.25–0.25 cycles/min; Cycle of 300–2000 s	Brain tissue density and ventricular shape (1984/1989)
Measurement mentioned by Podlas[27]	2–9 cycles/min	Ultrasound (sinusoidal pressure wave)
Marier (1986)[28]	9.54 cycles/min	Measurement (1986)
McCatty (1988)[29]	10.4 cycles/min	Palpation in healthy adults
Herniou[30]	12 cycles/min	Piezoelectric measurement in sheep
Gunnergaard (1992)[31]	12 cycles/min	Measurement using Hall effect at maxillary arch (1992)
Norton, Sibley, Broder-Oldach (1992)[32]	3.89 cycles/min	Palpation (1992)
Allen (1993)[33]	6.34 cycles/min	Palpation in infants <1 month (1993)
Wirth-Patullo/Hayes (1994)[7]	3–9 cycles/min	Palpation (1994)
Greenman/McPartland (1995)[34]	7.2 cycles/min	Palpation in traumatic brain damage (1995)
McAdoo (1995)[35]	3–9 cycles/min	Palpation (1995)
Jealous[36]	2.5 cycles/min	Palpation
Zanakis et al. (1996–97)[37]	6.35 cycles/min	Motion testing video analysis system (1996–97)
Liem (1998)[13]	0.2 cycles/min	Palpation
Lewer-Allen, Bunt Sorek (2000)[14]	0.2 cycles/min	CT scans of brain density and ventricular shape

expansion and retraction, has still not been clearly and fully explained. One possibility being mentioned is that the phenomenon is synonymous with THM oscillations. Others put forward are links with Lundberg waves, 'third order waves', cycles in the systems of lymph or cerebrospinal fluid, or the basal rest and activity cycle (BRAC), etc.

Another possibility is that the primary respiration waves may be part of the general homeodynamic activity of all life forms and of life itself, which find expression in varying phenomena.

Table 0.3 summarizes a few of the hypotheses as to the origin of primary respiration.

The inspiration phase of primary respiration is characterized by an externally directed motion from the center out toward the periphery – an expansion. The expiration phase describes motion that returns inward toward the center (Table 0.4).

These rhythmic features and 'motions' can be found locally, in a particular tissue, or in the entire body. The osteopath can detect the phase of primary respiration where restrictions of motion or abnormal tensions occur, and assess whether the outward or inward direction predominates in the flow of the life force. Motion restrictions can be palpated in the light of the therapist's knowledge of all the tissues involved and the sutural joint surfaces, and can be evaluated and treated accordingly.

➤ The therapist should evaluate the naturally occurring 'disengagement' during each inspiration phase and the retraction, or drawing closer, of, e.g. the interosseous and intraosseous structures in each expiration phase.

Table 0.3 Explanations advanced for the PRM rhythm

Rhythmic motion of the ventricles[25–27]
Rhythmic motion of the brain[38–54]
Motion impulses deriving from embryology[55]
Effect of PRM on pulmonary respiration[56]
Pressurestat model[57]
Respiration/heart rhythm[45,46,48]
Rhythm as reaction of muscles to gravity[58]
Rhythm as a function of neuromuscular system[59]
Lymphatic pump[60,61]
Tissue pressure model[7,62,63]
Entrainment model according to McPartland and Mein[64–67]
Local venomotion model according to Farasyn[68,69]
Traube-Hering-Mayer oscillation[8,70–75]
External rhythm producing resonance in the body[76]

Table 0.4 Wave characteristics in the inspiration and expiration phases

Inspiration	Expiration
Expansion	Retraction*, collection
Natural disengagement	Drawing closer
Divergent motion	Convergent motion
Flexion, external rotation	Extension, internal rotation
Flow of life force from within to outside, toward periphery, centrifugal	Flow of life force from outside to inside, to the center, centripetal
Extraversion, moving out from the center, being beyond oneself, developing the self	Introversion, coming to the center, deepening toward the center, return to origin
Breadth, space, distance	Closeness
Redeveloping oneself anew	Regression
External world	Inner world
Expressive	Receptive
Interpersonal	Intrapsychological

*These ideas are intended to express a natural, spontaneous movement directed toward the center, which draws the structures closer. They do not mean 'retraction' in the sense of active compression, contraction, or tension, or any reaction involving drawing in or circumscribing, or calling a halt, which would hinder free flow and prevent an unconstrained body physiology. These are more characteristic of a dysfunction.

➤ The therapist notes the symmetry, frequency, amplitude, strength and ease of the variations in rhythmic motion or tension and the 'feel' on completion, and looks for any abnormal asymmetric motion during inspiration and expiration. If any change is sensed at a particular position on the body, this is a sign of a disorder in this area. The therapist can also sense tensions that hinder the free expression of primary respiration.

➤ The tissue reaction to pulmonary respiration can also be palpated. Deep breathing amplifies the motion.

Motion testing

Motion testing can also be used to examine sutures and tissues. It can be carried out at the same time as the primary respiration test or independently.

Active and passive testing of fascial tension

Dysfunctions can create tension in the fasciae.

➤ General passive testing is done using the hands to detect possible tensions. Passive testing of an individual fascia can also be carried out. This is done by establishing hand contact with the tissue to be tested, and may detect tensile force operating in the fascia in the direction of the dysfunction.

> Active testing involves applying gentle traction. The fascia normally yields and slides along with the traction. Compare the mobility, evaluating its symmetry and trying to sense whether and where there is any resistance to the mobility of the fascia. The resistance increases as you approach the disturbance.

Adhesions, fibroses, inflammation and other dysfunctional processes reduce the mobility of the fascia, i.e. hinder its capacity to slide.
This method can be used to examine all locations on the body.

Differential diagnosis of the dysfunction level by palpation

In this diagnosis, the osteopath differentiates whether the motion restriction and hardness in the tissue originates from the bone, dura, brain tissue or fluid. Another option is to establish a resonance with electromagnetic fields.

Differential diagnosis by palpation

This method of differential diagnosis (Table 0.5) can be used to examine whether the motion restriction of a particular structure (e.g. hyoid bone) is caused by another body tissue (e.g. liver).

> Support one of the two structures (e.g. the liver) and establish a point of balance.
> Then examine the hyoid bone to see whether the inherent motion or mobility of this bone has changed. If any normalization or

Table 0.5 Methods of manual diagnosis
Thermodiagnosis
Palpation of shape
Palpation of density
Palpation of tissue elasticity
Tenderness to local pressure
Palpation of rhythmic expressions of primary respiration with breathing and/or compression
Motion testing in synchrony with primary respiration independently of primary respiration
Palpation of fascial tensions Passive Active
Differential diagnosis of the dysfunction level by palpation
Differential diagnosis by palpation
Palpation of fluid motion
Detecting spatial organization
Palpation of tissue 'potency'

improvement is felt, this indicates that the liver is affecting the hyoid bone.

A deterioration indicates a compensation situation in which the hyoid bone is affecting the liver.

Palpation of fluid motion

➤ Concentrate your attention on the fluid colloid properties of the patient's body, taking up a contact as if your hand is resting on the surface of some water. Sense a slight flow or direction drawing your hand along with it. This is related to the direction from which the traumatic force impacted on the patient's body.

Detecting spatial organization

● How is the structure organized, e.g. the temporal bone in terms of its intraosseous elasticity?
● How is the temporal bone organized in terms of its immediate location, e.g. its sutural, fascial and ligamentous attachments?
● How is the temporal bone organized in terms of its regional location, e.g. in relation to the head as a whole?
● How is the temporal bone organized in terms of the rest of the body?

Palpation of potency

➤ Draw your hands swiftly upward from the feet to the various regions of the patient's body, placing them on each region in turn, but without allowing your hands to remain for too long in any one place. Assess the vitality of the tissue at each location, a sort of fine oscillatory motion characteristic of all living tissue. Treat first the areas that exhibit the lowest potency.

PRINCIPLES AND METHODS OF TREATMENT

Contraindications

There are few contraindications to the use of cranial techniques, because the force applied is so slight.

The following, however, are absolute contraindications: acute fractures, acute traumatic head injuries, acute cerebral bleeding or risk of cerebral bleeding.

Care should be taken when treating epileptic patients not to trigger a seizure.

Complications of treatment

No scientific studies have been carried out on complications following cranial treatment. Isolated cases of the following complications have been reported. These have mainly been transient and were resolved by rest or by CV-4 technique[77]:

- Nausea[34,77]
- Vertigo[77,78]
- Vomiting[34]
- Diarrhea[34]
- Cardiac palpitations[34]
- Psychiatric disturbances[34]
- Cases of depression[78]
- Confusion[78]
- Diplopia[78]
- Loss of consciousness[78]
- Trigeminal nerve damage[78]
- Hypopituitarism[78]
- Brainstem dysfunction[78]
- Opisthotonus[78, 79]
- Tonic-clonic seizure[78]
- Possible miscarriage of a 12-week pregnancy[78]
- Two cases of pituitary dysfunction following treatment by an unqualified therapist was reported. This was resolved with further cranial and hormonal treatment.[77, 78]
- One case of aggravation of traumatic brain injury.[34]
- Also dizziness, headache, loss of appetite, and sleep disturbances.

Recognition of normal function

It is fundamentally important in any therapeutic intervention to be able to recognize normal function, normal patterns of tension and their normal elasticities or ranges of motion. This involves sensing and recognizing the difference between bones, membrane or ligament, fluid, soft tissue, electromagnetism, 'potency', and other features, as well as a dynamic stillness in the patient, and enables the osteopath to distinguish between healthy and sick tissues and between normal and abnormal tension patterns. The ability to recognize and differentiate the expression of the various body rhythms is not only necessary in examination and localization, but also plays a role in treatment.

Stillness is, according to R Becker, the key to understanding the patient. He sees the ability to consciously recognize stillness as an essential skill in treatment, indeed as the factor that actually brings about a change during treatment.[80]

THE STAGES OF TREATMENT AND THE FULCRUM

The first step in treatment involves taking up contact with the inherent stillness in the patient and the homeodynamic forces in the body. The second is to examine the abnormal tension patterns and the finer energy patterns and to find the fulcrum around which they organize themselves (or are organized). The third step involves establishing a fulcrum about which motion/energy can organize itself in such a way that resolution of the abnormal tension and energy patterns can take place. In effect, you copy exactly the abnormal tension/energy pattern and establish a new therapeutic state of balance that copies the suspended automatic shifting fulcrum of a healthy system. This newly established fulcrum enables the inherent homeodynamic forces to transform the abnormal tension/energy state into a freer state of balance. This releases the forces that were bound by the abnormal tension/energy pattern to re-integrate themselves into the physiological activity of the body.

The new fulcrum is not only an expression of the local resolution of underlying tensions; it is at the same time related to the entirety of the forces acting within the body which are responsible for maintaining local and global homeodynamic processes. This means that the establishment of a new fulcrum will not necessarily be a complete return to an absolute ideal state of balance, with a total restoration of health and the resolution of all symptoms, but the best possible state of balance at that time.

Fulcrums are not limited to the dural membrane. A bony fulcrum at the SBS, a membranous fulcrum at the straight sinus and a fulcrum of the nervous system at the laminae terminales have been described. Sutherland also detected a fulcrum in the fluctuations of the CSF.[81]

A procedure for establishing a fulcrum or point of balanced membranous tension is described below. A point of balance can be induced in the fluid and in the potency in a similar way. Sutherland spoke of also identifying the fulcrum, the 'still point,' in the fluctuations of the CSF and maintaining the reciprocal tension membrane and the fluid fluctuation at the 'balance point'.[82]

Sutherland describes the potency in the CSF as a fundamental principle in the functioning of the PRM[83]; he also goes further and makes clear that the potency in the fluctuation of the CSF can be used in diagnosis and therapy.

Sutherland/Magoun even accord the CSF an intelligence of its own.[84] The treatment principles described below can be applied in all the techniques presented in this book.

Jim Jealous's 'neutral of the patient'

Like an orchestral concert in which the notes of the individual instruments blend into the music being played, the reciprocal tensions in the body and the aspects of body, mind and spirit combine in the neutral state into a homogeneous mind-body-spirit unity. In the neutral state the whole person of the patient is particularly receptive; interaction between the 'Breath of Life' and the patient can take place most effectively, and the patient is best able to react directly with the 'tides'. The neutral state creates the best and easiest conditions for healing and changing dysfunctional patterns, and the amount of force that the therapist needs to apply to carry out a technique is at its least in this state. It is also easier to sense how much force is necessary to perform the technique and when it has been completed. Negative consequences are minimized and patients themselves can sense the change brought about in their bodies more clearly.

Procedure: ➤ Place your hands on the patient's head or other part of the body. Act as a passive observer, concentrating with a gentle attentiveness. Do not follow any motion or dysfunction pattern. The moment will come when the various motion impulses and tensions in the patient's tissues become still, and you will detect a rhythm of around 2.5 cycles per min. The various body tissues, body fluids and potency can be sensed as an undifferentiated, homogeneous density. The neutral state can be palpated as a kind of point of balance of the reciprocal tensions present in the body, at which body, mind and spirit become integrated, felt to be a unity in its best possible state of balance of that moment.

➤ Maintain your contact with this neutral state throughout the whole of the ensuing treatment.

There are rare instances when the neutral state is not achieved. This usually happens after loss of consciousness or extreme use of force, resulting in an extreme dissociation between body, mind and spirit. Jealous states that in such cases a gentle EV-4 is indicated.

The establishment of a point of balance leads to the release of the bound forces in the dysfunction, enabling the tissues to resolve their relationship to one another. Inherent homeodynamic forces in the dysfunction come into effect, a dynamic balance is re-established and, in contact with the dysfunctional fulcrums, sets healing processes in motion. In other words, the bound energy plays its part again in the working of the homeodynamic forces of the body as a whole, and the dysfunctional fulcrums either dissipate or diminish. The tissues and their innate forces can reorganize themselves in the direction of the natural fulcrum.

Induction of the point of balanced membranous tension (PBMT)

The PBMT is the position in which the tension in the dural membrane and between the structures involved is in its optimum state of even distribution.

➤ If a mobility restriction lies within the physiological range of movement, the right approach is to allow yourself to be led to the PBMT. If it lies outside the physiological range of movement, the therapist should encourage the structures concerned toward the PBMT.

➤ With increasing experience the therapist will usually find that less and less force is needed to induce the correction that is right for that patient's body. This is in accordance with Sutherland's method of procedure as his own experience increased. Sutherland places special importance on the idea that it is not so much the direction by the therapist as the fluid fluctuations of the PRM that lead the structures to the PBMT. The therapists' role is rather to allow themselves to be led by the fluctuations to the point of balanced tension (PBT).

'... we do not have to find the point of balance in the reciprocal tension membranes because the cerebrospinal fluid tide will do it for us. We merely initiate the movement and follow it as the fulcrum shifts. These membranes maintain a constant reciprocal tension for whatever pattern exists in the osseous elements of the cranial mechanism. If permitted by the proper manual application in the technic approach the tide will carry the mechanism to the balance point in that particular pattern. When the balance point is reached the cerebrospinal fluid has found its proper fulcrum and it is at this time that the correction takes place'.[85]

Maintaining the PBMT

➤ Once the point of membranous balance has been achieved, the therapist's task is to maintain the balance until a correction of the abnormal tension in the dural membrane has occurred and the tidal motion of the cerebrospinal fluid has brought about a correction in the affected structures. This involves holding them in PBMT with the gentlest possible touch until the motion of the structures has ceased.[85]

Point of balanced membranous tension: variation according to Jealous

➤ Another way of establishing a point of balance is by synchronization with primary respiration. According to Jealous, about 90% of your attention should reside with the primary respiration while 10% is directed toward the tensions present. The usual method is to follow the expressions of tension during the inspiration phase and enhance them to the slightest possible extent.
➤ A spontaneous disengagement may occur at the end of the inspiration phase. During the next expiration, inherent correcting forces may arise spontaneously and lead the affected tissue out of the dysfunction.
➤ A lateral fluctuation at the level of the affected tissue may be felt. There may also be a transition to a still point.

Balanced fluid tension

This is a less well known type of point of balance, although Sutherland himself made some mention of it, saying for example that attention should not only be paid to the fulcrum in the reciprocal tension membrane, but also the 'fulcrum point', the still point in the fluctuation of the CSF, and that the reciprocal tension membrane and the fluctuation of the fluid should be maintained at balance point. He also said that the therapist is led to the point of balance by the fluid fluctuations. Jim Jealous in particular has developed this approach. The technique is directed toward the fluid aspect of the body.

Balanced fluid tension according to Jealous

➤ Establish a resonance with the fluid pattern in the dysfunction. Do not address any tissue restrictions or barriers in the dysfunction. Follow the physiological 'motion' of the fluids with your hands and remain within it.

➤ Synchronize your hands with the motion of the fluids, with the speed of these motions and with the inherent, spontaneously occurring disengagement. A balance point for the fluids becomes established.

➤ Note the interaction of the local fluid pattern with the whole fluid body. Broaden your attention to include the field around the body.

Induction of a local, regional and global point of balanced tension (PBT)

This should be done in three stages.

➤ First establish a local PBT, e.g. in the coronal suture.

➤ Then a regional PBT should be established between this suture and the cranium.

➤ When this has been done, a global PBT can be established between this suture and the body as a whole.

Methods of achieving a point of balanced tension

The following techniques can be used to help achieve a PBMT: exaggeration, direct technique, opposite physiological motion, disengagement and molding.

These maneuvers are like an invitation to the tissue and part of a dialogue with the tissue. The tissue is not forced in a particular direction; rather, opportunities are presented to it and the therapist must respect the response of the tissue when it complies or does not.

The techniques are both a means of diagnosis, by which the osteopath senses the response of the tissue to these 'invitations' and can also be used as a means of treatment to achieve a new dynamic balance of tension.

The techniques described below have the character of spontaneous healing reactions in the tissue. The maneuvers are not movements that the osteopath tries to induce; the therapist's task is rather to assist the naturally occurring homeodynamic activity in the tissue by means of resonance, synchronization and focusing of attention.

Exaggeration

➤ In this technique, the therapist follows the motion of the bone or tissue in the direction away from the restriction, that is, in the 'direction of ease' (i.e. of greater motion) without confronting motion barriers. Very gently the tissue is moved out of the field of tension. The therapist stays within the range of motion, meaning that he avoids confronting the motion barriers directly. The tissue dynamics are just perceived without intervention. In the end a new equilibrium of tension will establish itself. Structural approaches on the other hand move the tissues towards the physiological motion barriers. Wait for a release of the tissue, when it will regain motility, then guide it on further to the point where it reaches a physiological barrier again.

➤ Repeat this procedure until you no longer sense tensions being released.

The following are relative contraindications: children below age 5–8, and acute traumatic injuries.

Direct technique

➤ Direct technique is used to guide the affected tissue in the direction of restricted motion. The force applied is very slight, remaining below the threshold at which the structures involved react by counter-contracting. In this case too, the tissue is moved out of the field of tension very gently, without confronting motion barriers.

This technique is indicated in children below age 4–7 and in acute dysfunctions of traumatic etiology. Indirect and direct approaches can be applied in combination.

Opposite physiological motion. Example: occipitomastoid suture

Opposite physiological motion is indicated for some severe traumatic dysfunctions.

➤ Achieve the point of balance by following the occipital bone further in the direction of ease (indirect technique), for example, into flexion. At the same time the temporal bone is moved or held or followed in internal rotation (direct technique).

This treatment principle should whenever possible be applied (or may occur spontaneously) in synchrony with primary respiration; the occipital bone moves into flexion during the inspiration phase, whereas the temporal bone moves into internal rotation. In the expiration phase, in contrast, both bones move into extension and internal rotation.

Disengagement

➤ This technique involves gently separating two structures. If possible it should be performed in harmony with primary respiration.

The point of balance can then be attained.

Alternative method I: ➤ Hold one of the bones of the joint and gently draw the other away. Establish a point of balance.

➤ Then hold the other component of the joint and repeat the corresponding process.

Alternative method II: ➤ The therapist induces the disengagement simply by focusing attention on disengagement and the inherent correcting forces connected with this, during the inspiration phase. This separation is not designed to eliminate the forces operating, but to make it possible to experience their operation and internal order, to expose the underlying fulcrums, and to bring about the activity of these forces in the point of balance.

Treatment using this principle is indicated when the traumatic injuries underlying the dysfunction mean that the forces present cause more constriction and density than can be resolved by a point of balance. Examples are: sutural compressions, especially at pivot points, at limb joints, in traumatic and severe chronic restrictions, fibroses of the dural membrane, and to stretch fascial or muscular structures.

Compression

Compression can be used to help create a context in which the relationship between tissues is intensified and hidden conflicts become visible.

➤ Two adjacent components of a joint are gently moved closer together.
➤ This should be done in harmony with primary respiration if possible.
➤ The point of balance can then be attained.
➤ Focus your attention on the activity of the inherent homeodynamic forces.

Alternative method I: ➤ Hold one component and draw the other gently closer.
➤ Establish a point of balance.
➤ Then hold the other component and repeat the corresponding process.

Alternative method II: ➤ The therapist induces the compression simply by focusing attention on the convergent movement and on the inherent correcting forces connected with this, during the expiration phase.

Note: Compression may also become necessary in order to make contact with very early tissue dynamics. The dynamics of embryological tissue development, for example, as well as those of the birth process are usually linked with compression. Therefore, according to Heede, the cranium reacts to compression induced by the therapist by adopting its original rotation pattern, and indicates a fulcrum/mechanical point of balance for this pattern.[84]

Combined compression and decompression

➤ The joint is first of all compressed, that is, moved further into the lesion, with the intention of then decompressing it in the opposite direction. This is a combination of direct and indirect technique. It is like freeing a jammed drawer by first pushing it further in, making it possible to pull out the drawer without forcing it.

Molding: Molding involves the attempt to affect the shape and pliancy of a bone by applying external pressure or traction.

Taking the example of the parietal tuber, this may appear too prominent or too flat on one side. In molding, energy is directed to lower the parts that are too prominent and make the excessively flat parts more prominent.

Indications are intraosseous dysfunctions, particularly in young children, but also in adults.

Molding can be assisted by fluctuations of the cerebrospinal fluid, by pulmonary breathing, and by the myofascial system.

Fluid impulse (direction of energy)

Also known as the V-spread, this technique uses the inherent forces of fluid fluctuations to release even the most stubborn restrictions in an extremely gentle way. It is based on the fluid crystalline properties of body tissues.

➤ The exact position of the fingers is located by placing the middle and index fingers in a V-formation on the structure that is either restricted or is to be tested. A slight pulsation is palpated at the position opposite this, where the vector of the V formed by your fingers leaves the cranium. This is the ideal position from which to direct energy toward the restricted suture.

➤ To test the suture, use one finger of the hand in the position opposite the V to direct energy in a fine fluid impulse toward the suture to be tested, during the inspiration phase. If the fingers that are arranged in a V sense the suture opening, then the suture is free. The sensation is like a wave running up onto a sandy beach. The suture is restricted if no opening is felt.

➤ To free the suture, direct a gentle fluid impulse toward the blocked suture from the finger opposite the suture, during each inspiration phase. Simultaneously, you should also spread the suture using the fingers forming the V and applying minimal force. Another method is to direct a continuous fluid impulse toward the restricted suture. This need not be synchronized with the inspiration phase.

The V-spread can also be applied in the following ways:

➤ Another part of the hand or body (e.g. the stomach) can be used instead of just the finger to direct the fluid impulse. A fluid impulse can also be directed from the opposite foot or from the sacrum in order to release restrictions in the cranium. In addition, the patient may be asked to assist the treatment by dorsal flexion of one or both feet or by holding the breath, either when breathing in or when breathing out.

Any part of the body, for example the shoulder, can be treated using this direction of energy method. Sutherland stated that simple force of will can influence body fluids, without direct body contact.

TREATMENT OF ELECTRODYNAMIC FIELDS

Dysfunctions can arise as a result, for example, of unequally polarized fields.

Position at start of treatment: ➤ Place your hand above the skin of the patient, level with the structure to be treated. Let your hand sink down until you sense a resistance.

> An alternative is to place one hand behind the structure to be treated and one in front of it. In this case the resistance is felt as an inflated balloon or spherical field.

Method: ➤ Your hands should continue to hold the detected field.
➤ Permit all the types of motion by this field until they come to rest (unwinding) or until you sense a symmetrical motion.
➤ Finally, induce a PBET using the equivalent method to that for establishing PBMT.

Complex wave forms according to Abehsera

Modern physics encountered the paradox that matter, at its minutest level, can be seen as being composed of particles, but can equally be viewed as consisting of a field of energy waves. According to Abehsera this insight can be transferred to the human body, each part of which can then be seen as a collection of tiny particles or as complex wave forms, for example, a wave-like liver.

These complex wave forms cannot be palpated directly with the hands, so the position of the hands is not critical.

> To establish contact the osteopath creates a holographic image of the structure concerned (suture, ligament, joint, or organ of the patient), and projects this image, created as it were of pure thought waves, so that it is held in the osteopath's hands. There the osteopath can sense rhythms, abnormal dysfunctional patterns of the dysfunctional structure, via the holographic image, and can correct them according to the therapeutic principles already described, applying these to the holographic image.

Abehsera found that the more precise the creation of the hologram, the more successful the results. Sensing at this level makes it easier to register and influence the interaction of the organ with other parts of the body. The great advantage of this approach is that the flow of information between organs can be influenced directly.

Sensing the health of the patient

It is an important requirement for therapists to be able to sense in themselves what is taking place in the body of the other person. It is essential for them to be in contact with the flow within themselves and with their own original nature, and develop a consciousness for their own immediate process of feeling. They should also develop the capacity to admit closeness and intimacy and allow things to happen without having to intervene. The extent to which they themselves are in contact with this original nature and flow is the extent to which they will be able to establish this same contact with the patient.

Method: ➤ Direct your attention first to your own flow or sense of being 'in' the flow; then begin to direct caring, non-invasive awareness, but without losing contact with your own flow.

➤ Pass your hands over the patient's body and direct your attention – not only through your hands, but with all your senses – to the areas of the body that are most alive. Where is there motion? Vitality? Pulsation?

➤ Once you have found or been led to this area, begin to take up the contact with the patient here.

➤ Place your hand on this area and give the patient your attention and empathy. Simply doing this will strengthen the living, flowing element in the patient. Permit whatever you find happening at this point of greatest health, whether it is expressed through the medium of the tissues or beyond.

➤ Then sense the region of the body where the free flow encounters resistance, restrictions to motion and contractions. It is important to identify this place precisely. You are not looking for the place where the immobility is greatest but the place where there is still a good degree of flow, rhythmic pattern and pulsation, the place that forms a sort of borderline between flexibility and rigidity: the place where rigidity and immobility have not yet fully developed. This is the exact point at which the therapy should be applied, because health can spread more easily from it and soften the resistances and restrictions to motion. Encourage the inherent rhythmic pattern and flow here.

It is no use either to remain at the place of greatest vitality and rhythmic flow (because there is already free flow here) or to try to intervene where the immobility is most pronounced (because this would be invasive and too much like the use of force). It would be active intervention if the therapist intervened at the most immobile point, instead of letting the patient's own body perform the process – 'doing' instead of 'allowing to do'.

The natural endeavor of the vitality in the body to spread and extend softens motion restrictions and this is where healing takes place from the inside outward. Patients experience their own health and flow. Touch of this sort is a direct reflection of the remark by Still that our main task is to find health; anyone can find disease.

Below is a possible treatment procedure (Table 0.6)

➤ 1 Neutral of the patient according to Jim Jealous

➤ 2 Resonance: Here the therapist entrains his hands with the tension and oscillation of the structure to be treated: bone, fascia/membrane, fluids (viscera, brain/spinal cord, etc.), electrodynamic field.

➤ 3 Point/state of balance

➤ 4 Fluid impulse: this can be used as a form of assistance or may occur spontaneously.

Table 0.6 Treatment methods

Neutral of the patient according to J. Jealous
Point of balanced tension (PBT): PBMT, PBLT, PBFT
Induction of a local, regional and global PBT
Methods of achieving PBT: exaggeration, direct technique, opposite physiological motion, disengagement of joint facets, molding
Assistance by: fluctuation of CSF and extracellular fluids, pulmonary breathing, myofascial system
Enhancing entrainment of CRI between the practitioner and patient
Electrodynamic fields
Unwinding, PBET
Complex wave forms
Sensing the health of the patient

Point of balanced fluid tension (PBFT)

Once the PBMT has been induced, the rhythmic motions of the primary respiratory mechanism (PRM) are able to take effect. At first a kind of increasing unrest in the fluid components usually becomes evident to palpation. This comes to a point of rest when a PBMT (also called a fulcrum) is established in the fluids. This is the moment when the correction takes place, and the therapist senses a softening of hardened structures and a resolution of tissue resistance. There is a change in the fluctuations of the cerebrospinal fluid, and a kind of new balance can be sensed in the tissue.

Fluctuations

➤ Finally the fluctuations of the cerebrospinal fluid increase slightly once more, and the therapist can sense that the rhythmic expansion of the fluctuations is now no longer hindered by any tissue restrictions. There is a marked increase in the amplitude, strength and symmetry of the fluctuations.

Final phase of correction

➤ In the final phase of the correction the fluctuations may be felt to come to a spontaneous rest, very much as they do in a CV-4. Other, slower rhythmic patterns may become evident to palpation.

ASSESSMENT OF THE COURSE OF TREATMENT

Self-organizing systems that participate in a constant exchange of energy with the outside world are continually active. There is entropy, which has a dissipating effect. When these systems are close to a state of equilibrium they become disordered, but when they are far from equilibrium they maintain a state of order, and new order may be established by passing through instability.[86]

Human beings too, in their somatic-emotional unity, seem to pass from an ordered state to a disordered one and spontaneously back again to order. There is a tendency toward order and stability with periods of disorder which are necessary for a new order to develop.

Similar processes can be observed during the therapeutic process. The patient passes through a stage of instability so that old patterns of order which are no longer adequate can disintegrate and a new structure or order can develop. The disorder is a necessary precursor of the new order.

Superficially, this process can seem like disintegration on the part of the patient. The therapist should not make the mistake of remaining on the superficial level; the task is not to support the patient in reorganizing and stabilizing the dysfunctional pattern of order. Instead, therapists can make contact with the homeodynamic forces present and encourage the spontaneous process of reorganization. An improvement in general wellbeing (despite possible temporary symptoms such as withdrawal symptoms, the reappearance of former, suppressed symptoms, or regression of chronic disorders/emotions to an acute stage) and a development tending to bring greater clarity or enlightenment, sense and security, are typical of a process leading toward health.

Important: The way in which these techniques are performed will vary to some extent from one therapist to another, from one patient to another and according to the time of treatment.

The reason for this is certainly that the manner of performing a technique emerges from a dialog directly with the tissue, the forces at work and the body as a whole. It is the tissue that tells us what it needs and what we should do. Establishing a point of balance, for example, may require exaggeration on one occasion, on another a direct technique, opposite physiological motion, disengagement, compression, or a combination of the treatment categories listed.

(There are a few general principles such as the one that it is better to use direct techniques to treat young children, but there are no hard and fast rules.) Some prominent osteopaths, for instance, exert far more force on the cranium than is normally said to be applicable; some, such as Jean Pierre Barral, use almost exclusively indirect methods (with great success), even with small children. So allow yourself to gather your own experience. Do this in humility and empathy, respecting the uniqueness of the body and its tissues, but do not allow yourself to be limited by dogma. Test various models of working and use them according to what the experience of your palpation tells you.

The specific reaction of a tissue to traumatic force also provides indications as to the type of therapeutic touch that it needs.

● Every technique varies in addition according to its synchronization with primary respiration: whether its use is partly or fully synchronized, and which frequency of primary respiration the therapist has chosen for synchronizing the treatment. (There is a danger of distancing oneself too much from immediate experience, so any too dogmatic classification of frequencies – whether based on biomechanical or metaphysical models – should be avoided at present. Further experimental and clinical research is needed.)

- Each of the techniques that follow can be performed dynamically in synchronicity with primary respiration, so that a given motion is gently supported only during the inspiration phase or only during the expiration phase. This can be done as either a direct or an indirect technique.
- Similarly, the execution of techniques to treat dysfunctions may differ significantly according to whether motion barriers are encountered during therapy, or the therapist is entirely allowing the activity of the Breath of Life to guide the therapy. Every structure can be treated without tackling a motion barrier. Particular attention should be paid in these cases to the naturally occurring disengagement during each inspiration phase.
- Go with the disengagement of the structures involved by supporting it physically in varying degrees or mentally giving space to it in an empathetic way, or purely focusing your attention on the process.
- The retraction and 'drawing closer' in the tissue can likewise be encouraged by providing physical support to whatever degree is necessary, or empathetic mental encounter with the forces at work in drawing closer, or pure focus of attention on the process occurring.
- With experience, the therapist will usually be able to sense more clearly when in the course of treatment the inherent regulating and correcting forces of primary respiration come into the foreground. Palpation will encourage the spontaneous occurrence of a local or systemic still point, e.g. in the form of a CV-4, EV-4 or CV-3. It must be carried out in a state of relaxed, non-invasive attention and empathy and the therapist should synchronize it with the inherent homeodynamic forces and rhythmic patterns. This focus by the therapist on the inherent homeodynamic processes and on the health within the patient is one of the most important fundamental points on which therapy is based.
- The way a technique is performed, on the other hand, depends on more than just the therapist's perception of the rhythms of primary respiration. Therapists' awareness of their own physical, intellectual and spiritual experience, the forces and the worlds acting within them and the dynamic interaction of their inner and outer world are also involved.
- All the techniques presented in this manual can and should be adapted through a process of dialog with the tissue.

Note: Nomenclature of dysfunctions:
The dysfunctions of all the bones are named for the direction in which the bone moves more – the 'direction of ease'. For example,

when there is motion restriction of the temporal bone in internal rotation and greater ease of motion in external rotation, this is called an external rotation dysfunction.

- The terms 'inspiration' and 'expiration' are used in this book to refer to the rhythmic phases of the primary respiratory mechanism (PRM).
- Where the rhythmic motion of pulmonary respiration is referred to, the terms 'inhalation' ('in-breath') and 'exhalation' ('out-breath') are used. The word 'pulmonary' is generally added where necessary to make quite clear that breathing with the lungs is meant.
- The patient is assumed to be supine unless otherwise stated.
- The therapist should adopt a position with elbows resting on the table whenever possible to provide a fixed point. Both feet should be placed on the floor to create a fulcrum in combination with the ischial tuberosities when sitting to treat the patient. Therapists should sit upright, in no way supporting themselves on the patient. Physical and psychological support are both to be avoided.
- If it is necessary to stand to carry out the treatment the therapist can also lean against the table as a support.
- Whenever bilateral contact needs to be made, you should create a link by means of a fulcrum if at all possible (usually by placing the thumbs of your two hands in contact with each other).
- Robert Fulford has pointed out in recent years that it can be important for treatment for the therapist to touch the left side of the patient with the right hand and to use the left hand for the right side of the patient. This aspect of energy polarity has not been taken into account in the description of the techniques, but this might be done if required by having the therapist stand, and face the patient when taking up hand contact.[87]
- Where the motion of the cranial bones is described on the basis of sutural, dural, muscular (and fluid) structures, this book uses the term 'biomechanical' palpation. The term 'biodynamic' is used to denote palpation where the motion of the cranial bones is described on the basis of embryological development. The description of the motion impulses is of course only roughly approximate to the reality. The above-mentioned explanation, too, is purely hypothetical. Most important for the therapist's approach is to stand aside from theory and trust the experience of the palpation in as unprejudiced a way as possible.
- The bones of the viscerocranium, unlike those of the neurocranium, are not attached to each other by means of the dural membranes. This means that a PBMT cannot be established there as it can for the neurocranium. Despite this, Sutherland does also mention the PBT as a form of treatment for the bones of the viscerocranium. The explanation for this lies partly in Sutherland's own palpation experience and partly in the way the sutures themselves are constructed, with fibrous structures within the intrasutural joint. According to KE Graham DO, 'point of balanced

fascial tension' would be a more comprehensive choice of term, as every structure in the body is surrounded by fascia. Bony dysfunctions are also treated using PBT. It is possible to induce a PBMT because the bone lies in a periosteal membrane, as well as a PBFT, because the bone itself consists of around 70% fluid, or a point of balanced electrodynamic tension (PBET).

ABBREVIATIONS

ER = external rotation
IR = internal rotation
PBT = point of balanced tension
PBMT = point of balanced membraneous tension
PBLT = point of balanced ligamentous tension
PBFT = point of balanced fluid tension
PBET = point of balanced electrodynamic tension
The PBET is not mentioned for every technique in the text. However, if the osteopath has acquired this type of palpation, the PBET should be incorporated into the treatment of the tissue as appropriate (see also Glossary).

LANDMARKS OF THE SKULL (FIG. 0.2)

- Nasion: mid-point of the frontonasal suture
- Glabella: smooth area between the eyebrows at the lower part of the metopic suture
- Ophryon: point above the glabella
- Bregma: junction of the sagittal and coronal sutures
- Vertex: topmost point of the skull
- Lambda: junction of the sagittal and lambdoid sutures
- Inion: external occipital protuberance

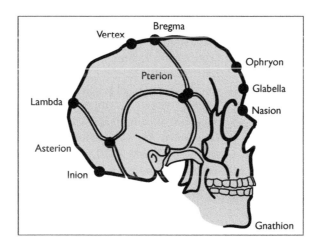

- Pterion: junction of the frontal, sphenoid, temporal and parietal bones
- Asterion: junction of the parietal, occipital and temporal bones
- Basion: middle point of the anterior margin of the foramen magnum
- Opisthion: middle point of the posterior margin of the foramen magnum
- Gnathion: the most inferior point of the mandible, centrally located at the tip of the chin.

References

1 Guillaume JP. Entwicklungen und Perspektiven der kraniofascialen Osteopathie. Osteopath Med 2002; 2:9–12.

2 Woods JM, Woods RH. A physical finding related to psychiatric disorders. J Am Osteopath Assoc 1961; 60:988–993.

3 Magoun HI. Osteopathy in the Cranial Field. 3rd edn. Kirksville: Journal Printing Company; 1976; 25.

4 Becker RE. Craniosacral trauma in the adult. Osteopath Ann 1976; 4:43–59.

5 Lay E. Cranial Field. In: Ward RC., ed. Foundations for Osteopathic Medicine. Baltimore: Williams and Wilkins; 1997; 901–913.

6 Lay EM, Cicorda RA, Tettambel M. Recording of the cranial rhythmic impulse. J Am Osteopath Assoc 1978; 78:149.

7 Wirth-Patullo V, Hayes KW. Interrater reliability of craniosacral rate measurements and their relationship with subjects' and examiner's heart and respiratory rate measurements. Phys Ther 1994; 74:908–920.

8 Nelson KE, et al. Cranial rhythmic impulse related to the Traube-Hering-Mayer oscillation: comparing laser-Doppler flowmetry and palpation. J Am Osteopath Assoc 2001; 101:163–173.

9 Becker R. Life in Motion: The Osteopathic Vision of Rollin E Becker. Brooks, RE., ed. Portland: Stillness Press 1997:120.

10 Upledger J, Vredevoogt JD. Craniosacral Therapy. Seattle: Eastland Press 1983; 243.

11 Jealous J. Emergence of originality. A biodynamic view of osteopathy in the cranial field. Course manual 1997:12, 35, 36.

12 Michael DK, Retzlaff EW. A preliminary study of cranial bone movement in the squirrel monkey. J Am Osteopath Assoc 1975; 74:886–889.

13 Liem T. Lecture: Vortrag OFM. 1998; Munich.

14 Lewer-Allen KL, Bunt EA, Lewer-Allen CM. Hydrodynamic Studies of the Human Craniospinal System. London: Janus Publishing Company; 2000:5.

15 Wallace WK et al. Ultrasonic techniques for measuring intracranial pulsations. Research and clinical studies. Neurology 1966; 16(4):380–382.

16 Lewer-Allen KL, Goldmann H. Phasic pressure characteristics of the cerebrospinal system. J S Afr Surg 1967:151.

17 Baker EG. Alteration in width of maxillary arch and its relation to sutural movement of cranial bones. J Am Osteopath Assoc 1970; 70:559–564.

18 White DM, Jenkins CO, Campbell JK. The compensatory mechanism for volume changes in the brain. 23rd Annual Conference on Engineering in Medicine and Biology November 1970:15–19.

19 Jenkins CO, Campbell JK, White DM. Modulation resembling Traube-Hering waves recorded in human brain. Eur Neurol 1971; 5:1–6.

20 Frymann VM. A study of the rhythmic motions of the living cranium. J Am Osteopath Assoc 1971; 70:928–945.

21 Life in Motion: The Osteopathic Vision of Rollin E Becker. Brooks, RE., ed. Portland: Stillness Press 1997:122.

22 Upledger JE, Karni Z. Mechanical electrical patterns during craniosacral osteopathic diagnosis and treatment. J Am Osteopath Assoc 1979; 78:782–791.

23 Brookes D. Lectures on Craniosacral Osteopathy. Northampton: Thorsons Publishers Ltd; 1981:58.

24 Upledger JE, Vredevoogt JD. Craniosacral Therapy. Seattle: Eastland Press; 1983:275–281.

25 Podlas H, Lewer-Allen K, Bunt EA. Computed tomography studies of human brain movements. S Afr J Surg; 1984; 22(1):57–63.

26 Lewer-Allen K, Bunt EA. Slow oscillation of compliance and pressure rate in the naturally closed craniospinal system. In: Hoff JT, Betz AL, ed. Intracranial Pressure III. Berlin: Springer-Verlag; 1989; 251–254.

27 Lewer-Allen K, Bunt EA, Lewer-Allen CM. Hydrodynamic Studies of the Human Craniospinal System. London: Janus Publishing Company; 2000; 5, 150, 158.

28 Druelle P. Allgemeine und craniale Osteopathie bei Neugeborenen und Kleinkindern. Skript des Deutschen Osteopathie Kolleg; 40.

29 McCatty RR. Essentials of Craniosacral Osteopathy. Bath: Ashgrove Press; 1988.

30 Herniou JC. Studies of the structures and mechanical properties of the cranium. In: Upledger JE, ed. Research and Observations Support the Existence of a Craniosacral System. Florida: UI Enterprises;1995:2.

31 Gunnergaard K. Rhythmische und nicht rhythmische Veränderungen der Dimensionen des menschlichen Schädels. Dtsch Zschr f biol Zahnm 1992; 8:160–169.

32 Norton JM, Sibley G, Broder-Oldach RE. Quantification of the cranial rhythmic impulse in human subjects. J Am Osteopath Assoc 1992; 92:1285.

33 Allen D. Observations from normal newborn osteopathic evaluations. Kirksville, MO: Kirksville Osteopathic Medical Center; Residency project report 1993:19.

34 Greenman PE, McPartland JM. Cranial findings and iatrogenesis from craniosacral manipulation in persons with traumatic brain injury. J Am Osteopath Assoc 1995; 95:182–191.

35 McAdoo J, Kuchera ML. Reliability of cranial rhythmic impulse palpation. Unpublished data 1995.

36 Jealous J. Emergence of originality. A biodynamic view of osteopathy in the cranial field. Course notes 1997:12, 35, 36.

37 Zanakis MF, Marmora M, Dowling T et al. Cranial mobility in humans. J Am Osteopath Assoc 1996/97.

38 Magoun HI. Osteopathy in the Cranial Field. 3rd edn. Kirksville: Journal Printing Company 1976:24.

39 Woolley DW, Shaw EN. Evidence for the participation of serotonin in mental processes. Ann NY Acad Sci 1957; 66:649–665.

40 Clark LC. Discussion of evidence for the participation of serotonin. Ann NY Acad Sci 1957; 66:668.

41 Hyden H. Satellite cells in the central nervous system. Sci Am 1961; 205:62.

42 Pomerat CM. Rhythmic contraction of Schwann cells. Science 1959; 130:1759.

43 Lumsden CE, Pomerat CM. Normal oligodendrocytes in tissue culture. Exp Cell Res 1951; 2:103–114.

44 Retzlaff EW, Mitchell FL. The Cranium and its Sutures. Berlin: Springer-Verlag 1987:14.

45 Feinberg DA, Mark AS. Human brain motion and cerebrospinal fluid circulation demonstrated with MR velocity imaging. Radiology 1987; 163:793–799.

46 Du Boulay G, O'Connell J, Currie J, Bostick T, Verity P. Further investigations on pulsatile movements in the cerebrospinal fluid pattern. Act Rad Diagn 1972; 13:496–523.

47 Sutherland WG. The Cranial Bowl. The Free Press Company, USA; 1939; 51, 55.

48 Greitz D, Wirestam R, Franck A, et al. Pulsatile brain movement and associated hydrodynamics studied by magnetic resonance phase imaging. Neuroradiology 1992; 34:370–380.

49 Greitz D, Franck A, Nordell B. On the pulsatile nature of intracranial and spinal CSF circulation demonstrated by MR imaging. Acta Radiol 1993; 34:321–328.

50 Gröschel-Stewart U, Unsicker K, Leonhardt H. Immunohistochemical demonstration of contractile proteins in astrocytes, marginal glial and ependymal cells in rat diencephalon. Cell Tiss Res 1977; 180(1):133–137.

51 Scordilis SP, et al. Characterisation of the myosin-phosphorylating system in normal murine astrocytes and derivative SV 40 wild-type and A-mutant transformants. J Cell Biol 1977; 74:940–949.

52 Fifkova E. Actin in the nervous system. Brain Res Rev 1985; 9:187–215.

53 Alonso G, et al. Ultrastructural organisation of actin filaments in neurosecretory axons of the rat. Cell Tiss Res 1981; 214:323–341.

54 Kimura A, et al. Tissue-specific and non-tissue-specific heavy-chain isoforms of myosin in the brain as revealed by monoclonal antibodies. Biochim Biophys Acta 1991; 1118(1):59–69.

55 Magoun HI. Osteopathy in the cranial field. 1st edn. Kirksville: 1951; 24.

56 Sears TA. Investigations on respiratory motoneurones of the thoracic spinal cord. Prog Brain Res 1964; 259–272.

57 Upledger JE, Vredevoogt JD. Craniosacral therapy. Seattle: Eastland Press; 1983:11.

58 Upledger JE, Vredevoogt JD. Craniosacral Therapy. Seattle: Eastland Press; 1983:13.

59 Ferguson A. Cranial osteopathy: a new perspective. Acad Appl Osteopath 1991; 1:12–16.

60 Degenhardt B, Kuchera M. Update on osteopathic medical concepts and the lymphatic system. J Am Osteopath Assoc 1996; 96:97–100.

61 Kinmonth J, Taylor G. Spontaneous rhythmic contraction in human lymphatics. J Physiol 1956; 133–136.

62 Norton JM. A tissue pressure model for palpatory perception of the cranial rhythmic impulse. J Am Osteopath Assoc 1991; 91:975–994.

63 Norton JM. Failure of a tissue model to predict cranial rhythmic impulse frequency. J Am Osteopath Assoc 1992; 92:1285.

64 McPartland J, Mein J. Entrainment and the cranial rhythmic impulse. Alt Ther Hlth Med 1997; 3:40–45.

65 Tiller WA, McCraty R, Atkinson M. Cardiac coherence: a new, noninvasive measure of autonomic nervous system order. Alt Ther 1996; 2:52–65.

66 McCraty R, Atkinson M, Tiller WA. New electrophysiological correlates associated with intentional heart focus. Subtle Energies 1995; 4:251–268.

67 Vern BA, Schuette WH, Leheta B, Juel VC, Radulovacki M. Low-frequency oscillations of cortical oxidative metabolism in waking and sleep. J Cereb Blood Flow Metab 1988; 8:215–226.

68 Farasyn A. New hypothesis for the origin of craniosacral motion. J Bodywork Move Ther 1999; 3:229–237.

69 Farasyn A, Vanderschueren F. The decrease of the cranial rhythmic impulse during maximal physical exertion: an argument for the hypothesis of venomotion? J Bodywork Move Ther 2001; 5(1):56–59.

70 Traube L. Über periodische Tätigkeits-Äusserungen des vasomotorischen und Hemmungs-Nervenzentrums. Cbl Med Wiss 1865; 56:881–885.

71 Hering E. Über Atembewegungen des Gefässsystems. Sitz Ber Akad Wiss Wien Mathe-Naturwiss Kl Anat 1869; 60:829–856.

72 Meyer S. Über spontane Blutdruckschwankungen. Sitz Ber Akad Wiss Wien Mathe-Naturwiss Kl Anat 1876; 67:282–305.

73 Sergueef N, Nelson KE, Glonek T. Changes in the Traube-Hering wave following cranial manipulation. J Am Osteopath Assoc 2001; 11:17.

74 Sergueef N, Nelson KE, Glonek T. The effect of cranial manipulation on the Traube-Hering-Meyer oscillation as measured by laser-Doppler flowmetry. Alt Ther Hlth Med 2002; 8(6):74–76.

75 Nelson KE, Sergueef N, Glonek T. The cranial rhythmic impulse and the Traube-Hering-Meyer oscillation. In: Proceedings of the International Research Conference in celebration of the 20th anniversary of the Osteopathic Center for Children (Frymann VM, Director), San Diego California, 6–10 February, 2002.

76 Jealous J. Personal course notes from the biodynamic course; 1997.

77 DiGiovanna EL, Kuchera ML, Greenman PE. Efficacy and complications. In: Ward RC, ed. Foundations for Osteopathic Medicine. Baltimore: Williams and Wilkins 1997:1015–1023.

78 McPartland JM. Side effects from cranial-sacral treatment: case reports and commentary. J Bodywork Move Ther 1996; 1(1):2–5.

79 Greenman PE, McPartland JM. Cranial findings and iatrogenesis from craniosacral manipulation in patients with traumatic brain syndrome. J Am Osteopath Assoc 1995; 95:182–192.

80 Becker R. The Stillness of Life. Brooks RE, ed. Portland: Stillness Press 2000:66, 67, 69.

81 Sutherland WG. Contributions of Thought. Sutherland Cranial Teaching Foundation 1967:153, 208.

82 Sutherland WG. Contributions of Thought. Sutherland Cranial Teaching Foundation 1967:244.

83 Sutherland WG. Contributions of Thought. Sutherland Cranial Teaching Foundation 1967:166.

84 Heede PVD. Der Natürliche Geburtsvorgang. Osteopath Med 2001; 4:10–12.

85 Magoun HI. Osteopathy in the Cranial Field. 1st edn. Kirksville: Journal Printing Company; 1951:76.

86 Jantsch E. Die Selbstorganisation des Universums. Vom Urknall zum menschlichen Geist. Munich: Hanser Verlag 1992; 61–63.

87 Commeaux Z. Robert Fulford DO and the Philosopher Physician. Seattle: Eastland Press 2002.

1 The sphenobasilar synchondrosis

The sphenobasilar synchondrosis (spheno-occipital synchondrosis) (also called the sphenobasilar joint or junction, or SBJ) occupies a central position in the cranium; it lies in the midline. Its position and its function as the attachment for muscles and fasciae make it an important fulcrum. This region also has a great influence on the growth of the face and skull.

Ossification of the SBS is complete between the 13th and 17th years of life,[1-3] and it seems unlikely that any motion or mobility can be found in the ossified SBS in adults. Mobility is however proven in the sutures of the cranial vault. Such mobility as is found at the SBS in adulthood consists of changes in elasticity and density and a capacity to adapt to certain forces. Further clarification is needed as to how far rhythmic intraosseous changes in elasticity occur in this region in response to primary respiration or form part of these rhythmic phenomena. The extent to which it is possible to palpate the assumed intraosseous adaptation due to primary respiration or trauma and the clinical significance of the SBS in adulthood, also remain to be fully clarified.

The question is, then, what is it that we sense when we palpate, indirectly, the region of the SBS? What can we detect by doing so? Are the classical descriptions still adequate or do they need to be translated into other terms based on more suitable models, or even abandoned?

It seems at least possible that the position of this region as a central point in the midline of the skull and as the attachment for many fascial structures may enable it to serve as a fulcrum even in later years.

ROHEN'S CONCEPT OF THE METAMORPHOSIS OF VERTEBRAE INTO THE CRANIAL BASE

The evolutionary developments associated with upright gait mean that the cranial base lies at an angled position in humans as compared with mammals in general, and so the viscerocranium lies more beneath the vault of the skull.[4]

The idea that the bones of the cranium were metamorphosed vertebrae, dates back to an insight by Goethe, the German poet and polymath, in 1790, and this idea was taken up by the researcher and philosopher Oken some years later.

The sphenoid and occipital bone are closely linked to each other in the base of the skull. Taken together they exhibit all the formal elements of a vertebra, except that in the cranial bones these formal elements appear in reverse. The seven spinous processes, which in the vertebra reflect the three dimensions of space, find their equivalent in the processes of the body of the sphenoid: lateral to the body of the sphenoid are the greater wings, superiorly the lesser wings, inferiorly the pterygoid processes, and anteriorly the sphenoidal rostrum.

The occipital bone is the equivalent of the body of the vertebra. An account of individual elements such as that given by Mees[5] does not greatly assist the understanding of the structures. The functional dynamics of the tissue are more important.

Rohen sees the basilar bone (occipital bone and sphenoid) as representing not simply the vertebra but the vertebral column of the skull, appearing to have the formal elements of all vertebrae and so of the spine as a whole, which it integrates in one ideal form. This means a complete reversal at the craniocervical transition zone: anterior and posterior are exchanged and a new space is created.

For Rohen,[6] the spongy substance of the extremities, which ossifies intracartilaginously from inside and in relation to the physical substance and blood vessels (adapted through its trajectories to static stresses) metamorphoses into the viscerocranium. The compact substance, meanwhile, which ossifies periosteally from the outside, gives shape to the long bones, (and is closely linked with the system of locomotion via its many muscle attachments) he sees as metamorphosing into the cranial vault. Viewed in this way the base of the skull represents the link between the cranial vault, with its cosmic orientation, and the terrestrially oriented viscerocranium.

The sensory nerves, located particularly at the base of the skull, are the route by which the external world impinges on the brain; in return, individuality communicates itself to the external world by means of language and facial expression. It is above all at the cranial base that this interchange, or, we might say, these countercurrents occur. Stone[7] sees the sphenoid as the positive pole of the coccyx.

LOCATION, CAUSES AND CLINICAL PRESENTATION OF OSTEOPATHIC DYSFUNCTIONS OF THE SBS

Disturbances may affect all the structures linked to the occiput or sacrum.

Osseous dysfunction

Occipital bone

a) Lambdoid suture: The squamous interdigitated suture prevents overlapping of the bones, but can be compressed by a fall or blow.

b) Occipitomastoid suture and the condylo-squamoso-mastoid pivot point (CSMP):

Causes:
- Bilateral compression: fall or blow to the occipital squama.
- Unilateral compression: fall or blow to the side of the occipital squama or mastoid process.

This forces the squama in an anterior direction, the basilar part of the occiput inferiorly and the temporal bones into internal rotation. The concave mastoid border of the occipital bone is forced anteriorly and superiorly, wedging it into the convex posterior edge of the mastoid process of the temporal bone, which moves posteriorly and medially.

● Whiplash injuries and direct thrust techniques to the back of the head can also result in compression of this suture.

Compression at this suture leads to opposite motion of the temporal bone relative to the occipital bone. In other words, the occiput moves into flexion and the temporal bone into internal rotation.

Clinical presentation: Abnormal tensions of the tentorium cerebelli, venous congestion of the sigmoid sinus, disturbances in the fluctuation of the cerebrospinal fluid (with possible disturbance to the cranial nerve nuclei at the 4th ventricle), disturbances to the cerebellum, medulla oblongata or other centers of the brain, and of the vagus nerve (nausea, vomiting, etc.).

Sequelae: Dysfunction of the SBS and a change in the frequency and amplitude of PRM rhythm, impairing homeostasis of the body as a whole.

c) Petro-occipital fissure (petro-occipital synchondrosis; this fissure is also known as the petrobasilar suture): The lateral margins of the base of the occipital bone form a ridge, which articulates with a groove on the lower posterior portion of the petrous part of the temporal bone. This construction enables a turning and sliding motion.

Causes: In association with the occipital bone: usually as a result of trauma, e.g. tooth extraction with mouth wide open.

Clinical presentation: Disturbance of the jugular foramen and foramen lacerum and the nerves and blood vessels that pass through these (Figs 1.1, 1.2).

d) Petrojugular suture: The jugular process of the occipital bone articulates with the jugular articular surface of the petrous part of the temporal bone. This location can be seen as a pivot point from which the motion of the occiput is transmitted to the temporal bone.

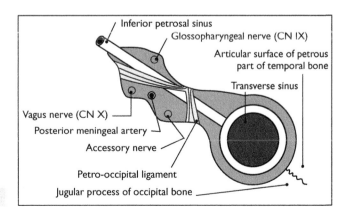

Figure 1.1 Jugular foramen

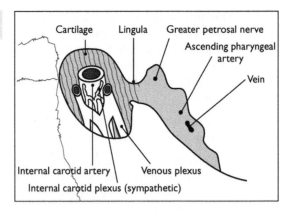

Figure 1.2 Foramen lacerum

Causes and clinical presentation: See petro-occipital fissure (petro-occipital synchondrosis) (above).

e) Atlanto-occipital joint: The many neural, vascular, muscular and fascial associations and attachments mean that this region is responsible for a large number of symptoms.

Causes: Birth trauma, falls and blows. Secondary lesions can result from dysfunctions of the SBS or sacrum, hypertonus of the splenius muscles, abnormal fascial tensions, psychological tension, stress, abnormal asymmetric loads, poor working position, etc.

Clinical presentation: Upper cervical syndrome, pain in the nuchal area.

- Headache and other functional disturbances of the brain (obstruction of drainage of the jugular vein).
- Stenosis of the vertebral artery with disturbance of the sympathetic fibers of the inferior cervical ganglion.
- Disturbances of the salivary glands and eyes (superior cervical ganglion).
- Cranial nerve symptoms (see below) (disturbance of the vagus nerve, glossopharyngeal nerve, accessory nerve and hypoglossal nerve).
- Disturbance of fine motor function and motor skills (decussation of pyramids).
- Dysfunction of the medulla oblongata.
- Spinal scoliosis.
- Disturbance of the hypophysis, thyroid and parathyroid.
- Possible dull pain in the lower half of the body (irritation of fibers of the spinal cord).
- Abnormal dural tensions, sometimes accompanied by compression of the SBS or sacrolumbar transition zone, etc.

Sphenoid

a) The mobility of the orbits may be disturbed, and restriction of the fine mobility and position of the sphenoid may impair the muscles and nerves of the eye and the optic nerve.

Clinical presentation: Visual disturbances.

b) Sphenosquamous suture and sphenosquamous pivot point (SSP)

Causes: Primary trauma as a result of a fall or blow to the cheek or mastoid process of the temporal bone on the same side. Secondary lesions can result from dysfunctions of the sphenoid or viscerocranium or hypertonus of the temporalis muscle (in psychological stress or temporomandibular syndrome).

Clinical presentation:
- At the vertical portion of the suture: middle meningeal artery → migraine.
- At the horizontal portion of the suture: greater and lesser petrosal nerves. From the greater petrosal nerve to the pterygopalatine ganglion: disturbance of the lacrimal gland, dry or irritated mucosa of the nose, nasopharynx, and palate, allergic rhinitis (see also pterygopalatine fossa). Lesser petrosal nerve: disturbance of the parotid gland.
- Functional disturbance of neighboring parts of the brain.

Sequelae: Dysfunction of the SBS and a change in the frequency and amplitude of the PRM rhythm, impairing homeostasis of the body as a whole.

c) Sphenopetrosal synchondrosis

Causes: Tooth extraction from the upper jaw can produce an ipsilateral dysfunction of the petrosphenoidal ligament. Tooth extraction from the lower jaw can cause a contralateral dysfunction of the ligament. The III, IV and VI cranial nerves (controlling the eye muscles) run beside the body of the sphenoid, close to this ligament. The VI cranial nerve in particular is susceptible to tensions arising from the tentorium and the ligament, because it is linked by fibers to the petrosphenoidal ligament and runs through an osteofibrous channel formed by the ligament and the temporal bone.

Clinical presentation: Disturbances of the eye, fatigue-related strabismus in young children, etc. Twisting of the medial two-thirds of the Eustachian tubes with tinnitus or deafness. Maxillary malalignment with nose and throat symptoms.

d) Sphenoparietal suture

e) Sphenofrontal suture

Clinical presentation: The mobility of the SBS can be restricted by force to the suture.

f) Sphenozygomatic suture

Causes: A fall or blow to the cheek and SBS dysfunctions.

Clinical presentation: The zygomatic bone is an important integration point for influences arriving from the occipital bone, sphenoid and viscerocranium. Traumatic injuries can impair this important integrative function. Maxillary sinusitis, disturbance of the orbits.

g) Sphenoethmoidal suture

Clinical presentation: Dysfunctions of the SBS, sphenoid and ethmoid bones can disturb the transmission of motion from the spine of the sphenoid to the ethmoid bone, and the drainage of the nasal cavities.

h) Sphenovomerine suture

i) Sphenopalatine suture

The tips of the pterygoid processes of the sphenoid move within grooves on the back of the small palatine bones. The pterygoid processes converge anteriorly and separate posteriorly, so that the sphenoid spreads the palatine bones in the inspiration phase and moves them into external rotation. According to Sutherland this slight pendulum motion between the tips of the pterygoid processes of the sphenoid and these grooves on the palatines is particularly important for the effective transmission of motion to the palatine and maxillary bones, and also for its function as a 'speed reducer'. This mechanism is frequently disturbed, for example in SBS dysfunctions or in traumatic injuries to the face.

Clinical presentation: Disturbance of motion transmission to the maxillary complex, motion restriction of the maxillary complex, disturbance of the pterygopalatine ganglion.

j) Intraosseous dysfunctions

Between the complex of the body of sphenoid and lesser wings, and the complexes of the greater wing and pterygoid process (ossification around the 7th month of life).

Causes: Primary trauma as a result of direct force to the sphenoid during birth or traumatic injury in infancy; secondary lesion caused by dysfunction of the sacrum.

Sequelae: Reduced pliancy of the bone, SBS dysfunction, development of scolioses, disturbances of the foramen lacerum and jugular foramen, and impairment of the function of all structures involved.

Note: Sutherland observed that prenatal disturbances in the fusing of pre- and post-sphenoid can be expressed in the course of development in a slanting orbit, a typical feature of Down syndrome. (The pre- and post-sphenoid fuse in about the 8th month of fetal development.)[1]

Muscular dysfunction

Occipital bone

a) Tonus of all nuchal muscles can impair the mobility of the occiput and thus the SBS

b) Sternocleidomastoid muscle

Clinical presentation: Hypertonus: Motion restriction of the occipitomastoid suture, migraine or hemicranial headache.

The XI cranial nerve runs through the jugular foramen, which can be impaired by hypertonus of the sternocleidomastoid or trapezius muscle. This in turn can lead to further increase in muscle tonus via the XI cranial nerve.

c) Trapezius muscle

Clinical presentation: Headache affecting the back of the head, pain and stiffness of the shoulder, aggravation of pain in the muscles of mastication.

● Bilateral hypertonus: flexion dysfunction of the SBS.

d) Semispinalis capitis muscle

Clinical presentation: ● Headache affecting the back of the head; temporal headache.
● Bilateral hypertonus: flexion dysfunction of the SBS.
● Unilateral hypertonus: torsion dysfunction of the SBS.

e) Hypertonus of the splenius capitis muscle can lead to headache affecting the nape of the neck, the back of the head, and the parietal region

f) Longus capitis and rectus capitis anterior muscles
Clinical presentation: ● Bilateral hypertonus: extension dysfunction of the SBS.
● Unilateral hypertonus: torsion dysfunction of the SBS.

g) Rectus capitis lateralis muscle
Clinical presentation: ● Venous reflux to the inside of the cranium and disturbances of the IX, X, and XI cranial nerves.
● Unilateral hypertonus: torsion dysfunction of the SBS.

h) Rectus capitis posterior major and minor muscles
Clinical presentation: ● Headache affecting the back of the head.
● Bilateral hypertonus: flexion dysfunction of the SBS.
● Unilateral hypertonus: torsion of the SBS.

Muscle atrophy: ● Possible slight compression of spinal cord due to connective tissue link between the rectus capitis posterior minor muscle and the posterior part of the dura mater.[8]

i) Obliquus capitis superior muscle
Clinial presentation: ● Headache affecting the back of the head.
● Bilateral hypertonus: flexion dysfunction of the SBS.
● Unilateral hypertonus: side-bending/rotation dysfunction of the SBS.

j) Superior pharyngeal constrictor muscle
Clinical presentation: ● Pain and dysfunction of the floor of the mouth and pharynx.
● In the case of hypertonus: via the pharyngeal raphe, flexion and extension dysfunctions of the SBS.

Sphenoid

a) Masticatory muscles: Temporalis muscle, lateral pterygoid muscle, medial pterygoid muscle
Clinical presentation: Dental malocclusion; grinding of teeth, temporomandibular joint pain, headache, pain in the upper jaw, central region of the face, floor of the mouth, or ear.

b) Muscles of the eye
● Superior rectus muscle, inferior rectus, medial rectus and lateral rectus, superior oblique muscle.
● Dysfunction of the sphenoid, of the rest of the orbits, or of innervation produces changes in tension of these muscles resulting in visual disturbances.

c) Tensor veli palatini muscle
Affects the auditory tube and soft palate.

d) Palatopharyngeus and superior pharyngeal constrictor muscles

Clinical presentation: Disturbances in swallowing.

Ligamentous dysfunctions

Occipital bone

a) Abnormal tension of the nuchal ligaments can impair the mobility of the occiput

b) Posterior atlanto-occipital membrane
The vertebral artery and suboccipital nerve pierce this membrane. Tensions in the membrane can therefore impair their function.

c) Other ligaments in the occipital area may also be involved in any dysfunctions:

The anterior atlanto-occipital membrane, anterior longitudinal ligament, apical ligament of the dens, alar ligaments, tectorial membrane, and posterior longitudinal ligament.

Sphenoid

a) Petrosphenoidal ligament (Gruber's ligament) at the petrosphenoidal suture (fissure)

Causes: Dysfunction of the petrous part of the temporal bone, tooth extractions, and ossification of the ligament.
   Magoun states that tooth extraction from the upper jaw can lead to ipsilateral dysfunction of the petrosphenoidal ligament.[9]
   Tooth extraction from the lower jaw can lead to dysfunction of the ligament and a separation of the sphenopetrosal synchondrosis on the opposite side.[10]

Clinical presentation: Abducent nerve (CN VI) symptoms. Twisting of the medial two-thirds of the Eustachian tubes with tinnitus or deafness. Maxillary malalignment with nose and throat symptoms.

b) Excessive strain of the sphenomandibular ligament can occur unilaterally as a result of dental surgery[10]

Fascial dysfunction

Occipital bone

a) Investing layer of cervical fascia: extending to the superior nuchal line

b) Prevertebral layer of cervical fascia: extending from its attachment to the pharyngeal tubercle to the occipitomastoid suture

c) Pharynx: at the pharyngeal tubercle

Sphenoid

a) Interpterygoid aponeurosis: at the spine of the sphenoid and anterior border of the foramen ovale and foramen spinosum *b)* Pterygo-temporo-mandibular aponeurosis: from the lateral pterygoid plate to the foramen ovale

c) Palatine aponeurosis: at the medial pterygoid plate

d) Orbital fascia

e) Superficial layer: over the muscular and ligamentous attachment to the styloid process

f) Body cavity and pharynx: at the medial pterygoid plate and foramen lacerum.
Dysfunctions may be caused by hypertonus muscular tension, dysfunctions of the locomotor system and internal organs (e.g. esophagus, stomach, lung).

Sequelae: ● Motion restrictions of the SBS, dysfunctions of involved structures.

Dysfunction of intracranial and extracranial dural membranes

Falx cerebri, tentorium cerebelli, falx cerebelli, spinal dura mater

a) A torsion dysfunction causes a twisting distortion of the falx cerebri on account of its anterior attachments to the frontal bone and posterior to the occipital bone. Anteriorly the falx is shifted away from the raised greater wing, whereas posteriorly it moves closer to the side of this greater wing, that is, closer to the side of the lowered occiput.

The tentorium cerebelli moves caudad on the side where the occipital bone is lowered and cephalad on the opposite side. The spinal dura mater moves caudad on the side where the occipital bone is lowered.

b) A side-bending/rotation dysfunction causes the falx cerebri to bend toward the convex side, i.e. the side of the dysfunction. The tentorium also bends toward the side of the convexity. The spinal dura mater moves caudad on the side where the occipital bone is lowered.

Clinical presentation: Disturbance of venous drainage and drainage of the choroid plexus, and the cranial nerves where they run along and are sheathed in the dura.

Disturbances to nerves and parts of the brain

All the cranial nerves are susceptible. The symptoms and sequelae correspond to the nerve affected.

a) Olfactory nerve (CN I)
Causes: At the level of the lesser wing of the sphenoid; main cause is dysfunction of the ethmoid bone.
Clinical presentation: Disturbance of sense of smell.

b) Optic nerve (CN II)

Causes: Abnormal dural tension in the optic canal or alteration in the position of the body of the sphenoid.

Clinical presentation: Disturbance of vision.

c) The motor nerves of the eye, e.g. oculomotor (CN III), trochlear (CN IV) abducent (CN VI), and ophthalmic nerve (CN V 1)

Causes: Abnormal tension in the petrosphenoidal ligament (see also CN VI), tentorium or superior orbital fissure; often found in vertical strain.

Clinical presentation: CN III: Lateral deviation of the eyeball, horizontal double vision, divergent strabismus, restriction of the line of sight upward, downward and medially.
CN III, autonomic: Mydriasis, ptosis of the eyelid and diminution of the photomotor reflex.
CN IV: Upward and medial deviation of the eyeball, reduced downward, lateral movement, vertical or oblique double vision, convergent strabismus.
CN V 1: Altered sensitivity and pain in the skin of the forehead and upper eyelid, the mucous membrane of the frontal sinus and the connective tissue membrane, limitation of the corneal reflex (CN V 1), pain in the eye and lacrimation (the trigeminal nerve contains some parasympathetic fibers).
CN VI: Horizontal double vision, convergent strabismus, medial deviation of the eyeball, restriction of the lateral line of sight, tendency to hold the head turned to one side to compensate for the deficiency.

d) Trigeminal nerve (CN V)

Causes: Abnormal dural tension of the tentorium cerebelli and the dura of the trigeminal ganglion, alteration in the position of the temporal bone, tensions and stasis in the wall of the cavernous sinus (CN V 1, V 2), abnormal dural tension at the foramen rotundum (CN V 2) or foramen ovale (CN V 3). The foramen ovale lies close to the spine of the sphenoid, which according to Magoun[11] is the point of maximum motion of the sphenoid, making it susceptible to dysfunctions.
The application of force to the face or a dysfunction of the temporomandibular joint with hypertonus of the lateral and medial pterygoid muscles may produce disturbances of the junction between the palatine and the sphenoid bones and in some circumstances affect the pterygopalatine ganglion in the sphenopalatine foramen. SBS dysfunctions can also impair the functioning of the pterygopalatine ganglion.

Clinical presentation: Trigeminal neuralgia.
CN V 1: see above.
CN V 2: Disturbances of sensation affecting the center of the face, restriction of the sneezing reflex.
CN V 3: Disturbances of sensation affecting the lower face, disturbance of masticatory muscle function.
Trigeminal ganglion: all listed symptoms of the trigeminal branches.
Pterygopalatine ganglion: secretory disturbances of the lacrimal gland and the mucous membranes of the nose and palate.

e) Facial nerve (CN VII) and intermediate nerve (CN VII)
Pass through the internal acoustic meatus in the facial canal; unite at geniculate ganglion; branch of sensory fibers in the chorda tympani supplies sensation (taste); main part of nerve through the stylomastoid foramen.

Causes: Dural tensions of the internal acoustic meatus and stylomastoid foramen.

Clinical presentation:
- Facial nerve (CN VII): disturbance of facial expression.
- Intermediate nerve (CN VII): disturbance of saliva secretion; taste disturbances of the anterior three-quarters of the tongue, functional disturbance of the lacrimal gland, nasal and palatine glands (via greater petrosal nerve).

f) Vestibulocochlear nerve (CN VIII)
Through the internal acoustic meatus to the organs of hearing and balance.

Causes: Abnormal dural tension of the internal acoustic meatus, dysfunction of the petrojugular suture.

Clinical presentation: Disturbances of hearing and balance.

g) Glossopharyngeal nerve (CN IX), vagus nerve (CN X), accessory nerve (CN XI)
at the jugular notch, together with the intrajugular process.

Causes: Dural tensions at the jugular foramen, dysfunction of the occipital and temporal bones, occipitomastoid suture, petrojugular suture and petro-occipital fissure (petrobasilar suture; petro-occipital synchondrosis).

Clinical presentation: CN IX: Disturbances of swallowing (fibers supplying sensation to the pharynx), taste disturbances, dry mouth (parasympathetic fibers serving parotid gland).
CN X: Functional disturbances of the heart, digestion, pulmonary respiration, speaking and swallowing.
CN XI: Torticollis.

h) Greater and lesser petrosal nerves in groove for the nerve of that name.

Causes: Abnormal dural tension in groove; the greater petrosal nerve runs along its groove to the foramen lacerum, an opening in the sphenopetrosal synchondrosis. Vertical strain in particular can impair this nerve (a parasympathetic branch of the intermediate nerve).

Clinical presentation:
- Greater petrosal nerve: dysfunction of the lacrimatory and nasal glands and of the palate.
- Lesser petrosal nerve: dysfunction of the parotid gland.

i) Hypoglossal nerve (CN XII)

Causes: Dural tensions of the hypoglossal canal.

Clinical presentation: Restriction of mobility of the tongue, disturbances in sucking.

j) Basal ganglia

Causes: Disturbance in supply and drainage of the basal ganglia; the basal ganglia are drained through the cavernous sinus and straight sinus, which are directly linked with the sphenoid, occiput and tentorium.

Clinical presentation: Disturbances of movement and trembling.

k) Mesencephalon
Causes: The mesencephalon has to pass through the opening in the tentorium above the SBS, as do all links between the spinal cord and cerebral cortex. Torsions and side-bending dysfunctions can cause disturbance of these structures.

l) Hypothalamus
Causes: Side-bending/rotation dysfunction of the SBS.
Clinical presentation: Disturbances of temperature regulation, water balance, endocrine system, and emotional disturbances.

m) Cortical regions
Clinical presentation: Dysfunction of the greater wing of the sphenoid can cause impairment of the taste cortex, olfactory cortex and auditory cortex. Dysfunction of the lesser wing can impair the speech cortex.

n) Cerebral aqueduct and interventricular foramen
Causes: The aqueduct is situated between the 3rd and 4th ventricles and can be twisted as a result of torsion or bent by side-bending dysfunction of the SBS, leading to hydrocephalus.
  The interventricular foramen between the lateral and 3rd ventricles can become constricted in SBS dysfunctions.

o) CSF fluctuation in the subarachnoid space
Causes: Occurs particularly in torsion or side-bending dysfunctions of the SBS.

Vascular disturbances

a) Internal carotid artery
Causes: Abnormal dural tension in the carotid canal, foramen lacerum and cavernous sinus, and alteration in the position of the sphenoid (especially in torsion and side-bending dysfunctions of the SBS).
Clinical presentation: Disturbance of the sympathetic nervous system brought about by impingement of the internal carotid plexus, disturbance of the voluntary control of the muscular system (the frontal lobe center that controls this is supplied by the middle cerebral artery, a terminal branch of the internal carotid artery).

b) Middle meningeal artery
Causes: Compression of the sphenosquamous suture and the sphenosquamous pivot point (SSP), abnormal tension of the dura mater in the middle cranial fossa.
Clinical presentation: Migraine and raised intracranial pressure.

c) Occipital artery
Causes: Dural tensions in the occipital groove, medial to the mastoid notch.

d) Jugular vein (responsible for drainage of about 95% of the venous blood that leaves the head).

Causes: Abnormal dural tension at the jugular foramen, dysfunction of the occipital and temporal bones, occipitomastoid and petrojugular sutures and petro-occipital fissure (petrobasilar suture; petro-occipital synchondrosis). The jugular foramen is like a broad suture between the occiput and temporal bone and so liable to be impaired when there is any dysfunction of these two bones.

Clinical presentation: Venous congestion within the cranium → headache, memory disturbances and impairment of brain function.

e) Dural venous sinuses
Sigmoid sinus, superior and inferior petrosal sinus, transverse sinus, cavernous sinus, superior and inferior sagittal sinus, occipital sinus, confluence of sinuses.

Causes: Compression, abnormal dural tension in the jugular foramen, foramen magnum, tentorium cerebelli, falx cerebri and falx cerebelli, motion restriction of the sphenoid and occipital bone.

Sequelae: *Sigmoid sinus:* Congestion affecting the confluence of sinuses and superior petrosal sinus.
Superior and inferior petrosal sinuses: Congestion affecting the cavernous sinus and basilar venous plexus, the ophthalmic veins, and the veins of the medulla, pons, inferior surface of the cerebellum and other segments of the brain.

Clinical presentation:
- Region of the sigmoid sinus → pain behind the ear.
- Region of the transverse sinus → pain in the temporal region or ipsilateral front of the head or the eye.
- Confluence of sinuses → pain in the ipsilateral front of the head and in the eye.
- Region of the superior petrosal sinus → pain in the temporal region.
- Cavernous sinus → pain in the ipsilateral eye and maxillary region.
- Region of the superior sagittal sinus and veins serving this area → pain in the frontoparietal region and region of the eye.
- Venous stasis affecting particular segments of the brain → headache, impairment of relevant brain functions.
- Venous stasis affecting the eyes → visual disturbances, sensation of pressure.

Endocrine disturbances

Hormonal control is centered in the hypophysis, which is located in the sella turcica of the sphenoid. Any alteration in the fine mobility of the sphenoid, abnormal dural tension of the diaphragma sellae, and tensions in the lateral walls of the cavernous sinus impair the function of the hypophysis.

Note: The opening in the diaphragma sellae is thought to enlarge during the inspiration phase of PRM for the stalk of the hypophysis, and to become smaller again during the expiration phase.

The occipital bone

Examination and techniques

- History-taking
- Visual assessment
- Palpation of the position
- Palpation of the PRM rhythm
- Motion testing
- Active
- Passive
- O-A
- Intraosseous techniques: cranial base-occiput-foramen-magnum technique in young children, platybasia technique, occipital squama technique
- CV-4
- EV-4

Sutures

- Lambdoid suture, see under parietal bone
- Lambda, see under parietal bone
- Occipitomastoid suture, see under temporal bone
- Petro-occipital fissure (petrobasilar suture; petro-occipital synchondrosis) and petrojugular suture, see under temporal bone

Visual assessment

Occipital squama bent: occiput in flexion
Occipital squama flattened: occiput in extension

Palpation of the position of the atlanto-occipital joint (Fig. 1.3)

Patient position: Supine.

Therapist: Take up a position at the head of the patient.

Hand position: ➤ Place your hands underneath the patient's head, to each side of the occiput.
➤ Place the index and middle fingers as close as possible to the occipital condyles.

Method: ➤ Compare the two sides.
➤ The side that is lying farther anterior and inferior than the other may be the side where the compression is present, if any.

Palpation of the position of the occipital bone

➤ Supraoccipital part: inferior (ER) or superior (IR).
➤ The angle of the squama and condyles: reduced or enlarged.
➤ External occipital protuberance: whether or not laterally displaced.
➤ Condylar part: compressed anterior-posterior or mediolaterally.

Figure 1.3 Palpation of the position of the atlanto-occipital joint

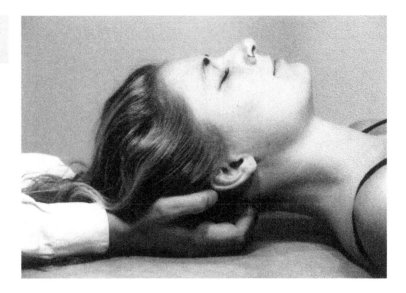

➤ Lambda: depressed, e.g. primary traumatic injury due to force, or elevated.
➤ Occipitomastoid suture: depressed or elevated.
➤ Flexibility of the occipital bone: pliant or hard.

Palpation of primary respiration

● Biomechanical/biodynamic palpation; motion test as necessary.
● If a motion restriction is discovered on palpation, the therapist may induce motion in the direction of restricted motion. This will emphasize the restriction and make it clearer to identify. The therapist will be able to sense which structure is the origin of the motion restriction:

1. intraosseous tension
2. sutural/osseous restriction relative to adjoining bones
3. dural restriction
4. fascial or ligamentous restriction
5. muscular restriction
6. vascular effect
7. neuronal activity.

Therapist: Take up a position at the head of the patient (Fig. 1.4).
Hand position: ➤ Place your hands under the patient's head, one each side, so that the occiput is cradled in your hands. Place your index and middle finger as close as possible to the occipital condyles.

Biomechanical approach
Inspiration phase of primary respiration, normal finding (Fig. 1.5):

➤ The joint articulations with the atlas move anteriorly.
➤ The inferior lateral parts of the occipital squama move inferiorly and anteriorly.
➤ Lambda and the cranial part of the occipital squama move posteriorly and inferiorly.

Figure 1.4 Palpation of primary respiration of the occipital bone

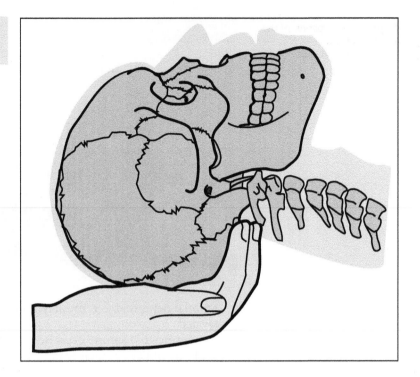

Figure 1.5 PR inspiration phase: biomechanical

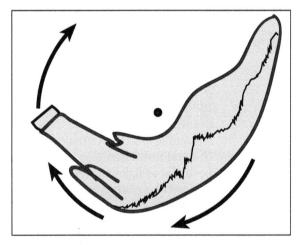

➤ The peripheral, lateral parts of the occiput at the asterion move inferiorly and laterally in an external rotation motion.

(The mastoid border (of the occipital with the temporal bone) moves anteriorly. The basilar part of the occipital bone moves superiorly and anteriorly.)

Expiration phase of the PR, normal finding:

➤ The joint articulations with the atlas move posteriorly.
➤ The inferior lateral parts of the occipital squama move superiorly and posteriorly.

> Lambda and the cranial part of the occipital squama move anteriorly and superiorly.
> The peripheral, lateral parts of the occiput at the asterion move superiorly and medially in an internal rotation motion.

(The mastoid border (of the occipital with the temporal bone) moves posteriorly. The basilar part moves inferiorly and posteriorly.)

Biodynamic/embryological approach
Inspiration phase of PR, normal finding (Fig. 1.6):

> The occipital squama moves centrifugally (outward motion).
> The convexity of the squama is reduced: the squama flattens.

Expiration phase of PR, normal finding:

> The occipital squama moves centripetally.
> The convexity of the squama increases.
> Compare the amplitude, strength, ease and symmetry of the motions of the occiput.

Motion testing

Hand position: As above.
Method: > Apply slight cephalad traction to the occiput to test the motion of the atlanto-occipital joint.
> Restrictions or compression may be unilateral or bilateral.
> Compare the amplitude and ease of movement of the occiput, or the amount of force required to produce motion.

TREATMENT OF THE OCCIPITAL BONE

Atlanto-occipital joint

Bilateral release of the atlanto-occipital joint and decompression of the occipital condylar region (Figs 1.7a,b)

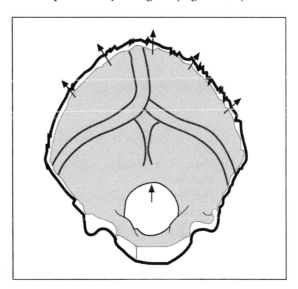

Figure 1.6 PR inspiration phase: biodynamic

Figure 1.7 (a,b) Bilateral release of the atlanto-occipital joint and decompression of the occipital condylar region

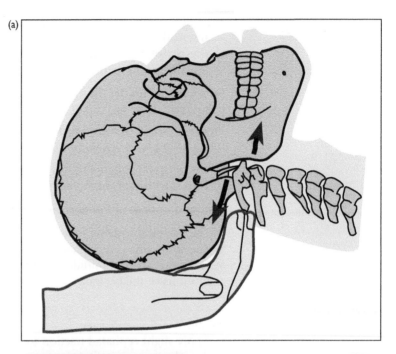

(a)

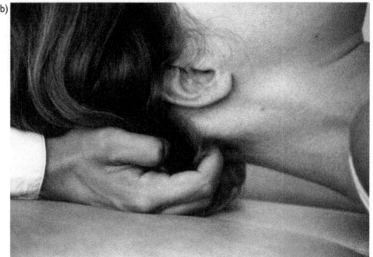

(b)

Therapist: Take up a position at the head of the patient.

Hand position: ➤ Place both hands underneath the occiput with the palms facing anterior.
➤ The patient's head should at this stage be resting in the palms of your hands.
➤ Bend your fingers upward at a right angle so that they are pointing directly anterior.
➤ Place your fingers immediately by the inferior palpable border of the occiput, very close to the arch of the atlas. (During the course

of the treatment, when the nuchal muscles relax, your fingers will rest on the posterior arch of the atlas.)

Method:
- ➤ Do not apply any additional pressure with your fingers. The weight of the skull alone, with your fingers acting as a lever, is used to release the nuchal muscles.
- ➤ Readjust your fingers into the upright position as often as necessary if the release of the nuchal muscles causes them to shift to an oblique angle.
- ➤ As the nuchal muscles relax it will gradually become possible to feel the bony arch of the atlas.
- ➤ At the end of treatment the skull will no longer be resting on your palms but will be supported at the atlas by your fingers alone.
- ➤ After releasing the nuchal muscles you can also go on to release the occipital condyles from the atlas. To do this, hold the arch of the atlas in place with your middle fingers alone and using the ring fingers and little fingers to draw the cranium gently cephalad.
- ➤ Then decompress the occipital condyles transversally. Continue to point your fingers toward the foramen magnum at a 45° angle corresponding to the arrangement of the occipital condyles. Draw your elbows together so that your fingers move outward at the occipital condyles. Continue until you sense a softening and inherent motion of the tissues.

Contraindications:
- ➤ Fracture of the dens axis, e.g. as a result of whiplash injury.
- ➤ Risk of intracranial bleeding, in acute aneurysm or cerebrovascular accident.
- ➤ Fracture of the cranial base.

Bilateral release of the atlanto-occipital joint *(Figs 1.8a,b)*

Therapist: Take up a position at the head of the patient.

Hand position:
- ➤ Grasp the arch of the atlas with the thumb and index finger of one hand.
- ➤ Hold the occiput with the other hand, placing your thumb and little finger on the lateral parts of the occiput.
- ➤ Place your index and middle finger next to the inion, on the superior nuchal line.

Method:
- ➤ Begin by palpating the motion of the occiput in extension and flexion (phases of PR).
- ➤ Then hold the atlas firmly in position.
- ➤ As you do so, go with the occiput in the direction of greater ease (indirect technique).
- ➤ Establish a position of the occiput (in terms of flexion or extension, side-bending and rotation) that achieves the best possible balance of ligamentous and membranous tensions in the joint (PBLT and PBMT).
- ➤ This position will enable the ligamentous/membranous tensions to normalize.
- ➤ Now you should also draw the head gently cephalad, to disengage the joint.

Figure 1.8 (a,b) Bilateral release of the atlanto-occipital joint

(a)

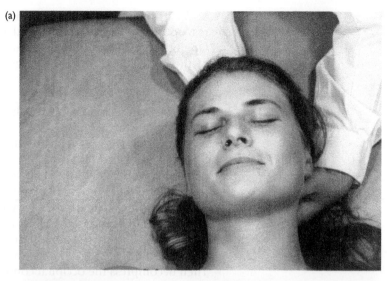

(b)

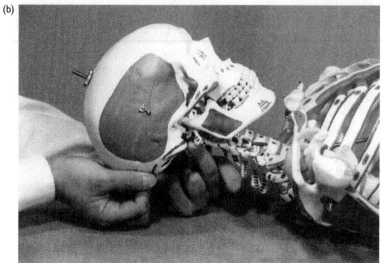

➤ Allow all further unwinding of the tissue, without slackening the gentle cephalad traction to the occipital bone and all the time maintaining the PBLT and PBMT.

➤ Maintain the PBT of the atlanto-occipital joint until you sense that the unwinding of the tissues is complete and that a release of the motion restriction has occurred.

Sutherland's technique for condyloatlantal dysfunctions *(Fig. 1.9)*

Therapist: Take up a position at the head of the patient.

Hand position: ➤ Place the tip of your middle finger on the posterior tubercle of the atlas.

➤ Place your other hand on the frontal bone with your fingers pointing caudad.

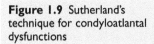

Figure 1.9 Sutherland's technique for condyloatlantal dysfunctions

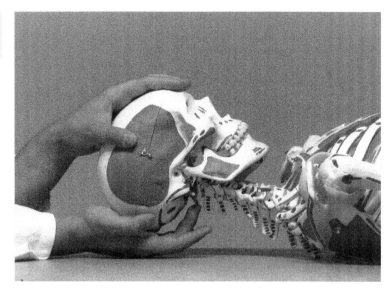

Method:
- ➤ Hold the atlas anterior and prevent it from moving posterior.
- ➤ Ask the patient to make a slight nod of the head.
- ➤ The anteriorly directed pressure of your finger on the atlas prevents bending anywhere other than at the atlanto-occipital joint, involving the rest of the cervical spine.
- ➤ The nodding movement releases the occipital condyles from the atlas. At the same time there is an increase in tension of the atlanto-occipital ligaments.
- ➤ Induce a PBLT (and PBMT). The point of balanced tension (PBT) is the position in which the tension in the ligaments (dural membranes) between the occiput and the atlas is as balanced as possible.
- ➤ Maintain the PBT until the ligamentous/membranous tension is normalized.
- ➤ Breathing assistance: ask the patient to hold an inhalation or exhalation for as long as possible at the end of an in or out-breath. The moment just before the patient has to draw the next involuntary breath (or has to breathe out) is when release of the motion restriction usually occurs.

Note: As strictly defined, Sutherland's technique is only concerned with the ligamentous tension of the atlanto-occipital joint. However, in view of the fact that the dura mater spinalis is attached at the foramen magnum and C2 and that there is also some attachment at C1, a PBMT should also be induced.

Unilateral release of the atlanto-occipital joint *(Fig. 1.10)*

If the above technique fails to release a condyle, it can be treated individually.

Patient position: Supine.

The patient's head should be aligned at an angle of 45° toward the side of the restricted condyle.

Figure 1.10 Unilateral release of the atlanto-occipital joint

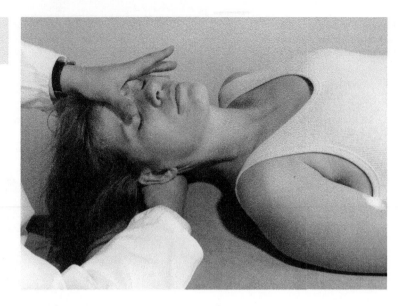

Therapist: Take up a position at the head of the patient.

Hand position:
- Place the hand that is on the same side as the restricted condyle under the atlas, supporting the hand on the little finger, the side of which should rest on the table.
- Align the basal joint of the index finger so that it provides the main contact with the articular surface of the atlas that is obstructed. Place the thumb to the side of the cranium, but do not exert any pressure.
- Place the other hand on the patient's forehead.

Method:
- The patient's head should not be in contact with the table. Support it entirely on the hand that is underneath the atlas.
- Apply gentle posterior pressure with the hand on the frontal bone, from the contralateral side to the obstructed joint, in the direction of that joint.
- Maintain this pressure until the occiput moves posterior on the articular surfaces of the atlas, so that the restricted joint opens.

Unilateral release of the atlanto-occipital joint using the V-spread (fluid impulse) technique to direct energy *(Fig. 1.11)*

Place the finger that is to direct the energy on the frontal tuber.

Intraosseous dysfunctions

Cranial base-occiput-foramen-magnum technique in young children (Fig. 1.12)

Therapist: Take up a position at the head of the patient.

Hand position:
- Place the index and middle fingers of one hand on the occipital squama and between the atlas and occiput. The thumb should be placed a little higher on the occipital squama.

Figure 1.11 Unilateral release of the atlanto-occipital joint using the V-spread (fluid impulse) technique. The sending finger is placed on the frontal tuber

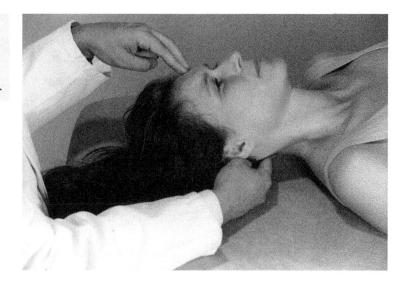

Figure 1.12 Cranial base-occiput-foramen magnum technique in young children

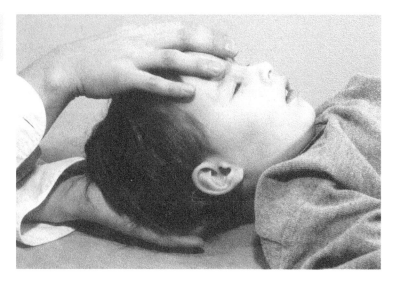

> Place the other hand on the frontal bone with the index finger lying along the metopic suture.

Method: Anterior-posterior decompression of the SBS and anterior intraoccipital synchondrosis between the lateral and basilar parts of the occipital bone:

> Apply traction in an anterior direction with the hand on frontal bone.

Posterior-anterior decompression of the posterior intraoccipital synchondrosis between the squama and the lateral part of the occipital bone (and to the anterior intraoccipital synchondrosis):

> Apply traction in a posterior direction to the occipital squama, using the index and middle fingers.

Lateral decompression of the lateral parts of the occipital bone:

➤ Spread the index and middle fingers, focusing your attention to the lateral parts of the occipital bone.

Rotation of the occipital squama:

➤ Rotate the occipital squama against the restriction, using the thumb that is placed on the squama (direct technique).
➤ Establish the PBMT.

In addition the other hand, which is placed on the frontal bone, can be used to direct a fluctuation wave in the direction of the restriction.

Platybasia technique *(Fig. 1.13)*

Therapist: Take up a position at the head of the patient.

Hand position:
➤ Place your thumbs on the greater wings of the sphenoid.
➤ Your index fingers should be positioned on the temporal bones anterior to the occipitomastoid suture.
➤ Position your middle, ring and little fingers on the occiput.

Method: Anterior-posterior decompression of the sphenobasilar synchondrosis

➤ With your thumbs on the greater wings of the sphenoid, apply traction in an anterior direction.

Decompression of the occipitomastoid suture

➤ Separate your index and middle fingers.

Posterior-anterior decompression

➤ Apply traction to the occiput in a posterior direction with your middle, ring and little fingers, so as to decompress the squama from

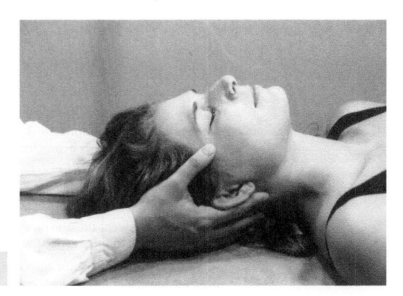

Figure 1.13 Platybasia technique

the lateral parts of the occipital bone, the lateral from the basilar parts and the basilar parts of the occipital bone from the sphenoid.

➤ Establish the PBMT and PBFT.

Occipital squama technique *(Fig. 1.14)*[12]

Therapist: Take up a position at the head of the patient.

Hand position:
➤ Place your hands symmetrically on each side of the patient's head.
➤ Position your little fingers bilaterally on the interparietal occiput.
➤ Position your ring fingers posterior to the lambdoid suture.
➤ Position your middle fingers anterior to the lambdoid suture.
➤ Let your index fingers rest lightly on the parietal bones, without exerting any pressure.
➤ Your thumbs should be touching each other above the vertex, but not in contact with the patient's head.

Method:
➤ Decompress the lambdoid suture by spreading the middle and ring fingers.
➤ Harmonize intraosseous tensions with your little finger and ring finger.
➤ Treat the occipital squama.

Testing: Test the motion of the squama in rotation, flexion, extension and side-bending. Encourage the particular motion that you are testing, using your little finger and ring finger, and compare the amplitude, ease and symmetry of this motion.

Treatment:
➤ Using your little finger and ring finger, guide the squama in the direction of the motion restriction and wait for the release of the tissue (direct technique).
➤ Alternatively, guide the squama in the direction of ease (indirect technique).
➤ Establish the PBMT and PBFT.

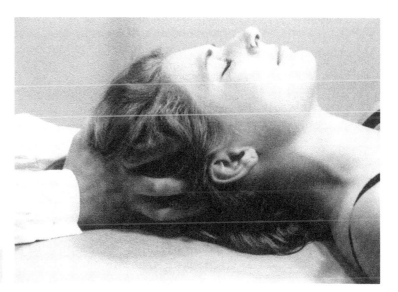

Figure 1.14 Occipital squama technique

Figure 1.15 Alternative hand position: fronto-occipital palpation

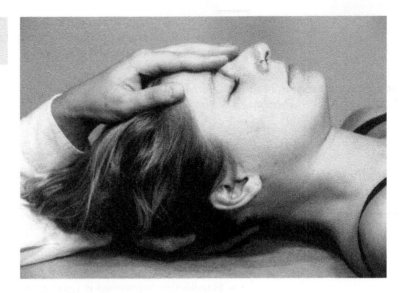

Alternative hand position: Fronto-occipital palpation (Fig. 1.15)

➤ Place your upper hand on the frontal bone, with the fingers pointing caudad.
➤ Position your middle finger on the metopic suture above the nasion.
➤ Your ring and index fingers should rest laterally beside it, above the arch of the eyebrows.
➤ Place your thumb and little finger on the frontal bone near the coronal suture.
➤ Place your other hand under the patient's head, so that the occipital squama rests on the palm.

Compression of the 4th ventricle (CV-4) *(Figs 1.16a–c)*

Explanation of effect: Compression applied to the sides of the occiput reduces the accommodation of the occipital squama to the changes in pressure of the intracranial fluid. This produces a rise in intracranial pressure and leads to an increase in the motion and exchange of fluid.[13]

As a result, the CSF flows not only through the larger openings but also penetrates right into the smallest reaches of its distribution, to the sheaths of nerves and blood vessels, to the tubuli of the fasciae and to the extracellular and intracellular fluid. The overall effect is an improved supply to the cells, an improved motion of the lymph and a regeneration of the tissue, as well as the stimulation of the cranial nerve centers in the region of the 4th ventricle. The biodynamic, bioelectric and biochemical qualities of the CSF mean that all the body's exchange processes are stimulated.[13–15]

Effect and indication: ➤ Normalization of PRM rhythm.
➤ Tonus reduction of the sympathetic nervous system, with positive effects on stress symptoms, anxiety states, and insomnia.[15,16]
➤ Tonus reduction of the entire connective tissue system. It is

Figure 1.16 (a) CV-4 technique. The arrows indicate the direction of extension/internal rotation. (b) CV-4 technique (side-view) (c) CV-4 technique: hand position

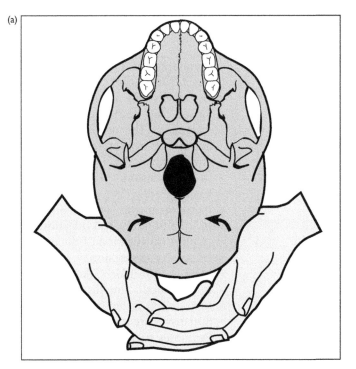

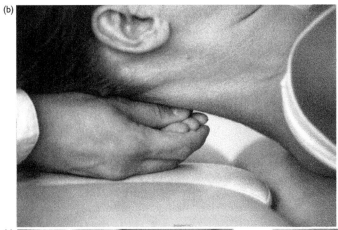

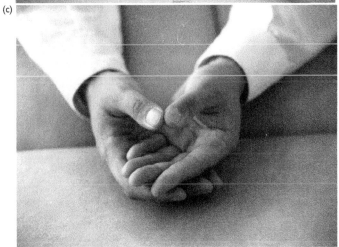

therefore indicated in acute and chronic muscular disturbances, degenerative joint disorders and period pains.

➤ Lowers fever by up to 2°C within 30–60 min.[16]

➤ Raises core body temperature in compression of the occipital squama.[17] (The author is aware that the finding of this study appears to contradict a previously reported and acknowledged effect of the CV-4.)

➤ In hypertension.

➤ In tachycardia.[18]

➤ In edema due to venous congestion.[19]

➤ In inflammation and infections.[19]

➤ In poor calcification of the bones (promotes ossification).[20]

➤ In cases of depression.

➤ In cases of headache due to disturbances of venous drainage.[19]

➤ In neuroendocrine disturbances.[20]

➤ In cases of thyroid hyperactivity.

➤ Epilepsy (care must be taken not to trigger a seizure).

➤ Promotes uterine contraction and so aids the birth process and induction of labor.

➤ Arthritic disorders.[16,19]

➤ Can release secondary, slight dysfunctions of the spinal column.[21]

➤ Lymphatic pump effect.[22]

➤ This technique can reveal primary dysfunctions elsewhere in the body so that they can be recognized.[20]

➤ Universal technique: 'When you do not know what else to do, compress the 4th ventricle' (Sutherland).[23] The CV-4 can also be used to counteract the negative effects of another technique.

➤ Lowers blood sugar.[15]

Contraindications: ➤ Where there is a risk of cerebral bleeding, e.g. in acute cerebrovascular accident or aneurysm, and malignant hypertension (on account of the increase in intracranial pressure).

➤ Fractures of the base of the skull, head injuries, especially fractures of the occipital bone.

➤ Pregnancy from the 7th month onward, as there is a risk of inducing labor. (However, Frymann, a leading authority on newborns, is of the view that the effect of CV-4 on the birth is homeostatic only.)

➤ In much-weakened elderly patients, as they may lack the strength to come back out of the expiration phase/emptying phase. It is better to induce a still point in the inspiration phase in such patients.

Therapist: Take up a position at the head of the patient.

Hand position: ➤ Place your slightly cupped hands one on top of and resting in the other, and place the tips of your thumbs together in the form of a letter V.

➤ Position the tips of your thumbs roughly at the spinous process of the patient's second or 3rd cervical vertebra, pointing distally.

➤ The ball of your thumbs should lie medially on the occipital squama.

Caution: Do not position them over the occipitomastoid suture: according to Magoun, this could predispose to fracture.

Method: Direct your attention throughout the procedure to the fluid in the 4th ventricle.

> ➤ During the expiration phase, follow the narrowing motion of the occipital squama with the ball of the thumbs.
> ➤ In the inspiration phase, hold the ball of the thumbs so as to prevent the external rotation or broadening of the occipital squama. This is achieved, according to Magoun, by contraction of the flexor digitorum profundi muscles alone.[24]
> ➤ In the next expiration phase, follow the occiput further into internal rotation with your hands, and resist it once more as it tries to broaden in the following inspiration phase.
> ➤ After a few cycles, the pressure against your thumbs in the inspiration phase will be felt to reduce. This means that the flexion/extension motion has stopped: the still point has been reached.
> ➤ Keep your hands on the occiput during the still point, following any minor motion of the nuchal muscles if this occurs. This motion is a kind of unwinding and release of the fasciae, muscles and bones.
> ➤ The still point may last anywhere from a few seconds to several minutes.
> ➤ The signs of a successfully induced still point are: deeper breathing; slight sweat formation on the forehead; reduction in muscle tonus; patient falling asleep.
> ➤ End of the still point: the therapist will sense a strong, even pressure on each side of the occiput, in the direction of external rotation. Follow this motion passively, noting the quality of the rhythm.
> ➤ Once you have assessed the quality of the craniosacral rhythm, you will be able to decide whether it is necessary to induce a further still point.

The CV-4 can be done in several ways:

1. Perform the technique so as to influence the 4th ventricle via the bone and the dura. As you do this you will sense the changes in elasticity of the bone during the inspiration and expiration phases and the effects of your treatment on the dura, or, more precisely, on the tentorium cerebelli.
2. Direct your attention straight toward the intracranial fluid, visualizing the cranium and 4th ventricle as a water-filled balloon and applying the technique to this fluid.
3. Direct your attention to the region around the 4th ventricle, but sense the effect taking place synchronously at all levels of density. Gently encourage expiration and retraction, without altering the tempo of the motion and without preventing inspiration or expansion. Passively follow inspiration. Continue with this procedure until a still point is established.

4. Follow just the tissue qualities that are present, with relaxed, non-invasive attention and empathy. Synchronize with the inherent homeodynamic forces and rhythmic patterns. It is the inherent regulatory system (or primary respiration) that decides whether a CV-4 or an EV-4 is established. The role of the osteopath is 'only' as a fulcrum, going with these processes. This method demands no meeting of tissue resistance and no confrontation with it. Nor does it require the exercising of resistance in a phase of primary respiration.

5. Korth sees a CV-4 as focusing the attention during palpation on the center of fluid structures or fluid patterns (this includes intraosseous techniques).

Expansion of the 4th ventricle (EV-4) according to Jim Jealous *(Fig. 1.17)*

Effect and indication CV-4 works centripedal, EV-4 works centrifugally.

Contraindications: See CV-4.

Therapist: Take up a position at the head of the patient.

Hand position: ➤ Let the patient's occiput rest on the palms of your hands.
➤ Your fingertips should meet in the middle. Direct the fingertips anteriorly.

Method: ➤ During the inspiration phase, go with the occipital squama into external rotation.

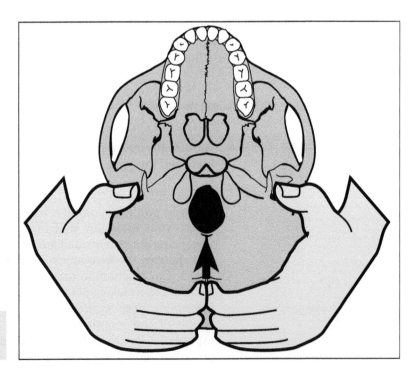

Figure 1.17 Expansion of the 4th ventricle (EV-4) according to Jim Jealous

> In the expiration phase, resist the extension and internal rotation of the occipital squama by applying gentle pressure with your fingertips in an anterior direction at the midline of the occiput.
> In the next inspiration phase, go with the occipital squama further into external rotation.
> Continue as for CV-4.

Biodynamic approach

It is the body itself that sets the healing processes in motion through the medium of mechanisms such as spontaneous local or system-wide still points, e.g. as a CV-4 or EV-4. The therapist can encourage these processes by synchronization with the inherent homeodynamic forces and rhythmic patterns. This method demands no meeting of tissue resistance and no confrontation with it. Nor does it require the exercising of resistance in a phase of primary respiration.

DIAGNOSIS OF THE SPHENOBASILAR SYNCHONDROSIS

(See Table 1.1).

TREATMENT OF THE SPHENOBASILAR SYNCHONDROSIS (SPHENO-OCCIPITAL SYNCHONDROSIS) (SBS)

SBS (See Figs 1.20, 1.23, 1.24)

With experience and practice, it is possible to treat SBS dysfunctions together rather than individually. When doing so, however, it is important to deal with the dysfunctions in order of severity. If, for example, palpation has revealed the following SBS dysfunctions: right torsion dysfunction, left side-bending/rotation, superior vertical strain, the first step in the correction must be to establish the PBMT of the superior vertical strain, then the PBMT of the left side-bending/rotation and finally the PBMT of the right torsion dysfunction.

Cranial vault hold

> Place your index fingers on the greater wings of the sphenoid on each side, behind the lateral orbital margin.
> Position your middle fingers in front of the ear and your ring fingers behind it, on the temporal bone.
> Position your little fingers on the occiput.
> If possible, place your thumbs in contact with each other on the top of the patient's head, to act as a fulcrum or fixed point.

Flexion: The amplitude of flexion motion is greater than that of extension (Fig. 1.18).

Correction: > With your index fingers, guide the greater wings in an inferior and anterior direction.
> With your little fingers, guide the lower part of the occipital squama in an inferior and anterior direction.

Table 1.1 SBS diagnosis – history-taking

Dysfunction	Axes	Causes	Clinical presentation	Severity
Flexion	Transverse 2	Compensatory, e.g. visceral disturbance Rarely traumatic (birth: pressure of the mother's pubic bone on the occiput). Adrenal or thyroid hyperactivity, hydrocephalus	Headache Endocrine disturbance Long-sightedness Sinusitis, rhinitis Masked allergy Weakness in lumbar spine and sacrum Extroversion	1
Extension	Transverse 2	Compensatory, e.g. visceral disturbance Rarely, prenatal or perinatal trauma Disturbance of hypophysis Micrencephaly	Severe migraine Asthma and sinusitis Short-sightedness Moodiness Loner behavior	1–2
Torsion	Longitudinal 1	Compensatory in disturbances of the myofascial-skeletal system, viscera etc. Rarely primary trauma	Severe migraine Pain syndromes Scoliosis Endocrine disturbance Visual disturbances Sinusitis, allergy Dyslexia Sense of inner conflict Disturbances of balance	2
Lat. flex.-rot.	Vertical 2	Compensatory in disturbances of the myofascial-skeletal system, viscera etc. Rarely primary trauma	Also: Dental malocclusion and TMJ syndrome Hypermobility of the upper cervical spine Mild psychological disturbances	2–3
Vertical strain	Longitudinal 1	Primary trauma Sup.vert. strain: force from above onto the basilar part or from behind onto the occiput Visceral disturbances Inf. vert. Strain: force from above onto the base of the sphenoid or from in front onto the frontal bone. Fall onto the pelvis or heels. Visceral disturbances	Endocrine disturbance Dental malocclusion TMJ syndrome Visual disturbances Headache and migraine Depression Schizoid states Inf. vert. strain: sinusitis, allergy Sup. vert. strain: Disturbances of hearing	3
Lateral strain	Transverse 2	Primary trauma Lateral force onto the greater wing or occiput, unilateral force from anterior onto the frontal bone or from behind onto the occiput Prenatal or perinatal Membranous	Visual disturbances Severe migraine and headache Endocrine disturbance Disturbances of balance Learning disturbances Severe psychological disturbances	4

table continued

table continued

Dysfunction	Axes	Causes	Clinical presentation	Severity
		Trauma to the temporal bone or occiput Orthopedic procedures to the jaw		
Compression	Vertical 2	Compression of: L5 –S1, O-A Membranous, sutural Prenatal or perinatal Emotional stress	Also: severe metabolic disturbance Neuropsychiatric problems Disturbances: depression	5

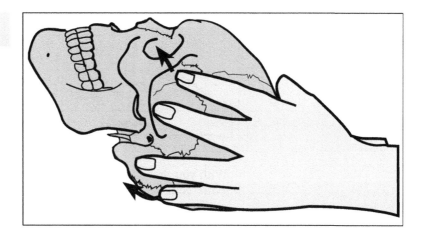

Figure 1.18 Flexion dysfunction of the SBS

> ➤ Breathing assistance by the patient: at the end of an in-breath, hold the inhalation for as long as possible, while dorsally flexing both feet. Repeat for several breathing cycles.

Extension: The amplitude of extension motion is greater than that of flexion (Fig. 1.19).

Correction: ➤ With your index fingers, guide the greater wings in a superior and posterior direction.
> ➤ With your little fingers, guide the lower part of the occipital squama in a superior and posterior direction.
> ➤ Breathing assistance by the patient: at the end of an out-breath, hold the exhalation for as long as possible, while performing a plantar flexing of the feet. Repeat for several breathing cycles.

Right torsion dysfunction *(Fig. 1.20)*

The amplitude of induced right torsion is greater than that of induced left torsion.

Correction: ➤ With your right index finger, guide the right greater wing of the sphenoid cephalad.
> ➤ With your right little finger, guide the right side of the occiput caudad.

Figure 1.19 Extension dysfunction of the SBS

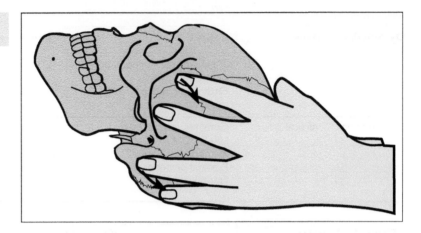

Figure 1.20 Right torsion dysfunction of the SBS

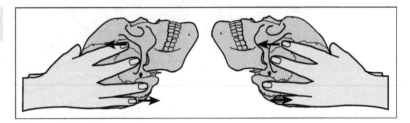

- ➤ With your left index finger, guide the left greater wing caudad.
- ➤ With your left little finger, guide the left side of the occiput cephalad.

Left torsion dysfunction *(Fig. 1.21)*

The amplitude of induced left torsion is greater than that of induced right torsion.

Correction:
- ➤ With your left index finger, guide the left greater wing of the sphenoid cephalad.
- ➤ With your left little finger, guide the left side of the occiput caudad.
- ➤ With your right index finger, guide the right greater wing caudad.
- ➤ With your right little finger, guide the right side of the occiput cephalad.

Right lateroflexion-rotation *(Fig. 1.22)*

The amplitude of induced right side-bending/rotation is greater than the amplitude of induced left side-bending/rotation.

Correction:
- ➤ Right hand: Move your index finger and small finger apart. Move your right hand caudad.
- ➤ Left hand: Move your index finger and small finger closer together. Move your left hand cephalad.

Left lateroflexion-rotation *(Fig. 1.23)*

The amplitude of induced left side-bending/rotation is greater than the amplitude of induced right side-bending/rotation.

Figure 1.21 Left torsion dysfunction of the SBS

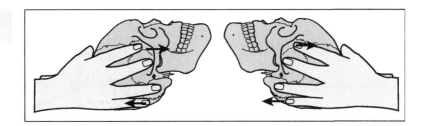

Figure 1.22 Right lateroflexion-rotation

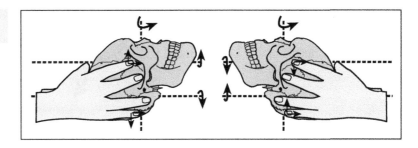

Figure 1.23 Left lateroflexion-rotation

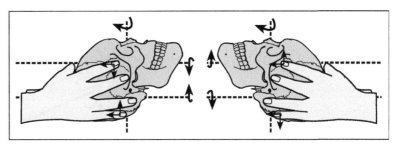

Correction: ➤ Left hand: Move your index finger and small finger apart. Move your left hand caudad.

➤ Right hand: Move your index finger and small finger closer together. Move your right hand cephalad.

Superior vertical strain *(Fig. 1.24)*

The amplitude of induced superior vertical strain is greater than that of induced inferior vertical strain.

Correction: ➤ With your index finger, guide the greater wings in an inferior and anterior direction (flexion).

➤ With your little fingers, guide the occipital squama in a superior and posterior direction (extension).

Inferior vertical strain *(Fig. 1.25)*

The amplitude of induced inferior vertical strain is greater than that of induced superior vertical strain.

Correction: ➤ With your index fingers, guide the greater wings in a superior and posterior direction (extension).

➤ With your little fingers, guide the occipital squama in an inferior and anterior direction (flexion).

Figure 1.24 Superior vertical strain

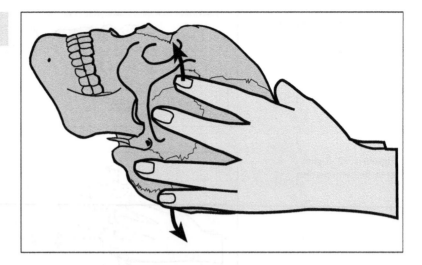

Figure 1.25 Inferior vertical strain

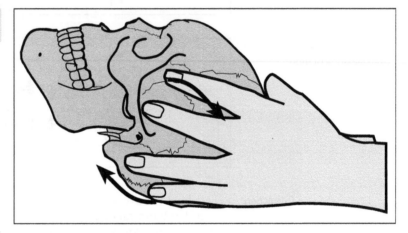

Lateral strain right *(Figs 1.26a,b)*

The amplitude of induced right lateral strain is greater than that of induced left lateral strain.

Correction:
➤ With your right index finger, guide the right greater wing in an anterior direction.
➤ With your right little finger, guide the right side of the occiput in an anterior direction.
➤ With your left index finger, guide the left greater wing in a posterior direction.
➤ With your left little finger, guide the left side of the occiput in a posterior direction.
➤ (Or, when treating the effect of extreme force without dysfunction axes: move your right and left index fingers to the right.)

Left lateral strain *(Fig. 1.27)*

The amplitude of induced left lateral strain is greater than that of induced right lateral strain.

Figure 1.26 (a) Right lateral strain (b) Right lateral strain (without axis of dysfunction)

(a)

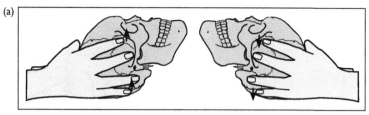

(b)

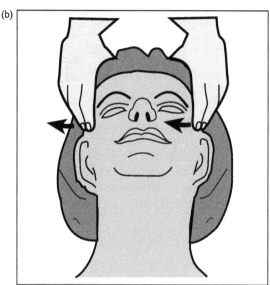

Figure 1.27 Left lateral strain

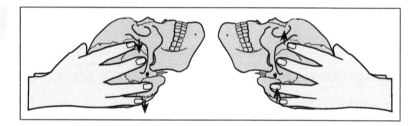

Correction: ➤ With your left index finger, guide the left greater wing in an anterior direction.
➤ With your left little finger, guide the left side of the occiput in an anterior direction.
➤ With your right index finger, guide the right greater wing in a posterior direction.
➤ With your right little finger, guide the right side of the occiput in a posterior direction.
➤ (Or when treating the effect of extreme force without dysfunction axes: move your left and right index fingers to the left.)

Compression of the SBS *(Figs 1.28, 1.29)*

Compression dysfunction: The sphenoid moves posteriorly, but not anteriorly, i.e. there is no motion away from the occiput.

Figure 1.28 Compression of the SBS

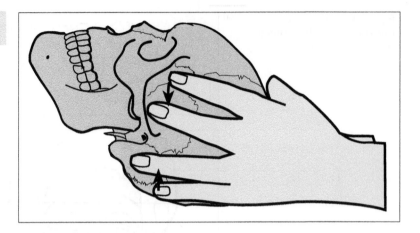

Correction: ➤ Compression: Begin by moving your index fingers in a posterior direction at the same time as your little fingers move anteriorly.
➤ Decompression: Then move your index fingers anteriorly while at the same time moving your little fingers posteriorly.
➤ Maintain this traction until the membrane tension is resolved.

The sphenoid

Examination and techniques

- Visual assessment
- Palpation of the position
- Palpation of the PRM rhythm
- Motion testing
- Active
- Passive
- SBS
- Intraosseous techniques: molding
- CV-3
- Sutural techniques
- Drainage of the sphenoidal sinus: see vomer pump technique
- Sphenosquamous suture, see Temporal bone
- Sphenopetrosal synchondrosis, see Temporal bone
- Sphenoparietal suture, see Parietal bone
- Sphenofrontal suture, see Frontal bone
- Sphenozygomatic suture, see Zygomatic bone
- Sphenoethmoidal suture, see Ethmoid bone
- Sphenovomerine suture, see Vomer
- Sphenopalatine suture, see Palatine bone
- Technique for the pterygopalatine ganglion
- Jealous's anterior dural girdle technique

Figure 1.29
Decompression of the SBS

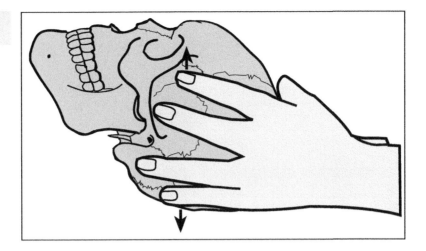

DIAGNOSIS

Palpation of the position

➤ Greater wing: lowered (ER) or elevated (IR).
➤ Temporal fossa: flat (ER) or depressed (IR).

Palpation of primary respiration

➤ Biomechanical/biodynamic palpation plus motion testing as required.
➤ If palpation reveals a restriction to motion, the therapist can induce motion in the direction of the restriction. This will emphasize the restriction and enable you to identify the structure from which the restriction originates.

Example: cranial vault hold *(Fig. 1.30)*

➤ Place your hands on each side of the patient's head.
➤ Position your index fingers on the greater wings, behind the lateral corners of the eyes.
➤ Position your middle fingers on the temporal bones, in front of the ears.
➤ Position your ring fingers on the temporal bones, behind the ears.
➤ Position your little fingers on each side of the occiput.
➤ Place your thumbs on top of the patient's head, if possible in contact with each other to act as an external fixed point.

Biomechanical approach

Inspiration phase of primary respiration, normal finding (Fig. 1.31):

➤ The greater wings move outward, anterior and inferior.
➤ (The lesser wings, which lie beneath the posterior horizontal portion of the frontal bone, slide anterior, inferior and outward. The pterygoid processes move posterior and outward.)

Figure 1.30 Cranial vault hold

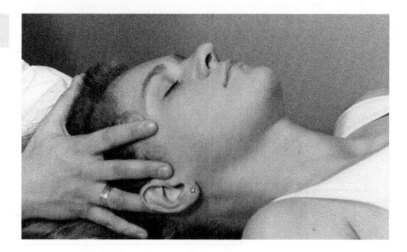

Figure 1.31 Inspiration phase of PR, biomechanical

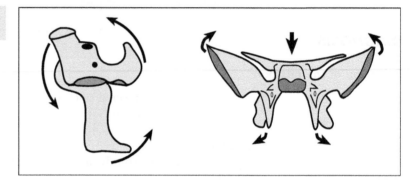

Expiration phase of PR, normal finding:

➤ The greater wings move inward, posterior and superior.
➤ (The lesser wings, which lie beneath the posterior horizontal portion of the frontal bone, slide posterior, superior and inward. The pterygoid processes move anterior and inward.)

Biodynamic/embryological approach
Inspiration phase of PR, normal finding (Fig. 1.32):

➤ The sphenoid moves anterior, the posterior part rises and the anterior part dips down.
➤ The greater wings move laterally.

Expiration phase of PR, normal finding:

➤ The sphenoid moves posterior, the posterior part dips down and the anterior part rises.
➤ The greater wings move medially.
➤ Compare the amplitude, strength, ease and symmetry of the motions of the sphenoid.

Motion testing
Hand position: As above.

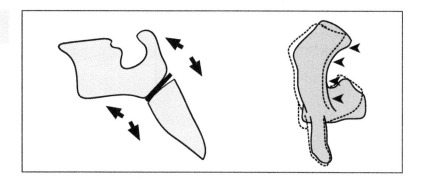

Figure 1.32 Inspiration phase of PR, biodynamic

Method: This differs from palpation of primary respiration only in that the motions of flexion/external rotation and of extension/internal rotation in harmony with primary respiration are now actively induced by the therapist.

➤ Compare the amplitude and ease of the motions of the sphenoid, or the strength needed to induce motion.

TREATMENT OF THE SPHENOID

Intraosseous dysfunctions

Molding

Between the presphenoid and postsphenoid.
Between the complex of the body of sphenoid and lesser wings, and that of the greater wings and pterygoid process.
The pre- and postsphenoid fuse around the eighth month of fetal development.

At birth, the sphenoid is composed of three parts:

- (1) body of the sphenoid and the two lesser wings;
- (2 and 3) the greater wings on each side, with their respective pterygoid process.

The sphenoid has ossified completely by around the 7th month of life.

According to Sutherland, malformations between the pre- and post-sphenoid during the early stages of development of the cranial base can be expressed in a slanting orbit such as is typical of Down syndrome.

Disturbances between the complex of the body of sphenoid and lesser wings, and that of the greater wings and pterygoid process can lead to disturbances in the development of the orbits and to disturbances of vision (CN II, III, IV, VI). The function of CN V 1 and the adjacent cavernous sinus can also be impaired.

Technique to release tensions between the pre- and post-sphenoid *(Fig. 1.33)*

Note: This technique is particularly indicated in newborns and small children.

Figure 1.33 Technique to release tensions between the pre- and post-sphenoid

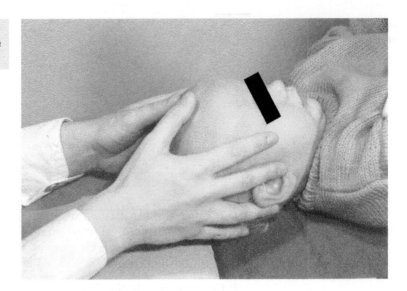

Patient position: Supine.
Therapist: Take up a position at the head of the patient.
Hand position: Cranial vault hold.

> Place your hands either side on the patient's head.
> Position your index fingers on the greater wings, behind the lateral corners of the eye.
> Position your middle fingers on the temporal bones, in front of the ears.
> Position your ring fingers on the temporal bones, behind the ears.
> Position your little fingers on the sides of the occiput.
> Your thumbs should if possible meet and touch above the head to act as a fulcrum or fixed point.

Method:
> Begin by sensing the tissue tension between the pre- and post-sphenoid.
> Move both parts of the bone in the direction of their motion restriction.
> Establish the PBMT and PBFT between the pre- and post-sphenoid.
> Maintain this position until you sense a release of tension between the pre- and post-sphenoid.

Cant hook technique for disengagement of the complex of the body of sphenoid and lesser wings from the complex of the greater wings and pterygoid process.

Cant hook technique

Note: Before carrying out this technique, ensure that the sphenofrontal suture is free to move.
Patient position: Supine.
Therapist: Take up a position at the patient's head, on the side opposite the dysfunction.

Hand position: Left hand:

> ➤ Place the little finger of your left hand intraorally, positioning it on the side of the right pterygoid process. To locate this position, pass your little finger back along the side of the alveolar part of the mandible until the front of your finger pad rests on the pterygoid process.
> ➤ Place the index finger of your left hand laterally on the greater wing.

Method: To free the sphenofrontal suture (Fig. 1.34):
Right hand:

> ➤ Grasp the two sides of the frontal bone by its lateral surface (zygomatic process) with your thumb and index finger.
> ➤ If possible the end of your left thumb (the distal phalanx) should rest on the left greater wing.
> ➤ With your left hand, hold the sphenoid firmly in position.
> ➤ Keep your right thumb immobile, and also your left thumb which is resting on the side opposite the dysfunction. Your right thumb is acting as the pivot around which the movement is organized.
> ➤ During the inspiration phase, begin to apply traction to the frontal bone in a superior and very slightly anterior direction with your middle finger (disengagement of the frontal bone from the greater wing).
> ➤ Without reducing the gentle disengagement, permit all motions and unwinding of the frontal bone.
> ➤ At each release of the tissues, seek the next limit of motion of the frontal bone in the superior direction on the side of the dysfunction.
> ➤ Allow yourself to be guided by the fluctuations of the PRM until you achieve the PBMT between the frontal bone and the greater

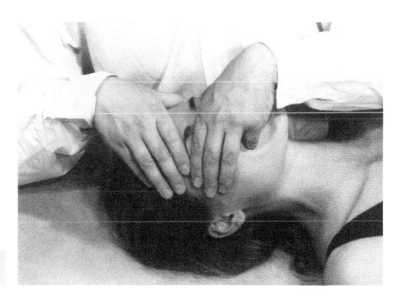

Figure 1.34 Freeing the sphenofrontal suture

wing. The PBMT is the position in which the dural membrane tension between the frontal bone and the greater wing is as balanced as possible.

➤ Maintain the PBMT until a correction of the abnormal membranous tension has been achieved and the inherent homeostatic forces (PRM rhythm, etc.) have brought this into effect and stabilized.

➤ When this has happened, begin – again during the inspiration phase – to apply traction in an anterior direction to the frontal bone, with your middle finger (disengagement of the frontal bone from the lesser wing).

➤ Continue as for the greater wing.

To disengage the complex of the body of the sphenoid and lesser wings from the complex of the greater wings and pterygoid process (Fig. 1.35).

➤ Now place the fingers of your right hand on the right superior orbital margin of the frontal bone, level with the lesser wing.

➤ Release your left thumb from the left greater wing.

➤ Use your right hand to sense the motion of the lesser wing.

➤ At the same time, use your left hand (which is in contact with the greater wing and pterygoid process) to sense the motion of the greater wing-pterygoid process complex.

➤ If you sense dysfunctional tensions, guide the two parts of the bone in the direction of motion restriction (direct technique).

➤ Permit minute unwinding motions of the tissue, but do not relax the gentle pressure in the direction of the restriction.

➤ Establish the PBMT between the complex of the body of the sphenoid and lesser wings from the complex of the greater wings and pterygoid process.

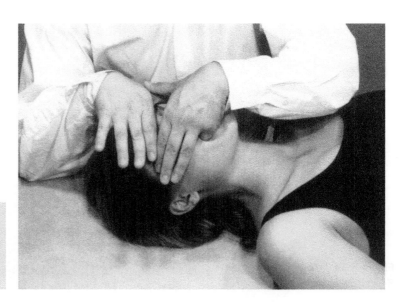

Figure 1.35 Release of the complex of the body of the sphenoid and lesser wings from the complex of the greater wings and pterygoid process.

> Maintain this position until you sense a release between the two parts of the bone.

Compression of the 3rd ventricle (CV-3) according to Jim Jealous (Fig. 1.36)

The 3rd ventricle is an important fulcrum during embryological development. It influences the development of the hemispheres of the brain, eyes, the epiphysis, the pituitary gland, the hypothalamus, the heart, the lungs, the diaphragm, the foregut and also the neuroendocrinological development.

Effects and indication: The CV-3 is the method of choice for:

- Restrictions in the 3rd ventricle.
- Asymmetries in the rhythmic rolling and unrolling of the cerebral hemispheres.
- Dysfunctions of the hypothalamus, hypophysis and epiphysis.
- Dysfunction of the lamina terminalis.
- The activation of the ignition system.

Therapist: Take up a position at the head of the patient.

Hand position:
- Place your index and/or middle finger on the greater wings.
- Your thumbs should rest on the coronal suture.

Method:
- You then synchronize yourself with the primary respiration.
- A neutral condition is established.
- First, be aware of and differentiate the movement or restriction at the bottom (the hypothalamus and pituitary stalk), the top (epiphysis) and at the anterior boarders of the 3rd ventricle.
- The CV-3 is done exactly at the moment when the 'long tide' meets the midline.

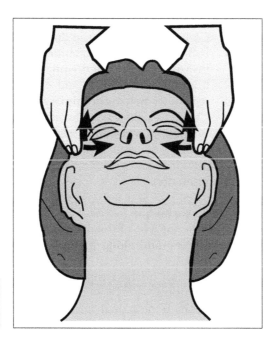

Figure 1.36 Compression of the 3rd ventricle (CV-3) according to Jim Jealous

➤ Only at that moment the 'spark' or the 'tide' is directed at the fulcrum of the 3rd ventricle.

➤ It is important to be careful and not to hold or fixate the tide or potency in the fulcrum of the 3rd ventricle or at midline. That would restrict the ignition system.

➤ Immediately afterwards, perceive how the inspiration phase expresses itself.

➤ When the spark hits the fulcrum in the 3rd ventricle, the ignition system is started and can reload.

➤ Then perceive how the tide spreads from the 3rd ventricle through the midline to the coccyx.

➤ Then assess the further consequences in the fluid, in the longitudinal fluctuation and in the tissue.

Important note: With the CV-3 you do not use or manipulate hydraulic pressure and fluid is not pressed into the 3rd ventricle or toward midline.

Note: The unfolding of the ignition system can also be done at every other part of midline.

There are various ways of performing this technique:

1. The osteopath can influence the 3rd ventricle via the bones and the dura.

2. The osteopath's attention can concentrate directly on the intracranial fluid. Visualize the cranium and 3rd ventricle as a water-filled balloon and perform the technique directly on the fluid.

3. The osteopath's attention can concentrate on the region around the 3rd ventricle but sense the effect taking place synchronously at all levels of density. Gently encourage expiration and retraction, without altering the tempo of the motion and without preventing inspiration or expansion. Passively follow inspiration. Continue with this procedure until a still point is established.

4. Follow just the tissue qualities that are present, with relaxed, non-invasive attention and empathy. Synchronize with the inherent homeodynamic forces and rhythmic patterns. It is the inherent regulatory system (or primary respiration) that decides whether a CV-3 is established. The role of the osteopath is 'only' as a fulcrum, going with these processes. This method demands no meeting of tissue resistance and no confrontation with it. Nor does it require the exercising of resistance in a phase of primary respiration.

Jim Jealous's anterior dural girdle technique *(see Figs 1.37, 1.38)*

The anterior fold of the dura runs along the posterior margin of the lesser wing and along the parietal bone, posterior to the coronal suture.

Indication: Dysfunction of the temporomandibular joint, migraine, abnormal dural tension.

Method: Palpation of the cranial 'dural sac' and anterior dural fold (Fig. 1.37).

Therapist: Take up a position at the head of the patient.

Figure 1.37 Palpation of the cranial dural sac and the anterior dural girdle

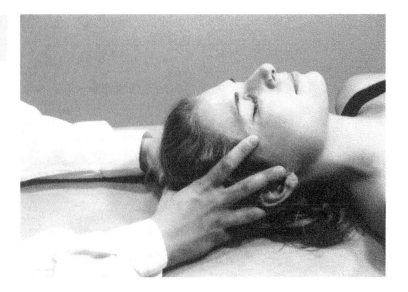

Figure 1.38 Anterior dural girdle and tentorium

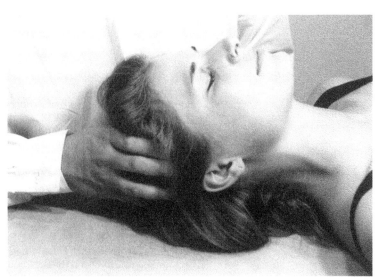

Hand position: ➤ Cranial vault hold according to Sutherland, but placing the thumbs on the patient's head, aligned along the anterior dural girdle, directly behind the coronal suture.
➤ Begin by sensing the entire dural sac and dural folds: sense the tension and primary respiration.
➤ Then sense primary respiration of the anterior dural girdle.
➤ Compare the tension, the amplitude, strength, ease and symmetry of motion of the anterior dural girdle.

Jealous states that the therapist should sense the reaction of the anterior dural girdle to the 'Breath of Life' and wait for the appearance of a lateral fluctuation.

Method: Anterior dural girdle and tentorium (Fig. 1.38)

Therapist: Take up a position beside the head of the patient.

Hand position (a):
➤ Hold the occiput with one hand so that the superior part of the transverse attachment of the tentorium lies in the palm of your hand.
➤ Place your other hand immediately behind the coronal suture, holding the anterior dural girdle. Place your thumb on one side and your fingers on the other, in the hollow often found posterior to the coronal suture.
➤ Establish the PBMT and PBFT.

Hand position (b):
➤ As for (a) except that the palm of the hand on the occiput should now hold the inferior part of the transverse attachment of the tentorium.

References

1 Schalkhausser A. Schließung und Mobilität der Synchondrosis sphenobasilaris. Munich: COE; 2000:26–27

2 Madeline LA, Elster AD. Suture closure in the human chondocranium. CT assessment. Radiology 1995; 196:747–756

3 Okamoto K, et al. High resolution CT findings in the development of the sphenooccipital synchondrosis. Am J Neuroradiol 1996: 17:117–120

4 Rohen JW. Morphologie des menschlichen Organismus. 2. Aufl. Stuttgart: Verlag Freies Geistesleben; 2002:362–365

5 Mees LCF. Das menschliche Skelett. Form und Metamorphose. Stuttgart: Verlag Urachhaus; 1981.

6 Rohen JW. Morphologie des menschlichen Organismus. 2. Aufl. Stuttgart: Verlag Freies Geistesleben; 2002:387.

7 Stone R. Polaritätstherapie. 2. Auflage Hugendubel; 1994:204.

8 Hack GD, et al. Anatomic Relation between the Rectus capitis posterior minor Muscle and the Dura Mater. Spine 1995; 20:2484–2486.

9 Magoun HI. Osteopathy in the Cranial Field. 3rd edn. Kirksville: Journal Printing Company; 1976:298.

10 Magoun HI. Osteopathy in the Cranial Field. 3rd edn. Kirksville: Journal Printing Company; 1976:295–299.

11 Magoun HI. Osteopathy in the Cranial Field. 3rd edn. Kirksville: Journal Printing Company: 1976:184.

12 Kasack A. Die osteopathische Behandlung für Kinder mit Down-Syndrom mit Schwerpunkt auf dem Os occipitale, Bonn: Diplomarbeit; 1998.

13 Lippincott HA. Compression of the bulb. J Osteopath Cranial Assoc Meridian, Idaho: Cranial Academy; 1948:51.

14 Bolet P. La compression du 4ème ventricule modifie-t-elle le profil ionique chez le patient. St. Etienne: Mémoire;1993.

15 Magoun HI. Osteopathy in the Cranial Field. 3rd edn. Kirksville: Journal Printing Company; 1976:112.

16 Upledger JE, Vredevoogd JD. Craniosacral Therapy. Seattle: Eastland Press; 1983:42.

17 Puylaert M. Der Einfluss der Kompression der Squama occipitalis auf die Erhöhung der Körperkerntemperatur. Diplomarbeit. München; 1988.

18 Courty F. Compression du IVème ventricule et rythme cardiaque. Marseille: Mémoire; 1988.

19 Magoun HI. Osteopathy in the Cranial Field. 3rd edn. Kirksville: Journal Printing Company; 1976:114.

20 Lippincott HA. Compression of the bulb. J Osteopath Cranial Assoc Meridian, Idaho: Cranial Academy; 1948:56.

21 Sutherland WG. Teachings in the Science of Osteopathy. Sutherland Cranial Teaching Foundation; 1991:204.

22 Magoun HI. Osteopathy in the Cranial Field. 3rd edn. Kirksville: Journal Printing Company; 1976:110.

23 Sutherland, WG. Teachings in the Science of Osteopathy. Sutherland Cranial Teaching Foundation: 1991:37.

24 Magoun HI. Osteopathy in the Cranial Field. 3rd edn. Kirksville: Journal Printing Company; 1976:111.

25 Mager J. Die osteopathische Behandlung cranialer Läsionen und deren Auswirkung auf die Konzentrationsfähigkeit bei Grundschulkindern. Thesis. Munich: 1998.

26 Frymann VM. Relation of disturbances of craniosacral mechanisms to symptomatology of the newborn, Study of 1250 Infants. J Am Osteopath Assoc 1966;65.

27 Frymann VM. Learning difficulties of children viewed in the light of the osteopathic concept. J Am Osteopath Assoc 1976;76.

28 Magoun HI. Osteopathy in the Cranial Field. 3rd edn. Kirksville: Journal Printing Company; 1976:283.

2 The ethmoid bone

THE MORPHOLOGY OF THE ETHMOID BONE [1]

The ethmoid occupies a key position, as important for the adjacent bones of the viscerocranium as the thorax is for the function of the pectoral girdle and upper limbs and for pulmonary respiration. It is the central point for the organization of the viscerocranium: the maxillae, frontal, palatine and lacrimal bones. It is through the ethmoid that breath is drawn into the olfactory region and respiratory tract, by way of the nasal conchae. The rhythm of pulmonary breathing may also be able to affect the cerebrospinal fluid system of the brain via the cribriform plate.

LOCATION, CAUSES AND CLINICAL PRESENTATION OF OSTEOPATHIC DYSFUNCTIONS OF THE ETHMOID BONE

Osseous dysfunction

Causes: Occurs particularly in dysfunctions of the sphenoid, frontal bone and maxilla.

a) Sphenoethmoidal suture

b) Vomeroethmoidal suture

c) Frontoethmoidal suture
The area where the cribriform plate of the ethmoid bone articulates with the ethmoidal notch of the frontal bone is particularly susceptible to dysfunctions.
    The following locations are especially susceptible:

d) Ethmoidonasal suture

e) Ethmoidomaxillary suture

f) Palatoethmoidal suture

g) Ethmoidolacrimal suture

h) Ethmoidoseptal suture

i) Ethmoidoconchal suture

Dysfunction of the falx cerebri

Causes: Occurs in dysfunctions of the ethmoid bone (crista galli), especially in combination with the frontal bone (frontoethmoidal suture).

Clinical presentation: Congestion of the anterior part of the superior sagittal sinus with functional disturbances in the corresponding parts of the brain; pain in the ipsilateral eye.

Disturbances of the nerves and parts of the brain

a) Olfactory nerves

Causes: In dysfunctions of the frontal and ethmoid bones, especially in the area where the cribriform plate of the ethmoid bone articulates with the ethmoidal notch of the frontal bone.

Clinical presentation: Disturbances of the sense of smell.

b) Anterior and posterior ethmoidal nerves (both branches of the nasociliary nerve, branch of the ophthalmic nerve V1).

Causes: See olfactory nerves.

Clinical presentation: Disturbances of sensation and pain in the mucosa and skin of the nose and mucosa of the sphenoidal sinus and posterior ethmoid air cells.

Vascular disturbances

a) Anterior and posterior ethmoidal artery

Causes: See olfactory nerves.

Clinical presentation: Sinusitis, rhinitis, allergic rhinitis, colds.

Anterior ethmoidal artery: Disturbances of the mucosa of the ethmoid air cells and frontal sinus, and disturbances of the nasal cavity.

Posterior ethmoidal artery: Disturbances of the mucosa of the ethmoid air cells and of the nasal cavity.

Causes of dysfunctions of the ethmoid bone

Primary dysfunction:

Intraosseous

● In disturbances of intrauterine development between the pre- and postsphenoid or disturbances of ossification between the complex of the body of the sphenoid and lesser wings and that of the greater wings and pterygoid process (Ossification around the 7th month of life).

Primary traumatic injury

● During early childhood and beyond, falls, blows and other examples of force to the sutures can cause posterior displacement of the ethmoidal notch in particular. This may be unilateral or bilateral, and leads to restriction of the ethmoid bone and tensions in the falx cerebri.

Secondary dysfunction:

Secondary motion restriction of the ethmoid bone can be brought about by dysfunction of the sphenoid (in SBS dysfunctions), the frontal bone, the maxilla, or the zygomatic bone, or by the transmission of tensions via the falx cerebri.

Examination and techniques
- History-taking
- Palpation of primary respiration
- Motion testing
- Intraosseous dysfunctions
- Flexion dysfunctions
- Extension dysfunctions
- ER/IR dysfunctions

Sutures
- Frontoethmoidal suture (cribriform plate – unilateral and bilateral)
- Perpendicular plate
- Lateral part, unilateral and bilateral
- Ethmoid pump technique
- Drainage of the ethmoid air cells, unilateral
- Drainage of the ethmoid air cells, self-help technique

DIAGNOSIS

History-taking

Sinusitis, rhinitis, allergic rhinitis, disturbances of the sense of smell, reddened eyes; always consider previous traumatic injury.

Palpation of the PRM rhythm *(Fig. 2.1)*

- Biomechanical/biodynamic palpation, motion testing as required.
- If palpation reveals a restriction, the therapist may induce motion in the restricted direction. This will emphasize the restriction, making it easier to sense which structure is the origin of the motion restriction.

Patient: Supine

Therapist: Take up a position beside the head of the patient.

Hand position: Cranial hand:
  ➤ Span the greater wings with your middle or index finger and your thumb.

Caudal hand:

  ➤ Place your middle finger below the nasion (the median point of the frontonasal suture) so as to rest on the internasal suture. Place your index finger on the glabella (between the arches of the eyebrows).

Figure 2.1 Palpation of primary respiration of the ethmoid bone

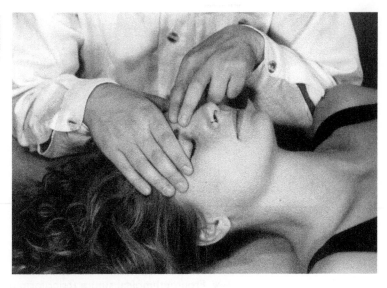

Biomechanical approach
Inspiration phase of PR, normal finding (Fig. 2.2):

➤ At the glabella (index finger), motion in a posterior (and superior) direction.
➤ At the internasal suture (middle finger), an anterior motion.

Expiration phase of PR, normal finding:

➤ At the glabella (index finger), motion in an anterior (and inferior) direction.
➤ At the internasal suture (middle finger) a posterior motion.

Biodynamic/embryological approach
Inspiration phase of PR, normal finding (Fig. 2.3):

➤ A force operating forward and downward.

Expiration phase of PR, normal finding:

➤ A force operating backward and upward.
➤ Compare the amplitude, strength, ease and symmetry of the motion of the ethmoid bone.

Other types of motion of the ethmoid bone may sometimes occur during the flexion and extension motion of the ethmoid bone: torsions, lateral shear and side-bending.

These provide an indication as to further dysfunctions of the ethmoid.

Motion testing

Hand position: As above.
Method: During the inspiration phase of PR:

➤ At the beginning of the inspiration phase, administer a slight impulse to posterior and cephalad motion with the index finger that is on the glabella.

Figure 2.2 PR inspiration phase/biomechanical

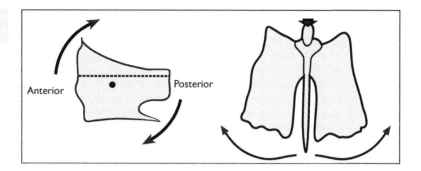

Figure 2.3 PR inspiration phase/biodynamic

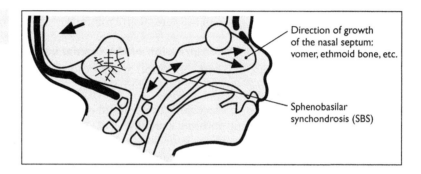

> ➤ With the middle finger that is on the internasal suture, you will sense a minute anterior motion (flexion of the ethmoid bone) in response to this pressure.

Remember: The lower part of the anterior surface of the ethmoid moves anteriorly during the inspiration phase.

During the expiration phase of PR:

> ➤ At the beginning of the expiration phase, administer a slight impulse in the posterior direction with the middle finger on the internasal suture.
> ➤ With the index finger that is on the glabella, you will sense a minute anterior motion (extension of the ethmoid bone) in response to this pressure.
> ➤ Compare the amplitude and ease of motion or the force needed to bring about motion.

TREATMENT OF THE ETHMOID BONE

The SBS, frontal bone and maxilla should also be examined and treated as required.

Intraosseous dysfunctions

At birth, the ethmoid bone is made up of two lateral parts and a perpendicular plate.

The perpendicular plate fuses with the cribriform plate and unites with the ethmoid air cells in the 2nd year of life.

Tensions between the pre- and postsphenoid can be transmitted to the ethmoid bone, affecting intraosseous organization.

Birth trauma, falls and blows (especially in early childhood) can also affect the ethmoid bone.

A fall onto the median line of the frontal bone, for example, causes flexion or extension dysfunctions of the frontal and ethmoid bones. Unilateral falls onto the frontal bone lead to side-bending/rotation or lateral strain dysfunctions. A side-bending/rotation dysfunction causes compression of the cranial bones on the side of the concavity.

It is important for the success of intraosseous techniques to ensure that all the sutural articulations of the ethmoid bone are free to move.

Decompression of the cranial base *(Fig. 2.4)*

Therapist: Take up a position at the head of the patient.

Hand position: Fronto-occipital cranial hold.

- ➤ Place your upper hand around the frontal bone, with your fingers pointing caudally.
- ➤ Place your lower hand around the occiput, with your fingers pointing caudally.

Method:
- ➤ During the inspiration phase, apply a gentle movement impulse to the frontal bone in an anterior direction, by pressing your elbow down onto the table.
- ➤ Direct your attention as you do this toward the articulations of the ethmoid: anteriorly with the frontal bone and posteriorly with the sphenoid and the sphenobasilar synchondrosis. Gently decompress the articulations with the ethmoid bone.
- ➤ Establish the PBMT and PBFT.

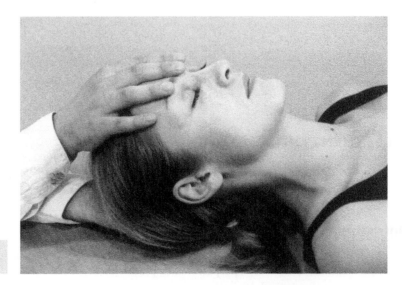

Figure 2.4 Decompression of the cranial base

Figure 2.5 Ethmoid V-spread technique

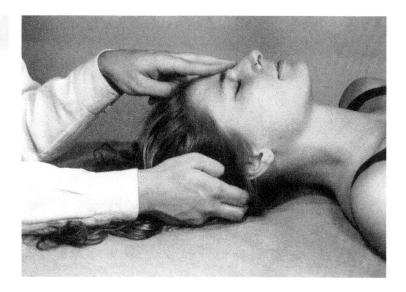

Ethmoid V-spread technique *(Fig. 2.5)*

➤ Place your index and middle finger each side of the metopic suture, between the nasion and glabella, forming a letter 'V' between your two fingers.
➤ Place the sending finger at the asterion on the side opposite the dysfunction.

Alternative: ➤ Position the sending finger at the inion and caudally on the midline.

Flexion and extension dysfunctions of the ethmoid bone

Flexion dysfunction of the ethmoid bone *(Fig. 2.6)*

The motion of the ethmoid bone into extension is reduced.

Therapist: Take up a position beside the head of the patient.

Hand position: ➤ Place one hand across the occipital bone, with the squama in the palm of your hand.
➤ Place the index finger of your other hand on the glabella, and the middle finger below the nasion on the internasal suture.

Method: **Indirect technique**

➤ Guide the occipital bone into flexion (caudally and anteriorly).
➤ Go with the ethmoid bone into the direction of the dysfunction, in other words, in the direction of greater motion (of ease). Apply slight pressure on the glabella with your index finger so as to guide the ethmoid into flexion.
➤ Establish the PBMT to find the position of the ethmoid bone that creates the best possible reciprocal balance of the abnormal intracranial membranous joint tensions – and PBFT.
➤ Maintain the PBT until a correction of the abnormal membranous tension has been achieved and the inherent homeostatic forces (PRM rhythm etc.) have brought this into effect and stabilized.

Figure 2.6 Flexion dysfunction of the ethmoid bone, indirect technique

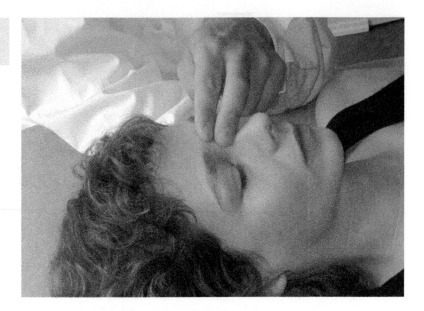

➤ Breathing assistance: The patient can assist as follows: at the end of an in-breath, hold the inhalation for as long as possible, while performing a plantar flexing of both feet. Repeat for several breathing cycles.
➤ A fluid impulse may be used to direct energy from the occiput towards the ethmoid bone.

Alternative indirect technique: in harmony with primary respiration

➤ During the inspiration phase of primary respiration, go with the occipital bone into flexion (in a caudal and anterior direction).
➤ At the same time, administer gentle pressure on the glabella to encourage the flexion motion of the ethmoid bone.
➤ During the expiration phase of primary respiration, you should just passively follow the motion of the occipital and ethmoid bones.
➤ In the next inspiration phase, again give an impulse at the occiput and ethmoid bone to encourage motion into flexion, and passively follow the motion during the expiration phase.
➤ Continue until you sense a release of the ethmoid bone.

Extension dysfunction of the ethmoid bone *(Fig. 2.7)*

The motion of the ethmoid bone into flexion is reduced.

Hand position: As for flexion dysfunction.

Method: **Indirect technique**

➤ Guide the occipital bone into extension (in a cranial and posterior direction).
➤ Go with the ethmoid bone in the direction of the dysfunction, in other words, into the direction of greater motion (direction of ease). With your middle finger, administer gentle pressure to the internasal suture to guide the ethmoid bone into extension.

Figure 2.7 Extension dysfunction of the ethmoid bone, indirect technique

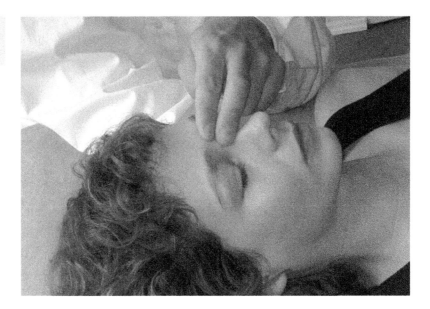

➤ Establish the PBMT and PBFT.
➤ Breathing assistance: The patient can also be asked to assist as follows: at the end of an out-breath, hold the exhalation for as long as possible, while dorsally flexing both feet. Repeat for several breathing cycles.
➤ A fluid impulse may be used to direct energy from the occiput toward the ethmoid bone.

Alternative indirect technique: in harmony with the PRM rhythm

➤ During the expiration phase of primary respiration, go with the occipital bone into extension (in a cranial and posterior direction).
➤ At the same time, administer gentle pressure with your middle finger on the internasal suture to encourage the extension motion of the ethmoid bone.
➤ During the inspiration phase, you should just passively follow the motion of the occipital and ethmoid bone.
➤ In the next expiration phase, again give an impulse at the occiput and ethmoid bone to encourage motion into extension, and passively follow the motion during the inspiration phase.
➤ Continue until you sense a release of the ethmoid bone.

Biodynamic approach
Encourage a spontaneous still point or correcting inspiration phase, flexion and expansion, or expiration phase, extension and retraction at the ethmoid bone by palpation, applied in a state of relaxed, non-invasive attentiveness and empathy, synchronizing with the inherent homeodynamic forces and rhythmic patterns. This approach involves no encounter or confrontation with tissue resistances, and it is unnecessary to exert resistance during any phase of primary respiration.

External and internal rotation dysfunction of the ethmoid bone

Testing: The mobility of the ethmoid bone in external and internal rotation is dependent on that of the frontal bone and maxilla. The free mobility of the perpendicular plate, for example, can be reduced by an internal rotation dysfunction of the maxilla.

Testing and treatment of the ethmoid is therefore done via the frontal bone and maxilla.

Palpation of primary respiration *(Fig. 2.8)*

Therapist: Take up a position at the head of the patient.

Hand position: Place your hands on each side of the frontal bone and maxilla, pointing in a caudal direction.

Method: ➤ During the inspiration phase, palpate the external rotation motion of the frontal bone and maxilla.
➤ During the expiration phase, palpate the internal rotation motion of the frontal bone and maxilla.
➤ Direct your attention toward the ethmoid bone.

Motion testing

This differs from palpation of primary respiration only in one feature: the external and internal rotation of the frontal bone and maxilla are actively induced by the therapist.

Compare the amplitude and ease of motion and the amount of force needed to elicit motion.

Rotation dysfunction of the frontal bone, in particular dysfunction in internal rotation

Aim: To spread the ethmoidal notch, create freedom of motion of the cribriform plate, release the surrounding sutures, release the falx cerebri, and improve drainage of the superior and inferior sagittal sinuses.

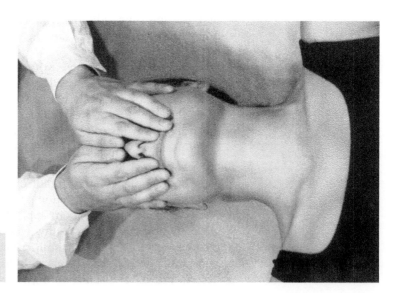

Figure 2.8 Palpation of the external and internal rotation of the ethmoid bone

Indication: Fall or blow to the frontal bone, rhinitis, sinusitis, and functional disturbances to the sense of smell.

Frontal bone spread technique *(Fig. 2.9)*

Therapist: Take up a position at the head of the patient.

Hand position:
- ➤ Hold the outside of the zygomatic processes of the frontal bone with your in-bent ring fingers to provide a firm purchase.
- ➤ Support your ring fingers with your little fingers.
- ➤ Position your middle and index fingers next to the midline of the frontal bone.
- ➤ Place your thumbs posteriorly, touching or crossing.

Method:
- ➤ Administer slight pressure in a posterior direction with your index fingers on the midline of the frontal bone.
- ➤ At the same time, move your ring fingers in an anterior, lateral and caudal direction.
- ➤ This widens the ethmoidal notch.
- ➤ Establish the PBMT and PBFT.
- ➤ A fluid impulse may be used to direct energy from the inion.
- ➤ If this technique is insufficient, a frontal bone lift may be performed.

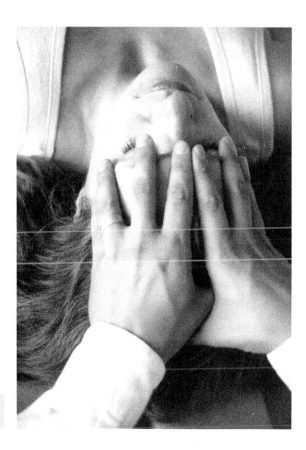

Figure 2.9 Frontal bone spread technique

Frontal bone lift technique *(Fig. 2.10)*

Therapist: As for spread technique.

Hand position: As for spread technique.

Method:
- ➤ During the expiration phase, begin to administer gentle pressure in a medial direction on the lateral surfaces of the frontal bone with your ring fingers, to release the frontal bone from the sphenoid (IR).
- ➤ As soon as the frontal bone begins to move anterior, you can relax the medial pressure of your ring fingers. It is very important to do this, as IR of the frontal bone would further narrow the ethmoidal notch.
- ➤ Replace this pressure with anterior, slightly cephalad traction. This traction is very gentle and is administered by pressing your elbows slightly down on the table, so that your fingers rise anteriorly. Never let the degree of force rise above the level where the tissue begins to contract in resistance.
- ➤ The weight of the cranium is sufficient to keep the occiput, the posterior point of attachment of the falx, in position on the table.
- ➤ At each release of the tissues, seek the new limit of motion of the frontal bone in the anterior direction.
- ➤ Permit all motions and tissue unwinding of the frontal bone, without reducing the gentle traction.

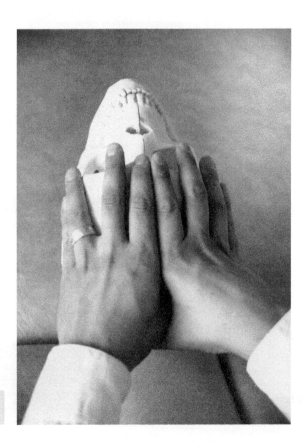

Figure 2.10 Frontal bone lift technique

> You will be able to sense the various stages of tissue release: first the sutural tensions, then the elastic and collagenous tensions of the falx cerebri (feels like cement or a rubber band or chewing gum).
> When the falx has been freed of its tension patterns (floating sensation), you can relax the anteriorly directed traction and remove your hands.
> To release the frontoethmoidal suture, focus your attention particularly on this suture.

Important: > The degree of tension applied in the lift should be judged by imitating the tension present; apply about 5 g of extra tension over and above the degree of tension you detect.
> Never lift your hands suddenly away from the bone while performing the technique.
> Take care to position your hands accurately. Incorrect positioning can cause the technique to be ineffective or in the worst case can exacerbate or give rise to symptoms, especially if your fingers are lying on the sutures.
> A fluid impulse may be used to direct energy from the inion.

Note: A further option is to encourage the flexion and extension motion of the frontal bone while administering the gentle anterior traction (in harmony with primary respiration).

Rotation dysfunction of the maxilla
Maxilla lift and spread technique *(Fig. 2.11)*

Aim: To release the ethmoidomaxillary, lacrimomaxillary and ethmoidolacrimal sutures and create freedom of motion of the perpendicular plate.

Therapist: Take up a position at the head of the patient.

Hand position: > Place your hands either side of the patient's head.

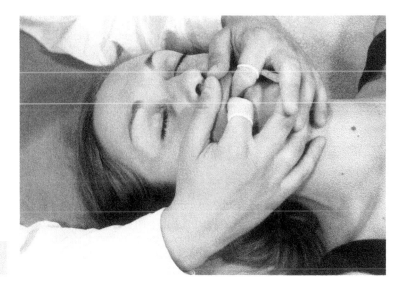

Figure 2.11 Maxilla lift and spread technique

➤ Place your thumbs outside or just above the alveolar process of the maxillae. Your thumbs should be medially oriented.

➤ Place your index fingers intra-orally on the alveolar process of the maxillae.

➤ This means that you are in effect grasping the maxillae between your finger and thumb, from inside and outside.

Method: **Maxilla lift technique**

➤ With your thumb and index finger, administer anterior and caudal traction to the two maxillary bones.

This frees the maxillae from the ethmoid bone.

Note: The medial border of the orbital surface of the maxilla is released from the bottom of the ethmoid air cells, the posterior border of the frontal process of the maxilla is freed from the anterior of the ethmoidal labyrinth and the ethmoidal crest on the medial side of the maxilla released from the middle nasal concha.

➤ A fluid impulse may be used to direct energy from the opposite lambdoid suture.

Maxilla spread technique

➤ When you sense a release at the ethmoidomaxillary sutures, you can go on to spread the maxillae away from each other.

➤ Without reducing the anterior and caudal traction, induce external rotation of the maxillae.

➤ Administer posterior pressure on the intermaxillary suture with your thumbs.

➤ With your index fingers, guide the alveolar process in a lateral and anterior direction.

➤ Establish the PBMT and PBFT.

➤ A fluid impulse may be used to direct energy from the opposite lambdoid suture.

Alternative technique to treat an internal rotation dysfunction of the maxillae *(Fig. 2.12)*

Aim: To release the ethmoidomaxillary suture and create freedom of motion of the perpendicular plate.

Therapist: Take up a position beside the patient's head.

Hand position: Cranial hand:

➤ Span the greater wings with your thumb and your middle or index finger.

Caudal hand:

➤ Place your middle and index finger intraorally, against the upper teeth on each side.

Method:

➤ During the inspiration phase, deliver a caudad impulse via the greater wings to induce flexion.

➤ At the same time, spread apart the fingers resting on the upper teeth (external rotation of the maxillae).

Figure 2.12 Alternative technique to treat an internal rotation dysfunction of the maxillae

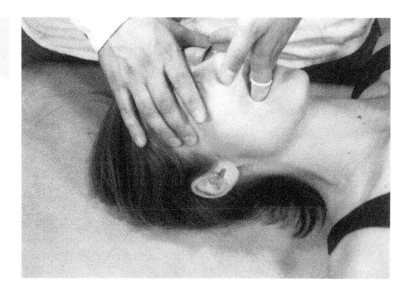

> During the expiration phase, passively follow the motion of the cranial bones.
> Repeat this procedure for several cycles, until the mobility of the perpendicular plate increases.

Technique to treat the cribriform plate

Suture margin of the frontoethmoidal suture: the cribriform plate articulates with the ethmoidal notch of the frontal bone.

Suture type: Plane suture.
Cribriform plate.
Technique: See frontal bone spread and lift.

Alternative technique to treat the cribriform plate *(Fig. 2.13)*

Therapist: Take up a position beside the patient's head.
Hand position: Cranial hand:

> Span the frontal bone with your thumb and middle finger (and/or index finger) by hooking the thumb and finger around the zygomatic processes of the frontal bone.
> Place the basal joint of your index finger on the glabella.

Caudal hand:

> Grasp the frontal processes of the maxillae with the middle and index fingers.
> Place your thumb and ring finger on the anterolateral surfaces of the maxillae.

Method: Direct technique:
Cranial hand:

> Administer posterior and superior pressure with the basal joint of the index finger on the glabella, while moving the outer inferior

Figure 2.13 Alternative technique to treat the cribriform plate

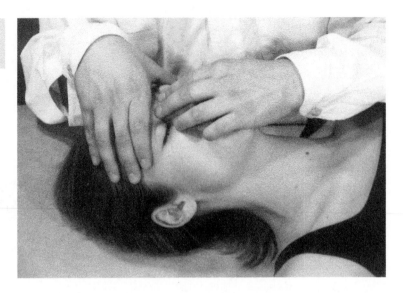

parts of the frontal bone anterior and laterally with your thumb and middle finger (external rotation of the frontal bone).

The overall effect is to move the frontal bone into a more shallow-angled position (flexion of the frontal bone).

➤ At the same time, induce external rotation of the maxillae with your caudal hand.
➤ Also administer inferiorly directed pressure on the frontal processes of the maxillae with the index and middle finger of your caudal hand, supporting these fingers with your thumb and ring finger.
➤ Establish the PBMT and PBFT at the frontal and ethmoid bones.
➤ Maintain the PBT until a correction of the abnormal membranous tension has been achieved and stabilized by the inherent homeostatic forces (primary respiration etc.), and you sense a release at the cribriform plate and ethmoidal notch, and at the ethmoidomaxillary sutures. Continue until the motion of the ethmoid and frontal bones has ceased.

Unilateral treatment of the cribriform plate *(Fig. 2.14)*

Therapist: Take up a position to the (left) of the patient's head, the opposite side to the dysfunction.

Hand position: Cranial hand:

➤ Span the frontal bone with your thumb and middle finger (and/or index finger), by hooking them around the outside of the zygomatic processes of the frontal bone. Place the basal joint of your index finger on the glabella.

Caudal hand:

➤ Place your index finger on the (right) frontal process of the maxilla.

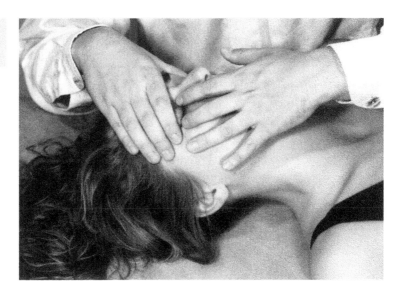

Figure 2.14 Unilateral treatment of the cribriform plate. Example: right

> Position your middle finger on the (right) anterior surface of the maxilla.
> Position your ring finger on the (right) zygomatic bone.

Method: Direct technique:
Cranial hand:

> Administer gentle posterior and superior pressure with the basal joint of the index finger on the glabella, while moving the outer inferior parts of the frontal bone anterior and laterally with your thumb and middle finger (external rotation of the frontal bone).

The overall effect is to move the frontal bone into a more shallow-angled position (flexion of the frontal bone).

> Guide the maxilla into external rotation with the index and middle finger of your caudal hand.
> With your ring finger, guide the zygomatic bone into external rotation.
> Establish the PBMT and PBFT at the frontal bone.
> Maintain the PBT until a correction of the abnormal membranous tension has been achieved and stabilized by the inherent homeostatic forces, and you sense a release at the cribriform plate and ethmoidal sutures, and at the ethmoidomaxillary sutures. Continue until the motion of the frontal bone has ceased.

Perpendicular plate

Aim: To create freedom of motion of the perpendicular plate and release the surrounding sutures.

Technique: See under external and internal rotation dysfunction of the ethmoid bone.

Ethmoidal labyrinth

Ethmoidal labyrinth (lateral mass of the ethmoid bone).

Indication: Motion restriction of the ethmoidal labyrinth, sinusitis.

Therapist: Take up a position beside the patient's head.

Hand position: Indirect technique (Figs. 2.15a,b):

Cranial hand:

➤ Span the frontal bone with your thumb and middle finger (and/or index finger), by hooking them around the outside of the zygomatic processes of the frontal bone. Place the basal joint of your index finger on the glabella.

Caudal hand:

➤ Place your index finger intraorally on the median palatine suture, posterior to the transverse palatine suture.

(a)

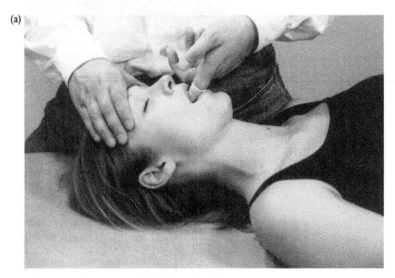

(b)

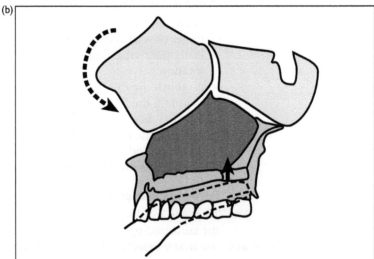

Figure 2.15 Ethmoidal labyrinth. (a,b) Indirect technique: Impulse by index finger to encourage motion of the ethmoid bone into extension

Method: Cranial hand:

> ➤ Deliver an impulse to the frontal bone to encourage motion into internal rotation and extension during the expiration phase.
> ➤ During the expiration phase, gently follow the anterior motion with the basal joint of your index finger on the glabella. Meanwhile use your thumb and middle finger to move the outer, inferior parts of the frontal bone posterior and medially (internal rotation of the frontal bone).

The overall effect is to move the frontal bone into a more steeply angled position (extension of the frontal bone).
Caudal hand:

> ➤ At the same time, administer pressure in a superior direction with your index finger. This encourages motion of the ethmoid bone into extension, via the vomer.

The effect of this is to guide the ethmoidal labyrinth into extension and internal rotation (narrowing of the ethmoidal labyrinth).

> ➤ Breathing assistance: You can also ask the patient to hold an exhalation at the end of an out-breath for as long as possible. Repeat for several breathing cycles.
> ➤ Establish the PBMT and PBFT at the frontal bone, vomer and ethmoid bone.
> ➤ Maintain the PBT until a correction of the abnormal membranous tension has been achieved, the inherent homeostatic forces (primary respiration etc.) have brought this into effect, and you sense a release of the ethmoidal labyrinth. Continue until the motion of the ethmoidal labyrinth and frontal bone has ceased.

Hand position: Direct technique (Figs. 2.16a,b):
Cranial hand:

> ➤ Span the frontal bone with your thumb and middle finger (and/or index finger), by hooking them around the outside of the zygomatic processes of the frontal bone. Place the basal joint of your index finger on the glabella.

Caudal hand:

> ➤ Place your index finger intraorally on the median palatine suture, anterior to the transverse palatine suture.

Method: Cranial hand:

> ➤ During the inspiration phase, follow the glabella in a posterior and superior direction with the basal joint of the index finger, while moving the outer inferior parts of the frontal bone anterior and laterally with your thumb and middle finger (external rotation of the frontal bone).

The overall effect is to move the frontal bone into a more shallow-angled position (flexion of the frontal bone).

Figure 2.16 Ethmoidal labyrinth. (a,b) Direct technique: Impulse by index finger to encourage motion of the ethmoid bone into flexion

(a)

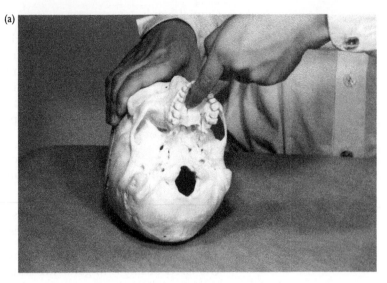

(b)

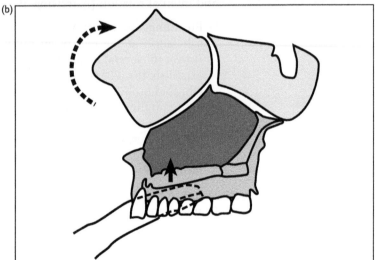

Caudal hand:

➤ At the same time, administer pressure in a superior direction. This encourages motion of the ethmoid bone into flexion, via the vomer.

The effect of this is to guide the ethmoidal labyrinth into flexion and external rotation (spreading of the ethmoidal labyrinth).

➤ Breathing assistance: You can also ask the patient to hold an inhalation at the end of an in-breath for as long as possible. Repeat for several breathing cycles.

➤ Establish the PBMT and PBFT at the frontal bone, vomer and ethmoid bone.

➤ Maintain the PBT until a correction of the abnormal membranous tension has been achieved and stabilized by the inherent homeostatic forces (PRM rhythm etc.), and you sense a release of the ethmoidal labyrinth. Continue until the motion of the ethmoidal labyrinth has ceased.

Note:
> Always make sure that the amount of force used is not so great as to cause additional tension of the tissue.
> Both in the direct and the indirect technique, you may deliver the therapeutic impulses only in harmony with the PRM rhythm.

Unilateral treatment of the ethmoidal labyrinth *(Fig. 2.17)*

Therapist: Take up a position to the (left) of the patient's head, the side opposite the dysfunction.

Hand position: Cranial hand:

> Span the frontal bone with your thumb and middle finger (and/or index finger), by hooking them around the outside of the zygomatic processes of the frontal bone. Place the basal joint of your index finger on the glabella.

Caudal hand:

> Place your index finger on the frontal process of the (right) maxilla.
> Place your ring finger intraorally, with the inner edge of the finger on the outside of the alveolar process of the maxilla.
> Place the thumb, and that of your cranial hand, externally on the zygomatic process of the frontal bone.

Method:
> Stabilize the (right) maxilla with your caudal hand.
> With the index and/or middle finger of your cranial hand, move the frontal bone on the affected side cephalad.
> With your thumbs, stabilize the other (left) side of the frontal bone in its position.

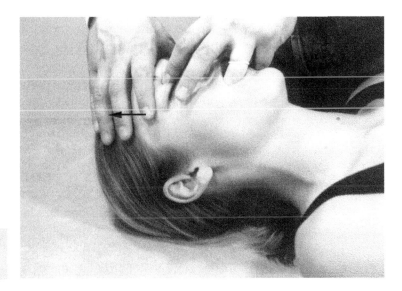

Figure 2.17 Unilateral treatment of the ethmoidal labyrinth. Example: right

> ➤ The effect is to release the frontal bone on the side of the dysfunction from the maxilla, so freeing the ethmoidal labyrinth, which lies between these two bones.
> ➤ Establish the PBMT and PBFT.

Drainage of the ethmoidal air cells
Ethmoid pump technique

Indication: Sinusitis.

Aim: To drain the ethmoidal air cells, to enable secretions to drain away.

This technique is very like the ethmoidal labyrinth release, except that the impulses are delivered in harmony with the PRM rhythm in the ethmoid pump technique.

Therapist: Take up a position beside the patient's head.

Hand position: (Figs 2.18a–c)

Cranial hand:

> ➤ Span the frontal bone with your thumb and middle finger (and/or index finger), by hooking them around the outside of the zygomatic processes of the frontal bone. Place the basal joint of your index finger on the glabella.

Caudal hand:

> ➤ Place your index finger intraorally on the median palatine suture, anterior to the transverse palatine suture.
> ➤ Position your middle finger intraorally on the median palatine suture, posterior to the transverse palatine suture.

Alternative hand position: (Fig. 2.19. See also Figs 3.1a, b):

> ➤ The index finger only is placed on the median palatine suture, both anterior and posterior to the transverse palatine suture. This method should only be used if you are able to sense and induce the flexion and extension of the vomer using this finger position.

Method: During the inspiration phase:

Cranial hand:

> ➤ With the basal joint of the index finger resting on the glabella, administer gentle pressure in a posterior and superior direction. As you do this, move the outer, inferior parts of the frontal bone anteriorly and laterally with your thumb and middle finger (external rotation of the frontal bone).
> ➤ The overall effect is to move the frontal bone into a more shallow-angled position (flexion of the frontal bone).

Caudal hand:

> ➤ At the same time apply pressure in a superior direction with the index finger of the caudal hand (superiorly directed impulse in front of the transverse palatine suture: flexion).

This encourages motion of the ethmoid bone into flexion, via the vomer.

Figure 2.18 (a–c) Ethmoid pump technique. Continuous arrows: impulse to ethmoid bone during inspiration phase. Dotted arrows: impulse to ethmoid bone during expiration phase

(a)

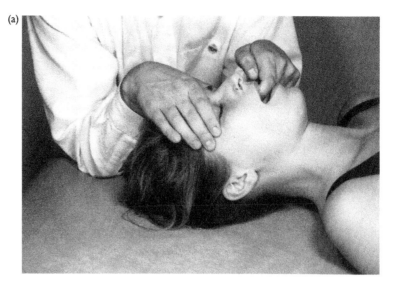

(b)

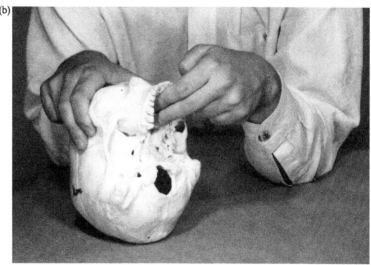

(c)

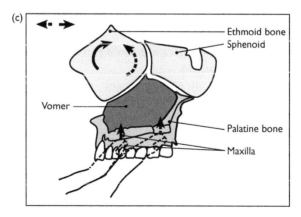

Ethmoid bone
Sphenoid
Vomer
Palatine bone
Maxilla

Figure 2.19 Alternative hand position: ethmoid pump technique

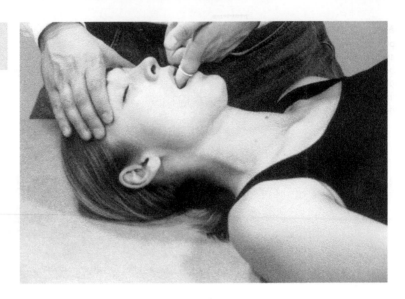

During the expiration phase:
Cranial hand:

➤ With the index finger resting on the glabella, gently follow the glabella anterior. As you do this, move the outer, inferior parts of the frontal bone in a posterior and medial direction using your thumb and middle finger (internal rotation of the frontal bone).

The overall effect is to move the frontal bone into a more steeply angled position (extension of the frontal bone).
Caudal hand:

➤ At the same time, administer pressure in a superior direction with your middle finger (superiorly-directed impulse behind the transverse palatine suture: extension).

This encourages motion of the ethmoid bone into extension, via the vomer.

➤ Repeat for several cycles of the PRM rhythm.

Alternative ethmoid pump technique (opposite physiological motion)

Method: ➤ With the basal joint of the index finger on the glabella, administer gentle pressure in a posterior and superior direction. As you do this, move the outer, inferior parts of the frontal bone in an anterior and lateral direction using your thumb and middle finger (external rotation of the frontal bone).

The overall effect is to move the frontal bone into a more shallow-angled position (flexion of the frontal bone).

➤ At the same time, deliver an impulse in a superior direction with the middle finger of your caudal hand (superiorly directed impulse behind the transverse palatine suture: extension).

> With the index finger resting on the glabella, gently follow the glabella anteriorly. As you do this, move the outer, inferior parts of the frontal bone in a posterior and medial direction using your thumb and middle finger (internal rotation of the frontal bone).

The overall effect is to move the frontal bone into a more steeply angled position (extension of the frontal bone).

> At the same time deliver an impulse in a superior direction with the index finger of the caudal hand (superiorly directed impulse in front of the transverse palatine suture: flexion).

Note: The frontal bone lift also brings about drainage of the ethmoidal air cells.

Additional techniques for the treatment of the ethmoidal cells
Zygomatic bone technique *(Fig. 2.20)*

Therapist: Take up a position at the head of the patient.
Hand position: > Place the index and middle fingers of both hands on the ipsilateral zygomatic bone.
Method: > Administer gentle medially directed pressure to the zygomatic bones with your fingers.
This puts gentle pressure on the maxillae and eases breathing.

Maxilla lift and spread technique

(see the maxillae)
Unilateral drainage of the ethmoid air cells (Figs 2.21a,b).
Therapist: Take up a position to the (left) of the patient's head, the side opposite the dysfunction.
Hand position: Cranial hand:

> Place the palm of your hand on the frontal bone (right-hand side).

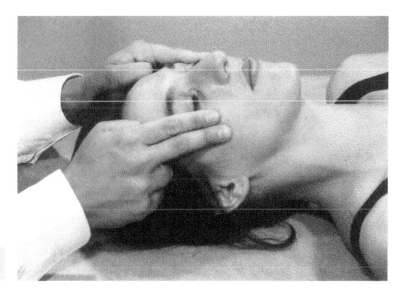

Figure 2.20 Zygomatic bone technique

Figure 2.21 (a,b) Unilateral drainage of the ethmoid air cells

(a)

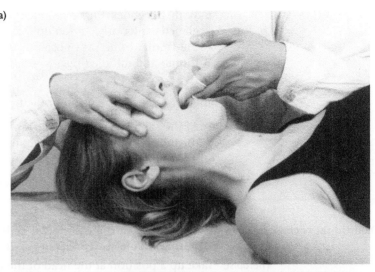

(b)

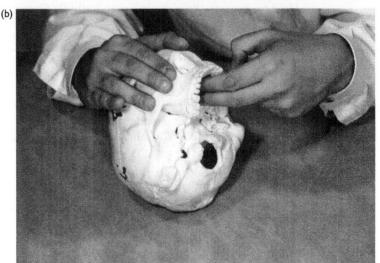

➤ Place your thumb on the opposite (left-hand) side of the frontal bone, resting on the side of the bone.

➤ Position your index finger on the frontal process of the (right) maxilla.

➤ Position your middle finger on the anterior surface of the (right) maxilla.

➤ Rest your ring finger and little finger on the (right) zygomatic bone.

Caudal hand:

➤ Place your index finger intraorally on the median palatine suture, anterior to the transverse palatine suture.

➤ Place your middle finger intraorally on the median palatine suture, posterior to the transverse palatine suture.

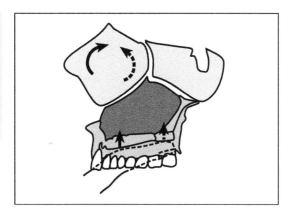

Figure 2.22 Alternative hand position: Unilateral drainage of the ethmoid air cells. Continuous arrows: Impulse to ethmoid bone during inspiration phase. Dotted arrows: Impulse to ethmoid bone during expiration phase

Alternative hand position: (Fig. 2.22)

> The index finger only is placed on the median palatine suture, both anterior and posterior to the transverse palatine suture. This method should only be used if you are able to sense and induce the flexion and extension of the vomer using this finger position.

Method: During the inspiration phase:

> Administer an impulse to the frontal bone, maxilla and zygomatic bone to encourage motion into external rotation.
> At the same time, administer pressure in a superior direction with the index finger of your caudal hand (superiorly directed impulse in front of the transverse palatine suture: flexion).

This encourages motion of the ethmoid bone into flexion, via the vomer.

During the expiration phase:

> Administer an impulse to the frontal bone, maxilla and zygomatic bone to encourage motion into internal rotation.
> At the same time, administer pressure in a superior direction with the middle finger of the caudal hand (superiorly directed impulse behind the transverse palatine suture: extension).

This encourages motion of the ethmoid bone into extension, via the vomer.

> Repeat for several cycles of the PRM rhythm.

Self-help technique for drainage of the ethmoid air cells (see Fig. 13.28)

Reference

1 Rohen JW. Morphologie des menschlichen Organismus. 2. Aufl. Stuttgart: Verlag freies Geistesleben; 2002:391.

3 Vomer

Causes of dysfunctions of the vomer

Primary traumatic dysfunction:
Blow or fall to the face.

Secondary dysfunction:
Dysfunction of the sphenoid (in SBS dysfunctions).

Examination and techniques

- History-taking
- Visual assessment and palpation of the position
- Palpation of PRM rhythm
- Motion testing
- Flexion dysfunction of the vomer
- Extension dysfunction of the vomer
- Torsion dysfunction of the vomer
- Lateral shear of the vomer
- Sphenovomerine suture
- Vomeromaxillary suture
- Decompression of the vomer
- Vomer pump technique

According to Magoun, the rhythmic motion of the vomer promotes drainage and circulation in the sphenoidal sinus[1] and nasal cavity. The growth of the vomer also has a considerable influence on the embryological development of the nasal cavity.

DIAGNOSIS

History-taking

Nasal problems (rhinitis, sinusitis).

Visual assessment and palpation of the position

Hard palate: lowered (possibly ER) or elevated (possibly IR).

107

Palpation

Palpation of primary respiration *(Figs 3.1a,b)*

Since there is a sutural articulation between the vomer and the hard palate, motion of the vomer can be palpated via a contact with the hard palate.

Therapist: Take up a position beside the head of the patient.

Hand position: Cranial hand:

> Span the greater wings with your thumb and your middle or index finger.

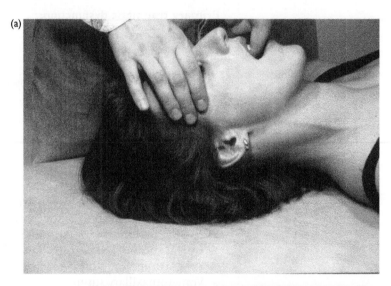

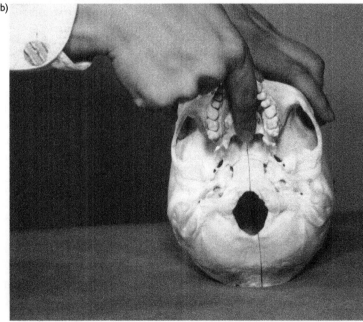

Figure 3.1 (a,b) Palpation of primary respiration of the vomer

Caudal hand:

> Place your index finger on the median palatine suture (both anterior and posterior to the transverse palatine suture).

Biomechanical approach
During the inspiration phase, the vomer descends overall, with the posterior part sinking lower than the anterior part.
Inspiration phase of the PR, normal finding (Fig. 3.2):

● A lowering of the posterior inferior border of the vomer can be palpated posterior to the transverse palatine suture.

(Anterior to the transverse palatine suture there is a cephalad motion of the anterior inferior border of the vomer.)
Expiration phase of the PR, normal finding:

● A cephalad motion of the posterior border of the vomer can be palpated posterior to the transverse palatine suture.

(Anterior to the transverse palatine suture there is a lowering of the anterior inferior border of the vomer.)

Biodynamic/embryological approach
Inspiration phase of PR, normal finding (Fig. 3.3):

> Force operating in an anterior and downward direction.

Expiration phase of PR, normal finding:

● Force operating in a posterior and upward direction.

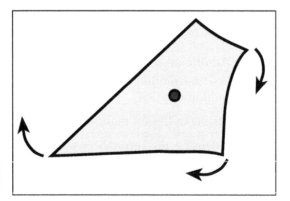

Figure 3.2 Inspiration phase of PR, biomechanical

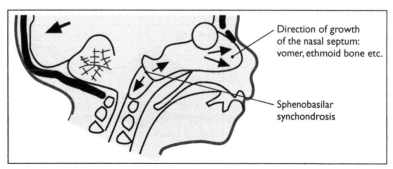

Direction of growth of the nasal septum: vomer, ethmoid bone etc.

Sphenobasilar synchondrosis

Figure 3.3 Inspiration phase of PR, biodynamic

➤ Compare the amplitude, strength and ease of motion of the vomer.
➤ Other types of motion of the vomer may occur during the flexion and extension motion: torsion, lateral shear, and side bending. These provide an indication about further dysfunctions of the vomer.

Motion testing

The only difference between motion testing and palpation of the PRM rhythm is that here the flexion and extension motion of the vomer is actively induced by the therapist.

Hand position: As above.
Method: Testing of flexion and extension.
During the inspiration phase:

➤ With the thumb and middle finger on the greater wings, administer an impulse in a caudal direction (flexion motion).
➤ You will sense a reaction to this pressure, via the index finger on the median palatine suture. This reaction is a minute caudad motion behind the transverse palatine suture (flexion motion of the vomer).

During the expiration phase:

➤ With the thumb and middle finger on the greater wings, administer an impulse in the cranial direction (extension motion).
➤ You will sense a reaction to this pressure, via the index finger on the median palatine suture. This reaction is a minute cephalad motion behind the transverse palatine suture (extension motion of the vomer).
➤ Compare the amplitude and ease of motion, or the amount of force needed to elicit motion.

Additional test options

Test the motion of the vomer by directly inducing the particular motion (Fig. 3.4).

Testing of flexion motion

➤ During the inspiration phase of primary respiration, move the posterior part of the vomer in a caudal direction and the anterior part cephalad.

Testing of extension motion

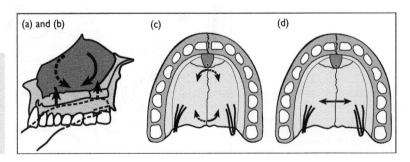

Figure 3.4 Testing of the vomer: (a) Testing of flexion motion: continuous line; (b) Testing of extension motion: dotted line; (c) Testing of torsion motion; (d) Testing of lateral shear.

➤ During the expiration phase, move the posterior part of the vomer cephalad and the anterior part caudally.

Testing of torsion motion

➤ Turn the vomer to the right and left while holding the greater wings in a neutral position.

Testing of lateral shear

➤ Shift the vomer to the right and left while holding the greater wings in a neutral position.
➤ Compare the amplitude and ease of motion, and the amount of force needed to elicit motion.

Test the vomer via the ethmoid bone

➤ Place your middle finger on the glabella and your index finger below the nasion on the internasal suture.
➤ Palpate the reaction of the vomer via induction of flexion and extension motion of the ethmoid bone.

TREATMENT OF THE VOMER

When treating the vomer it is usually advisable to treat the sphenoid and the maxillae first.

Flexion and extension dysfunctions of the vomer

Flexion dysfunction of the vomer

Therapist: Take up a position beside the patient's head.
Hand position: Cranial hand:

➤ Span the greater wings with your thumb and middle or index finger.

Caudal hand:

➤ Place your index finger on the median palatine suture (anterior and posterior to the transverse palatine suture).

Method: Indirect technique (exaggeration technique) (Fig. 3.5; see also Fig. 3.1a):

➤ During the inspiration phase, ease the greater wings in a caudal direction with your thumb and middle finger (flexion motion).
➤ At the same time, administer a cephalad impulse with the index finger on the median palatine suture, anterior to the transverse palatine suture (flexion motion of the vomer).
➤ Hold the sphenoid and vomer in flexion.
➤ Breathing assistance: Ask the patient to hold an inhalation for as long as possible at the end of an in-breath. Repeat for several breathing cycles.
➤ Establish the PBMT and PBFT.

Figure 3.5 Flexion dysfunction of the vomer. Continuous arrows: indirect technique. Go with the sphenoid into flexion and hold it there. Encourage motion of the vomer into flexion. Dotted arrows: . direct technique. Go with the sphenoid into extension and hold it there. Encourage the motion of the vomer into extension.

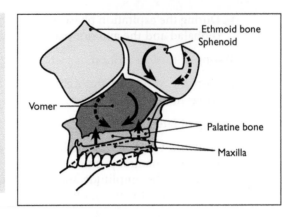

➤ A fluid impulse may be used to direct energy from the inion.

Direct technique (see Fig. 3.5):

➤ During the expiration phase, ease the greater wings cephalad with your thumb and middle finger (extension motion).
➤ At the same time, administer a cephalad impulse with the index finger on the median palatine suture, posterior to the transverse palatine suture (extension motion of the vomer).
➤ Hold the sphenoid and vomer in extension.
➤ Breathing assistance: Ask the patient to hold an exhalation for as long as possible at the end of an out-breath. Repeat for several breathing cycles.
➤ Continue as for indirect technique.

Extension dysfunction of the vomer *(Fig. 3.6)*

Hand position: As above.
Method: Indirect technique (exaggeration technique):

➤ During the expiration phase, ease the greater wings and vomer into extension and hold them there.
➤ Breathing assistance: Ask the patient to hold an exhalation for as long as possible at the end of an out-breath. Repeat for several breathing cycles
➤ Establish the PBMT and PBFT.
➤ A fluid impulse may be used to direct energy from the inion.

Direct technique:

➤ During the inspiration phase, ease the greater wings and vomer into flexion and hold them there.
➤ Breathing assistance: Ask the patient to hold an inhalation at the end of an in-breath for as long as possible. Repeat for several breathing cycles.
➤ Continue as for indirect technique.

Figure 3.6 Extension dysfunction of the vomer. Continuous arrows: indirect technique. Go with the sphenoid into extension and hold it there. Encourage the motion of the vomer into extension. Dotted arrows: direct technique. Go with the sphenoid into flexion and hold it there. Encourage the motion of the vomer into flexion.

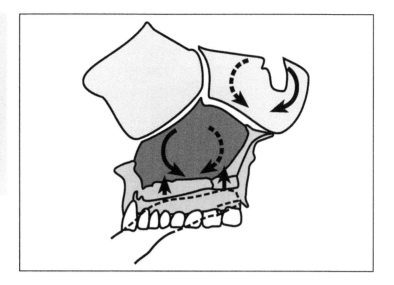

Alternative method to treat flexion or extension dysfunction

Indirect technique: Flexion dysfunction

> During the inspiration phase, deliver a gentle impulse to encourage motion into flexion.
> During the expiration phase, passively follow the motion of the vomer.
> In the next inspiration phase, again gently encourage motion into flexion.
> Continue until the restriction is released.

Biodynamic approach
Encourage the spontaneous occurrence of a still point or correcting motion at the vomer (an inspiration phase, flexion and expansion, or an expiration phase, extension and retraction) by means of palpation, carried out in a state of relaxed, non-invasive attention and empathy and in synchrony with the inherent homeodynamic forces and rhythmic patterns. This method requires no encounter or confrontation with tissue resistance and no resistance to a phase of primary respiration.

Torsion dysfunction of the vomer *(Fig. 3.7; see also Fig. 3.4)*

Hand position: As above
Method: Indirect technique (exaggeration technique):

> Hold the greater wings in a neutral position.
> At the same time, administer an impulse to encourage motion in the direction of ease of the torsion (right) with the index finger on the median palatine suture.
> Establish the PBMT and PBFT.
> A fluid impulse may be used to direct energy from the inion.

Figure 3.7 Torsion dysfunction of the vomer. Continuous line: indirect technique. Dotted line: direct technique.

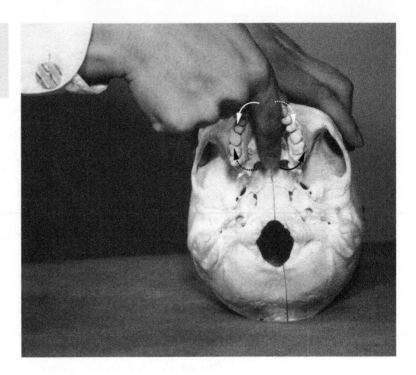

Direct technique:

➤ Hold the greater wings in a neutral position.
➤ At the same time, administer an impulse to encourage motion in the direction of restricted torsion (left) with the index finger on the median palatine suture.
➤ Continue as for indirect technique.

Lateral shear of the vomer *(Fig. 3.8; see also Fig. 3.4)*

Hand position: As above.

Method: Indirect technique (exaggeration technique):

➤ Hold the greater wings in a neutral position.
➤ At the same time, administer an impulse in the direction of lateral shear with greater ease of motion (right) with the index finger on the median palatine suture.
➤ Establish the PBMT and PBFT.
➤ A fluid impulse may be use to direct energy from the inion.

Direct technique:

➤ Hold the greater wings in a neutral position.
➤ At the same time, administer an impulse in the direction of restricted shear (left) with the index finger on the median palatine suture.
➤ Continue as for indirect technique.

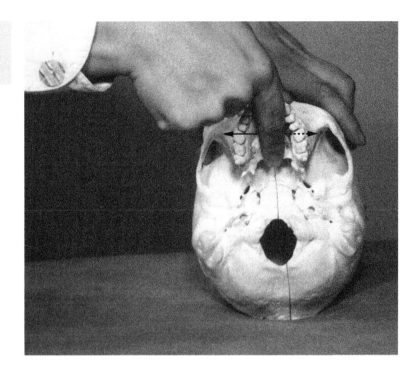

Figure 3.8 Lateral shear of the vomer. Continuous line: indirect technique. Dotted line: indirect technique

Sutural dysfunctions

Sphenovomerine suture

Suture margin: The rostrum of the sphenoid fits between the alae of the vomer.

Suture type: Schindylesis.

Hand position: As above.

Method: Indirect technique:

> ➤ Using your hands, go with the vomer and sphenoid in the direction of the dysfunction (i.e. the direction of greater ease of motion).
> ➤ Establish the PBMT and PBFT between the sphenoid and the vomer.
> ➤ Maintain the PBT until a correction of the abnormal tension has been achieved and stabilized by the inherent homeostatic forces (PRM rhythm etc.), and the motion of the vomer and sphenoid has ceased.
> ➤ Breathing assistance: Ask the patient to hold an inhalation for as long as possible at the end of an in-breath. Repeat for several breathing cycles.
> ➤ A fluid impulse may be used to direct energy from the inion.

Vomeromaxillary suture in internal rotation dysfunction of the maxillae *(Fig. 3.9)*

Suture margin: Inferiorly the anterior part of the vomer articulates with the nasal crest of the maxilla.

Suture type: Plane suture.

Aim: To release the vomeromaxillary suture and create freedom of motion of the vomer.

Figure 3.9
Vomeromaxillary suture in internal rotation dysfunction of the maxillae

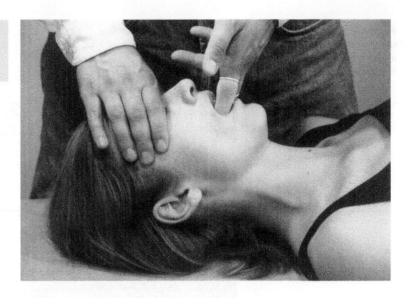

Therapist: Take up a position beside the patient's head.
Hand position: Cranial hand:

> ➤ Span the greater wings with your thumb and middle or index finger.

Caudal hand:

> ➤ Place your middle and index fingers on each side of the maxillae, resting on the teeth.

Method: ➤ During the inspiration phase, administer an impulse to induce flexion (in a caudal direction) via the greater wings (direct technique).
> ➤ At the same time, spread the fingers that are resting on the upper teeth (external rotation of the maxillae).
> ➤ During the expiration phase, passively follow the motion of the cranial bones.
> ➤ Repeat this procedure for several cycles, until the mobility of the vomer in the vomeromaxillary suture increases.

Decompression of the vomer *(Fig. 3.10)*

Therapist: Take up a position beside the patient's head.
Hand position: Cranial hand:

> ➤ Span the greater wings with your thumb and middle or index finger.

Caudal hand:

> ➤ Position your index finger intraorally, on the median palatine suture (anterior and posterior to the transverse palatine suture).
> ➤ Place your thumb externally below the nose, on the intermaxillary suture.

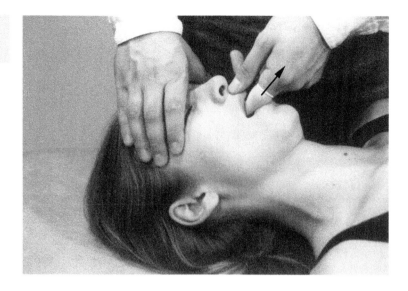

Figure 3.10
Decompression of the vomer

Method: ➤ Hold the greater wings in a neutral position.
➤ At the same time, administer traction in an anterior and inferior direction with the index finger and thumb of your caudal hand, at a roughly 45° angle.

Vomer pump technique *(Figs 3.11, 3.12)*

Indication Sinusitis.

Aim: Drainage of the sphenoidal sinus (sphenoid air cells), and to allow secretions to drain away.

Patient: Supine.

Therapist: Take up a position beside the patient's head.

Hand position: Cranial hand:

➤ Span the greater wings with your thumb and middle and/or index finger.

Caudal hand:

➤ Position your index finger intraorally, on the median palatine suture.

Method: To close the sinus:

➤ During the expiration phase, administer gentle pressure to the posterior part of the median palatine suture with your index finger (extension of the vomer).
➤ At the same time, guide the greater wings cephalad, using your thumb and middle finger (extension).
➤ Hold the vomer and sphenoid in extension, and ask the patient to hold an exhalation for as long as possible at the end of an out-breath. Repeat the procedure several times.

Note: Magoun asks patients to bend their head slightly forward. Your finger acts as the fulcrum for this movement, and as the patient's head

Figure 3.11 Vomer pump technique. To close the sinus. Dotted arrows: during the expiration phase, impulse to encourage the motion of the vomer into extension and of the sphenoid into extension. To open the sinus. Continuous arrows: during the inspiration phase, impulse to encourage the motion of the vomer into flexion and of the sphenoid into flexion.

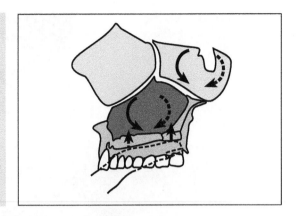

Figure 3.12 Vomer pump technique. Opposite physiological motion. Continuous arrows: during the inspiration phase, flexion of the sphenoid and extension of the vomer. Dotted arrows: during the expiration phase, extension of the sphenoid and flexion of the vomer.

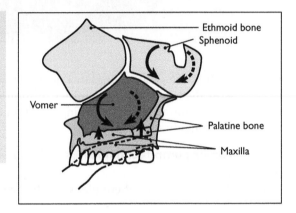

bends forward, the pressure is transmitted through the posterior part of the vomer to the rostrum of the sphenoid, moving it into extension.[2]

Method: To open the sinus:

➤ During the inspiration phase of primary respiration, administer pressure with your index finger to the anterior part of the median palatine suture (flexion of the vomer).
➤ At the same time, guide the greater wings caudad using your thumb and middle finger (flexion).
➤ Hold the vomer and sphenoid in flexion and ask the patient to hold an inhalation for as long as possible at the end of an in-breath. Repeat the procedure several times.

Method: Opposite physiological motion:
During the inspiration phase of primary respiration:

➤ Perform a caudad movement with your middle finger and thumb on the greater wings (flexion motion).
➤ At the same time, administer a cephalad impulse to the posterior part of the palatine suture with your index finger (extension motion of the vomer).

During the expiration phase:

> ➤ Perform a cephalad movement with your middle finger and thumb on the greater wings (extension motion).
> ➤ At the same time, administer a cephalad impulse to the anterior part of the palatine suture with your index finger (flexion motion of the vomer).
> ➤ In the next inspiration phase, again induce opposite physiological motion of the vomer.
> ➤ Continue until you sense a relaxation and release of the sphenoid sinuses.

Method: Finish this technique by re-synchronizing the motion of the vomer with that of the sphenoid, in harmony with the PRM rhythm.

> ➤ During the inspiration phase, go with the sphenoid and the vomer into flexion, and in the expiration phase, go with both sphenoid and vomer into extension.

References

1 Magoun HI. Osteopathy in the Cranial Field. 3rd edn. Kirksville: Journal Printing Company; 1976:57.
2 Magoun HI. Osteopathy in the Cranial Field. 1st edn. Kirksville: Journal Printing Company; 1951:172.

The temporal bones

THE MORPHOLOGY OF THE TEMPORAL BONE ACCORDING TO ROHEN[1]

There are striking similarities in shape between the embryonic hip bone and the temporal bone: the ilium can be compared with the temporal squama, the ischium and pubis to the mastoid zygomatic processes, and the acetabulum resembles the temporomandibular joint and the external acoustic meatus. For a real understanding of the structures, we need more than just a simple description of similarities between individual elements or homologous features. We need to understand the functional dynamics, including the motions and attitudes seen in the development and growth of the tissue. It is in motion that we gain a deeper understanding, because in motion we find the origin of form.

The temporal bone displays a remarkably similar dynamic to the pelvis, a similar 'gesture' or attitude in terms of its polarity as its form unfolds. We see this in the way the ilium opens its surface upward, separating itself from the space around it, rising up and expressing a lightness, while the developing character of the ischium is expressed in a downward thickening of the bone, fortifying, static, and incorporated into the space around it.

The temporal bone is similar in the way its development and appearance are expressed. The squamous part belongs to the cranial vault. It undergoes membranous ossification, beginning at a center, about level with the external auditory meatus, and spreading ray-like toward the cranial vault. Its outspread surface, opening to above, echoes that of the ilium.

The petrous or petromastoid part, in contrast, belongs to the cranial base and undergoes endochondral ossification. As it develops, it pushes downward and inward in a wedge-like way, into the skull. The petrous part envelops the organs of hearing and balance at a very early stage. It is the first part of the skull to ossify and is the hardest bone in the body. 'Petrous' (stone-like), is the perfect name for it. The mastoid process forms in a downward direction from the petrous part.

Between the squamous and petromastoid parts, the zygomatic process extends horizontally forward and provides a balance between these two polarities.

Just as the pelvis anchors and balances movements from above and below, so the temporal bone serves to unify these two polarities.

The pelvis establishes and maintains balance upward and downward, and is the point from which the dynamic of motion of the lower limbs originates, reaching out into the space around. In a way the hip joint is the gateway to the world outside. In a corresponding way, the process of hearing brings the inner nature of that world outside into the consciousness, so that the external acoustic meatus is the gateway to inside.

The pneumatization of the petrous part begins in the 8th month of intrauterine development. An epithelial anlage into the middle ear quickly grows and displaces the mesenchyme. This process is complete by the time of birth, but then continues into the inner ear region. In the course of development the petrous part dies off, in effect, to the point where it becomes the hardest, most lifeless bone in the body, which (unlike other intercartilaginous bones) is incapable of any further adaptive or transmutational processes.

LOCATION, CAUSES AND CLINICAL PRESENTATION OF OSTEOPATHIC DYSFUNCTIONS OF THE TEMPORAL BONE

Osseous dysfunction (including sutures and other joints)

a) Occipitomastoid suture and condylo-squamosomastoid pivot point (CSMP)

Causes:
- In the case of bilateral compression: fall or blow to the occipital squama.
- In the case of unilateral compression: fall or blow to the side of the occipital squama.

The effect is to force the squama in an anterior direction, the basilar part of the occiput in an inferior direction and the temporal bones into internal rotation. The concave mastoid border of the occiput is forced anteriorly and superiorly, wedging it into the convex posterior border of the mastoid part of the temporal bone and moving the mastoid part posteriorly and medially.

- Whiplash injury, and sometimes as a result of a direct thrust technique at the back of the head.
- Secondary to compression of the atlanto-occipital joint or dysfunction of the sphenopetrosal synchondrosis.

Compression of this suture leads to opposite motion of the temporal bone relative to the occipital bone, i.e. the occipital bone moves into flexion and the temporal bone into internal rotation.

Clinical presentation: Abnormal tensions of the tentorium cerebelli, venous congestion of the sigmoid sinus, disturbances in the fluctuation of cerebrospinal fluid, disturbances of the cerebellum, medulla oblongata or other centers of the brain, and of the vagus nerve (nausea, vomiting, etc.).

Sequelae: Dysfunction of the SBS and change in the frequency and amplitude of the PRM rhythm, affecting homeostasis of the body overall.

b) Sphenosquamous suture and sphenosquamous pivot point (SSP)

Causes: Primary injury caused by a fall or blow to the cheek or the ipsilateral mastoid process. Secondary: in connection with the sphenoid bone or hypertonus of the temporalis muscle (in psychological stress or temporomandibular joint syndrome).

Clinical presentation: At the vertical course of the suture: middle meningeal artery, migraine.[2]
At the horizontal course of the suture: greater and lesser petrosal nerves.
Greater petrosal nerve (to the pterygopalatine ganglion): disturbance of the lacrimal gland, dryness or irritation of the mucosa of the nose, nasopharynx and palate, allergic rhinitis (see also pterygopalatine fossa).
Lesser petrosal nerve: disturbance of the parotid gland.

● Functional disturbance of adjacent parts of the brain.

Sequelae: Dysfunction of the SBS and change in the frequency and amplitude of PRM rhythm, affecting homeostasis of the body overall.

c) Petrojugular suture and petro-occipital fissure (petro-occipital synchondrosis).

Causes: In connection with the occipital bone: primary traumatic, e.g. in tooth extractions with mouth wide open.
Leads to impairment of motion of the temporal bone.

Clinical presentation: All functions of structures linked with the temporal bone.

d) Sphenopetrosal synchondrosis

Causes: Tooth extraction from the upper jaw can cause ipsilateral dysfunction of the petrosphenoidal ligament, and tooth extraction from the lower jaw causes contralateral dysfunction of the ligament. Cranial nerves CN III, CN IV and CN VI (which supply the muscles of the eye) run alongside the body of the sphenoid, near this ligament. CN VI in particular is vulnerable to tensions originating in this ligament.

Clinical presentation: Disturbances of the eye, fatigue strabismus in young children, etc.

e) Temporozygomatic suture

Causes: A fall or blow to the cheek or SBS dysfunctions.

Sequelae: Impairment of motion of the zygomatic bone and of the integration between sphenoid and occipital bones.
A restriction of the temporozygomatic suture can mean that the zygomatic process of the temporal bone cannot glide outward and inferiorly with the temporal process of the zygomatic bone during the inspiration phase. This would fix the temporal bone in internal rotation during the inspiration phase.

Note: The zygomatic bone is mainly influenced by the sphenoid and the temporal bone by the occiput.

f) Parietomastoid suture

Causes: A fall or blow from above onto the ipsilateral parietal bone.

g) Temporomandibular joint

Sequelae: Unilateral and bilateral anomalies of dental occlusion, protrusion and retraction, etc.

- Disturbances to dental growth
- Bruxism (grinding of the teeth)
- Clicking due to dysfunction of the articular disk
- 'Popping'
- Disturbances of hearing (tinnitus, etc.) or of balance
- Eye disturbances, taste disturbances.

h) Pharyngotympanic (auditory) tube

Causes and clinical presentation: IR of the temporal bone → narrowing of the cartilaginous auditory tube → hissing, high-pitched sound.

ER of the temporal bone → widening of the auditory tube → pulsations, low-pitched sound.

Explanation: The sounds heard are probably produced by the blood flow in the internal carotid artery where it forms a bend inside the petrous part of the temporal bone. At this point it is separated from the inner ear only by a thin plate of bone, so that structural changes in this region can cause tinnitus.

i) Intraosseous dysfunctions
Between:

- Petromastoid part/tympanic plate
- Petromastoid part/squamous part
- Squamous part/tympanic plate.

Causes: Primary injury: by direct force to the temporal bone, especially during birth and infancy.

Secondary injury: through dysfunctions of other bones (occipital bone, sphenoid).

Sequelae: Reduced pliancy of the bone and functional impairment of all involved structures.

At birth the temporal bone consists of:

- the squamous part and tympanic ring (tympanic part)
- the petrous part.

Muscular dysfunction

Location: *a)* At the mastoid process
- Sternocleidomastoid muscle (SCM)

Clinical presentation: Headache, abnormal position of head

- Splenius capitis muscle
- Digastric muscle (posterior belly)

b) At the styloid process
- Stylohyoid muscle

Clinical presentation: Grinding of teeth, pain in the floor of the mouth, pharynx and larynx

- Styloglossus muscle
- Stylopharyngeus muscle

c) Masticatory muscles
- Temporalis muscle: at the temporal fossa
- Masseter muscle: at the zygomatic process of the temporal bone

d) Other muscles
- Levator veli palatini muscle: at the inferior opening of the carotid canal that passes through the petrous part
- Tensor tympani muscle: the tensor muscle of the tympanic membrane, in the canal for the tensor tympani muscle
- Stapedius muscle

Clinical presentation: Abnormal hearing sensitivity.

Ligamentous dysfunction

a) Petrosphenoidal ligament (Gruber's ligament) at the sphenopetrosal synchondrosis

Causes: Tooth extraction; ossification of the ligament.

Magoun states that tooth extraction from the upper jaw can cause dysfunction of the ipsilateral petrosphenoidal ligament.

Tooth extraction from the lower jaw can cause dysfunction of the suture on the opposite side.[3]

Clinical presentation: ● Abducent nerve (CN VI).

b) Stylomandibular ligament
Causes: Tooth extraction.

c) Stylohyoid ligament
Causes: Ossification of the ligament.
Sequelae: Motion restriction of the hyoid bone.

d) Anterior ligament of the malleus
From the anterior process of the hammer into the petrotympanic fissure, from where some fibers run to the spine of the sphenoid and on to the ramus of the mandible, together with the sphenomandibular ligament.

e) Pintus ligament
Not regular; from the hammer through the petrotympanic fissure to the head of the mandible.
Causes: Dysfunction of the temporomandibular joint.
Clinical presentation: Hearing disturbances.

Fascial dysfunction

a. Temporal fascia
b. Investing layer of cervical fascia
c. Prevertebral layer of cervical fascia
d. Interpterygoid aponeurosis

    e. The 'rideau stylien' (styloid apparatus and its adjacent tissues)

    f. Pharynx

    Caused by muscular, organic disturbances, etc.

Sequelae: Motion restrictions of the temporal bone, functional disturbances of involved structures.

Dysfunction of the tentorium cerebelli

Causes: Meningitis, cranial injury, motion restriction, etc.

Clinical presentation: Superior surface: Pain in the eye and the external frontal region. Inferior surface: Pain behind the ear, in the forehead and the eye. Obstruction to venous flow in the transverse sinus, sigmoid sinus, inferior and superior petrosal sinuses, headache, and motion restriction of the temporal bone.

Disturbances affecting nerves and parts of the brain

a) Temporal lobe

Causes: Dysfunctions in the middle cranial fossa and motion restrictions of the temporal bone, especially IR of the temporal bone.

b) Cerebellum

Causes: IR of the temporal bone, torsion of the tentorium cerebelli.

Clinical presentation: Disturbances of balance, of muscle tonus and of coordination of voluntary muscle activity.

c) Oculomotor (CN III) and trochlear (CN IV) nerves

Causes: Dural tensions at the attachment of the tentorium cerebelli to the posterior clinoid process, tensions and stasis at the walls of the cavernous sinus and dysfunctions at the superior border of the petrous part of the temporal bone.

Clinical presentation:
- CN III: lateral deviation of the eye, horizontal double vision, divergent strabismus, restriction of the line of vision upward, downward and medially.
- CN III, autonomic: mydriasis, ptosis and impairment of the photomotor reflex.
- CN IV: upward and medial deviation of the eye, vertical or oblique double vision, convergent strabismus.

d) Trigeminal nerve (CN V)

The trigeminal ganglion lies in a dural sac in the trigeminal impression on the anterior surface of the petrous part.

Causes: Dural tensions affecting the tentorium cerebelli, the meningeal dura of the trigeminal ganglion; change in the position of the temporal bone, tensions and stasis in the wall of the cavernous sinus (CN V1,V2).

    A dysfunction of the temporomandibular joint with tensions at the medial and lateral pterygoid muscles leads to disturbances of the junction of the sphenoid and palatine bones, which may sometimes affect the pterygopalatine ganglion (CN V2) in the sphenopalatine foramen.

Clinical presentation: Trigeminal cave: pain in the facial region.

Trigeminus neuralgia, disturbances of sensation affecting the face, functional disturbances of the masticatory muscles, inhibition of the sneezing reflex (CN V2) or corneal reflex (CN V1), pain and watering of the eye (CN V1, some parasympathetic fibers in trigeminal nerve).

e) Abducent nerve (CN VI)
At the apex of the petrous part of the temporal bone, between the petrous part and the petrosphenoidal ligament.

Causes: The VI cranial nerve is particularly vulnerable to tensions arising from the tentorium and the ligament because of the fibrous link with the petrosphenoidal ligament and the fact that it runs in an osteofibrous canal formed by this ligament and the petrous part of the temporal bone. If affected this can lead to disturbances of the eye, including fatigue strabismus in young children. Stasis and tensions in the wall of the cavernous sinus can also cause disturbances of the abducent nerve.

Clinical presentation: Horizontal double vision, convergent strabismus, lateral restriction of the line of vision, tendency to hold the head turned to one side to compensate for the functional deficiency.

f) Facial nerve (CN VII) and intermediate nerve (CN VII)
Pass through the internal acoustic meatus in the facial canal; unite at the geniculate ganglion; branch of sensory fibers in the chorda tympani supplies sensation (taste); main portion passes through the stylomastoid foramen.

Causes: Dural tensions at the internal acoustic meatus and stylomastoid foramen.

Clinical presentation:
- Facial nerve (CN VII): Disturbance of facial expression.
- Intermediate nerve (CN VII): Disturbance of saliva secretion, taste disturbances relating to the anterior two-thirds of the tongue, functional disturbance of the lacrimal, nasal and palatine glands (via the greater petrosal nerve).

g) Vestibulocochlear nerve (CN VIII)
Through the internal acoustic meatus to the organs of hearing and balance.

Causes: Dural tensions at the temporal bone and internal acoustic meatus, dysfunction of the petrojugular suture.

Clinical presentation: Disturbances of hearing, disturbances of balance.

h) Glossopharyngeal nerve (CN IX), vagus nerve (CN X), accessory nerve (CN XI)
At the jugular notch with the intrajugular process.

Causes: Dural tensions at the jugular foramen, dysfunction of the occipital and temporal bones, the occipitomastoid suture, petrojugular suture, and petro-occipital fissure (petro-occipital synchondrosis).

Clinical presentation:
- CN IX: Disturbances of taste, dry mouth (parasympathetic fibers supplying the parotid gland), disturbances of swallowing (fibers supplying sensation to the pharynx).

● CN X: Disturbances of cardiac, digestive and respiratory function, disturbances of speaking and swallowing.
● CN XI: Torticollis.

i) Greater and lesser petrosal nerves
In the groove of the same name.
Causes: Dural tensions in the groove.
Clinical presentation: Greater petrosal nerve: functional disturbance of the lacrimal, nasal and palatine glands.
Lesser petrosal nerve: functional disturbance of the parotid gland.

j) Parasympathetic fibers
Some parasympathetic fibers run together with the facial nerve (CN VII) and innervate part of the internal tympanic membrane.

Some parasympathetic fibers run together with the chorda tympani (CN VII) and then on with CN V3.

Some fibers run together with the glossopharyngeal nerve (CN IX) and on to the otic ganglion via the lesser petrosal nerve and then onward with CN V3.

Most together with the vagus nerve (CN X).

● Interactions can occur between the tympanic membrane and parasympathetic system, e.g. sounds affect the vagus nerve and may produce reactions within the autonomic system.[4]

k) Internal carotid plexus
Causes: Dural tensions at the carotid canal and foramen lacerum, and changes in position of the apex of the petrous part of the temporal bone, and abnormal tensions of the dura mater at the cavernous sinus.
Clinical presentation: Disturbances of the sympathetic system via effect on the internal carotid plexus etc.

Vascular disturbances

a) Internal carotid artery
Causes: Dural tensions at the carotid canal and at the foramen lacerum, and changes in position of the apex of the petrous part of the temporal bone, and abnormal tensions of the dura mater at the cavernous sinus.

The anterior and posterior margins of the foramen lacerum are formed by the posterior border of the greater wing of the sphenoid and the anterior portion of the petrous part of the temporal bone. The foramen lacerum is divided into two by the sphenoidal lingula. It is open on the outside, and closed with fibrocartilage inside. The internal carotid artery lies on this.
Clinical presentation: Disturbances of the sympathetic system via effect on the internal carotid plexus.

b) Middle meningeal artery

Causes: Compression of the sphenosquamous suture and sphenosquamous pivot, abnormal tensions of the dura mater in the middle cranial fossa.

Clinical presentation: Migraine and raised intracranial pressure.

c) Occipital artery

Causes: Dural tensions in the occipital groove, medial to the mastoid notch.

d) Jugular vein

Causes: Dural tensions at the jugular foramen, dysfunction of the occipital and temporal bones, the occipitomastoid suture, petrojugular suture and petro-occipital fissure (petrobasilar suture; petro-occipital synchondrosis). The jugular foramen resembles a widened suture between the occipital and temporal bones and so can easily be affected by dysfunctions of these bones.

Clinical presentation: Venous congestion in the cranium, headache, memory disturbances, impairment of brain function.

e) Venous sinus
- Sigmoid sinus: in the groove of the same name at the posterior, inferior corner of the petrous part.
- Superior petrosal sinus: in the groove of the same name, on the crest of the posterior border of the petrous part.
- Inferior petrosal sinus: in the groove of the same name, below the opening of the internal acoustic meatus.

Causes: Change in position of the apex of the petrous part of the temporal bone and abnormal tensions of the tentorium cerebelli.

Sequelae:
- Sigmoid sinus: congestion in the confluence of sinuses and superior petrosal sinus.
- Superior and inferior petrosal sinuses: congestion affecting the cavernous sinus and basilar venous plexus, ophthalmic veins and veins of the medulla, pons and inferior surface of the cerebellum as well as other regions of the brain.

Clinical presentation: Region of the sigmoid sinus → pain behind the ear.
Region of the superior petrosal sinus → pain in the temporal region of the head.
Venous congestion of regions of the brain → headache, impairment of the relevant function of the brain.
Venous congestion affecting the eyes → visual disturbances, sensation of pressure.

Disturbances of the endolymphatic ducts

Causes: Tensions at the endolymphatic sac hinder the drainage of endolymph into the dura.

Clinical presentation: Dizziness.

Causes of dysfunctions of the temporal bone

Primary dysfunction:

a. Intraosseous

The temporal bone forms part of the cranial base, where its embryonic structure is cartilaginous, and also part of the cranial vault, where the anlage is membranous.

Direct force to the temporal bone, especially during birth and in infancy, can result in dysfunctions between the petromastoid part/tympanic plate, between the petromastoid part/squamous part, and between the squamous part/tympanic plate.

b. Primary trauma

Perinatal, and as a result of falls, blows, tooth extraction, whiplash injury or other types of force affecting the sutures. These can cause motion restrictions of the temporal bone, e.g. compression of the occipitomastoid suture or condylo-squamomastoid pivot point (CSMP) can occur, producing asynchronous motion between the occipital bone and temporal bone. Falls onto the pelvis can also cause dysfunction of the temporal bone.

Secondary dysfunction:

Dysfunction of the occipital bone, e.g. SBS dysfunctions, transmission of tension via the tentorium cerebelli or extra-cranial tensions of muscles or fasciae (sternocleidomastoid muscle, trapezius muscle, overall nuchal muscle tonus etc.) and pelvis dysfunctions can all cause secondary motion restriction of the temporal bone.

Examination and techniques

- History-taking
- Visual assessment
- Palpation of the position
- Palpation of PRM rhythm
- Motion testing
  - External/internal rotation
  - Anterior and posterior rotation
- Intraosseous dysfunctions
  - Direct/indirect
  - Molding
- Dysfunction in external and internal rotation, unilateral
- Dysfunction in external and internal rotation, bilateral
- Dysfunction in anterior and posterior rotation, unilateral
- Dysfunction in anterior and posterior rotation, bilateral
- Temporal bone lift technique
- Petro-occipital fissure (petrobasilar suture; petro-occipital synchondrosis) and petrojugular suture
- Occipitomastoid suture
- Parietomastoid suture
- Squamoparietal suture

- Sphenosquamous suture: sphenosquamous pivot technique
- Sphenopetrosal synchondrosis
- Temporozygomatic suture
- Technique for the auditory ossicles
- 'Ear pull' technique
- 'Pussy foot' technique
- 'Father Tom' reanimation technique
- Auditory tube technique (see under Ear)

DIAGNOSIS

History-taking

The most common symptoms are deafness, tinnitus, dizziness, earache, otitis media, neuralgia (trigeminal neuralgia), migraine, headache, tic douloureux, problems of the temporomandibular joint ('clicking' of the joint, dental malocclusion, pain), and facial nerve paralysis. The temporal bone can also be involved in disturbances of the eye muscles, the nose, the oral cavity, in autism, and in shoulder-hand syndrome (reflex sympathetic dystrophy). Previous injury should always be considered.

Visual assessment

- Ear: protruding (ER) or close-lying (IR).
- Unilaterally protruding or close-lying ear: torsion or lateroflexion rotation of the SBS.

Palpation

Palpation of the position

- Mastoid process: postero-medial (ER) or anterolateral (IR).
- Mastoid part of temporal bone: anterolateral (ER) or postero-medial (IR).
- Squamoparietal suture: separated and displaced anterolaterally (ER) or approximated and displaced postero-medially (IR).

Palpation of primary respiration *(Fig. 4.1)*

- Biomechanical/biodynamic palpation; motion testing as required.
- If palpation reveals a motion restriction, an impulse in the restricted direction will emphasize the restriction and enable you to sense which structure is the origin of the restriction.

Therapist: Take up a position at the head of the patient.

Hand position: ➤ Place the thenar eminence on the mastoid part of the temporal bone on each side.
➤ Position your thumbs on the anterior tip of the mastoid process on each side.
➤ Place the palms of your hands on the occiput.
➤ Clasp your fingers together.
➤ Rest your elbows on the bench.

Figure 4.1 Palpation of primary respiration of the temporal bone

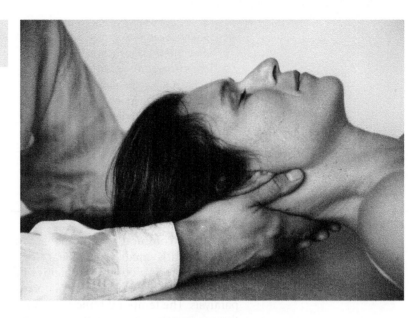

Figure 4.2 Inspiration phase of PR/biomechanical

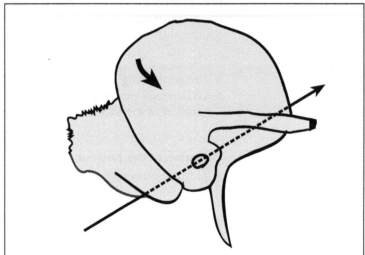

Biomechanical

An external rotation of the temporal bone occurs during the inspiration phase of the PR.

Inspiration phase of PR, normal finding (Fig. 4.2):

➤ Your thumbs, resting on the tips of the mastoid processes, will sense a postero-medial motion.
➤ With the thenar eminences, resting on the mastoid part of each temporal bone, you will sense an anterolateral motion.
➤ The palms of your hands will sense the flexion motion of the occiput.

(The zygomatic processes move laterally, with an additional anterior and inferior motion of the anterior portion.)

Expiration phase of PR, normal finding:

➤ Your thumbs, resting on the tips of the mastoid processes, will sense an anterolateral motion.
➤ With the thenar eminences, resting on the mastoid parts of the temporal bones, you will sense a postero-medial motion.
➤ The palms of your hands will sense the extension motion of the occiput.

(The zygomatic processes move medially, with an additional posterior and superior motion of the anterior portion.)

Biodynamic, embryological approach (Fig. 4.3)
Inspiration phase of PR, normal finding:

● The squamae of the temporal bones move centrifugally (outward motion).
● The convexity of the squamae becomes less, i.e. they become flatter.

Expiration phase of PR, normal finding:

● The squamae of the temporal bones move in a centripetal direction.
● The convexity of the squamae becomes greater.

➤ Compare the amplitude, strength, ease and symmetry of the motions of the temporal bones.
➤ Other types of motion of the temporal bone may sometimes occur during external and internal rotation. These provide an indication of any further dysfunctions of the particular temporal bone.

Motion testing

This resembles the palpation of primary respiration except that in motion testing the external and internal rotation motion of the temporal bones is actively induced by the therapist.

Hand position: As above.
Method: Testing of external and internal rotation:
During the inspiration phase:

➤ At the beginning of the inspiration phase, administer an impulse in a postero-medial direction with your thumbs positioned on the tips of the mastoid processes.

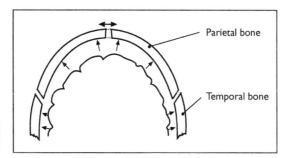

Figure 4.3 Inspiration phase of PR/biodynamic

During the expiration phase:

> At the beginning of the expiration phase, administer an impulse in a postero-medial direction with the thenar eminences of your thumbs, positioned on the mastoid parts of the temporal bones.
> Compare the amplitude and ease of motion or the amount of force needed to elicit movement.

Alternative hand position: (Fig. 4.4)

> Grasp the zygomatic process of each side between your thumb and index finger.
> Place your middle finger in the external ear canal of each side.
> Place your ring finger on the tip of the mastoid process each side.
> Position the little finger of each hand on the mastoid part of the temporal bone.
> Rest both elbows on the bench.

Method: Testing of external and internal rotation.

During the inspiration phase:

> At the beginning of the inspiration phase, administer an impulse in an inferior and lateral direction with your thumbs on the zygomatic processes.
> With your middle fingers in the external ear canal, administer an impulse to ease the temporal bones into anterior rotation and external rotation.
> At the same time, administer a postero-medial impulse with your ring fingers, on the mastoid processes.

During the expiration phase:

> At the beginning of the expiration phase, administer an impulse in a superior and medial direction with your index fingers on the zygomatic processes.

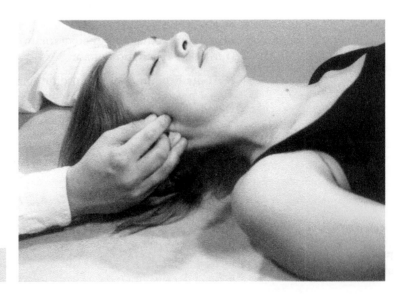

Figure 4.4 Alternative hand position

> With your middle fingers in the external ear canal, administer an impulse to ease the temporal bones into posterior rotation and internal rotation.
> At the same time, administer a postero-medial impulse with your little fingers on the mastoid parts of the temporal bone.

Hand position: Unilateral testing (Fig. 4.5)

> Hold the occiput in the palm of one hand.
> Position the fingers of the other hand on the temporal bone as described above:
>   • Thumb and index finger grasping the zygomatic process.
>   • Middle finger in the external ear canal.
>   • Ring finger on the tip of the mastoid process.
>   • Little finger on the mastoid part of the temporal bone.
> Rest both elbows on the bench.

Method: Testing of external and internal rotation.
During the inspiration phase:

> At the beginning of the inspiration phase, administer an impulse into flexion with the hand on the occiput.
> With your other hand, sense the reaction of the temporal bone.

Normal finding: External rotation of the temporal bone.

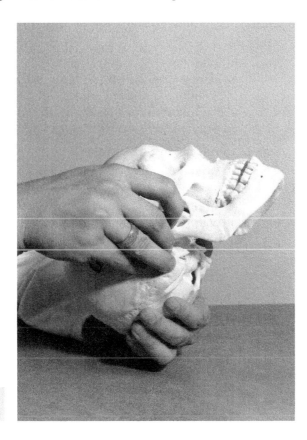

Figure 4.5 Unilateral testing

➤ Zygomatic process in an inferior, lateral and anterior direction (thumb and index finger).
➤ External ear canal into anterior rotation and external rotation (middle finger).
➤ Mastoid process in a postero-medial direction (ring finger).
➤ Mastoid part of temporal bone in an anterolateral direction (little finger).

During the expiration phase:

➤ At the beginning of the expiration phase, administer an impulse to encourage motion into extension with the hand on the occiput.
➤ With your other hand, sense the reaction of the temporal bone.

Normal finding: Internal rotation of the temporal bone.

➤ Zygomatic process in a superior, medial and posterior direction (thumb and index finger).
➤ External ear canal into posterior rotation and internal rotation (middle finger).
➤ Mastoid process in an anterolateral direction (ring finger).
➤ Mastoid part of the temporal bone in a postero-medial direction (little finger).
➤ Compare the amplitude and ease of motion and the amount of force needed to elicit movement.

Hand position: Test of anterior and posterior rotation (Fig. 4.6).

➤ Grasp the zygomatic process of each side between your thumb and index finger.
➤ Place your middle finger in the external ear canal on each side.
➤ Position the ring finger each side anterior to the mastoid process.
➤ Position the little finger each side posterior to the mastoid process.
➤ Rest both elbows on the bench.

Method: During the inspiration phase:

➤ At the beginning of the inspiration phase, administer an impulse in an inferior direction with your thumbs on the zygomatic processes.
➤ With your middle fingers in the external ear canal, administer an impulse to ease the temporal bones into anterior rotation.
➤ At the same time, with the ring fingers and little fingers on the mastoid processes, administer an impulse in a superior direction.

During the expiration phase:

➤ At the beginning of the expiration phase, administer an impulse in a superior direction with the index fingers on the zygomatic processes.
➤ With the middle fingers in the external ear canals, administer an impulse to ease the temporal bones into posterior rotation.
➤ At the same time, with the ring fingers and little fingers on the mastoid processes, administer an impulse in an inferior direction.

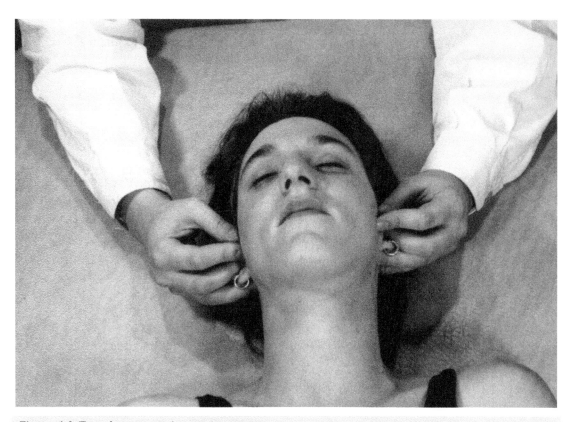

Figure 4.6 Test of anterior and posterior rotation

> ➤ Compare the amplitude and ease of motion and the strength needed to elicit movement.

TREATMENT OF THE TEMPORAL BONE[5]

Intraosseous dysfunctions

At birth, the temporal bone consists of:

- The squamous part and tympanic ring (tympanic part).
- The petrous part.
- The squamous part and the tympanic part are already partially joined at the time of birth. This gives rise to the petrosquamous fissure, which is a potential site for intraosseous dysfunctions.
- The squamous part, petrous part and styloid process fuse during the first year of life.
- The mastoid process does not develop until after the second year of life, so cannot yet be palpated in the newborn.
- The styloid process is still cartilaginous in the newborn. The proximal and distal parts do not unite until puberty.
- The mandibular fossa is still flat at birth and deepens only during the development of the articular tubercle.

- Primary intraosseous dysfunctions can be due to direct force to the temporal bone, especially during birth and in infancy.
- Secondary dysfunctions can occur as a result of dysfunctions of other bones (occipital bone, sphenoid).
- All the sutural junctions of the temporal bone should have free mobility to ensure the success of intraosseous techniques.
- Petromastoid part/tympanic part
- Petromastoid part/squamous part
- Squamous part/tympanic part

Petromastoid part/tympanic part. Example *(Fig. 4.7)*

Hand position ➤ Hold the occiput in your left hand, with your fingertips resting on the mastoid part and mastoid process.
➤ Place the little finger of your right hand in the external ear canal.

Alternative hand position: (Fig. 4.8)

➤ The patient's head is turned to the left.

Right hand:

➤ Place your thumb on the mastoid process.
➤ Place the thenar eminence on the mastoid part of the temporal bone.

➤ Hold the occiput in the remaining fingers of that hand.

Left hand:

➤ Place the little finger of your left hand in the external ear canal.

Petromastoid part/squamous part. Example *(Fig. 4.9)*

Hand position ➤ Hold the occiput in your left hand, with your fingertips resting on the mastoid part and mastoid process.

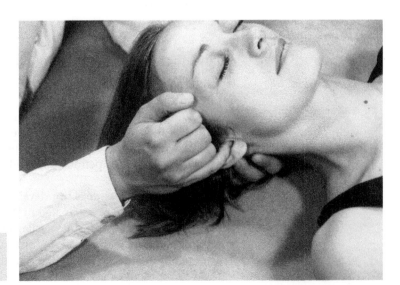

Figure 4.7 Petromastoid part/tympanic part. Example: right

Figure 4.8 Petromastoid part/tympanic part. Alternative hand position

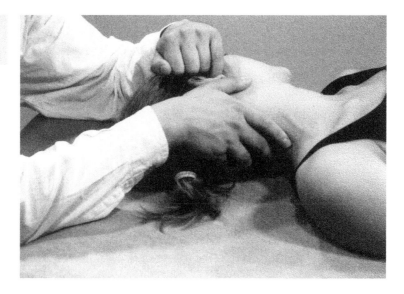

Figure 4.9 Petromastoid part/squamous part. Example: right

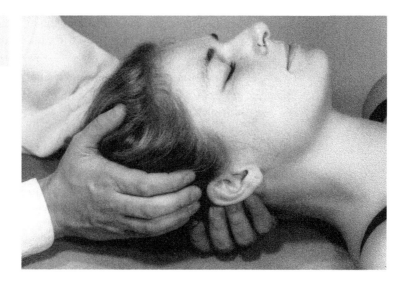

➤ Rest the index and middle fingers of your right hand, and also your ring finger if necessary, on the squamous part.

Alternative hand position: (Fig. 4.10)

➤ The patient's head is turned to the left.

Right hand:

➤ Place your thumb on the mastoid process.
➤ Place the thenar eminence on the mastoid part of the temporal bone.
➤ Hold the occiput in the remaining fingers of that hand.

Figure 4.10 Petromastoid part/squamous part. Alternative hand position

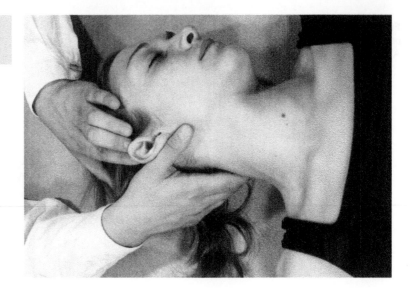

Left hand:

➤ Rest the index and middle fingers of your left hand, and also your ring finger if necessary, on the squamous part.

Squamous part/tympanic part. Example: right *(Fig. 4.11)*

Hand position: ➤ Rest the index and middle fingers of your left hand, and also your ring finger if necessary, on the squamous part.
➤ Place the little finger of your right hand in the external ear canal.

Method: Direct technique:

➤ Guide both portions of the bone in the direction of the restricted motion until you reach the motion barrier.
➤ Hold this position until tissue release or a still point occurs.

Indirect technique:

➤ Move both portions of the bone in the direction of the dysfunction, i.e. the direction of greater motion (direction of ease).
➤ Establish the PBMT and PBFT (the position that achieves the best possible balance between these two portions of the bone).
➤ Maintain this position until the tissues relax and mobility improves.

Molding *(Fig. 4.12)*

Indication: Asymmetrical convexity or flattening at the ossification centers.
Hand position: ➤ Draw the fingertips of one hand close together.
➤ Place them on the squama.

Method: a. To treat convexity:

➤ Administer centrifugal impulses with your fingers, to flatten the site of the convexity.

Figure 4.11 Squamous part/tympanic part. Example: right

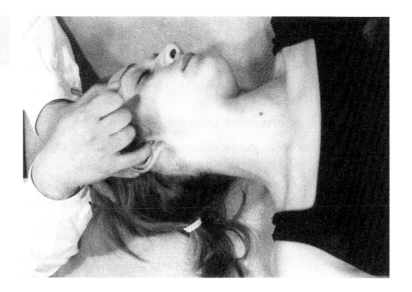

Figure 4.12 Molding

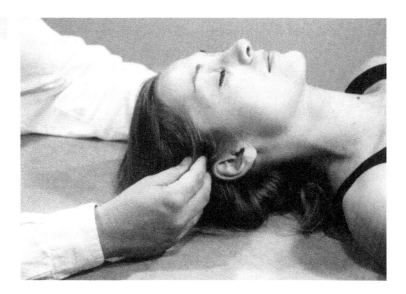

> You may supplement this with a fluid impulse to direct energy toward the borders of the temporal bone.

Important note: Gently release the adjacent bones from the temporal bone before beginning to apply this technique.

b. To treat a flattening of the bone:

> Administer centripetal impulses aimed at raising the profile at the flattened site.
> You may supplement this with a fluid impulse to direct energy toward the ossification center from the occipitomastoid suture on the opposite side.

c. To treat torsion tensions:

➤ Administer an impulse with your fingers, in the direction of the restricted motion.

d. Establish the PBMT and PBFT.

Dysfunction in external and internal rotation

Dysfunction in external and internal rotation, unilateral *(Fig. 4.13)*

Therapist: Take up a position at the head of the patient.

Hand position: ➤ Place the thenar eminences of your thumbs bilaterally on the mastoid parts of the temporal bone.
➤ Place your thumbs on the anterior tips of the mastoid processes.
➤ Place the palms of your hands on the occiput, with your fingers interclasped posteriorly at the upper cervical vertebrae.
➤ Rest both elbows on the bench.

Alternative hand position: (Fig. 4.14)

➤ Hand on the same side as the affected temporal bone:
➤ Grasp the zygomatic process between your thumb and index finger.
➤ Place your middle finger in the external ear canal.
➤ Place your ring finger on the mastoid process.
➤ Your little finger should rest on the mastoid part of the temporal bone.
➤ Hold the occiput in your other hand.

Dysfunction in external rotation, unilateral

(Motion restriction in direction of internal rotation)

Method: Indirect technique (Fig. 4.15)

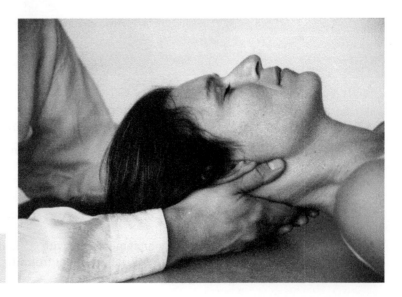

Figure 4.13 Dysfunction in external and internal rotation, unilateral

Figure 4.14 Dysfunction in external and internal rotation, unilateral. Alternative hand position

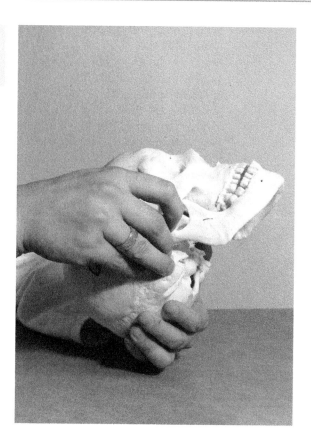

Figure 4.15 Dysfunction in external rotation. Example: right. Indirect technique

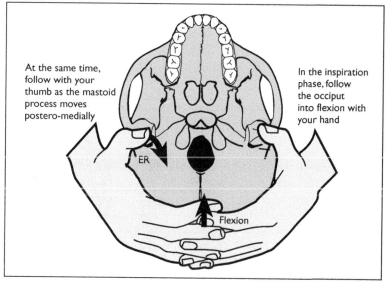

At the same time, follow with your thumb as the mastoid process moves postero-medially

In the inspiration phase, follow the occiput into flexion with your hand

ER

Flexion

> Left hand: In the inspiration phase, follow the occiput into flexion with your hand.
> Right hand: At the same time, follow with your thumb the tip of the mastoid process as it moves postero-medially (external rotation).

➤ Establish the PBMT and PBFT between the temporal bone and the occipital bone.

➤ Maintain the PBT until a correction of the abnormal tension has been achieved and stabilized by the inherent homeostatic forces (PRM rhythm, etc.).

➤ Breathing assistance: Ask the patient to hold an inhalation for as long as possible at the end of an in-breath. They may also perform plantar flexion of the opposite (left) foot at the same time. Repeat for several breathing cycles.

➤ You may supplement this with a fluid impulse to direct energy toward the affected temporal bone with your opposite (left) hand.

➤ This technique can also be carried out in harmony with PRM rhythm.

➤ During the inspiration phase, administer an impulse easing the occiput into flexion and right temporal bone into external rotation.

➤ During the expiration phase, passively follow the motion of these two bones.

➤ Continue until the mobility of the temporal bone in the direction of internal rotation improves.

Method: Direct technique:
See dysfunction in internal rotation, indirect technique (see Fig. 4.16).

Dysfunction in internal rotation, unilateral

(Motion restriction in the direction of external rotation)
Method: Indirect technique: (Fig. 4.16)
Left hand:

➤ In the expiration phase follow the occiput into extension with your hand.

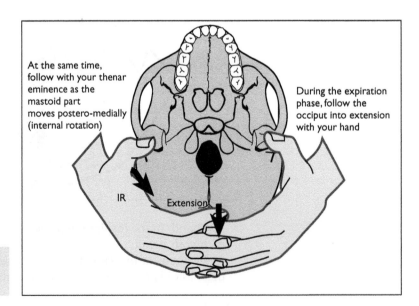

At the same time, follow with your thenar eminence as the mastoid part moves postero-medially (internal rotation)

During the expiration phase, follow the occiput into extension with your hand

IR   Extension

Figure 4.16 Dysfunction in internal rotation. Indirect technique

Right hand:

> ➤ At the same time, with your thenar eminence, follow the mastoid part of the temporal bone in a postero-medial direction (internal rotation).
> ➤ Establish the PBMT and PBFT.
> ➤ Breathing assistance: Ask the patient to hold an exhalation for as long as possible at the end of an out-breath. They may also perform dorsal flexion of the opposite (left) foot at the same time. Repeat for several breathing cycles.
> ➤ You may supplement this with a fluid impulse to direct energy toward the affected temporal bone with your opposite (left) hand.
> ➤ This technique can also be carried out in harmony with PRM rhythm.
> ➤ During the inspiration phase, passively follow the motion of these two bones.
> ➤ During the expiration phase, administer an impulse easing the occiput into extension and the right temporal bone into internal rotation.
> ➤ Continue until the mobility of the temporal bone in the direction of external rotation improves.

Method: Direct technique:
See dysfunction in external rotation. Example: right, indirect technique (see Fig. 4.15).

Dysfunction in external and internal rotation, bilateral

The technique described here is an indirect one. However, a direct technique can be used instead if necessary (e.g. when treating newborns and young children).

Therapist: Take up a position at the head of the patient.

Hand position:
> ➤ Place the thenar eminences of each hand bilaterally on the mastoid parts of the temporal bones.
> ➤ Place your thumbs on the anterior tips of the mastoid process of each side.
> ➤ Place the palms of your hands on the occiput.
> ➤ Interclasp your fingers.
> ➤ Rest both elbows on the bench.

Dysfunction in external rotation, bilateral *(Fig. 4.17)*

(Motion restriction in the direction of internal rotation)

Method: Indirect technique:

> ➤ During the inspiration phase, follow with your thumbs the tips of the mastoid processes as they move in a postero-medial direction (external rotation).
> ➤ Follow the occiput into flexion with the palm of your hand.
> ➤ Establish the PBMT and PBFT.
> ➤ Breathing assistance: Ask the patient to hold an inhalation for as long as possible at the end of an in-breath. They may also perform plantar flexion of both feet at the same time. Repeat for several breathing cycles.

Figure 4.17 Dysfunction in external rotation, bilateral. Indirect technique

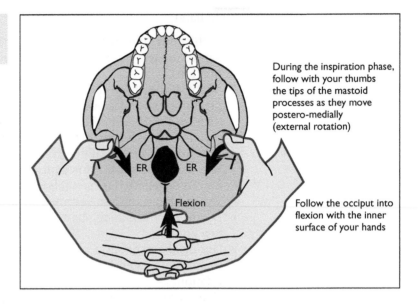

During the inspiration phase, follow with your thumbs the tips of the mastoid processes as they move postero-medially (external rotation)

ER   ER

Flexion

Follow the occiput into flexion with the inner surface of your hands

➤ This technique can also be carried out in harmony with PRM rhythm.
➤ During the inspiration phase, administer an impulse to ease the temporal bones into external rotation.
➤ During the expiration phase, passively follow the motion of the two bones.
➤ Continue until the mobility of the temporal bones in the direction of internal rotation improves.

Dysfunction in internal rotation, bilateral *(Fig. 4.18)*

(Motion restriction in the direction of external rotation)

Method: Indirect technique:
➤ During the expiration phase, follow the postero-medial motion of the mastoid parts of the temporal bones (internal rotation) with your thenar eminences.
➤ Follow the occiput into extension with the inner surface of your hands.
➤ Establish the PBMT and PBFT.
➤ Breathing assistance: Ask the patient to hold an exhalation for as long as possible at the end of an out-breath. They may also perform dorsal extension of both feet at the same time. Repeat for several breathing cycles.
➤ This technique can also be carried out in harmony with PRM rhythm.
➤ During the inspiration phase, passively follow the motion of the two bones.
➤ During the expiration phase, administer an impulse easing the temporal bones into internal rotation.
➤ Continue until the mobility of the temporal bones in the direction of external rotation improves.

Figure 4.18 Dysfunction in internal rotation, bilateral. Indirect technique

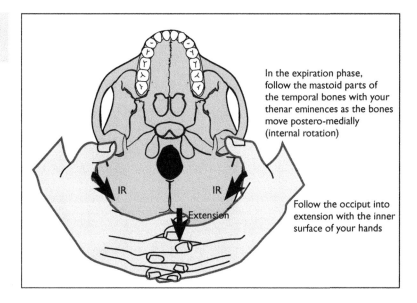

In the expiration phase, follow the mastoid parts of the temporal bones with your thenar eminences as the bones move postero-medially (internal rotation)

IR IR

Extension

Follow the occiput into extension with the inner surface of your hands

Biodynamic approach

Encourage the spontaneous occurrence of a still point or corrective external rotation and expansion or internal rotation and retraction of the temporal bone, by means of palpation, carried out in a state of non-invasive attention and empathy. Synchronize this treatment with the inherent homeodynamic forces and rhythmic patterns. This approach requires no encounter or confrontation with tissue resistances and no inhibition of any phase of primary respiration.

Dysfunction in anterior and posterior rotation

Dysfunction in anterior and posterior rotation, unilateral *(see Figs 4.19, 4.20)*

The technique described here is an indirect one. However, a direct technique can be used as necessary.

Hand position: Right hand:

➤ Grasp the zygomatic process between your thumb and index finger.
➤ Place your middle finger in the external ear canal.
➤ Position your ring finger anterior to the mastoid process.
➤ Position your little finger posterior to the mastoid process.
➤ Hold the occiput in your left hand.

Dysfunction in anterior rotation, unilateral. Example: *Fig. 4.19*

(Motion restriction in the direction of posterior rotation)

Method: Indirect technique:

➤ Right hand: anterior rotation of the temporal bone.
➤ During the inspiration phase, induce anterior rotation of the temporal bone.
➤ Administer an impulse in an inferior direction with the thumb on the zygomatic process.

Figure 4.19 Dysfunction in anterior rotation, unilateral. Example: right. Indirect technique

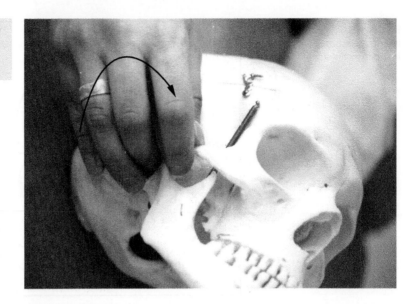

Figure 4.20 Dysfunction in posterior rotation, unilateral. Example: right. Indirect technique

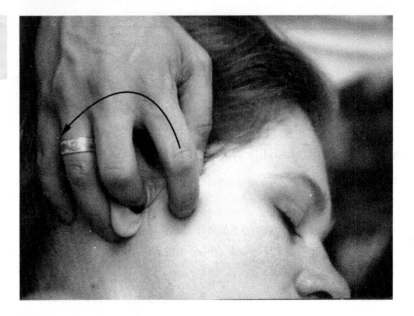

➤ With the middle finger in the external ear canal, administer an impulse to ease the temporal bone into anterior rotation.
➤ With the ring finger on the mastoid process, administer an impulse in a superior direction.
➤ Establish the PBMT and PBFT between the temporal bone and the occiput.
➤ Breathing assistance: Ask the patient to hold an inhalation for as long as possible at the end of an in-breath. They may also perform plantar flexion of both feet at the same time. Repeat for several breathing cycles.

Dysfunction in posterior rotation, unilateral. Example: *Fig. 4.20*

(Motion restriction in the direction of anterior rotation)

Method: Indirect technique:

Right hand:

➤ During the expiration phase, induce posterior rotation of the temporal bone.
➤ With the thumb on the zygomatic process, administer an impulse to ease it in a superior direction.
➤ With the middle finger in the external ear canal, administer an impulse easing it into posterior rotation.
➤ With the ring finger on the mastoid process, administer an impulse to ease it in an inferior direction.
➤ Establish the PBMT and PBFT between the temporal bone and the occiput.
➤ Breathing assistance: Ask the patient to hold an exhalation for as long as possible at the end of an out-breath. They may also perform dorsal flexion of both feet at the same time. Repeat for several breathing cycles.

Dysfunction in anterior and posterior rotation, bilateral *(Fig. 4.21)*

The technique described here is an indirect one. However, a direct technique can be used if necessary.

Hand position: ➤ Grasp the zygomatic processes between thumb and index finger.
➤ Place your middle fingers in the external ear canals.
➤ Position your ring fingers anterior to the mastoid processes.
➤ Position your little fingers posterior to the mastoid processes.

Dysfunction in anterior rotation, bilateral

(Motion restriction in the direction of posterior rotation)

Method: Indirect technique:

➤ At the beginning of the inspiration phase, administer an impulse with your thumbs on the zygomatic processes, easing the bones in an inferior direction.
➤ With your middle fingers in the external ear canal, administer an impulse into anterior rotation.
➤ At the same time administer a superiorly directed impulse with your ring fingers on the mastoid processes.
➤ Establish the PBMT and PBFT.
➤ Breathing assistance: Ask the patient to hold an inhalation for as long as possible at the end of an in-breath. They may also perform plantar flexion of both feet at the same time. Repeat for several breathing cycles.

Note: This technique can also be used to treat superior vertical strain of the SBS.

Dysfunction in posterior rotation, bilateral

(Motion restriction in the direction of anterior rotation)

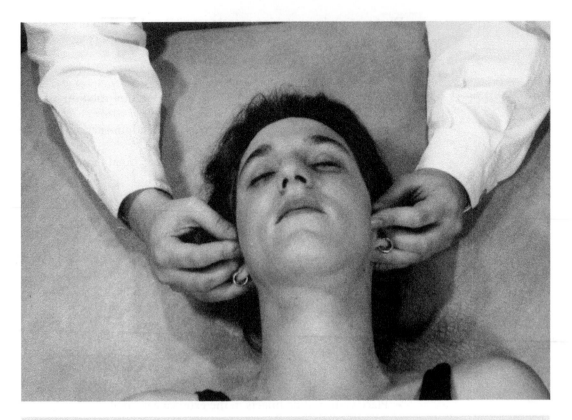

Figure 4.21 Dysfunction in anterior and posterior rotation, bilateral.

Method: Indirect technique:

> ➤ At the beginning of the expiration phase, administer an impulse with the thumbs on the zygomatic processes, easing the bones in a superior direction.
> ➤ With your middle fingers in the external ear canal, administer an impulse into posterior rotation.
> ➤ At the same time, administer an impulse in an inferior direction with the ring finger on the mastoid processes.
> ➤ Establish the PBMT and PBFT.
> ➤ Breathing assistance: Ask the patient to hold an exhalation for as long as possible at the end of an out-breath. They may also perform dorsal extension of both feet at the same time. Repeat for several breathing cycles.

Note: This technique can also be used to treat inferior vertical strain of the SBS.

Temporal bone lift technique *(Fig. 4.22)*

Indication: Tensions of the tentorium cerebelli, disturbances of the drainage of the inferior and superior petrosal sinuses, restrictions of the sutures of the temporal bone, etc.

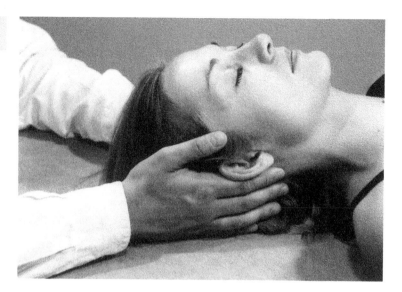

Figure 4.22 Temporal bone lift technique

Hand position: ➤ Place your index fingers on the mastoid processes.
➤ Rest your other fingers on the patient's head in a relaxed way.

Method: ➤ Administer gentle cephalad traction with your index fingers on the mastoid processes.
➤ Very gently the temporal bones are moved out of the field of tension, without confronting motion barriers. The tissue dynamics are just perceived without intervention.
➤ You will sense the various stages of tissue release: first the sutural tensions, then the elastic and collagenous tensions of the tentorium cerebelli (a sensation like cement, or like a rubber band or chewing gum).
➤ In the end a new equilibrium of tension will establish itself and a floating sensation may be perceived.

Important: Never remove your hands suddenly as this could cause dysfunctions.

Sutural dysfunctions

Petro-occipital fissure (petrobasilar suture; petro-occipital synchondrosis) (Fig. 4.23)

Suture margin: The lateral borders of the base of the occipital bone form a ridge that articulates with a groove on the posterior, inferior portion of the petrous part of the temporal bone (turning and sliding motion).

Suture type: Synchondrosis.

Petrojugular suture *(see Fig. 4.23)*

Suture margin: The jugular process articulates with the jugular articular surface of the petrous part of the temporal bone. This is a pivot point for the transmission of motion from the occipital bone to the temporal bone.

Suture type: Synchondrosis.

Figure 4.23 Petro-occipital fissure (petrobasilar suture; petro-occipital synchondrosis) and petrojugular suture. General technique

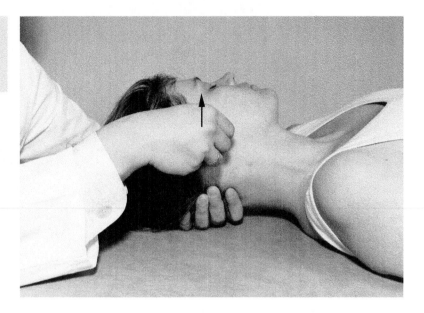

Hand position: General technique:
Right hand on the temporal bone on the affected side:

> ➤ Place the thumb in the external ear canal.
> ➤ Position your index and middle fingers behind the ear lobe, as close as possible to the temporal bone.
> ➤ Grasp the antitragus and ear lobe with your thumb and fingers.

Place your left hand across the occiput with your fingers pointing to the right.

Method: *Disengagement:*

> ➤ Administer traction to the temporal bone in an anterior direction.
> ➤ Hold the occiput in position in the opposite direction.
> ➤ Without reducing the traction, permit all motions/tissue unwinding of the bones that arise.

Hand position: Specific technique (Figs 4.24–4.26):
Right hand on the temporal bone on the affected side:

> ➤ Grasp the zygomatic process with your thumb and index finger.
> ➤ Place your middle finger in the external ear canal.
> ➤ Place your ring finger on the mastoid process.
> ➤ Place your little finger on the mastoid part of the temporal bone.

Place your left hand across the occiput with your fingers pointing to the right.

Method: Begin by releasing the temporal bone from the occiput using the disengagement technique (Fig. 4.24). Maintain the disengagement while seeking the PBMT and PBFT at the suture between the occiput and temporal bone.

Figure 4.24 Disengagement

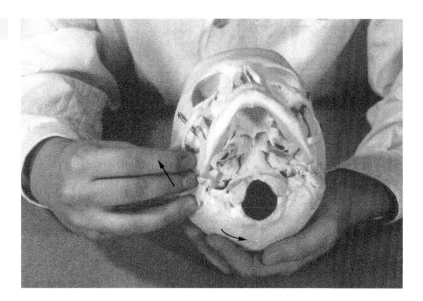

Figure 4.25 Petro-occipital fissure (petrobasilar suture; petro-occipital synchondrosis)

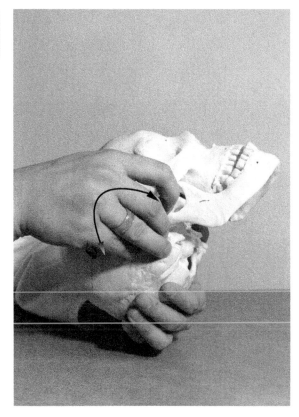

To treat the petro-occipital fissure (petrobasilar suture; petro-occipital synchondrosis) (Fig. 4.25):

➤ Move the occiput in a lateral direction to the opposite side (to the left) and hold it there.

Figure 4.26 Petrojugular suture

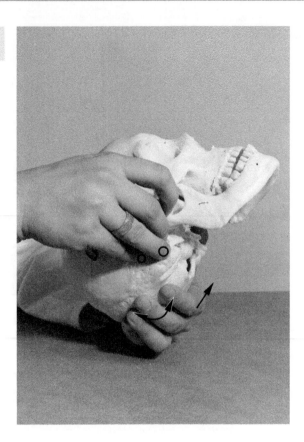

> Seek the PBMT and PBFT somewhere between the anterior and posterior rotation of the temporal bone.
> Also follow the occiput into flexion or extension depending on the tensions present, in order to establish the PBMT.

To treat the petrojugular suture (Fig. 4.26):

> Move the occiput laterally to the opposite side (to the left) and hold it there.
> Then seek the PBMT and PBFT somewhere between the external and internal rotation of the temporal bone.
> For external rotation, administer pressure in a medial and posterior direction with your ring finger on the mastoid process.
> For internal rotation, administer pressure in a medial and posterior direction with the little finger on the mastoid part of the temporal bone.
> Also follow the occiput into flexion or extension, according to the tensions present, in order to establish the PBMT.

Note: PBMT and PBFT for both sutures is normally sought simultaneously. The procedure has been subdivided here for the purpose of instruction only.

Alternative technique for the petro-occipital fissure (petrobasilar suture; petro-occipital synchondrosis) (right): opposite physiological motion according to Magoun *(Fig. 4.27):*

Hand position: As for previous technique.
Method: Opposite physiological motion.

➤ Move the occiput laterally to the opposite side (to the left) and hold it there.
➤ During the expiration phase, go with the occiput into extension and hold it there.
➤ During the inspiration phase, go with the right temporal bone into external rotation and hold it there:
➤ With your ring finger, administer pressure in a medial and posterior direction to the mastoid process.
➤ With your thumb and index finger, administer pressure in a lateral and inferior direction on the zygomatic process.
➤ Hold this position until release of the petro-occipital fissure (petrobasilar suture; petro-occipital synchondrosis) occurs.
➤ Conclude by resynchronizing the motion of the temporal bone and occiput with the PRM rhythm.

Occipitomastoid suture

Suture margin: The concave mastoid border of the occiput articulates with the convex posterior border of the mastoid part of the temporal bone. The suture

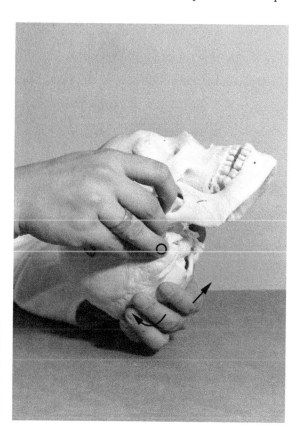

Figure 4.27 Alternative technique for the petro-occipital fissure (petrobasilar suture; petro-occipital synchondrosis) (right): opposite physiological motion according to Magoun

margin of the occipital bone is normally oriented outward; the inferior portion may be internally oriented. The changeover point is called the condylo-squamoso-mastoid pivot point (CSMP).

Suture type: Irregular suture.

The occiput and the mastoid part of the temporal bone normally move in opposing directions to each other: in the inspiration phase the border of the occiput moves in an anterior direction, while the border of the mastoid part slides posterior.

Compression of this suture can prevent the suture margins from moving in opposite directions in this way. If that happens the temporal bone is carried along with the border of the occiput in the inspiration phase, moving it into internal rotation. In the expiration phase the temporal bone is then moved into external rotation.

Notes: 1. A dysfunction of the occipitomastoid suture is often the result of compression of the atlanto-occipital joint. The atlanto-occipital joint should therefore be freed first. This often has the effect of releasing the dysfunction of the occipitomastoid suture as well.

2. A dysfunction of the petrosphenoidal (sphenopetrosal) fissure (suture) can be involved in a restriction affecting the occipitomastoid suture.

Hand position: (Fig. 4.28)

➤ Place the thumbs anterior to the mastoid processes.
➤ Place the thenar eminences on the mastoid parts of the temporal bones.
➤ Rest the other fingers on the occipital bone.

Method: Indirect technique, for a temporal bone in internal rotation (Fig. 4.29):

➤ With the thenar eminence on the dysfunctional side, administer pressure in a medial and posterior direction to the mastoid part of the temporal bone (IR).

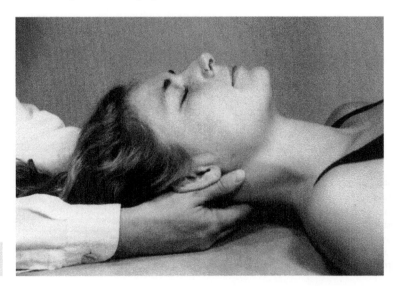

Figure 4.28
Occipitomastoid suture

Figure 4.29
Occipitomastoid suture. Indirect technique, right temporal bone in internal rotation

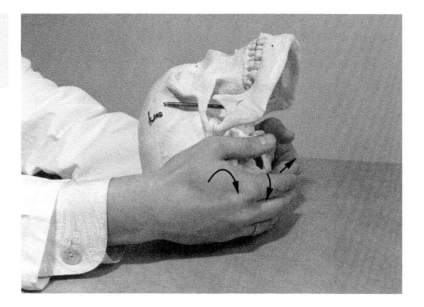

> With the other fingers, guide the occipital bone laterally, away from the suture and posteriorly, into extension.
> Breathing assistance: Ask the patient to hold an exhalation for as long as possible at the end of an out-breath.
> Establish the PBMT and PBFT.
> Maintain the PBT until a correction of the abnormal tension has been achieved and stabilized by the inherent homeostatic forces (PRM rhythm, etc.).
> A fluid impulse may be used to direct energy from the opposite frontal tuber.

Method: Direct technique, for a temporal bone in internal rotation (Fig. 4.30):

> During the inspiration phase, administer pressure in a medial and posterior direction to the mastoid process with the thumb on the dysfunctional side (ER).
> With the other fingers, guide the occipital bone laterally, away from the suture and anteriorly, into flexion.
> This draws the suture margins away from each other, which has the effect of opening the suture, especially the posterior portion.
> Breathing assistance: Ask the patient to hold an inhalation for as long as possible at the end of an in-breath.
> Establish the PBMT and PBFT.
> A fluid impulse may be performed to direct energy from the opposite frontal tuber.

Note: The indirect technique is usually applied first, followed by the direct technique.

Figure 4.30
Occipitomastoid suture.
Direct technique, right
temporal bone in internal
rotation

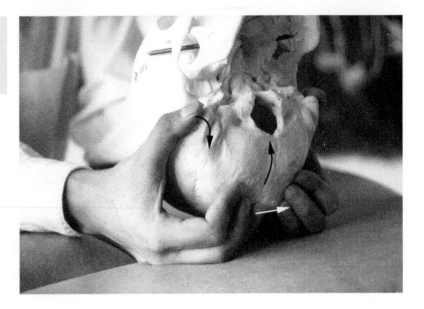

For a temporal bone in external rotation, the details are the exact opposite of the above:

Method: Indirect technique:

> The thumb on the dysfunctional side applies pressure in a medial and posterior direction to the mastoid process (ER).
> The other fingers guide the occipital bone posteriorly into extension.

Direct technique:

> With the thenar eminence on the dysfunctional side, exert pressure in a medial and posterior direction to the mastoid part of the temporal bone (IR).
> With the other fingers, move the occipital bone anteriorly, into flexion.

Opposite physiological motion according to Magoun

Method: Indirect technique:

If the petrous part of the temporal bone is in internal rotation: (Fig. 4.31)

> With the thenar eminence on the dysfunctional side, administer pressure in a medial and posterior direction to the mastoid part of the temporal bone (IR).
> With the other fingers, move the occipital bone anteriorly, into flexion.
> Breathing assistance: Ask the patient to hold an exhalation for as long as possible at the end of an out-breath.
> Establish the PBMT and PBFT.
> A fluid impulse may be used to direct energy from the opposite frontal tuber.

Figure 4.31
Occipitomastoid suture.
Opposite physiological
motion. Indirect technique,
right temporal bone in
internal rotation

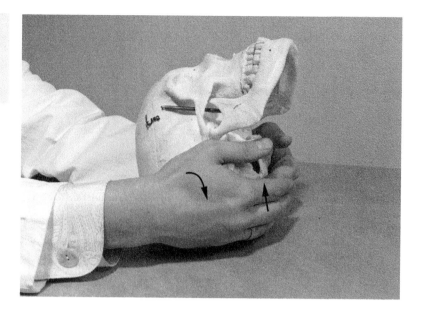

If the petrous part of the temporal bone is in external rotation:

➤ With the thumb on the dysfunctional side, administer pressure in a medial and posterior direction (ER).
➤ With the other fingers, guide the occipital bone posteriorly into extension.
➤ Breathing assistance: Ask the patient to hold an inhalation for as long as possible at the end of an in-breath.

Method: Direct technique (to follow indirect technique):
If the petrous part of the temporal bone is in internal rotation: (Fig. 4.32)

➤ With the thumb on the dysfunctional side, administer pressure in a medial and posterior direction (ER).
➤ With the other fingers, guide the occipital bone posteriorly into extension.
➤ Breathing assistance: Ask the patient to hold an inhalation for as long as possible at the end of an in-breath.
➤ Establish the PBMT and PBFT.
➤ A fluid impulse may be used to direct energy from the opposite frontal tuber.

If the petrous part of the temporal bone is in external rotation:

➤ With the thenar eminence on the dysfunctional side, administer pressure in a medial and posterior direction to the mastoid part of the temporal bone (IR).
➤ With the other fingers, move the occipital bone anteriorly, into flexion.
➤ Breathing assistance: Ask the patient to hold an exhalation for as long as possible at the end of an out-breath.

Figure 4.32
Occipitomastoid suture.
Opposite physiological
motion. Direct technique,
right temporal bone in
internal rotation

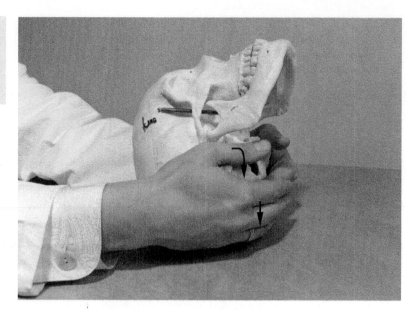

> Establish the PBMT and PBFT.
> A fluid impulse may be performed to direct energy from the opposite frontal tuber.

Parietomastoid suture *(Fig. 4.33)*

Suture margin: Margin of the mastoid process is inward-facing; margin of the parietal bone outward-facing.

Patient: The patient's head should be turned to the side opposite the dysfunction.

Hand position:
> Place the hand on the side of the dysfunction on the temporal bone: Your thumb should lie on the mastoid process, near the parietomastoid suture.
> Place the other hand on the parietal bone as follows: Place the thumb on the parietal bone near the suture.

Method:
> With the thumb on the parietal bone, administer pressure to the bone combined with cephalad traction.
> With the thumb on the mastoid process, administer caudad traction.
> Permit all motions/tissue unwinding that arise.
> Establish the PBMT and PBFT.
> A fluid impulse may be performed to direct energy from the opposite frontal tuber.

Alternative technique for a temporal bone in internal rotation *(Fig. 4.34)*

Patient: Supine, with head slightly turned to the opposite side.

Hand position: Place the hand on the side of the dysfunction on the temporal bone as follows:

> Position your thumb anterior to the mastoid process.

Figure 4.33 Parietomastoid suture

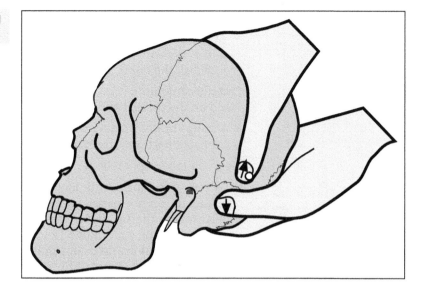

Figure 4.34 Parietomastoid suture. Alternative technique for a temporal bone in internal rotation

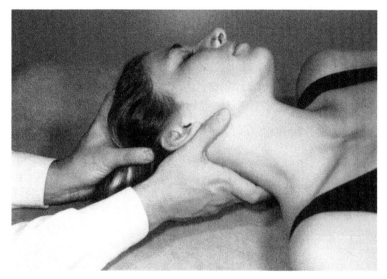

➤ Position the thenar eminence on the mastoid part of the temporal bone, immediately beside the parietomastoid suture.

Place your other hand on the parietal bone as follows:

➤ Position your thumb on the parietal bone near the parietomastoid suture.
➤ Hold the cranial vault with the fingers.

Method: Indirect technique:
Hand on the parietal bone:

➤ During the expiration phase, use the thumb next to the parietomastoid suture to begin to move that part of the parietal bone in an inferior, medial and posterior direction (IR).

Hand on the temporal bone:

➤ At the same time, with the thenar eminence, follow the mastoid part of the temporal bone in a postero-medial direction (IR).
➤ Establish the PBMT and PBFT.

Direct technique:
Hand on the parietal bone:

➤ During the inspiration phase, begin to administer anterior and cephalad traction (disengagement) with your thumb.

Hand on the temporal bone:

➤ At the same time, gently move the temporal bone downward to release it from the parietal bone (disengagement).
➤ Also follow the tip of the mastoid process in a postero-medial direction, using your thumb (ER).
➤ Permit all motions/tissue unwinding that arise.
➤ Establish the PBMT and PBFT.

Squamoparietal suture *(Fig. 4.35)*

Suture margin: Internally facing margin: parietal border of the squamous part of the temporal bone; externally facing margin: squamous border of the parietal bone.

Suture type: Squamous suture.

Patient: The patient's head should be turned toward the opposite side.

Hand position: Place the hand on the same side as the dysfunction on the temporal bone as follows:

➤ Position your thumb on the squama, beside and parallel to the squamoparietal suture.
➤ Position your other fingers on the patient's neck, pointing caudad.
➤ Arrange your thumb and fingers at right angles to each other.

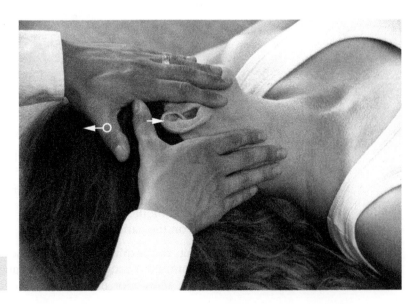

Figure 4.35 Squamoparietal suture

Place your other hand on the parietal bone as follows:

➤ Place your thumb on the parietal bone, beside and parallel to the squamoparietal suture.
➤ Point the other fingers caudad.
➤ Arrange your thumb and fingers at right angles to each other.

Method: Disengagement:

➤ Administer cephalad traction combined with medial pressure with the thumb on the parietal bone.
➤ With the thumb on the temporal bone, administer caudad traction.
➤ Permit all motions/tissue unwinding that arise.
➤ Establish the PBMT and PBFT.
➤ A fluid impulse may be used to direct energy from the pterion on the opposite side.

Alternative technique for a temporal bone in internal rotation
(Fig. 4.36)

Patient: The patient's head should be turned toward the opposite side to the dysfunction.

Hand position: Place the hand on the same side as the dysfunction on the temporal bone as follows:

➤ Position your thumb on the squama, beside and parallel to the squamoparietal suture.
➤ Position your index finger on the mastoid process.

Place your other hand on the parietal bone as follows:

➤ Place your thumb on the parietal bone, beside and parallel to the squamoparietal suture.
➤ Hold the cranial vault with your fingers.

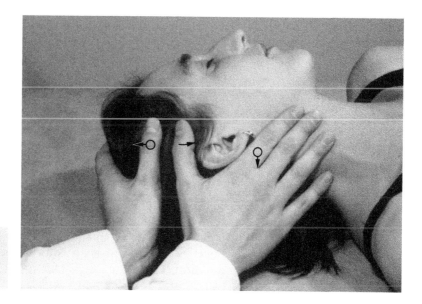

Figure 4.36 Squamoparietal suture. Alternative technique for a temporal bone in internal rotation

Method: Direct technique:

During the expiration phase:

➤ With the thumb on the parietal bone, by the squamoparietal suture, administer pressure in a medial direction (IR).

During the inspiration phase:

➤ With the thumb on the parietal bone, by the suture, perform an anterior, cephalad movement, without reducing the medial pressure.

➤ At the same time, with the index finger on the mastoid process, administer pressure in a posterior and medial direction. With the thumb on the squama of the temporal bone, perform a lateral, anterior and inferiorly directed movement (ER).

➤ Permit all motions/tissue unwinding that arise.

➤ Establish the PBMT and PBFT.

Sphenosquamous suture

Sphenosquamous pivot (Cant hook) technique *(Figs 4.37a,b)*

Suture margin: The anterior and inferior border of the squamous part of the temporal bone articulates with the posterior border of the greater wing.

The suture margin belonging to the temporal bone faces inward along its superior and anterior half. The inferior half faces outward. The suture margins of the sphenoid correspond. The point where the bevel changes is called the sphenosquamous pivot point (SSP).

Suture type: Squamoserrate.

Patient: The patient's head should be turned to the opposite side to the dysfunction.

Therapist: Take up a position beside the patient's head, on the opposite side to the dysfunction.

Hand position: Place the hand on the side of the dysfunction on the temporal bone as follows:

➤ Grasp the zygomatic process with your thumb and index finger.

➤ Place your middle finger in the external ear canal.

➤ Position your ring finger on the mastoid process.

➤ Position your little finger on the mastoid part of the temporal bone.

Place the other hand on the sphenoid as follows:

➤ Position your little finger intraorally on the outside of the lateral pterygoid plate.

➤ Position your middle and ring fingers on the greater wing.

Method: Disengagement:

During the inspiration phase:

➤ With your thumb and index finger, follow the zygomatic process as it moves in a lateral, anterior and inferior direction. With your ring finger, follow the mastoid process in a posterior and medial direction (ER).

Figure 4.37
(a,b) Sphenosquamous
pivot technique

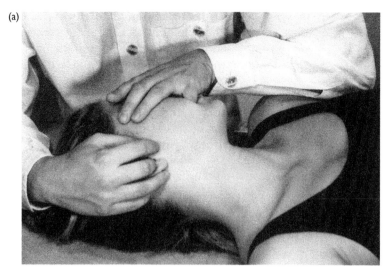

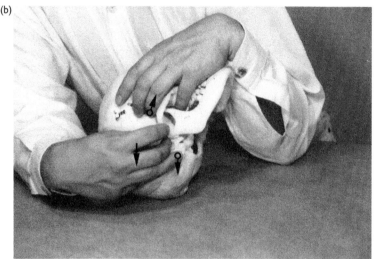

> ➤ Hold the temporal bone in external rotation.
> ➤ Also administer gentle posterior traction to the temporal bone.
> ➤ At the same time, with your middle and ring fingers, administer medial pressure and anteriorly directed traction to the greater wing.
> ➤ Permit all motions/tissue unwinding that arise.
> ➤ Continue to perform the disengagement until you sense a release at the suture.

PBT: ➤ Without reducing the disengagement, establish the PBMT and PBFT.
> ➤ A fluid impulse may be performed to direct energy from the opposite parietal tuber.

Sphenopetrosal synchondrosis (petrosphenoidal fissure) *(Fig. 4.38)*

Suture margin: The lateral part of the posterior wall of the hypophysial fossa articulates with the apex of the petrous part of the temporal bone by way of the petrosphenoidal ligament (Gruber's ligament) of the tentorium cerebelli. Also, the horizontal posterior, inferior border of the greater wing articulates with the anterior portion of the petrous part, although these do not actually join: between them lies the foramen lacerum, and they form the anterior and posterior border of the foramen opening.

Hand position: The initial position is as for the previous technique.

Method: Disengagement:

> With the middle and ring fingers on the greater wing, administer pressure in a medial direction and anteriorly directed traction.
> Also administer traction in an inferior direction to release the sphenopetrosal synchondrosis (below the SSP).
> With your thumb and index finger, follow the zygomatic process in a lateral, anterior and inferior direction. With your ring finger, follow the mastoid process in a posterior and medial direction (ER).
> Hold the temporal bone in external rotation.

PBT: > Without reducing the disengagement, establish the PBMT and PBFT between the sphenoid and the temporal bone.
> Maintain the PBT until a correction of the abnormal tension has been achieved and stabilized by the inherent homeostatic forces (PRM rhythm, etc.), and the motion of the sphenoid and the temporal bone has stopped.

Alternative technique according to E. Lay *(Figs 4.39a,b)*

Patient: The patient's head should be turned to the opposite side to the dysfunction.

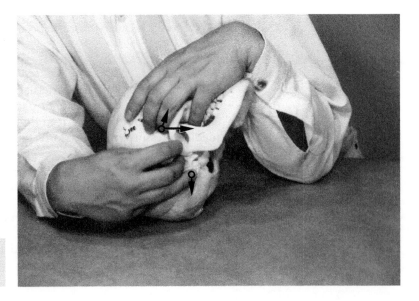

Figure 4.38 Sphenopetrosal synchondrosis (petrosphenoidal fissure)

Figure 4.39 (a,b)
Sphenopetrosal
synchondrosis. Alternative
technique according to E. Lay

(a)

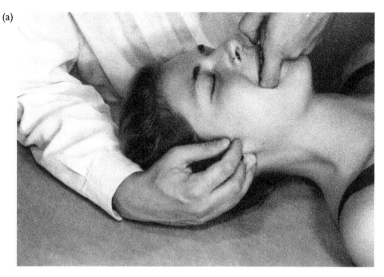

(b)

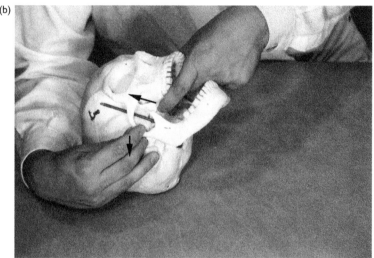

Therapist: Take up a position beside the patient's head, on the opposite side to the dysfunction.

Hand position: Place the hand on the side of the dysfunction on the temporal bone as follows:

➤ Grasp the zygomatic process with your thumb and index finger.
➤ Place your middle finger in the external ear canal.
➤ Position your ring finger on the mastoid process.
➤ Position your little finger on the mastoid part of the temporal bone.

Place your other hand on the sphenoid as follows:

➤ Place your index finger intraorally.
➤ The phalanx of the finger should lie on the upper molars.
➤ The tip of the finger should be bent and placed on the outside of the lateral pterygoid plate.

Method: Hand on the pterygoid process:

➤ Ask the patient to bite together.
➤ At the same time, move the pterygoid process in a superior direction with your index finger.

Hand on the temporal bone:

➤ At the same time, gently move the temporal bone in a posterior direction (disengagement).
➤ Without lessening the posterior traction, establish the PBMT (probably moving into IR) and PBFT at the temporal bone.
➤ Maintain the PBT until a correction of the abnormal tension has been achieved and stabilized by the inherent homeostatic forces (PRM rhythm, etc.), and the motion of the sphenoid and the temporal bone has stopped.
➤ At this point the patient's teeth can be unclenched.
➤ The temporal bone will probably now move into ER. Follow this motion.

Temporozygomatic suture *(Figs 4.40a,b)*

Suture margin: The process of the temporal bone articulates with the process of the zygomatic bone.

Suture type: Serrate suture.

Patient: The patient's head should be turned to the side opposite to the dysfunction.

Therapist: Take up a position beside the patient's head, on the opposite side to the dysfunction.

Hand position: Place the cranial hand on the temporal bone as follows:

➤ Grasp the zygomatic process with your thumb and index finger.
➤ Place your middle finger in the external ear canal.
➤ Position your ring finger on the mastoid process.
➤ Position your little finger on the mastoid part of the temporal bone.

Hand on the zygomatic bone:

➤ Grasp the temporal process of the zygomatic bone with the thumb and index finger of your caudal hand.

Method: Disengagement:

➤ With the index finger and thumb on the temporal bone, administer traction in a posterior direction.
➤ With the index finger and thumb on the zygomatic bone, administer traction in an anterior direction.
➤ Permit all motions/tissue unwinding that arise.

Direct technique:

➤ Without reducing the disengagement, move the temporal bone into ER.
➤ Move the zygomatic process of the temporal bone in a lateral, anterior and inferior direction.

Figure 4.40
(a,b) Temporozygomatic
suture

(a)

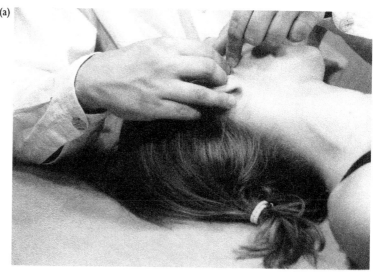

(b)

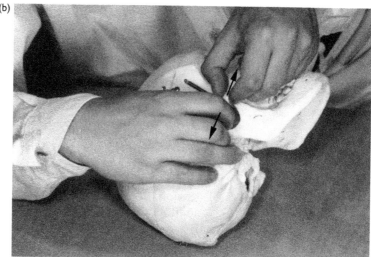

➤ Move the little finger on the mastoid part of the temporal bone in a posterior, medial direction.

Establish the PBMT and PBFT at the zygomatic bone:

➤ On concluding the technique, you should bring the motion of the zygomatic bone back into synchrony with that of the temporal bone, in harmony with the PRM rhythm.
➤ During the inspiration phase, go with the temporal bone and the zygomatic bone into ER, and during the expiration phase, go with the temporal bone and zygomatic bone into IR.
➤ A fluid impulse may be used to direct energy from the asterion on the opposite side.

Technique for the auditory ossicles *(Fig. 4.41)*

Indication: Tinnitus, deafness, syringitis.

Figure 4.41 Technique for the auditory ossicles

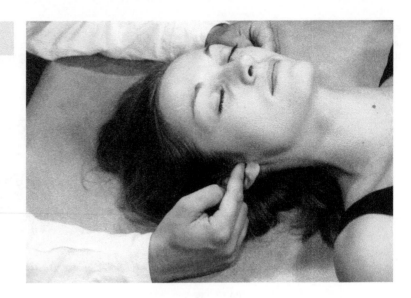

Patient: Jaw relaxed; masticatory surfaces of the teeth not in contact.

Therapist: Take up a position at the head of the patient.

Hand position: ➤ Place the tip of the index finger on the tragus.

Method: Indirect technique:

➤ With the index finger, administer pressure on the tragus in the direction of the external acoustic meatus.

➤ Without reducing the gentle pressure, rotate the index finger in an anterior or posterior direction and establish the PBMT.

➤ Direct your attention to the tympanic membrane, the tissue tension of the tympanic cavity in the middle ear and to the auditory ossicles.

➤ You may also follow the rotating motions/tissue unwinding that arise.

➤ A fluid impulse may be directed from the pterion on the opposite side.

J.E. Upledger's 'ear pull' technique *(Fig. 4.42)*

Indication: Tensions and fibrosis of the tentorium cerebelli, restrictions of the sutures of the temporal bone, disturbances of the ear or of balance, hindrances to the drainage of the superior and inferior petrosal sinuses, dysfunction at the foramen lacerum.

Hand position: ➤ Place your thumbs in the external acoustic meatus of each ear.

➤ Place your index and middle fingers behind the ear lobes, as close as possible to the temporal bones.

➤ Grasp the antitragus and lobe of each ear with your thumb and fingers.

Method: ➤ Apply traction in a lateroposterior superior direction and at an angle, roughly in a continuous line with the petrous parts.

➤ Gently very slowly increase the amount of force. A slightly greater application of force can sometimes be needed to release

Figure 4.42 J.E. Upledger's 'ear pull' technique

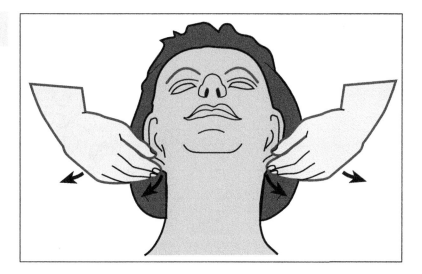

restrictions of the temporal bone, but this must always be kept below the point where the tissue reacts to the force of the traction and contracts against it.

➤ While administering the traction you can make constant slight adjustments to the angle of pull to correspond to the tension pattern of the tentorium and the sutures.

➤ Permit all motions/tissue unwinding of the tentorium by following the motions passively with your hands, without reducing the gentle traction.

➤ This traction first releases the sutural joints between the petrous part and the corresponding joint surfaces of the sphenoid and occiput, followed by the various membranous tensions of the tentorium (osseous release, elastic/collagen membrane and fluid release).

➤ When the tentorium has been released from its tension patterns, you can gradually relax the lateroposterior superior traction and then remove your hands.

Important: When performing the release technique, never remove your hands suddenly from the bone. Doing so can cause dysfunctions.

H.i. Magoun's 'Pussy-foot' technique *(Fig. 4.43)*[6]

Effect and indication:
● Induction of transverse fluctuation by moving the tentorium, brought about by induction of motion at the temporal bones.
● Energizing technique: stimulation of PRM rhythm and enhancement of its amplitude.
● Calming technique: sedation of PRM rhythm and reduction in the amplitude, e.g. to calm excited, nervous, anxious patients.
● In severe dysfunctions of the body.
● In restrictions of the temporal bone sutures.
● In chronic side-bending/rotation dysfunctions of the spheno-occipital (sphenobasilar) synchondrosis (SBS).

Figure 4.43 H.I. Magoun's 'pussy-foot' technique

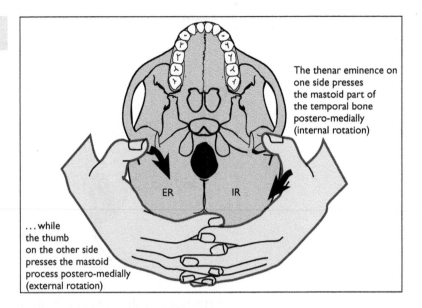

The thenar eminence on one side presses the mastoid part of the temporal bone postero-medially (internal rotation)

...while the thumb on the other side presses the mastoid process postero-medially (external rotation)

ER   IR

- According to Lippincott, lateral motion of the cerebrospinal fluid can restore a harmonious rhythm to the fluctuation.[7]
- According to Magoun, this technique is also indicated for insomnia, over-excitement, hypertension, spasms of cerebral vessels, headache, epilepsy, hypertonus, shock (of the CNS) following injury, excessive fluctuations from iatrogenic causes as a result of overstimulation of the centers in the medulla oblongata and the cranial nerve nuclei on the floor of the fourth ventricle.[8]

Therapist: Take up a position at the head of the patient.

Hand position:
- ➤ Position the thenar eminences bilaterally on the mastoid parts of the temporal bones.
- ➤ Place your thumbs bilaterally on the anterior tips of the mastoid processes.
- ➤ Position your other fingers under the upper cervical vertebrae and interclasp your fingers.
- ➤ Rest both elbows on the bench.

Method:
- ➤ Externally rotate the temporal bone of one side, by transferring your weight onto the elbow of that same side. This has the effect of moving the thumb on the mastoid process in a medial and posterior direction.
- ➤ As you transfer your weight from your other elbow, you move the other temporal bone into internal rotation. Your hand automatically moves in such a way that you exert medial and posterior pressure with the thenar eminence on the mastoid part of the temporal bone.
- ➤ Internal rotation of the right temporal bone/external rotation of the left temporal bone and external rotation of the right temporal bone/internal rotation of the left temporal bone.
- ➤ Change direction in step with PRM rhythm, so that you alternate the movement of the temporal bones, moving them in opposite directions to each other. If you are unable to find the PRM rhythm,

you can alternate the movement in time with pulmonary breathing instead.

> ➤ Once the motion restriction has been released and the primary respiratory mechanism has taken over the induction of opposite motion, just follow passively and wait for the opposite motion to come to rest.
> ➤ After a short pause, a natural symmetrical motion will re-establish itself, of its own accord.

Note: Lippincott instructs the therapist to roll the middle fingers back and forth to create the movement of the thumbs that induces the external and internal rotation of the temporal bones.[9]

Energizing: The method is the same as for the 'pussy-foot' technique described above, except that the rhythm of the opposite (external and internal rotation) motion in the rhythm of pulmonary breathing is accelerated and the amplitude of the motion performed is increased.

Calming: The method is the same as for the 'pussy-foot' technique described above, except that the rhythm of the opposite (external and internal rotation) motion and the amplitude with which it is performed are reduced.

Alternative method: Perform the procedure at the sacrum or another cranial bone.

Biodynamic approach

Palpation, carried out in a state of relaxed, non-invasive attention and empathy, and in synchrony with the inherent homeodynamic forces and rhythmic patterns, will assist the emergence of a spontaneous local or global still point in the body, or a particular integrating fluctuation. This approach requires no encounter or confrontation with tissue resistances and no inhibition of any phase of primary respiration.

W.G. Sutherland's 'Father Tom' reanimation technique
(Fig. 4.44)[10]

Effect: Forces the entire craniosacral system and the body as a whole into flexion/external rotation/inspiration phase.

Indication: Shock; life-threatening situations, when the PRM rhythm has become almost undetectable.

In anesthetic-induced breathing disturbances in newborns.

This technique stimulates the sympathetic nervous system.

> ● When performed more gently, this technique can bring about deeper breathing on the part of the patient and release restrictions at the occipitomastoid suture.

It can also be used at the end of a treatment session to neutralize undesired effects of therapy.

Therapist: Take up a position at the head of the patient.

Hand position:
> ➤ Place the thenar eminences bilaterally on the mastoid parts of the temporal bones.
> ➤ Rest the thumbs on the anterior tips of the mastoid processes.
> ➤ Interclasp your other fingers under the upper cervical vertebrae.

Method:
> ➤ Bring both temporal bones into external rotation by pressure of your thumbs in a medial and posterior direction on the tips of the mastoid processes.

Figure 4.44 W.G. Sutherland's 'Father Tom' reanimation technique

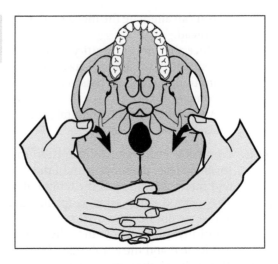

➤ Maintain this pressure for a few seconds and then release it. Repeat several times until the rhythm can once more be sensed and pulmonary breathing resumes.

➤ This is the only craniosacral technique for which very strong force is applied!

➤ If necessary this technique can be combined with other reanimation techniques. When doing this, bring the temporal bones into external rotation during the inspiration phase.

➤ The gentler version differs from the reanimation technique in that less force is used.

References

1 Rohen JW. Morphologie des menschlichen Organismus. 2 Aufl. Stuttgart: Verlag Freies Geisteslebsen; 2002:370.

2 Magoun HI. Osteopathy in the Cranial Field. 3rd edn. Kirksville: Journal Printing Company; 1976:76, 176, 282.

3 Magoun H I. Osteopathy in the Cranial Field. 3rd edn. Kirksville: Journal Printing Company; 1976:296, 298.

4 Tomatis AA. Der Klang des Lebens. Reinbek: Rowohlt; 1987:22.

5 Frymann VM, Nordell BE. Effects of temporal manipulation of respiration. J AM Osteo Assoc 1981; 80:751.

6 Kravchenko T I. The principles of osteopathic techniques efficacy monitoring. In: The first Russian-French Symposium: Fundamental aspects of Osteopathy. St. Petersburg: 12.7.96.

7 Lippincott HA. Lippincott RC. A manual of cranial technique. Cranial Academy, 1995; 22.

8 Magoun HI. Osteopathy in the Cranial Field. 1st edn. Kirksville: Journal Printing Company; 1951:87.

9 Lippincott HA, Lippincott RC. A manual of cranial technique. Cranial Academy; 1995:23.

10 Ohanian M. Father Tom et asthme. Paris: Mémoire; 1994.

5 The frontal bone

THE MORPHOLOGY OF THE FRONTAL BONE

The motion dynamics of the frontal bone with its plate-like structure correspond to those of the shoulder blade, which is also plate-like. Just as the shoulder blade enables the arm to be raised above the space that lies horizontally about it, so the frontal bone reflects the human self in the concept developed by Rohen, and expresses in spatial terms the connection with the world of the mind and spirit.

LOCATION, CAUSES AND CLINICAL PRESENTATION OF DYSFUNCTIONS OF THE FRONTAL BONE

Osseous dysfunction

a) Coronal suture
Sequelae: Restriction of mobility of the SBS, frontal bone and parietal bone.
Clinical presentation: Functional impairment of the corresponding parts of the brain; sometimes spasticity in the case of compression.

b) Sphenofrontal suture
Clinical presentation: A fall or blow to the suture can restrict the mobility of the SBS.

c) Frontoethmoidal suture
Sequelae: Restriction of mobility of the ethmoid bone; in particular restriction of the falx cerebri; also dysfunction of the anterior and posterior ethmoidal nerves.

d) Frontomaxillary suture

e) Frontozygomatic suture
Clinical presentation: Disturbance of the orbits, resulting in visual disturbances.

f) Frontonasal suture
Causes: A fall or blow to the suture can restrict the mobility of the nasal bone.

g) Frontolacrimal suture

h) Intraosseous dysfunction
Clinical presentation: Dysfunction of the related parts of the brain and the frontal sinus.

Muscular dysfunction

a. Traumatic injury in infancy can lead to disturbances of the muscles of the eye by affecting the III, IV and VI cranial nerves. Contact between the superior oblique muscle of the eye and the frontal bone is created by a connective tissue loop at the trochlear fovea.

b. Unilateral spasm of the anterior part of the temporalis muscle can move or fix the frontal bone to one side.

Fascial dysfunction

Temporal fascia, e.g. in dysfunction of the jaw or adjacent tissues.

Dysfunction at the falx cerebri

Causes: In dysfunctions of the frontal bone, especially involving the ethmoid bone (frontoethmoidal suture).

Clinical presentation: Congestion in the anterior portion of the superior sagittal sinus with functional disturbances in the corresponding parts of the brain; pain in the ipsilateral eye.

Disturbances of nerves and parts of the brain

a) Frontal lobe

Causes: Dysfunctions of the frontal bone and dysfunctions in the anterior cranial fossa.

Clinical presentation: Personality changes; irresponsible and inappropriate behavior; functional disturbances of the intellect, voluntary motor system, expression, and olfactory center.

b) Olfactory nerve (CN I)

Causes: Dysfunctions of the frontal bone, especially the frontoethmoidal suture and the cribriform plate of the ethmoid bone.

Clinical presentation: Disturbances of the sense of smell.

Symptoms affecting the following nerves as a result of dysfunctions of the frontal bone occur rarely:

c) Frontal nerve (CN V1), supraorbital nerve, lateral and medial branches

Causes: Dysfunction of the frontal bone, especially disturbances located at the roof of the orbit, the supraorbital foramen and the frontal notch.

Clinical presentation: Disturbances of sensation and pain affecting the skin of the forehead, the upper eyelid, the mucosa of the frontal sinus and connective tissue membrane.

d) Lacrimal nerve (CN V1)

Causes: Dysfunction of the frontal bone, especially disturbances affecting the lateral wall of the orbit.

Clinical presentation: Disturbances of sensation and pain affecting the skin of the lateral corner of the eye; disturbance of the lacrimal gland (parasympathetic fibers from the pterygopalatine ganglion and sympathetic fibers from the carotid plexus supplying the lacrimal gland run via the lacrimal nerve).

e) Nasociliary nerve (CN V1)

Causes: Dysfunction of the frontal bone, especially disturbances at the medial wall of the orbit and tensions of the common tendinous ring of extraocular muscles.

Clinical presentation: Disturbances of sensation and pain affecting the mucosa of the frontal sinus, and in the region of the ethmoidal air cells and anterior part of the nasal cavity, disturbance of pupil dilation (sympathetic fibers supplying the dilator pupillae muscle).

Vascular disturbances

a) Superior sagittal sinus

Causes: Dysfunction of the frontal bone, especially along the sinus, at the foramen cecum and frontal crest.

Clinical presentation: Superior sagittal sinus and the veins draining into this: pain in the frontoparietal region and region of the eye.

Symptoms affecting the following blood vessels, caused by dysfunctions of the frontal bone, occur rarely.

b) Ophthalmic artery

Clinical presentation: Disturbances at the wall of the orbit, the lacrimal gland, the external muscles of the eye and sometimes the eyeball.

c) Supraorbital and supratrochlear arteries

Clinical presentation: Disturbances of the skin and the muscles of the frontal region.

Causes of dysfunctions of the frontal bone

Primary dysfunction:

a. Intraosseous
   - As a result of direct force to the frontal bone, especially during birth and in infancy.
b. Primary traumatic injury
   - During early childhood and beyond, falls or blows or other force to the sutures can lead to motion restrictions of the frontal bone and surrounding bones.

Secondary dysfunction:

   - Secondary motion restriction of the frontal bone can be caused by dysfunction of the sphenoid, e.g. SBS dysfunctions or transmission of tension via the falx cerebri.

Examination and techniques

- History-taking
- Visual assessment
- Palpation of the position

- Palpation of primary respiration
- Motion testing
  External/internal rotation
  Flexion/extension
- Molding
- Dysfunction in external and internal rotation: indirect and direct
- Frontal bone lift technique
- Sphenofrontal suture: Cant hook technique
- Cranial vault hold
- Coronal suture
- Bregma, see under parietal bones
- Frontomaxillary suture: Cant hook technique
- Frontozygomatic suture: Cant hook technique
- Frontoethmoidal suture
- Frontonasal suture
- Frontolacrimal suture

EXAMINATION

History-taking

Headache affecting the frontal region, inflammation of the nasal cavity, disturbances of the eye, abnormalities of social behavior, previous traumatic injury.

Visual assessment

- Metopic suture: indented (ER) or convex (IR)
- Forehead: sloping (ER) or prominent (IR)
- More pronounced vertical supranasal furrow (IR of the affected side)
- Lateral corner: displaced anteriorly (ER) or posteriorly (IR)
- Bregma: indented, e.g. in the case of primary traumatic injury through force to bregma, or prominent
- Frontal tuber: convex or flat (intraosseous dysfunction)

Palpation of the position (see under visual assessment)

Palpation of primary respiration *(Fig. 5.1)*

- Biomechanical/biodynamic palpation, motion testing as required.
- If a motion restriction is discovered on palpation, an impulse in the restricted direction can be induced. This will emphasize the restriction and enable you to sense more easily which structure is the origin of the motion restriction.

Therapist: Take up a position at the head of the patient.
Hand position: ➤ Place your ring fingers on the outside of the zygomatic processes of the frontal bone.

Figure 5.1 Palpation of primary respiration of the frontal bone

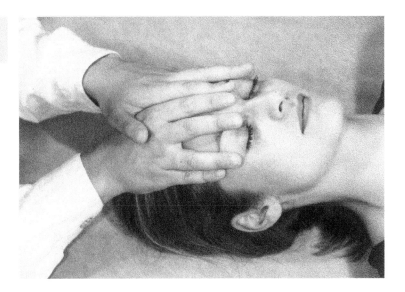

➤ Position your little fingers alongside the ring fingers.
➤ Place your middle and index fingers to the side, by the midline of the frontal bone.
➤ Your thumbs should be either crossed or touching, posteriorly.

Biomechanical approach
● During the inspiration phase of PR, flexion and external rotation of the frontal bone occur.
● The metopic suture flattens and the glabella moves in a posterior and superior direction.
● The zygomatic process of the frontal bone moves in an anterior, inferior and lateral direction.
● Bregma sinks downward.

Inspiration phase of PR, normal finding (Fig. 5.2):

➤ With the ring fingers on the zygomatic processes of the frontal bone you will be able to palpate a motion in an anterior, lateral and inferior direction.
➤ With the index fingers on the metopic suture, you will palpate a flattening.
➤ The overall motion is a flattening of the frontal bone, which slopes back at a shallower angle.

Expiration phase of PR, normal finding:

➤ With the ring fingers on the zygomatic processes of the frontal bone you will be able to palpate a motion in a posterior, medial and superior direction.
➤ With the index fingers on the metopic suture you will palpate an outward curving.
➤ The overall motion is a steepening of the frontal bone, which becomes more vertical.

Figure 5.2 Inspiration phase of PR/biomechanical

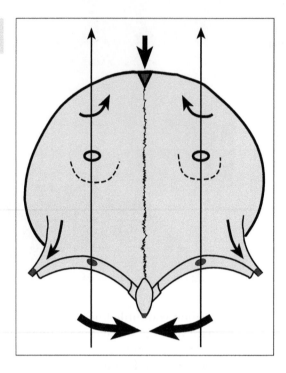

Biodynamic/embryological approach
Inspiration phase of PR, normal finding (Fig. 5.3):

➤ You will sense an expansive anteriorly directed force with your hands on the frontal bone.
➤ The motion is centrifugal (outward). Convexity lessens.

Expiration phase of PR, normal finding:

➤ You will sense a retracting, posteriorly directed force with your hands on the frontal bone.
➤ The motion is centripetal. Convexity increases.
➤ Compare the amplitude, strength, ease and symmetry of the motions of the frontal bone.
➤ Other types of motion of the frontal bone may sometimes occur during external and internal rotation. These provide an indication of further dysfunctions of the frontal bone.

Motion testing

Hand position: As above.
Method: Testing of external and internal rotation:
During the inspiration phase:

➤ At the beginning of the inspiration phase, administer a posteriorly directed impulse with your index fingers on the metopic suture.
➤ With your ring fingers on the zygomatic processes of the frontal bone, administer an impulse in an anterior, lateral (and inferior) direction.

Figure 5.3 Inspiration phase of PRM/biodynamic

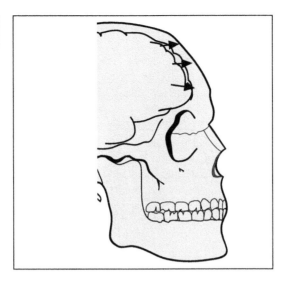

During the expiration phase:

➤ At the beginning of the expiration phase, administer an impulse in a posterior, medial (and superior) direction with the ring fingers on the zygomatic processes of the frontal bone.

➤ Compare the amplitude and ease of motion and the degree of force needed to elicit motion.

Method: Testing of flexion and extension motion:
During the inspiration phase:

➤ At the beginning of the inspiration phase, administer an impulse with your hands aimed at imparting a more shallow-angled slope to or flattening the frontal bone.

During the expiration phase:

➤ At the beginning of the expiration phase, administer an impulse with your hands aimed at making the frontal bone more vertical.

➤ Compare the amplitude and ease of motion or the degree of force needed to elicit motion.

➤ External rotation and flexion of the frontal bone can be tested at the same time, as can internal rotation and extension.

TREATMENT OF THE FRONTAL BONE

Intraosseous dysfunction

Molding *(Fig. 5.4)*

Indication: Asymmetric convexity or flattening, and torsion tensions at the ossification centers, usually as a result of birth trauma or a fall in early childhood.

Figure 5.4 Molding of the frontal bone

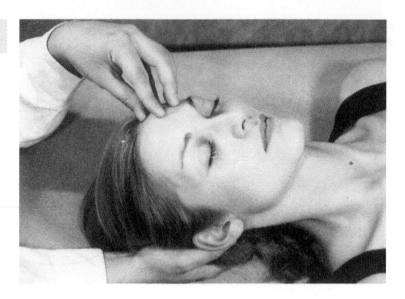

Hand position: ➤ Draw the fingertips of one hand close together.
➤ Place them on the frontal tuber.

Method: ➤ In the case of a convexity: Administer centrifugal impulses with your fingers, aimed at flattening the site.

This treatment may be augmented by using a fluid impulse to direct energy toward the borders of the frontal bone.

Note: It is important to release the surrounding bones gently from the frontal bone before beginning this technique.

➤ In the case of flattening: Administer centripetal impulses with your fingers, aimed at making the flattened site more prominent.

This treatment may be augmented by using a fluid impulse to direct energy from the opposite occipitomastoid suture toward the center of the frontal tuber.

➤ In the case of torsional tensions: Administer an impulse with your fingers in the direction of the restriction.
➤ Establish the PBMT and PBFT.

Spreading of the metopic suture *(Fig. 5.5)*

Indication: Compression of the suture by transverse forces during the birth process.

Therapist: Take up a position at the head of the patient.

Hand position: ➤ Cross your thumbs over the metopic suture, so that they rest next to the suture on the opposite side of the frontal bone.
➤ Place the palms of your hands on the ipsilateral cranial vault each side.
➤ With your thumbs, administer diverging lateral traction, so as to spread the metopic suture.
➤ Permit all motions/tissue unwinding that arise.

Figure 5.5 Spreading of the metopic suture

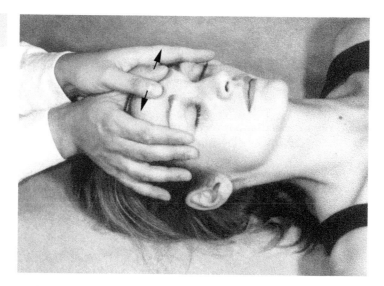

Figure 5.6 Spreading of the metopic suture. Alternative hand position

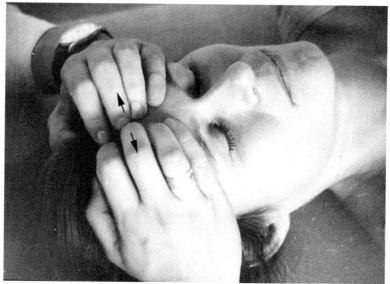

> Establish the PBMT and PBFT.
> Maintain PBMT until a correction of the abnormal tension has been achieved and stabilized by the inherent homeostatic forces (PRM rhythm, etc.).
> This treatment may be augmented by using a fluid impulse to direct energy from the inion.

Alternative hand position: (Fig. 5.6)
Method: Disengagement:
> Place the fingers of both hands bilaterally on the metopic suture.
> Administer diverging lateral traction with your fingers, so as to spread the metopic suture.
> Permit all motions/tissue unwinding that arise.
> Establish the PBMT and PBFT.

> ➤ Maintain PBMT until a correction of the abnormal tension has been achieved and stabilized by the inherent homeostatic forces (PRM rhythm, etc.).
> ➤ This treatment may be augmented by using a fluid impulse to direct energy from the inion.

Dysfunction in external and internal rotation
Dysfunction in external rotation

(Restricted internal rotation of the frontal bone.)

Hand position:
> ➤ Place your ring fingers on the outside of the zygomatic processes of the frontal bone.
> ➤ Grasp these securely from outside with your inbent fingers, to provide a firm hold.
> ➤ Place your little fingers beside your ring fingers.
> ➤ Position your middle and index fingers laterally adjacent to the midline of the frontal bone.
> ➤ Your thumbs should lie posteriorly, either crossed or touching.

Method: Indirect technique, frontal bone spread technique (Fig. 5.7):

> ➤ At the beginning of the inspiration phase, begin to apply gentle posteriorly directed pressure with your index fingers on the midline of the frontal bone (ER).
> ➤ With your ring fingers, administer an impulse in an anterior, lateral (and inferior) direction to the zygomatic processes of the frontal bone (ER).
> ➤ This reduces the antero-posterior diameter of the falx, reducing the membrane tension.
> ➤ Try to find the position in which the membrane tension on the frontal bone is most balanced (PBMT).
> ➤ Maintain PBMT until a correction of the abnormal tension has been achieved and stabilized by the inherent homeostatic forces (PRM rhythm, etc.).
> ➤ Breathing assistance: Ask the patient to hold an inhalation at the end of an in-breath for as long as possible.
> ➤ A fluid impulse may be directed from the inion or further caudad in the midline.

Direct technique (Fig. 5.8):

> ➤ At the beginning of the expiration phase, begin to administer an impulse in a posterior, medial (and superior) direction with your ring fingers on the zygomatic processes of the frontal bone (IR).
> ➤ Maintain the PBMT until no further release can be sensed, or the fluctuation of the cerebrospinal fluid has stopped and the frontal bone wants to move into external rotation.
> ➤ Breathing assistance: Ask the patient to hold an exhalation for as long as possible at the end of an out-breath.

Figure 5.7 Dysfunction in external rotation. Indirect technique. Frontal bone spread technique

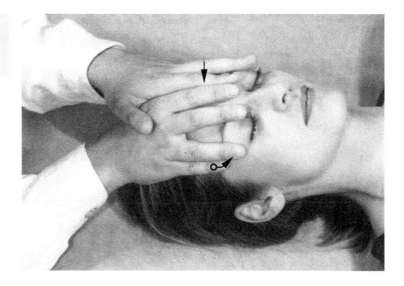

Figure 5.8 Dysfunction in external rotation. Direct technique

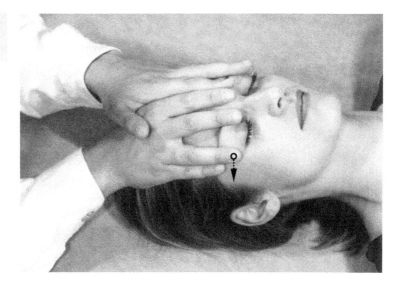

➤ A fluid impulse may be used to direct energy from the inion or further caudad in the midline.

Biodynamic approach
Palpation performed in a state of relaxed, non-invasive attentiveness and empathy, and in synchrony with the inherent homeodynamic forces and rhythmic patterns, will encourage the spontaneous occurrence of a still point or a correcting inspiration phase, flexion, external rotation and expansion or of an expiration phase, extension, internal rotation and retraction at the frontal bone. This approach does not require any encounter or confrontation with tissue resistances and does not impede any phase of primary respiration.

Dysfunction in internal rotation

(Restricted external rotation of the frontal bone.)

Method: Indirect technique:

> At the beginning of the expiration phase, begin to administer an impulse in a posterior, medial (and superior) direction with your ring fingers on the zygomatic processes of the frontal bone (IR).

> Maintain the PBMT until no further release can be sensed, or the fluctuation of CSF has stopped and the frontal bone wants to move into external rotation.

> Breathing assistance: Ask the patient to hold an exhalation at the end of an out-breath for as long as possible.

> A fluid impulse may be used to direct energy from the inion or further caudad in the midline.

Direct technique, frontal bone spread technique:

Method: > At the beginning of the inspiration phase, begin to administer a posteriorly directed impulse with your index fingers on the metopic suture (ER).

> With your ring fingers on the zygomatic processes of the frontal bone, administer an impulse in an anterior, lateral (and inferior) direction (ER).

> Maintain the point of balance until no further release can be sensed, or the fluctuation of the CSF has stopped and the frontal bone wants to move into internal rotation.

> Breathing assistance: Ask the patient to hold an inhalation for as long as possible at the end of an in-breath.

> A fluid impulse may be directed from the inion or further caudad in the midline.

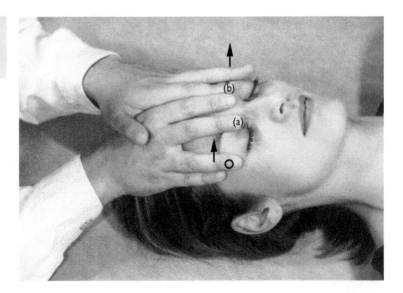

Figure 5.9 Frontal bone lift technique (a) Medial pressure. (b) Anterior and slightly cephalad traction

Frontal bone lift technique *(Fig. 5.9)*[1]

Indication: In combination with the spread technique.

Tensions and fibrosis of the falx cerebri, disturbances of the drainage of the superior and inferior sagittal sinuses, restrictions of the sutures of the frontal bone, rhinitis, sinusitis, functional disturbances of the sense of smell.

Hand position: Use the same position as for the spread technique.

Method:
➤ During the expiration phase, begin to apply gentle pressure in a medial direction with the ring fingers on the lateral surface of the frontal bone so as to release it from the sphenoid (IR).
➤ As soon as the frontal bone begins to move anteriorly you can relax the medial pressure of your ring fingers.
➤ Replace this pressure with an anterior, slightly cephalad traction. Induce the anterior traction by pressing your elbows slightly down into the table, so that your fingers lift anterior. Very gently the frontal bone is moved out of the field of tension. The therapist stays within the range of motion, meaning that he avoids confronting the motion barriers directly.
➤ The weight of the skull is enough to hold the occiput, the posterior attachment of the falx, in position on the table.
➤ The tissue dynamics are just perceived without intervention.
➤ You can sense the various stages of tissue release: first the sutural tensions, then the elastic and collagenous tensions of the falx cerebri (a sensation like cement, or a rubber band, or chewing gum).
➤ In the end a new equilibrium of tension will establish itself and a floating sensation may be perceived.

Important notes:
● Never remove your hands suddenly from the bone during the technique.
● Always take care to position your hands accurately. Failure to do so would mean that at best the technique would be ineffective. In the worst case, especially if your fingers are on the sutures, this could worsen or even give rise to symptoms.
● As an alternative you may assist the flexion and extension motions of the frontal bone (in harmony with the CRI) during the gentle anterior traction. Structural approaches imitating the amount of tension present and move the tissues towards the physiological motion barrier, but always below the threshold where the tissue reacts by contracting.

Alternative hold for the frontal bone lift technique I (Fig. 5.10):

➤ Grip bilaterally behind the edges of the temporal lines and behind the zygomatic processes of the frontal bone, with the ball of the little finger.
➤ Interclasp your fingers and support your elbows on the table slightly caudad and lateral to your hands.

Figure 5.10 Alternative hold for the frontal bone lift technique I

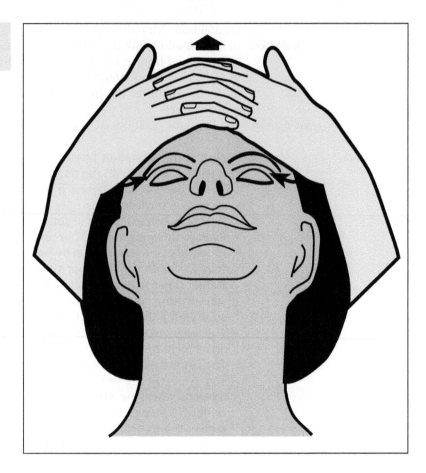

Method: ➤ Apply gentle medial pressure with the ball of your hands on the sides of the frontal bone. V.M. Frymann refined this method by drawing her fingertips apart laterally to produce the gentle medial compression. This internal rotation of the frontal bone causes a disengagement of the sutural articulations with the sphenoid.
➤ When the frontal bone begins to move slightly in an anterior direction, the cranial bones are released from each other.
➤ Then administer anterior traction to the frontal bone and so to the falx cerebri. An alternative way of performing this traction is to stretch your fingers gently in an anterior direction.

Alternative hold for the frontal bone lift technique II (Fig. 5.11):

Fronto-occipital cranial hold: This hold offers the advantage that you can check the nuchal muscles and the whole of the cranium together. The disadvantage, especially if you have small hands, is first that you cannot grasp the frontal bone adequately and second, that the anterior traction force applied to the frontal bone is generally more awkward and involves more tension of the hands and shoulders.

In this method, as previously, the anterior traction is induced by pressing the elbows in the direction of the table.

Figure 5.11 Alternative hold for the frontal bone lift technique II

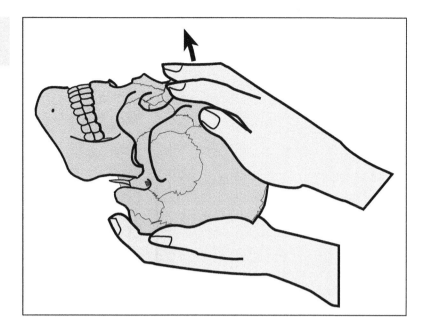

Sphenofrontal suture

Suture margin:
- Greater wing: inward facing margin (L-shaped); frontal bone: outward-facing margin (rocking motion; limits sphenoid motion).
- Lesser wing: usually outward-facing border; frontal bone: usually lies above (gliding motion).

Suture type: Squamoserrate suture.

Cant hook technique

Aim: To free the L-shaped joint surface of the greater wing from the frontal bone. This dysfunction is common. Also to release the lesser wing from the frontal bone.

Therapist: Take up a position beside the head of the patient, on the side opposite to the dysfunction.

Hand position: Caudal hand:

➤ Place your little finger intraorally, laterally on the pterygoid process. It will sometimes be necessary to ask patients to move their jaw to that side to make room for your finger.
➤ Position your index and middle finger externally on the greater wing on the side being treated.
➤ Place your thumb on the outside of the opposite greater wing if possible.

Cranial hand:

➤ Position your middle finger (or index finger) laterally on the frontal bone on the side of the dysfunction (directly above the sphenofrontal suture).

Figure 5.12 Cant hook technique. Suture between the greater wing of the sphenoid and the frontal bone

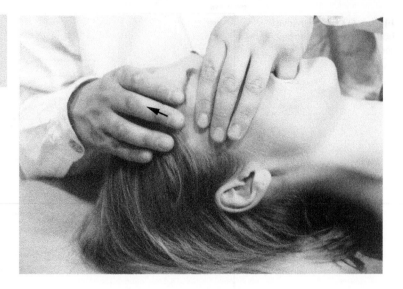

➤ Position your thumb laterally on the frontal bone on the opposite side. Do not move it; it provides the fixed point around which the motion is organized.
➤ It should be touching the thumb of the other hand.

Method: Disengagement:
Suture between the greater wing of the sphenoid and the frontal bone (Fig. 5.12):

➤ With your caudal hand, hold the sphenoid in place.
➤ Do not move the thumb on the side opposite the dysfunction. It is the hub around which the motion is organized.
➤ During the inspiration phase, begin to apply traction in a superior and very slightly anterior direction (disengagement of the frontal bone from the greater wing) with the middle finger on the frontal bone.
➤ Without reducing the gentle disengagement, permit all motions/unwinding of the frontal bone that arise.
➤ Establish the PBMT and PBFT.
➤ A fluid impulse may be used to direct energy from the opposite parietal tuber.
➤ Alternative option: without reducing the gentle disengagement, assist the flexion and extension motions of the greater wings in harmony with the PRM rhythm, either in synchrony with the flexion and extension motions of the frontal bone or as opposite physiological motion (flexion of the sphenoid with extension of the frontal bone and vice versa).

Suture between the lesser wing of the sphenoid and the frontal bone, Fig. 5.13):

➤ Do not move the thumb on the opposite side to the dysfunction. It is the hub around which the motion is organized.

Figure 5.13 Cant hook technique. Suture between the lesser wing of the sphenoid and the frontal bone

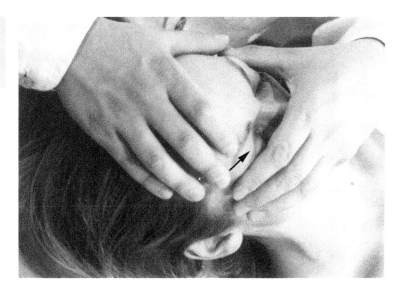

➤ During the inspiration phase, begin to administer anterior traction (disengagement of the frontal bone from the lesser wing) with the middle finger on the frontal bone.

➤ Without reducing the gentle disengagement, permit all motions/ tissue unwinding of the frontal bone that arise.

➤ Establish the PBMT and PBFT.

➤ A fluid impulse may be used to direct energy from the opposite lambdoid suture.

➤ Alternative option: without reducing the gentle disengagement, assist the flexion and extension motions of the wings of the sphenoid in harmony with the PRM rhythm, either in synchrony with the flexion and extension motions of the frontal bone or as opposite physiological motion (flexion of the sphenoid with extension of the frontal bone and vice versa).

Alternative technique with cranial vault hold *(Fig. 5.14)*

Hand position:
➤ Place your index fingers laterally on the frontal bone and on the zygomatic processes of the frontal bone.

➤ Place your middle fingers laterally on the greater wings of the sphenoid.

➤ In small children: Place your ring fingers and little fingers on the lateral parts of the occiput.

➤ In adults, place your ring fingers on the mastoid process.

Method: Disengagement:
➤ During the inspiration phase, begin to administer traction in a posterior direction with your ring fingers on the lateral parts of the occiput.

This applies posterior traction to the sphenoid (via the anterior attachment of the tentorium to the sphenoid).

Figure 5.14 Sphenofrontal suture. Alternative technique

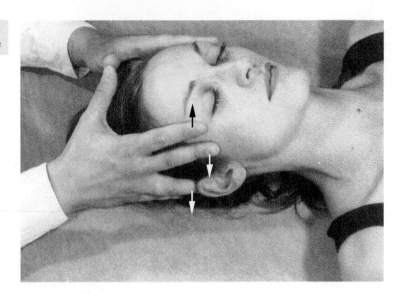

➤ Additionally, apply posterior traction with your middle fingers on the greater wings.

Take care: the greater wing has an inward-facing border at the sphenofrontal suture. Medial pressure to the greater wing compresses the suture.

➤ Administer anterior traction with your index fingers on the frontal bone.
➤ Permit all motions/tissue unwinding that arise.
➤ Without reducing the disengagement, establish PBMT between the sphenoid, occipital bone and frontal bone – the position in which the abnormal joint tensions are in the best possible state of balance one to another.
➤ Maintain the PBMT until a correction of the abnormal tension has been achieved and stabilized by the inherent homeostatic forces (PRM rhythm, etc.), and the motion of the sphenoid and the frontal bone has stopped.

Coronal suture (left) *(Fig. 5.15)*

Suture margin: ● Medial: frontal bone: inward-facing margin; parietal bone: outward-facing margin.
● Lateral: frontal bone: outward-facing margin; parietal bone: inward-facing margin.

Suture type: Squamoserrate suture.
Patient: The patient's head should be turned to the opposite side to the dysfunction.
Therapist: Take up a position beside the patient's head on the opposite side to the dysfunction.

Figure 5.15 Coronal suture (left)

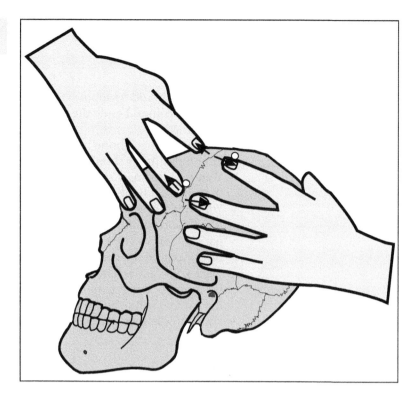

Hand position: ➤ Place the index and middle fingers of your left hand on the parietal bone, near the coronal suture.
➤ Position your index finger medially to the pivot point and your middle finger laterally to it.
Hand on the side opposite to the dysfunction.
➤ Place the index and middle fingers of your right hand on the frontal bone, near the coronal suture.
➤ Position the index finger medially to the pivot point and your middle finger laterally to it.

Method: Disengagement:

➤ Hand on the frontal bone: Administer anteriorly directed traction on the frontal bone with your index and middle fingers. Also apply pressure to the bone with the middle finger positioned below the pivot point.
➤ Hand on the parietal bone: Administer posterior traction on the frontal border of the parietal bone with your index and middle fingers. Also apply pressure on the bone with the index finger positioned above the pivot point.
➤ Without reducing the gentle disengagement, permit all motions/unwinding of the frontal bone that arise.
➤ Establish the PBMT and PBFT between the frontal bone and parietal bone – the position in which the abnormal tensions in the joint are in the best possible state of balance with each other.

➤ A fluid impulse may be used to direct energy from the opposite asterion.

Alternative technique: *(Fig. 5.16)*

Patient: The patient should be supine.

Therapist: Take up a position beside the patient's head, on the opposite side to the dysfunction.

Hand position: ➤ Hold the parietal bone in your cranial hand:
➤ Your index finger should point toward the pterion.
➤ Your middle finger should point toward the zygomatic process of the temporal bone.
➤ Your ring finger should point toward the asterion.
➤ Place the basal joints of your fingers on the axis of motion of the parietal bone, so that the basal joint of your index finger lies on the pivot point of the coronal suture.
➤ Place your caudal hand on the frontal bone.
➤ Position your index, middle and ring fingers directly anterior to the coronal suture and pointing toward it.
➤ Your middle finger should be on the pivot point of the coronal suture.

Method: Disengagement:
As for the previous technique.

➤ Administer posterior traction on the frontal border of the parietal bone.
➤ At the same time apply pressure to the medial part of the frontal border.
➤ Administer anterior traction to the parietal margin of the frontal bone.

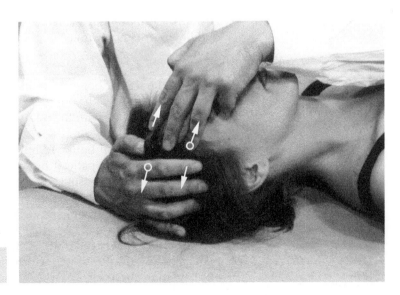

Figure 5.16 Coronal suture: Alternative technique

> At the same time apply pressure to the lateral part of the parietal margin of the frontal bone with your ring finger.
> Without reducing the gentle disengagement, permit all motions/unwinding of the frontal bone that arise.
> Establish the PBMT and PBFT.
> A fluid impulse may be used to direct energy from the opposite asterion.

The frontal bone lift is a general technique for the release of the coronal suture; see earlier.

Frontomaxillary suture

Cant hook *(Figs 5.17, 5.18)*

Suture margin: The lateral portion of the nasal part articulates with the frontal process of the maxilla.

Suture type: Serrate suture.

Cant hook technique

Therapist: Take up a position beside the patient's head, on the opposite side to the dysfunction.

Hand position: Cranial hand:

> Span the frontal bone between your thumb on one side and the middle and index fingers on the other.
> Place your middle finger laterally on the frontal bone on the side of the dysfunction (directly above the frontozygomatic suture).
> Position your thumb laterally on the frontal bone on the opposite side.

Caudal hand:

> Place your index finger on the frontal process of the maxilla.

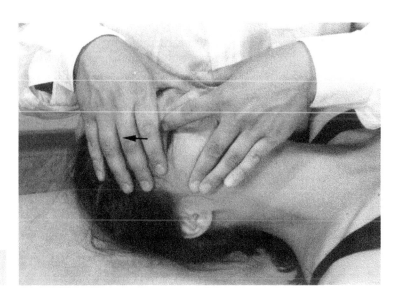

Figure 5.17 Frontomaxillary suture: Cant hook technique

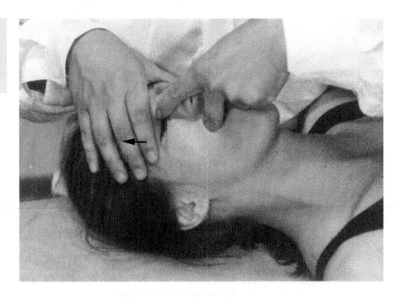

Figure 5.18 Frontomaxillary suture: Cant hook technique. Middle finger on the alveolar part of the maxilla, intraorally

➤ Place your middle finger externally or intraorally on the lateral surface of the alveolar part of the maxilla.

Method: Disengagement:
Caudal hand:

➤ Hold the maxillary bone in position with your index and middle fingers.

Cranial hand:

➤ Do not move the thumb on the opposite side to the dysfunction. It is the fixed point around which the motion is organized.
➤ Administer traction in a superior direction with the index finger on the lateral part of the frontal bone (disengagement of the frontal bone from the maxilla).
➤ Without reducing the gentle disengagement, permit all motions/ unwinding of the frontal bone that arise.
➤ Establish the PBMT and PBFT.
➤ A fluid impulse may be used to direct energy from the opposite parietal bone.

Frontozygomatic suture

Suture margin: The zygomatic process articulates with the frontal process of the zygomatic bone.
Suture type: Serrate suture.

Cant hook technique *(Figs 5.19, 5.20)*

Therapist: Take up a position beside the patient's head, on the opposite side to the dysfunction.

Figure 5.19
Frontozygomatic suture:
Cant hook technique

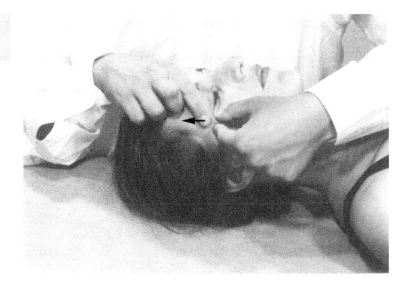

Figure 5.20
Frontozygomatic suture:
Cant hook technique,
intraoral hold

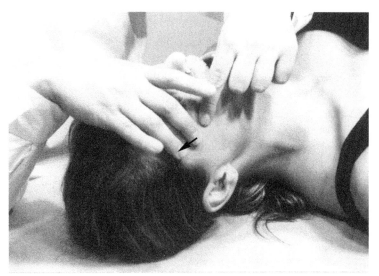

Hand position: Cranial hand:

> ➤ Span the frontal bone between thumb and index finger.
> ➤ Place your index or middle finger laterally on the frontal bone on the side of the dysfunction (directly above the frontozygomatic suture).
> ➤ Place your thumb laterally on the frontal bone on the opposite side.

Caudal hand:

> ➤ Grasp the frontal process of the zygomatic bone with your thumb and index finger.

(Alternatively you may hold the zygomatic bone with your thumb from inside (intraorally) and your index finger from outside.)

Method: Disengagement:
Caudal hand:

➤ Hold the zygomatic bone in place with the index finger and thumb of your caudal hand.

Cranial hand:

➤ Do not move the thumb on the opposite side to the dysfunction. It is the fixed point around which the motion is organized.
➤ Administer traction in a superior direction with your index finger on the zygomatic process of the frontal bone (disengagement of the frontal bone from the zygomatic bone).
➤ Without reducing the gentle disengagement, permit all motions/unwinding of the frontal bone that arise.
➤ At each release of the tissue, seek the new limit to motion of the frontal bone in the superior direction on the side of the dysfunction.

Direct technique:
In the case of a restriction of the frontozygomatic suture with a dysfunction of the frontal bone in internal rotation.

➤ Guide the frontal bone into flexion and external rotation.
➤ During the inspiration phase, gently move the frontal process of the zygomatic bone laterally with your thumb and index finger.
➤ Breathing assistance: Ask the patient to hold an inhalation for as long as possible at the end of an in-breath. Repeat for several breathing cycles.

Establish the PBMT:
➤ Maintain the gentle disengagement. At the same time follow the zygomatic bone into the position in which the tension between IR and ER is in the best possible state of balance.
➤ A fluid impulse may be used to direct energy from the opposite parietal tuber.

Frontoethmoidal suture

See technique to treat the cribriform plate, frontal bone spread and frontal bone lift techniques.

Frontonasal suture *(Fig. 5.21)*

Therapist: Take up a position at the head of the patient.
Hand position: Cranial hand:

➤ Place your thumb and index finger on the superciliary arch of the frontal bone.
➤ Place the basal joint of the index finger on the glabella (the area between the superciliary arches).

Caudal hand:
➤ Grasp the two nasal bones with your thumb and index finger.

Figure 5.21 Frontonasal suture

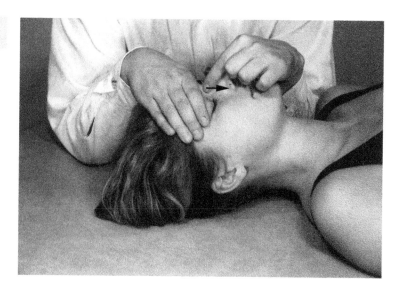

Method: ➤ During the inspiration phase, begin to apply a more angled tilt to the frontal bone (flexion) with your index and middle finger, while applying posterior and superior pressure to the glabella with the basal joint of your index finger (ER).
➤ Hold the frontal bone in flexion and ER.
➤ At the same time, move the nasal bones caudad (disengagement).
➤ Without reducing the gentle traction, permit all motions/unwinding of the frontal and nasal bones that arise.
➤ Establish the PBMT and PBFT.
➤ Breathing assistance: Ask the patient to hold an inhalation for as long as possible at the end of an in-breath. Repeat for several breathing cycles.

Note: Alternatively you may administer impulses easing the nasal bone into ER and IR in harmony with PRM rhythm, without reducing the disengagement.

Frontolacrimal suture (Fig. 5.22)

Therapist: Take up a position beside the head of the patient.
Hand position: ➤ Place the index and middle fingers of your cranial hand on the superior orbital margin, as close as possible to the frontolacrimal suture.
➤ Place the index finger of your caudal hand on the lacrimal bone.
Method: ➤ During the inspiration phase, begin to apply a more angled tilt to the frontal bone (flexion) with your index and middle finger, and to apply posterior and superior pressure to the glabella (ER).
➤ Hold the frontal bone in flexion and ER.
➤ At the same time, move the lacrimal bone caudad (disengagement).
➤ Without reducing the gentle traction, permit all motions/unwinding of the lacrimal bone that arise.
➤ Establish the PBMT and PBFT.

Figure 5.22 Frontolacrimal suture

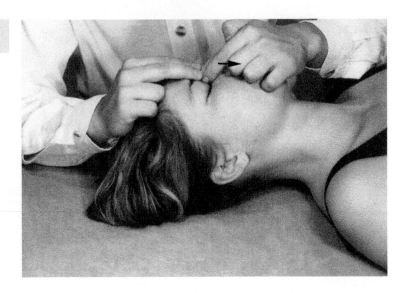

Note: Alternatively you may administer impulses easing the lacrimal bone into ER and IR in harmony with the PRM rhythm, without reducing the disengagement.

References

1 Kostopoulos D, Keramidas G. Changes in the magnitude of relative elongation of the falx cerebri during the application of external forces on the frontal bone of an embalmed cadaver. J Craniomand Practice 1992; 10:9–12.

6 The parietal bones

THE MORPHOLOGY OF THE PARIETAL BONES AND CRANIAL VAULT ACCORDING TO ROHEN[1]

The parietals, like the rest of the cranial vault, undergo membranous ossification from the outside in a similar way to the compact substance of the long bones. The difference is that the process begins from an ossification center in the bones of the cranial vault, rather than as a surrounding 'sleeve' of bone. Rays of bone spread outward, linking the ossification centers in the shape of a pentagon, which Rohen sees as expressing dominating strength of form.

Whereas the powers of the will in the case of the limbs find their outworking in movement, in the case of the head this outworking is in the powers of thought. These powers of the will can be found on the skull's exterior and reflected in the brain within, which Rohen sees as a complete reversal from the limbs to the head region.

Stone[2] sees the parietal bone as exhibiting the energetic polar reflexes of the sides of the body.

LOCATION, CAUSES AND CLINICAL PRESENTATION OF DYSFUNCTIONS OF THE PARIETAL BONES

Osseous dysfunction

Simultaneously occurring motion restrictions of the parietal bones and the thoracic cage are quite frequently found.

a) Coronal suture

Sequelae: Restriction of mobility of the SBS, frontal bone and parietal bones.

Clinical presentation: Functional impairment of the corresponding parts of the brain; sometimes spasticity in the case of compression.

b) Sagittal suture, bregma and lambda

Causes: A fall, blow or other force to the suture.

- Force to bregma → compression in the anterior region of the sagittal suture.
- Force to vertex → compression in the central region of the sagittal suture.
- Force to lambda → compression in the posterior region of the sagittal suture.

Occurrence: Frequently in asthmatic, hyperactive children or children with sleep disturbances.

Clinical presentation: Disturbances of drainage in the superior sagittal sinus with functional disturbances in the corresponding parts of the brain; pain in the frontoparietal and eye regions; sometimes spasticity in the case of severe compression.

Sequelae:
- *Force to bregma*: compression in the anterior region of the sagittal suture with posterior displacement of the occipital condyles and a lateral movement of the posterior inferior angles of the parietal bones.
- *Force to vertex*: compression in the central region of the sagittal suture with ER of the temporal bones and a flexion dysfunction of the SBS.
- *Force to lambda*: compression in the posterior region of the sagittal suture with impaction of the occipital condyles into the atlas and flexion dysfunction of the occipital bone and SBS, and ER of the temporal bones.

c) Lambdoid suture

The squamoserrate suture type prevents the bones from overlapping but can be compressed by a fall or blow.

d) Squamoparietal suture

Causes: A blow or fall from above onto the ipsilateral parietal bone; severe hypertonus of the temporalis muscle.

e) Parietomastoid suture

Causes: A blow or fall from above onto the ipsilateral parietal bone.

f) Sphenoparietal suture

g) Intraosseous dysfunction

Clinical presentation: Functional impairment of the parietal lobe.

Muscular dysfunction

a) Temporalis muscle

Dysfunction of the temporomandibular joint

Sequelae: Restriction of mobility of the parietal bone and squamoparietal suture.

Fascial dysfunction

Temporal fascia and superficial layer.

Dysfunction of the falx cerebri and the tentorium cerebelli

Causes: Motion restriction, sutural compression and change in position of the parietal bones, especially in conjunction with the occipital bone, temporal bones, and dysfunctions of the SBS.

Clinical presentation: ● Falx cerebri: disturbances of drainage in the superior sagittal sinus with functional disturbances in the corresponding parts of the brain; pain along the falx cerebri.

● Tentorium cerebelli: congestion in the transition from the transverse sinus/sigmoid sinus at the parietomastoid suture.

Disturbances of nerves and parts of the brain

Parietal lobe

Causes: Motion restriction, sutural compression and change in position of the parietal bones, especially in conjunction with the occipital bone, temporal bones and dysfunctions of the SBS.

Clinical presentation: Functional impairment of the motor and sensory centers, disturbances of attention in the field of visual and tactile perception,[3] aggressive behavior.

Vascular disturbances

a) Middle meningeal artery

Causes: Dysfunction of the parietal bones and sphenoparietal suture (especially in the case of compression of the sphenosquamous suture between the temporal bone and sphenoid).

Clinical presentation: Migraine and raised intracranial pressure.

b) Superior sagittal sinus

Causes: Compression of the sagittal suture, dysfunction of the parietal bones.

Sequelae: The greatest number of arachnoid villi is to be found in the superior sagittal sinus. Disturbances can affect the fluctuation of cerebrospinal fluid.

Clinical presentation: Pain in the frontoparietal and eye regions.

c) Sigmoid sinus

Causes: Compression of the parietomastoid suture.

Clinical presentation: Signs and symptoms of congestion; pain in the temporal region.

d) Middle meningeal veins
At the internal surface of the bone.

Causes of dysfunctions of the parietal bones

Primary dysfunction:

Intraosseous
● Direct force to the parietal bone, especially before or during birth and in infancy.

Primary trauma
● During early childhood and beyond, falls, blows or other force to the sutures can cause motion restrictions of the parietal and adjacent

bones. A fall onto the feet or pelvis can also affect the parietal bones.

Secondary dysfunction:

Dysfunction of the occipital bone, temporal bone, temporomandibular joint (via the temporalis muscle), SBS dysfunctions or transmission of tension via the falx cerebri can cause a secondary motion restriction of the parietal bones. The commonest secondary dysfunction is IR of the parietal bone.

Examination and techniques

- History-taking
- Inspection
- Palpation of the position
- Palpation of primary respiration
- Motion testing
    External/internal rotation
- Intraosseous dysfunctions
    Molding
- Dysfunction in external and internal rotation, bilateral
- Parietal spread technique
- Parietal lift technique
- Coronal suture, see under frontal bone
- Sphenoparietal suture
- Squamoparietal suture, see Temporal bone
- Parietomastoid suture, see Temporal bone
- Lambdoid suture
- Sagittal suture
- Bregma
- Lambda
- Pterion
- Asterion

EXAMINATION

History-taking

Headache, especially in the parietal region, idiopathic epilepsy, previous traumatic injury.

Visual assessment

- Mastoid angle: anterolateral (ER) or postero-medial (IR).
- Squamosal border: anterolateral (ER).
- Sagittal suture: flattened (ER), e.g. as a result of traumatic force, or convex (IR).
- Lambdoid suture: indented (ER), e.g. as a result of primary traumatic force, or convex (IR).
- Coronal suture: Depressed at bregma and displaced laterally in an anterior and outward direction (ER) or elevated at bregma and displaced laterally in a posterior and inward direction (IR).

● Parietal tuber: convex or flat (intraosseous dysfunction).

Palpation of the position (see under visual assessment)

Palpation of primary respiration *(Fig. 6.1)*

● Biomechanical/biodynamic palpation, motion testing as necessary.
● If palpation reveals a motion restriction, an impulse can be administered in the direction of restricted motion. This will emphasize the restriction and enable you to sense more easily which structure accounts for the origin of the motion restriction.

Therapist: Take up a position at the head of the patient.
Hand position: Sutherland's cranial vault hold.

➤ The tips of your thumbs should be touching at the sagittal suture but without resting on the suture.
➤ Place the palms of both hands on the parietal tubers.
➤ With the basal or proximal joints of your fingers, take up contact with the lateral borders of the parietal bones.
➤ Position the basal or proximal joints of your index fingers on the sphenoidal angles (anterior inferior angles of the parietal bones).
➤ Position the basal or proximal joints of your middle fingers above the roots of the zygomatic processes of the temporal bones.
➤ Position the basal or proximal joints of your ring fingers on the mastoid angles (posterior inferior angles of the parietal bones).

Biomechanical
In the inspiration phase of the PR there is an external rotation of the parietal bone.
Inspiration phase of the PR, normal finding (Fig. 6.2):

➤ The sagittal suture flattens.
➤ The lateral borders move in an anterior and lateral direction.

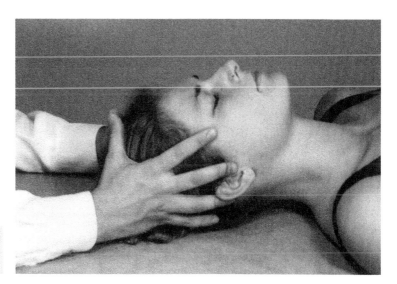

Figure 6.1 Palpation of primary respiration of the parietal bone

Figure 6.2 Inspiration phase of PR/biomechanical

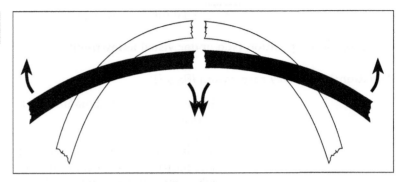

Figure 6.3 Inspiration phase of PR/biodynamic

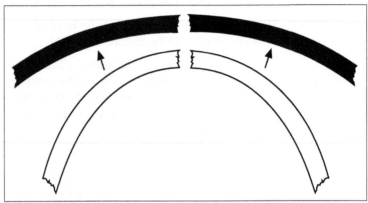

Expiration phase of the PR, normal finding:

➤ The sagittal suture moves cephalad.
➤ The lateral borders move in a posterior and medial direction.

Biodynamic/embryological approach
Inspiration phase of the PR, normal finding (Fig. 6.3):

➤ With your hands on the parietal bones, you will sense an expansive cephalad and lateral force.
➤ There is a centrifugal (outward) motion. The convexity becomes less.

Expiration phase of the PR, normal finding:

➤ With your hands on the parietal bones, you will sense a retractive caudad and medial force.
➤ There is a centripetal motion. The convexity increases.
➤ Compare the amplitude, strength, ease and symmetry of the motions of the parietal bones.
➤ During the external and internal rotation, other types of motion of the parietal bones may sometimes arise. These give an indication of further dysfunctions of the particular parietal bone.

Motion testing

The only difference between the palpation of primary respiration and motion testing is that when testing, the therapist actively induces the external and internal rotation motion of the parietal bones.

Hand position: As above, except:

> When testing the external rotation you should cross your thumbs so that they lie on the parietal bone on the opposite side.

Method: Testing of external and internal rotation:
During the inspiration phase:

> At the beginning of the inspiration phase, administer a caudad impulse with your thumbs.
> At the same time administer an impulse in the anterior and lateral direction with the basal or proximal joints of your fingers on the lateral borders of the parietal bones.

During the expiration phase:

> At the beginning of the expiration phase, administer an impulse in a posterior and medial direction with the palms of your hands on the lateral borders of the parietal bones.
> Compare the amplitude and ease of the motions of each parietal bone or the amount of force needed to elicit movement.

TREATMENT OF THE PARIETAL BONES

The SBS, occiput, temporal bones and atlanto-occipital transition zone should also be examined, and treated as necessary.

Intraosseous dysfunctions

Molding *(Fig. 6.4)*

Indication: Asymmetric convexity or flattening; torsion tensions at the ossification centers.

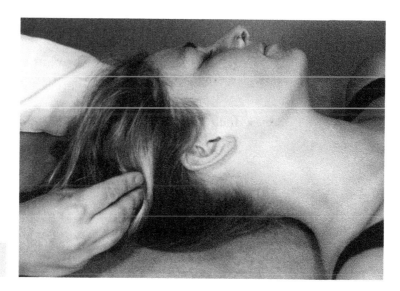

Figure 6.4 Molding of the parietal bone

Hand position: ➤ Draw the fingertips of one hand close together.
➤ Place them on the parietal tuber.

Method: ➤ To treat a convexity: Administer centrifugal impulses with your fingers aimed at flattening the raised part.
➤ This treatment can be augmented using a fluid impulse to direct energy toward the borders of the parietal bone.

Note: It is important to release the adjacent bones gently from the parietal bone before commencing treatment.

➤ To treat a flattening: Administer centripetal impulses, aimed at making the flattened part more prominent.
➤ A fluid impulse may be used to direct energy from the opposite lateral border of the occiput to the center of the parietal tuber.
➤ To treat torsion tensions: Administer an impulse in the direction of the motion restriction.
➤ Establish the PBMT and PBFT.

Dysfunction in external and internal rotation

Dysfunction in external rotation, parietal spread technique *(Figs 6.5a,b)*

(Motion restriction in the direction of internal rotation)

Indication: Tensions and fibrosis of the falx, disturbances of drainage of the superior and inferior sagittal sinuses and lateral ventricles, restrictions of the sutures of the parietal bone; according to Magoun, in the case of idiopathic epilepsy, where the suture is frequently fixed in the extension position.[4]

Hand position: ➤ Place the palms of both hands on the parietal tubers.
➤ Cross your thumbs to lie on the parietal bone on the opposite side.
➤ Place your index fingers on the sphenoidal angles (anterior inferior angles of the parietal bones).
➤ Position your middle fingers above the roots of the zygomatic processes of the temporal bones.
➤ Position your ring fingers on the mastoid angles (posterior inferior angles of the parietal bones).
➤ Place the basal or proximal joints of your index, middle and ring fingers on the parietal bones. Position them on the lateral borders of the parietal bones.

Method: Indirect technique:

➤ At the beginning of the inspiration phase, begin to administer gentle caudad and lateral pressure with the pads of your thumbs so that the sagittal suture spreads and becomes lower.

This reduces the membrane tension in the craniocaudal course of the falx.

➤ At the same time, with the basal or proximal joints of your fingers, administer an anterior and lateral impulse to the inferior and lateral borders of the parietal bones.

Figure 6.5 (a,b)
Dysfunction in external
rotation, parietal spread
technique

(a)

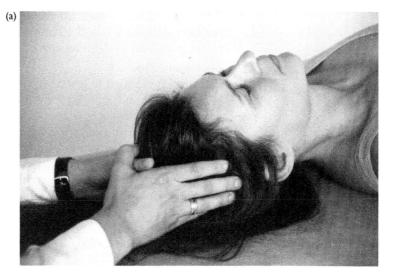

(b)

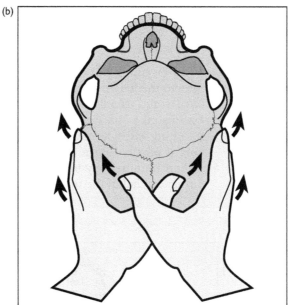

> ➤ Establish the PBMT of the parietal bones – the position in which
> the tension of the dural membrane is in the best possible state of
> balance – and the PBFT.
> ➤ Maintain the PBT until a correction of the abnormal tension has
> been achieved and stabilized by the inherent homeostatic forces
> (PRM rhythm, etc.), and the motion of the parietal bone has
> stopped.
> ➤ Breathing assistance: Ask the patient to hold an inhalation for as
> long as possible at the end of an in-breath.
> ➤ A fluid impulse may be used to direct energy from the inion or
> further caudad in the midline.

Note: If this technique is used for the release of the sagittal suture, it is considered to be a direct technique, as the impulse is designed to produce motion in the direction of the restriction.

Biodynamic approach

Palpation performed in a state of relaxed, non-invasive attentiveness and empathy, and in synchrony with the inherent homeodynamic forces and rhythmic patterns, will encourage the spontaneous occurrence of a still point or a correcting inspiration phase, external rotation and expansion or of an expiration phase, internal rotation and retraction at the parietal bones. This approach does not require any encounter or confrontation with tissue resistances and does not impede any phase of primary respiration.

Dysfunction in internal rotation *(Fig. 6.6)*

(Motion restriction in the direction of external rotation)

Hand position: As above, except:

> ➤ The tips of your thumbs should touch each other at the sagittal suture, but without resting on the suture.

Method: Indirect technique:

> ➤ At the beginning of the expiration phase, begin to administer a postero-medial impulse with the palms of your hands at the inferior and lateral borders of the parietal bones.
> ➤ Establish the PBMT and PBFT.
> ➤ Breathing assistance: Ask the patient to hold an exhalation for as long as possible at the end of an out-breath.
> ➤ A fluid impulse may be used to direct energy from the inion or further caudad in the midline.

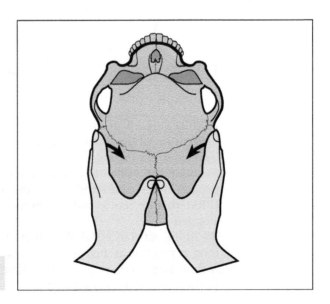

Figure 6.6 Dysfunction in internal rotation

Note: Internal rotation dysfunctions of the parietal bones are frequently caused by a dysfunction of the sagittal suture, so this treatment should be followed by a direct technique.

Biodynamic approach

Palpation performed in a state of relaxed, non-invasive attentiveness and empathy, and in synchrony with the inherent homeodynamic forces and rhythmic patterns, will encourage the spontaneous occurrence of a still point or a correcting inspiration phase, external rotation and expansion or of an expiration phase, internal rotation and retraction at the parietal bones. This approach does not require any encounter or confrontation with tissue resistances and does not impede any phase of primary respiration.

Parietal spread technique, alternative special technique for the superior sagittal sinus *(Fig. 6.7)*

Hand position: As for the parietal spread technique.

Method:
- ➤ Place your thumbs at the posterior end of the sagittal suture at lambda.
- ➤ During the inspiration phase, administer gentle caudad and lateral pressure with the pads of your thumbs at the sagittal borders of the parietal bones, so that the sagittal suture spreads and becomes lower.
- ➤ When release of the suture at this point occurs, move your thumbs slightly anterior and begin again with the same procedure until your thumbs reach the anterior end of the suture at bregma.

Parietal lift technique *(Figs 6.8, 6.9)*

Indication, in combination with the spread technique

Tensions and fibrosis of the falx cerebri, disturbances of drainage of the superior and inferior sagittal sinuses, restrictions of the sutures of

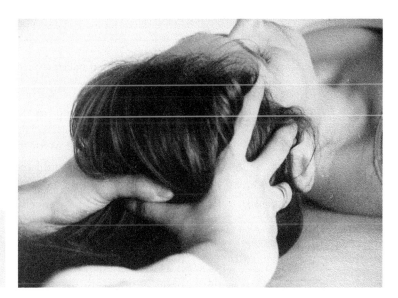

Figure 6.7 Parietal spread technique, alternative special technique for the sagittal suture and superior sagittal sinus

Figure 6.8 Parietal lift technique

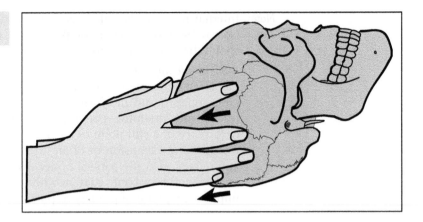

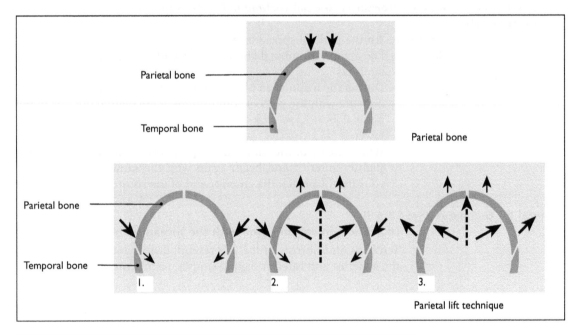

Figure 6.9 Diagrammatic representation of the parietal spread and lift technique

the parietal bone; according to Magoun also insomnia and hypertonus.[3]

Hand position: The hand position is the same as for the spread technique, except:

> The tips of your thumbs should touch each other at the sagittal suture, but without resting on the suture.

Method: > During the expiration phase, begin to administer gentle medial pressure with your index, middle and ring fingers on the inferior lateral borders of the parietal bones, to release them from the temporal bones (IR).

> As soon as the parietal bones begin to move cephalad (release of the parietal bones from the temporal bones), you can relax the medial pressure of your fingers.

➤ Replace this with cephalad traction with your fingers.
➤ At the same time, without reducing the cephalad traction, you can administer slight posterior traction to release the parietal bones from the frontal bone, and then slight anterior traction to release the parietal bones from the occipital bone.
➤ Very gently the parietal bones are moved out of the field of tension. The therapist stays within the range of motion, meaning that he avoids confronting the motion barriers directly.
➤ The tissue dynamics are just perceived without intervention.
➤ You will be able to sense the various stages of tissue release: first the sutural tensions, then the elastic and collagenous tensions of the falx cerebri (a sensation like cement, or a rubber band, or chewing gum).
➤ In the end a new equilibrium of tension will establish itself and a floating sensation may be perceived.

Important note: ● Never remove your hands suddenly from the bone during the technique.
● Always take care to position your hands accurately. Failure to do so would mean that at best the technique would be ineffective. In the worst case, especially if your fingers are on the sutures, this could worsen or even give rise to symptoms.

Note: Another option is to assist the flexion and extension motions of the parietal bones (in harmony with the PRM rhythm) during the gentle cephalad and slightly posterior traction. Structural approaches imitating the amount of tension present and move the tissues towards the physiological motion barrier, but always below the threshold where the tissue reacts by contracting.

Sphenoparietal suture, Cant hook *(Figs 6.10a,b)*

Suture margin: Outward-facing margin: sphenoidal angle of the parietal bone, inward-facing margin: greater wing of the sphenoid.
Suture type: Squamous suture.
Therapist: Take up a position beside the patient's head, on the opposite side to the dysfunction.
Hand position: Caudal hand:

➤ Place your little finger intraorally, laterally positioned on the pterygoid process.
➤ Position your middle finger externally on the greater wing on the side of the dysfunction.
➤ If possible place your thumb externally on the greater wing on the opposite side to the dysfunction.

Cranial hand:

Cranial hand: ➤ Span the parietal bones with your thumb and your index and/or middle finger.

Figure 6.10 (a,b)
Sphenoparietal suture

(a)

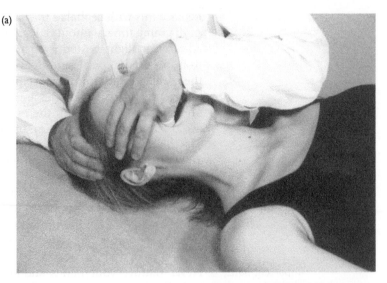

(b)

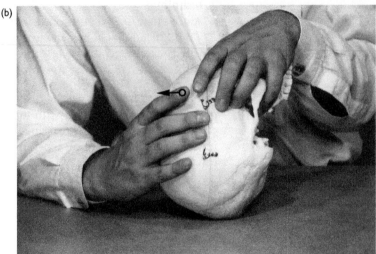

Method:

> Position your middle finger on the sphenoidal angle of the parietal bone on the side of the dysfunction.
> Hold the sphenoid in position with your caudal hand.
> Apply medial pressure and superiorly directed traction on the sphenoidal angle of the parietal bone with the index finger of your cranial hand.
> Without reducing the disengagement, permit all motions/unwinding of the parietal bone that arise.
> Establish the PBMT and PBFT between the sphenoid and the parietal bone.
> A fluid impulse may be used to direct energy from the opposite lambdoid suture or caudal to it.

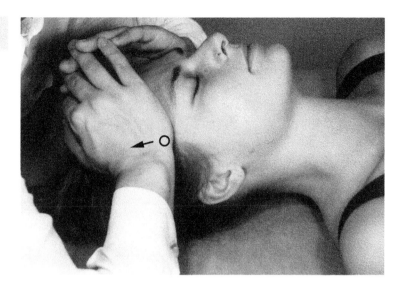

Figure 6.11 Sphenoparietal suture. Alternative technique

Alternative technique *(Fig. 6.11)*

Therapist: Take up a position at the head of the patient.

Hand position: ➤ Place the ball of your two little fingers on the sphenoidal angles of the parietal bones.
➤ Interclasp your fingers and support your elbows on the table slightly caudad and lateral to your hands.

Method: ➤ During the expiration phase, apply medial pressure with the ball of your little fingers on the sphenoidal angles of the parietal bones.
➤ Induce this pressure by drawing your fingertips apart laterally. The internal rotation of the parietal bones causes the disengagement of the sutural articulations with the sphenoid.
➤ During the next inspiration phase, move the sphenoidal angles cephalad, without reducing the medial pressure.
➤ Without reducing the disengagement, permit all motions/unwinding of the parietal bones that arise.
➤ At each release of the tissues, seek the new limit to motion of the parietal bones in the superior direction.
➤ Establish the PBMT and PBFT.
➤ A fluid impulse may be used to direct energy from the opposite lambdoid suture or caudad to it.

Lambdoid suture (right) *(Fig. 6.12)*

Suture margin: The suture margin of the occipital bone is inward-facing in its upper medial half, while the lower lateral half is outward-facing.

Suture type: Squamoserrate suture.

Therapist: Take up a position on the left, on the opposite side to the suture that is to be treated.

Hand position: ➤ Place your hands on the right-hand side of the cranium, overlapping and with your fingers pointing posteriorly.

Figure 6.12 Lambdoid suture (right)

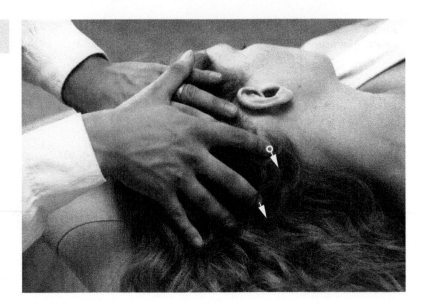

> Position the index and middle fingers of your left hand on the parietal bone anterior to the suture.
> Position the index and middle fingers of your upper hand posterior to the suture, on the occipital bone.

Method: > With your fingers on the parietal bone, administer traction in an anterior direction. Also apply pressure to the bone (occipital border of the parietal bone) with the index finger above the pivot point.
> With the fingers on the occipital bone, administer posterior traction.
> Also apply pressure to the bone (parietal border of the occipital bone) with the index finger below the pivot point.
> Then establish the PBMT and PBFT and maintain this until release of the suture occurs and mobility improves.
> A fluid impulse may be used to direct energy from the opposite frontal tuber or from pterion.

Lambdoid suture (right)

Sagittal suture *(Fig. 6.13)*

(Equivalent to the parietal spread technique)

Suture margin: The digits become longer toward the rear of the suture. This means that spreading of the suture can be wider here than at the front.

Suture type: Serrate suture.

Hand position: > Place your thumbs, crossing, on the parietal bones. Place your fingers on the sides of the parietal bones.

Method: > During the inspiration phase, begin to administer caudal and lateral traction with your thumbs on the sagittal borders of the parietal bones.

Figure 6.13 Sagittal suture

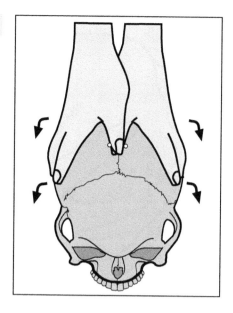

➤ Establish the PBMT and PBFT.
➤ A fluid impulse may be used to direct energy from the inion or further caudad in the midline.

Bregma *(Fig. 6.14)*

Suture margin: At bregma: frontal bone: inward-facing margin; parietal bone: outward-facing margin.

Therapist: Take up a position at the head of the patient.

Hand position:
➤ Place your index finger on the frontal bone.
➤ Place your thumbs next to the sagittal suture, crossing and each resting on the opposite parietal bone.
➤ Place your other fingers on the side of the cranium.

Method:
➤ With your index fingers, move the frontal bone in an anterior direction.
➤ At the same time, move the parietal bones posterolaterally with your thumbs.
➤ Without reducing the gentle disengagement, permit all motions/unwinding of the frontal bone that arise.
➤ With each release of the tissues, seek the new limit to motion of the frontal bone in the anterior direction and of the parietal bones in the posterior and lateral direction.
➤ Establish the PBMT and PBFT.
➤ A fluid impulse may be used to direct energy from the inion or further caudad in the midline.

Lambda *(Figs 6.15a,b)*

Suture margin: At lambda: occipital bone: inward-facing margin; parietal bone: outward-facing margin.

Figure 6.14 Bregma

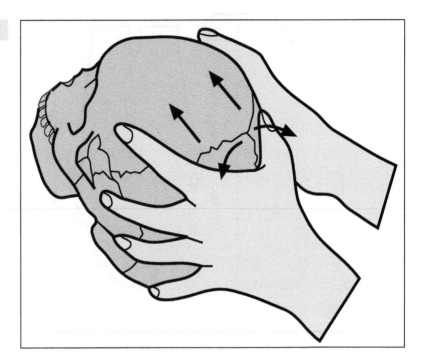

Hand position:	➤ Place your thumbs next to the sagittal suture, crossing so that each rests on the opposite parietal bone. ➤ Position your little fingers on the occipital squama, fingertips touching. ➤ Place your other fingers on each side of the cranium, on the parietal bones.
Method:	➤ With your little fingers, move the occipital bone caudad. ➤ At the same time, guide the parietal bones in an anterior and lateral direction with your thumbs. ➤ Your other fingers should remain passive. ➤ Without reducing the gentle disengagement, permit all motions/unwinding of the parietal bones that arise. ➤ At each release of the tissues, seek the next limit to anterolateral motion of the parietal bones and to caudad motion of the occiput. ➤ Establish the PBMT and PBFT.
Alternative hand position:	The three finger technique.
	➤ Place the index and middle fingers of one hand on the two parietal bones, and the thumb of the same hand on the occipital bone. Simultaneously move the thumb caudad and the middle and index fingers in an anterior and lateral direction.

Pterion *(Fig. 6.16)*

Sutures:	Four bones overlap at this point. Working outward, these are: The frontal bone, parietal bone, sphenoid, and temporal bone.

Figure 6.15 (a,b) Lambda

(a)

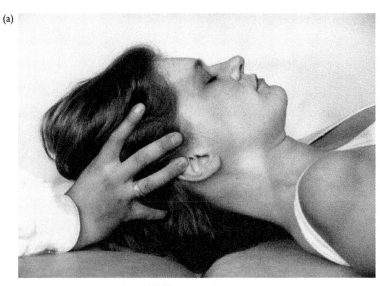

(b)

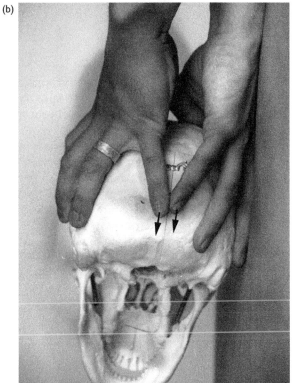

Hand position:
> ➤ Place all your fingers close to pterion.
> ➤ Place your index finger on the frontal bone.
> ➤ Place your thumb on the parietal bone.
> ➤ Place your middle finger on the sphenoid.
> ➤ Place your ring finger on the temporal bone.

Figure 6.16 Pterion

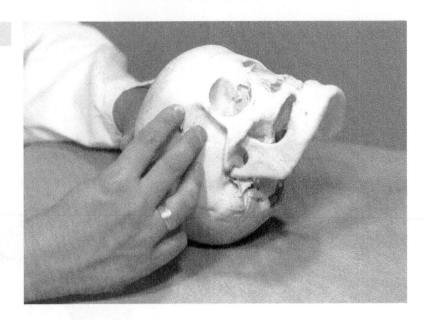

Method: ➤ With your index finger, apply gentle pressure to the frontal bone together with anterior and superior traction.
➤ When the frontal bone begins to disengage from the other bones, apply gentle pressure with your thumb, together with traction in a superior and slightly posterior direction.
➤ When the parietal bone begins to disengage from the other bones, apply gentle pressure with your middle finger on the sphenoid, together with anterior and slightly caudad traction.
➤ When the sphenoid begins to disengage from the other bones, apply caudad and posterior traction with your ring finger on the temporal bone.
➤ End by administering centrifugal traction with all your fingers to the respective bones.
➤ Establish the PBMT and PBFT.

Asterion *(Fig. 6.17)*

Sutures: Three bones meet at this point: the occipital bone, temporal bone and parietal bone.
Patient: The patient's head should be turned to the opposite side.
Hand position: ➤ Place all your fingers close to asterion.
➤ Place your thumb on the parietal bone.
➤ Place your index finger on the temporal bone.
➤ Place your middle finger on the occipital bone.
Method: ➤ Apply gentle pressure to the occipital bone with your middle finger, together with posterior traction.
➤ Then apply pressure to the parietal bone with the thumb positioned there, together with cephalad traction.

Figure 6.17 Asterion

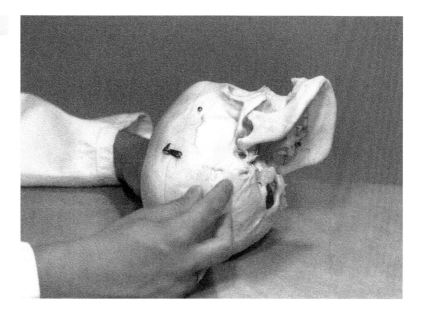

> ➤ Then with your index finger on the temporal bone, together with your middle finger and thumb, administer centrifugal traction to the respective bones.
> ➤ Establish the PBMT and PBFT.

References

1 Rohen JW. Morphologie des menschlichen Organismus. 2 Aufl. Stuttgart: Verlag freies Geistesleben; 2002:387.
2 Stone R. Polaritätstherapie. 2. Auflage. Hugendubel: 1994:207.
3 Magoun H I. Osteopathy in the Cranial Field. 3rd edn. Kirksville: Journal Printing Company; 1976:176.
4 Magoun H I. Osteopathy in the Cranial Field. 1st edn. Kirksville: Journal Printing Company; 1951:147.

7 The maxillae

THE MORPHOLOGY OF THE MAXILLAE ACCORDING TO ROHEN[1]

The dynamics of motion of the upper limbs is reflected in the global organization of the maxilla.

When man began to walk upright, the upper extremities gained the full range of movement between the fully raised and the fully lowered positions. For Rohen, two primal gestures are manifested in the hand: the clenched fist, which has currency in the world, i.e. in the earthly sphere, and the open hand, expressing a gesture of opening up and of receiving.

This paradoxical motion dynamic is also apparent in the design of the maxilla, with its four processes.

The narrow, upwardly sweeping frontal process corresponds to the open hand and has a role in the formation of the nasal root, which is located in the region of greatest concentration of the ego consciousness. In enclosing the nasal cavity, it is also involved in the rhythmic system.

At the base, the maxilla develops into the alveolar process. This structure accommodates the teeth and is thus involved in chewing, that is, in the processing of material aspects. The gesture of the clenched fist is discernible in the alveolar process.

The medially oriented palatine process and the laterally oriented zygomatic process are positioned between these two polarities. For Rohen, the palatine process is the diaphragm of the head in that it separates the oral cavity from the nasal cavity, while the zygomatic process links the visceral cranium with the cerebral cranium.

However, the integrative expressivity of the maxilla is achieved only through its being supported toward the rear on the cranial base via the zygomatic bone and toward the top on the skull-cap via the frontal bone.

For Stone,[2] the maxilla reflects polarity reflexes of the pelvis anteriorly and of the hips laterally.

LOCATION, CAUSES AND CLINICAL PRESENTATION OF MAXILLARY DYSFUNCTIONS

Osseous dysfunction

A high palatine arch (IR of maxilla) with vertical alignment of the frontal process is usually combined with narrow nasal cavities and

223

disturbances of the nasal septum. This can lead to functional impairment of the vascular, nervous and lymphatic structures, as well as to mouth breathing, nasal problems, etc.

a) Frontomaxillary suture

b) Ethmoidomaxillary suture
Dysfunctions of the maxilla have a usually direct influence on the mobility of the ethmoid bone, and may even lead to a restriction of the SBS.

c) Zygomaticomaxillary suture
Causes: Falling, or blows to the face.
Clinical presentation: Orbital disturbance, disturbance of the maxillary sinus resulting in sinusitis.

d) Lacrimomaxillary suture

e) Transverse palatine suture

f) Palatomaxillary suture

g) Nasomaxillary suture

h) Vomeromaxillary suture

i) Conchomaxillary suture

j) Median palatine suture
The mobility of the median palatine suture is often restricted by the use of dental braces.

k) Incisive suture
This suture, between the incisive bone (premaxilla) and the maxilla, ossifies between the 12th and the 18th month of life. It is often motion-restricted, due either to early traumatic influences or to the use of dental braces.

l) Inferior orbital fissure (infraorbital nerve, communications between the inferior ophthalmic vein and the pterygoid plexus)
Narrowness of the fissure can impair venous drainage.

m) Dental malocclusions

n) Dental dystopia
Causes: SBS dysfunction, dysfunction of the incisive suture, malnutrition, poor corrective dentistry, and dental surgery.

Muscular dysfunction

Although the maxilla is the site of attachment of many minor muscles, dysfunctions of these muscles affecting the upper jaw are not often encountered. To give one example, spasm of the masseter could be capable of moving the upper jaw in a posterior direction. Other masticatory muscles may impair the maxilla in conjunction with a dysfunction of the temporomandibular joint.

Disturbances of the nerves

a) Maxillary nerve (V2): The maxillary nerve emerges through the foramen rotundum into the pterygopalatine fossa, where it subdivides further.

b) Infraorbital nerve (V2) runs through the inferior orbital fissure into the infraorbital canal, and on through the infraorbital foramen.

Clinical presentation: e.g. following traumatic injury to the orbital floor: disturbances of sensitivity, or pain in the skin of the mid-facial region, and in the mucosae and upper teeth.

c) Superior alveolar nerves (V2) in the alveolar canals on the back of the infratemporal surface. From the infraorbital nerve in the pterygopalatine fossa, the branches which supply the teeth and gums branch off on the maxilla.

Clinical presentation: Toothache and painful gums.

d) Major palatine nerves

Clinical presentation: Disturbances of sensitivity and pain in the mucosa of the hard palate.

e) Sympathetic fibres from the deep petrosal nerve, via the pterygopalatine ganglion, the sensory root of the pterygopalatine ganglion, the maxillary nerve, the zygomatic nerve to the lacrimal nerve (lacrimal gland)

Clinical presentation: Disturbance of the lacrimal gland.

f) Zygomatic nerve

Clinical presentation: Disturbances of sensitivity and pain in the skin around the temporal and zygomatic bones.

g) Pterygopalatine ganglion

Clinical presentation: Secretory disturbances of the lacrimal gland and of the nasal and palatine mucosa, with reduced resistance of the nose, oral cavity and pharynx, possibly ocular disturbances and olfactory impairment (due to dryness of the nasal mucosae).

Vascular disturbances

a) Infraorbital artery and vein

Clinical presentation: Metabolic disturbance of the front teeth, and of the bones and gingivae of the upper jaw.

b) Anterior superior alveolar arteries

Clinical presentation: Metabolic disturbance of the anterior teeth.

c) Posterior superior alveolar artery

Clinical presentation: Functional disturbance of the maxillary sinus and upper molars, and of the bones and gingivae of the upper jaw.

d) Descending palatine artery in the greater palatine canal

Clinical presentation: Functional disturbance of the pharyngeal mucosa, gingivae of the front teeth, and soft palate.

e) Effects may be seen in the retromandibular and facial veins

Ocular disturbance

Displacement of the eye, e.g. following traumatic injury to the orbital floor.

Causes of maxillary dysfunctions

Primary dysfunction
- Intraosseous
- Traumatic injury: falls, blows, dental extractions, poor masticatory habits, or other examples of force affecting the maxillae can lead to restrictions both of the maxilla itself and of the bones which surround it, in particular the palatine bone, as well as of the pterygopalatine ganglion.

Secondary dysfunction
- Due to dysfunction of the sphenoid, e.g. in association with SBS dysfunctions (torsion of the SBS leads to relative restriction of one maxilla in IR and one maxilla in ER), dental braces, myofascial tension.
- Developmental disturbances of the cranial base at the embryonic stage lead to disturbances of maxillary development.

Examination and techniques
- History-taking
- Visual assessment
- Palpation of the position
- Palpation of primary respiration
- Motion testing
- Rotation dysfunction of the maxilla
- Maxilla lift and spread technique
- Global rotation dysfunction about a vertical axis
- Global lateral strain
- Decompression of the maxillary complex at the pterygopalatine suture
- General decompression of the maxillary complex
- Transverse palatine suture
- Palatomaxillary suture
- Frontomaxillary suture, see The Frontal bone
- Incisive suture
- Zygomaticomaxillary suture
- Median palatine suture
- Nasomaxillary suture, see The Nasal bone

DIAGNOSIS

History-taking

Nasal, oral or pharyngeal symptoms, ocular symptoms, dental dystopia and dental malocclusions, sometimes allergic rhinitis and asthma via the pterygopalatine ganglion, dental braces.

Visual assessment

- Nasolabial fold: lowered (ER) or flat (IR).
- Incisors: posteriorly positioned and widely spaced, whereas the remaining upper teeth appear inclined to one side (ER).
- Incisors: anteriorly positioned and close together, whereas the remaining teeth appear inclined inward (IR).
- Anterior teeth: protruding (possibly intraosseous dysfunction, IR of the premaxilla).

Palpation of the position

- ➤ Orbital process: tilted (ER) or straight (IR).
- ➤ Palatine process: lowered (ER) or elevated (IR).
- ➤ Alveolar process: externally rotated (ER) or vertically aligned (IR).

Palpation of primary respiration *(Fig. 7.1)*

- ➤ Biomechanical/biodynamic palpation, motion testing as required.
- ➤ If palpation reveals a restriction, the therapist may induce an impulse in the direction of the restriction. This will emphasize it, making it easier to sense from which structure it originates.

Therapist: Take up a position at the head of the patient.
Hand position:
- ➤ Position your index fingers on both sides of the nose, on the alveolar arches of the two maxillae.
- ➤ Place the other fingers beside the index fingers, on the alveolar arches of the two maxillae.

Alternative hand position I: (Fig. 7.2)
- ➤ Place your index fingers intraorally, and your thumbs outside on the alveolar arches of the two maxillae. Grasp the alveolar arches with your thumbs and index fingers.

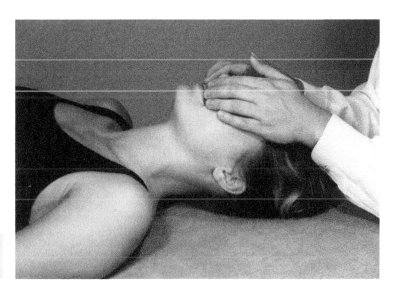

Figure 7.1 Palpation of primary respiration of the maxillae

Figure 7.2 Alternative hand position I

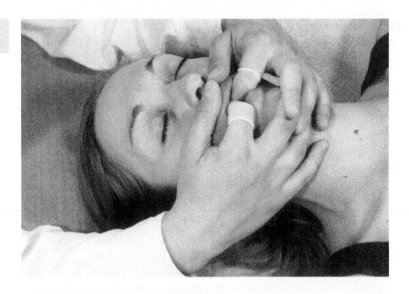

Figure 7.3 Alternative hand position II

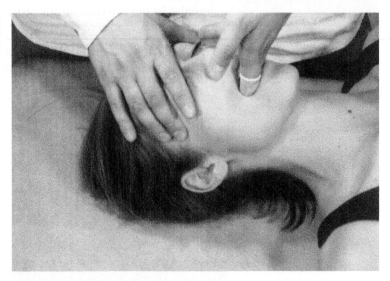

Alternative hand position II: (Fig. 7.3)

Take up a position beside the patient's head.

➤ Grasp the greater wings with the middle finger and thumb of your cranial hand.
➤ Place the index finger and middle finger of the other hand on the upper teeth on each side.

Alternative hand position III, unilateral: (Fig. 7.4)

Take up a position beside the patient's head, on the opposite side to the one being tested.

➤ Place the index finger of your caudal hand intraorally on the alveolar part.

Figure 7.4 Alternative hand position III

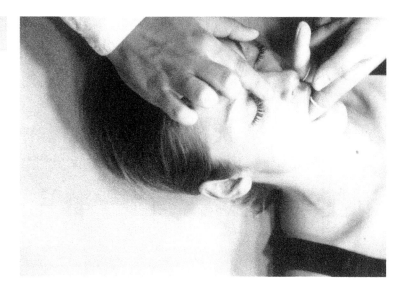

➤ Place the index finger of your cranial hand on the frontal process of the maxilla.

Biomechanical approach
During the inspiration phase, an external rotation of the maxilla occurs.

➤ The maxilla moves in parallel with the frontal bone.
➤ The zygomatic process of the maxilla moves in a superior, anterior direction.
➤ The median palatine suture and the palatine arch move inferior.
➤ The alveolar process widens on the lateral side.
➤ The intermaxillary suture moves posterior.

Inspiration phase of PR, normal finding (Fig. 7.5):

➤ The alveolar arch widens on the lateral side.
➤ The intermaxillary suture moves posterior.
➤ The palatine arch moves down.

Expiration phase of PR, normal finding:

➤ The alveolar arch narrows on the lateral side.
➤ The intermaxillary suture moves anterior.
➤ The palatine arch moves in the cranial direction.

Biodynamic/embryological approach
Inspiration phase of PR, normal finding (Figs 7.6, 7.7):

➤ The hands may perceive a force on the maxillae in an anterior, inferior direction.

Expiration phase of PR, normal finding:

➤ The hands may perceive a force on the maxillae in a posterior, superior direction.

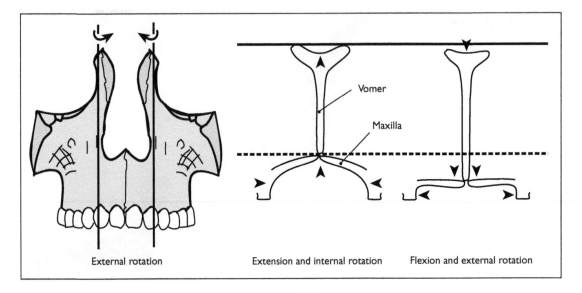

External rotation   Extension and internal rotation   Flexion and external rotation

Figure 7.5 PR inspiration phase: biomechanical approach

Figure 7.6 PR inspiration phase: biodynamic

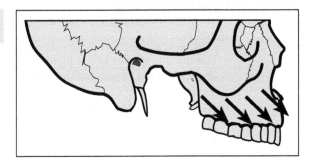

Figure 7.7 PR inspiration phase, biodynamic. Effects on the maxillary complex

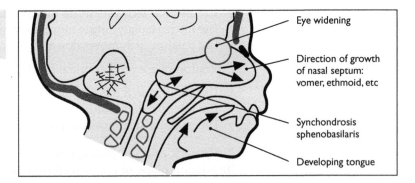

➤ Compare the amplitude, strength, ease and symmetry of the motion of the maxillae.
➤ Other types of motion of the maxillae may sometimes occur during external and internal rotation. These provide an indication as to further dysfunctions of the particular maxilla involved.

➤ Maxillary dysfunctions may be unilateral or bilateral, symmetrical or asymmetrical.

Motion testing

This differs from palpation of the PRM rhythm only in one feature: the external and internal rotation of the frontal bone and maxilla are now actively induced by the therapist.

Hand position: As above.

Method: Testing of external and internal rotation:
During the inspiration phase:

➤ At the beginning of the inspiration phase, with your index fingers, direct an impulse in a posterior direction on the intermaxillary suture.
➤ At the same time, direct an impulse laterally on the posterior region of the alveolar arches with your other fingers.

During the expiration phase:

➤ At the beginning of the expiration phase, with your ring fingers and little fingers, deliver a medially-directed impulse on the posterior region of the alveolar arches.
➤ At the same time, follow the intermaxillary suture anterior with your index fingers.
➤ Compare the amplitude and the ease of the respective maxillary motion, or the force needed to bring about motion.

TREATMENT OF THE MAXILLAE

Rotation dysfunction of the maxillae

Maxilla lift and spread technique *(Figs 7.8, 7.9)*

Aim: To release the ethmoidomaxillary, lacrimomaxillary and ethmoidolacrimal sutures and create freedom of motion of the maxilla and perpendicular plate.

Therapist: Take up a position at the head of the patient.

Hand position: ➤ Place your hands either side of the patient's head.
➤ Place your thumbs on the outside, on or slightly above the alveolar arches of the maxillae. Your thumbs should be medially oriented.
➤ Place your index fingers intraorally on the alveolar arches of the maxillae.
➤ This means that you are in effect grasping the maxilla between your index finger and thumb, from inside and outside.

Method: ➤ With your thumb and index finger, administer traction to the two maxillary bones anterior and caudad. This frees the maxillae from the ethmoid bone.

(The medial border of the orbital surface of the maxilla is released from the bottom of the ethmoid air cells, the posterior border of the maxillary frontal process is freed from the anterior of the ethmoidal labyrinth, and the ethmoidal crest on the medial side of the maxilla is released from the middle nasal concha of the ethmoid.)

Figure 7.8 Maxilla lift and spread technique

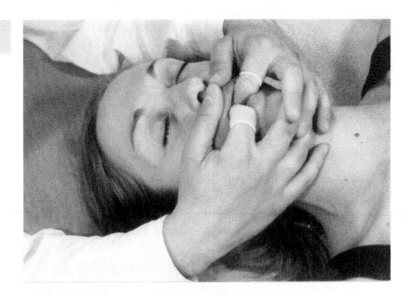

Figure 7.9 Maxilla lift and spread technique; (a) lift technique; (b) spread technique

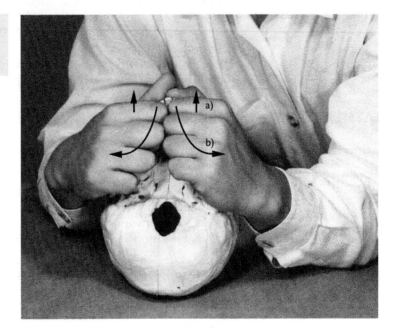

➤ When you perceive a release at the ethmoidomaxillary suture, you can go on to spread the maxillae away from one another.
➤ Do not relax the anterior and caudal traction, but instead induce external rotation of the maxillae.
➤ Administer posterior pressure on the intermaxillary suture with your thumbs.
➤ With your index fingers, guide the alveolar arches in a lateral and anterior direction.
➤ Establish the PBMT and PBFT.

Alternative technique to treat an internal rotation dysfunction of the maxilla
(Fig. 7.10, see also Fig. 7.3)

Aim: To release the ethmoidomaxillary suture and create freedom of motion of the maxilla and perpendicular plate.

Therapist: Take up a position beside the patient's head.

Hand position: Cranial hand:

> ➤ Span the greater wings with your thumb and your middle or index finger.

> Caudal hand:

> ➤ Place your middle and index finger against the upper teeth, one on each side.

Method: ➤ During the inspiration phase, direct an impulse caudad via the greater wings to induce flexion.
> ➤ At the same time, spread apart the fingers resting on the upper teeth (external rotation of the maxillae).
> ➤ During the expiration phase, passively follow the motion of the cranial bones.
> ➤ Repeat this procedure for a few cycles, until the mobility of the maxillae increases.

External and internal rotation dysfunction

External rotation dysfunction, bilateral: direct technique *(Fig. 7.11)*

Therapist: Take up a position at the head of the patient.

Hand position: ➤ Position your index fingers on the two sides of the nose, on the alveolar arches of the two maxillae.
> ➤ Place the other fingers beside the index fingers on the alveolar arches of the two maxillae.

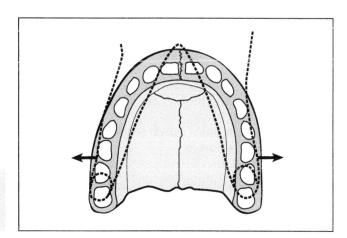

Figure 7.10 Alternative technique to treat an internal rotation dysfunction of the maxillae

Figure 7.11 External rotation dysfunction, bilateral: direct technique

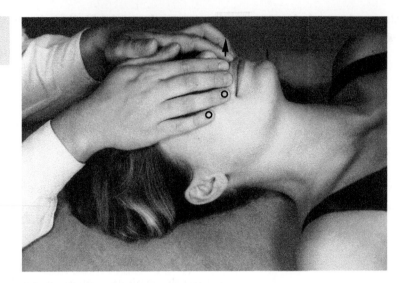

Method: Direct technique:
> ➤ Administer slight, laterally directed traction on the maxillae with your fingers (disengagement).
> ➤ At the beginning of the expiration phase, with your ring fingers and little fingers deliver an impulse medially on the posterior region of the alveolar arches (IR).
> ➤ At the same time, with the index fingers follow the intermaxillary suture anterior.
> ➤ Establish the PBMT and PBFT.
> ➤ Maintain the PBT until a correction of the abnormal tension has been achieved and the inherent homeostatic forces (PRM rhythm, etc.) have stabilized.

Biodynamic approach

Encourage the spontaneous occurrence of a still point or corrective inspiration phase, external rotation and expansion or expiration phase, internal rotation and retraction of the maxillae, by means of palpation, carried out in a state of relaxed, non-invasive attention and empathy. Synchronize this treatment with the inherent homeodynamic forces and rhythmic patterns. This approach requires no encounter or confrontation with tissue resistances and no inhibition of any phase of primary respiration.

Internal rotation dysfunction, bilateral: direct technique *(Fig. 7.12a)*

Hand position: As above.

Method: Direct technique:
> ➤ Administer slight, laterally-directed tension on the maxillae with your fingers (disengagement).
> ➤ With your index fingers on the intermaxillary suture, deliver an impulse posterior (ER).

Figure 7.12 (a) Internal rotation dysfunction, bilateral: direct technique. (b) External rotation dysfunction, unilateral: direct technique

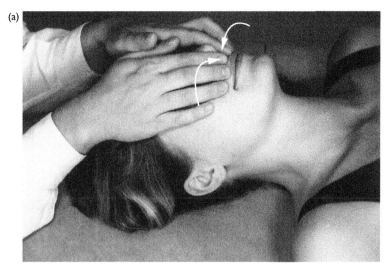

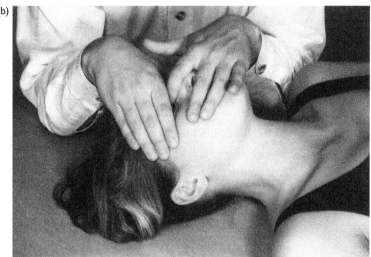

➤ At the same time, deliver a laterally-directed impulse on the posterior region of the alveolar arches with your ring fingers and little fingers (ER).

➤ Establish the PBMT and PBFT.

Alternative hand position I: (see Fig. 7.2):

➤ Place your index fingers intraorally and your thumbs outside on the alveolar arches of the two maxillae. Grasp the alveolar arches with your thumbs and index fingers.

Method: Direct technique:

External rotation dysfunction, bilateral:

➤ The method already described may be supplemented by applying cranially-directed pressure to the palatine processes of the maxillae using the index fingers (IR).

Internal rotation dysfunction, bilateral:

➤ The method already described may be supplemented by encouraging the lowering of the palatine processes of the maxillae using the index fingers (ER).

Alternative hand position II: (see Fig. 7.3)
Take up a position beside the patient's head.
Cranial hand:

➤ Span the greater wings with your middle or index finger and your thumb.

Caudal hand:

➤ Place the index finger and middle finger of one hand against the upper teeth, one on each side.

Method: Direct technique:
External rotation dysfunction, bilateral:

➤ The greater wings are moved into extension.
➤ Move the index finger and middle finger resting on the teeth closer together (IR).

Internal rotation dysfunction, bilateral:

➤ The greater wings are moved into flexion.
➤ Spread your index finger and middle finger on the teeth (ER).

External rotation dysfunction, bilateral: indirect technique

Therapist: Take up a position at the head of the patient.

Hand position: ➤ Position your index fingers on both sides of the nose, on the alveolar arches of the two maxillae.
➤ Place the other fingers beside the index fingers on the alveolar arches of the two maxillae.

Method: Indirect technique:

➤ With your fingers, administer slight, laterally directed traction on the maxillae (disengagement).
➤ At the beginning of the inspiration phase, direct an impulse posterior on the intermaxillary suture with your index fingers (ER).
➤ At the same time, deliver a laterally-directed impulse to the posterior region of the alveolar arches using your ring fingers and little fingers (ER).
➤ Establish the PBMT and PBFT.

Internal rotation dysfunction, bilateral: indirect technique

Hand position: As above.
Method: Indirect technique:

➤ With your fingers, administer slight, laterally directed traction on the maxillae (disengagement).

➤ At the beginning of the expiration phase, deliver an impulse medially on the posterior region of the alveolar arches with your ring fingers and little fingers (IR).

➤ At the same time, follow the intermaxillary suture in an anterior direction with your index fingers.

➤ Establish the PBMT and PBFT.

Alternative hand position I: ➤ Place your index fingers intraorally and your thumbs outside on the alveolar arches of the two maxillae. Grasp the alveolar arches with your thumbs and index fingers.

Method: Indirect technique:
External rotation dysfunction, bilateral:

➤ The method already described may be supplemented by encouraging the lowering of the palatine processes of the maxillae using your index fingers (ER).

Internal rotation dysfunction, bilateral:

➤ The method already described may be supplemented by applying cranially-directed pressure to the palatine processes of the maxillae using your index fingers (IR).

Alternative hand position II: Take up a position beside the patient's head.
Cranial hand:

➤ Span the greater wings with your thumb and your middle or index finger.

Caudal hand:

➤ Place your middle and index finger against the upper teeth, one on each side.

Method: Indirect technique:
External rotation dysfunction, bilateral:

➤ Go with the greater wings into flexion.
➤ Spread the index finger and middle finger, which are resting on the teeth on each side (ER).

Internal rotation dysfunction, bilateral:

➤ Go with the sphenoid wings into extension.
➤ Move the index finger and middle finger on the teeth closer together (IR).

External rotation dysfunction, unilateral: direct technique *(Fig. 7.12b)*

Therapist: Take up a position beside the patient's head, on the opposite side to the dysfunction.

Hand position: Cranial hand:

➤ Span the greater wings with your thumb and your middle or index finger.

Caudal hand:

➤ Place your ring finger or middle finger on the alveolar arches.
➤ Place your index finger on the frontal process of the maxilla.

Method: Direct technique:

➤ Using your ring or middle finger, deliver an impulse in the medial direction on the posterior region of the alveolar arches (IR).
➤ At the same time, using your index finger deliver an impulse on the frontal process in the vertical alignment direction (IR).
➤ Establish the PBMT and PBFT.
➤ A fluid impulse may be used to direct energy from the opposite lambdoid suture.

Biodynamic approach
Encourage the spontaneous occurrence of a still point or corrective inspiration phase, external rotation and expansion or expiration phase, internal rotation and retraction of the maxillae, by means of palpation, carried out in a state of relaxed, non-invasive attention and empathy. Synchronize this treatment with the inherent homeodynamic forces and rhythmic patterns. This approach requires no encounter or confrontation with tissue resistances and no inhibition of any phase of primary respiration.

Global rotation dysfunction about a vertical axis *(Fig. 7.13)*

Possible cause: ● Effect of a force from the side on the maxillae.
● The maxillae move in conjunction with the palatine bones and the sphenoid.

Possible sequelae: Lateral strain of the sphenobasilar synchondrosis.
Therapist: Take up a position beside the patient's head.
Hand position: Cranial hand:

➤ Span the greater wings with your middle or index finger and your thumb.

Caudal hand:

➤ Place the middle finger and the index finger of one hand against the upper teeth, one on each side.

Motion test:

➤ With your index finger and middle fingers, induce a global rotation of the two maxillae while holding the sphenoid firmly in the neutral position.
➤ Compare the amplitude and ease of the maxillary global rotation.
Method: ➤ The sphenoid is held firmly in the neutral position.
Exaggeration: ➤ With your index and middle fingers, induce a global rotation of the two maxillae in the direction of greater motion (of ease).

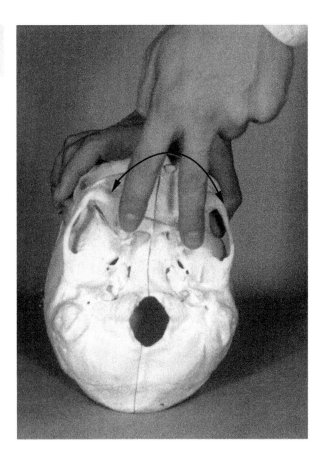

Figure 7.13 Global rotation dysfunction about a vertical axis

Direct technique:

➤ With your index and middle fingers, induce a global rotation of the two maxillae in the direction of the restriction.
➤ Establish the PBMT and PBFT.

Global lateral strain *(Fig. 7.14)*

Possible cause: ● Effect of a force from the side on the maxillae.
● The maxillae move relative to the palatines and sphenoid.

Sequelae: Curvature of the nasal septum, including the vomer.
Therapist: Take up a position beside the patient's head.
Hand position: Cranial hand:

➤ Span the greater wings with your thumb and your middle or index finger.

Caudal hand:

➤ Place the index and middle finger of one hand against the upper teeth, one on each side.

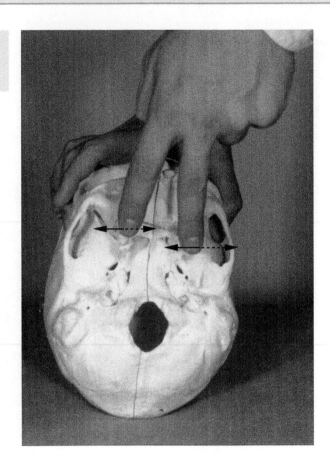

Figure 7.14 Global lateral strain, e.g. exaggeration to the right, solid arrow; direct technique, dotted arrow

Motion test:

> Using your index finger and middle finger, exert a global lateral strain on the two maxillae, while holding the sphenoid firmly in the neutral position.
> Compare the amplitude and ease of the maxillary global lateral strain.

Method: > The sphenoid is held firmly in the neutral position.

Exaggeration: > Using your index and middle fingers, induce a lateral displacement of the two maxillae in the direction of greater motion (of ease).

Direct technique:

> With your index and middle fingers, induce a lateral displacement of the two maxillae in the direction of the restriction.
> Establish the PBMT and PBFT.

Decompression of the maxillary complex *(Fig. 7.15)*

(See also technique for the pterygopalatine ganglion)

Indication: Dysfunction of the pterygopalatine ganglion following a fall or a blow to the face, compression of the pterygopalatine and palatomaxillary sutures.

Therapist: Take up a position beside the patient's head.

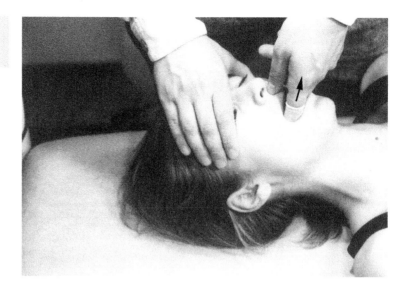

Figure 7.15
Decompression of the maxillary complex

Hand position: Cranial hand:

> Span the greater wings with your thumb and your middle or index finger.

Caudal hand:

> Place the index and middle finger of one hand on the upper teeth on each side and hook them firmly on the posterior surface of the maxillary alveolar arches.
> Position your thumb outside beneath the nose, on the intermaxillary suture.

Method:
> During the inspiration phase, go with the greater wings into flexion.
> Hold the greater wings in the flexion position.
> With your thumb, index finger and middle finger, simultaneously administer traction on the bones of the maxilla in an anterior direction.
> Decompression occurs first of all at the palatomaxillary suture, and then at the pterygopalatine suture.
> Permit all motions and unwindings of the maxillary complex, without reducing the decompression movement.
> With each release of the tissues, seek the new limit of motion of the maxillary complex anterior.
> Establish the PBMT and PBFT.
> A fluid impulse may be used to direct energy from the opposite parietal tuber.

Decompression of the maxillary complex I *(Fig. 7.16)*

Aim: To release the frontomaxillary, palatomaxillary, pterygopalatine and incisive sutures.

Figure 7.16
Decompression of the
maxillary complex I

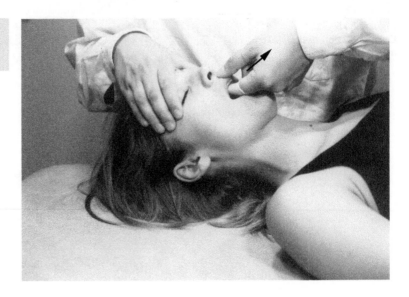

Hand position: Cranial hand:

> Span the greater wings with your thumb and your middle or index finger. Place the basal joint of your index finger on the frontal bone glabella.

Caudal hand:

> Position your index finger intraorally, immediately behind the incisors.
> Position your thumb outside beneath the nose, on the intermaxillary suture.
> Grasp the incisive bone with these two fingers.

Method: Cranial hand:

> Hold the greater wings and the frontal bone firmly in the neutral position.
> With the index finger and thumb of your caudal hand, simultaneously administer traction in an anterior, inferior direction at an angle of about 45°.
> This frees the frontomaxillary, palatomaxillary and pterygopalatine sutures. Decompression of the incisive suture also occurs.
> Establish the PBMT and PBFT.

Transverse palatine suture *(Figs 7.17a–c)*

Suture margin: Posterior margin of the palatine process of the superiorly orientated margin of the maxilla, anterior margin of the horizontal plate of the inferiorly orientated margin of the palatine bone.

Suture type: Serrated suture.

Therapist: Take up a position beside the patient's head.

Figure 7.17 (a–c)
Transverse palatine suture.
Solid arrows: impulse from
the fingers on to the maxilla
and palatine bone. Dotted
arrow: cranially-directed
pressure from the index
finger on the anterior region
of the maxillary palatine
process causes the posterior
region to move caudad.

(a)

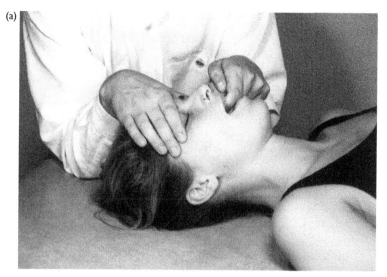

(b)

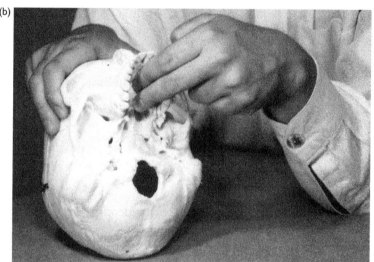

(c)

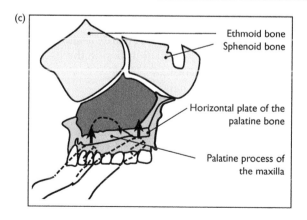

Ethmoid bone
Sphenoid bone

Horizontal plate of the
palatine bone

Palatine process of
the maxilla

Hand position: Cranial hand:

➤ Span the greater wings with your thumb and your middle or index finger.

Caudal hand:

➤ Intraoral.
➤ Position your index finger on one side, on the palatine process of the maxilla, immediately behind the anterior incisors.
➤ Position your middle finger on one side, on the horizontal plate of the palatine bone, immediately behind the transverse palatine suture.

Method: Direct technique:

➤ During the expiration phase, go with the greater wings into extension and hold them there.

Caudal hand:

➤ Apply pressure superior with your two fingers. This moves the horizontal plate of palatine bone in a superior direction and the posterior margin of the horizontal plate of the maxilla inferior.
➤ Establish the PBMT and PBFT.
➤ A fluid impulse may be used to direct energy from the opposite lambdoid suture.

Palatomaxillary suture *(Figs 7.18a,b)*

Suture margin: The posterior medial side of the orbital surface of the maxilla articulates with the anterior part of the orbital process of the palatine bone.

Suture type: Plane suture.

The posterior margin of the maxillary sinus articulates with the lateral edge of the perpendicular plate of the palatine bone.

Suture type: Plane suture.

The lower roughened area of the posterior margin of the maxilla articulates with the pyramidal process of the palatine bone.

Suture type: Irregular.

Possible causes of sutural compression: This suture is frequently disturbed by falls or blows to the face.

Therapist: Take up a position beside the patient's head, on the same side as the dysfunction.

Hand position: Cranial hand:

➤ Span the greater wings with your thumb and your middle or index finger.

Caudal hand:

➤ Intraoral.
➤ Position your index finger on the horizontal plate of the palatine bone, immediately behind the transverse palatine suture.
➤ Place the distal phalanx of your middle finger on the posterior surface of the maxillary alveolar arch. The middle phalanx of the middle finger is positioned on the first molar.

Figure 7.18 (a,b)
Palatomaxillary suture

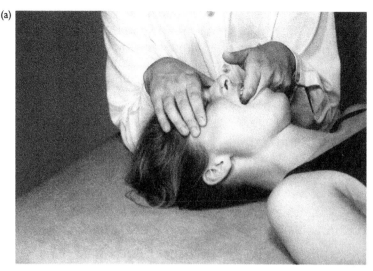

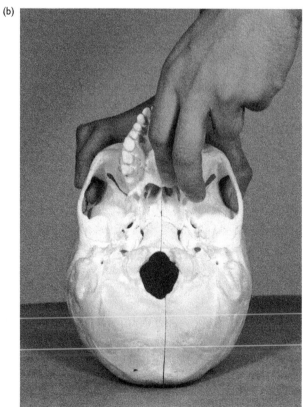

Method: Direct technique:

> ➤ During the expiration phase, go with the greater wings into extension in the cranial direction and hold them there.
> ➤ At the same time, with the index finger of your caudal hand apply pressure in a superior direction and traction medially on the horizontal plate (IR).

➤ During the subsequent inspiration phase, hold the position of the sphenoid and palatine bone.

➤ At the same time, move the alveolar arch of the maxilla laterally (and slightly anteriorly) with your middle finger (ER).

➤ Permit all motions and unwindings of the maxilla without reducing the gentle traction.

➤ With each release of the tissues, seek the new limit of motion of the alveolar arch on the side of the dysfunction in the lateral direction (ER).

➤ Establish the PBMT and PBFT.

➤ A fluid impulse may be used to direct energy from the opposite lambdoid suture.

Frontomaxillary suture (see also Frontal bone) *(Fig. 7.19)*

Suture margin: The frontal process of the maxilla articulates with the external lateral portion of the nasal part of the frontal bone.

Suture type: Serrated suture.

Therapist: Take up a position beside the patient's head.

Hand position: Cranial hand:

➤ Span the frontal bone with your thumb and middle finger or index finger, and hook them fast laterally.

➤ Place the basal joint of your index finger on the glabella, above the frontomaxillary suture.

Caudal hand:

➤ Grasp the frontal processes of the maxillae with your middle and index fingers, beneath the frontomaxillary sutures.

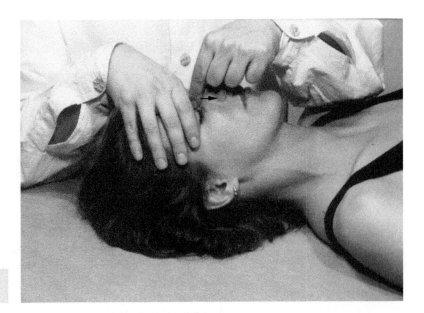

Figure 7.19
Frontomaxillary suture

Method: Disengagement:

> During the inspiration phase, go with the frontal bone into external rotation and hold it there.
> At the beginning of the inspiration phase, using the basal joint of your index finger begin to apply slight pressure posteriorly on the midline of the frontal bone and traction in a superior direction (ER).
> Using your thumb and middle finger or index finger, deliver an impulse on the zygomatic processes of the frontal bone in an anterolateral direction (ER).
> The overall effect is to move the frontal bone into a flattened position (flexion).
> The frontal bone is immobilized in flexion and ER.
> With the index finger and thumb, simultaneously administer traction caudad on the frontal processes of the maxillae.
> Permit all motions/unwinding of the maxillae without reducing the gentle disengagement.
> With each release of the tissues, seek the new limit of motion of the frontal processes in an inferior direction.
> Establish the PBMT and PBFT.
> A fluid impulse may be used to direct energy from the opposite occipital squama.

Alternative hand position: (Fig. 7.20)
Cranial hand:

> Span the frontal bone with your thumb and middle finger or ring finger, hooking fast laterally thereon.

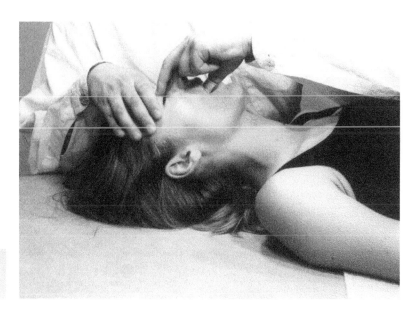

Figure 7.20
Frontomaxillary suture.
Alternative hand position

Caudal hand:

> ➤ Position your thumb intraorally, behind the anterior incisors.
> ➤ Place your index and middle fingers one on each side, on the frontal processes of the maxillae.

Method: As described.

Incisive suture *(Fig. 7.21)*

Aim: To release the incisive bone (premaxilla) from the maxilla.

Diagnosis: When an incisive bone is in ER and the maxilla in IR, the canine tooth is usually prominent.

When the incisive bone is in IR and the maxilla in ER, the canine tooth is usually posteriorly displaced.

Therapist: Take up a position beside the patient's head.

Hand position: Cranial hand:

> ➤ Span the greater wings with your thumb and middle finger or index finger.

Caudal hand:

> ➤ Position your thumb intraorally on the incisive bone, immediately behind the anterior incisors.
> ➤ Place your thumb on the outside beneath the nose, on the intermaxillary suture.

Method: ➤ Hold the greater wings firmly in the neutral position.
> ➤ At the same time, administer traction in an anterior direction with the index finger and thumb of your caudal hand.
> ➤ Permit all movements/unwindings of the incisive bone without reducing the gentle disengagement.

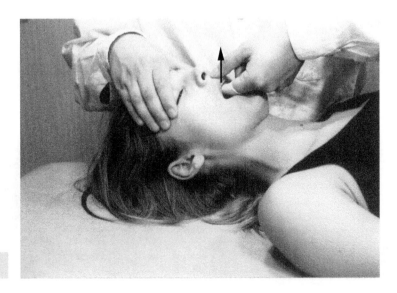

Figure 7.21 Incisive suture

> With each release of the tissues, seek the new limit of motion of the incisive bone in an anterior direction.
> A fluid impulse may be used to direct energy from the lambda.

Zygomaticomaxillary suture *(Fig. 7.22a)*

Suture margin: The zygomatic process of the upper jaw articulates with the anterior and lower margin of the zygomatic bone.

Suture type: Regularly formed suture.

Possible causes of sutural compression:
- A fall or a blow to the face.
- Sutural compression can result in orbital disturbances.

Therapist: Take up a position beside the patient's head, on the opposite side to the dysfunction.

Hand position: Caudal hand:

> Position the index finger intraorally on the inner surface of the zygomatic bone.
> Place your thumb outside against the zygomatic bone and, using your index finger, grasp the zygomatic bone.

Cranial hand:

> Place the palm of your hand passively on the frontal bone. Position your index finger along the course of the frontal process of the affected maxilla.

Method: Disengagement:

> With your caudal hand, administer traction laterally on the zygomatic bone. As you do this, hold the maxilla firmly in position with the index finger of the cranial hand.

Establish the PBMT:

> Maintain the gentle disengagement. At the same time, follow the zygomatic bone into the position that creates the best possible balance of the tension between the zygomatic bone and maxilla.
> A fluid impulse may be used to direct energy from the opposite lambdoid suture.

Alternative hand position: (Fig. 7.22b)
Cranial hand:

> Grasp the zygomatic bone with your thumb and index finger. Position your thumb on the orbital margin of the zygomatic bone. Place your index finger on the lower margin of the zygomatic bone.

Caudal hand:

> Position your index finger intraorally beneath the zygomatic process of the maxilla.

Method: As above.

Figure 7.22
(a) Zygomaticomaxillary suture.
(b) Zygomaticomaxillary suture. Alternative hand position

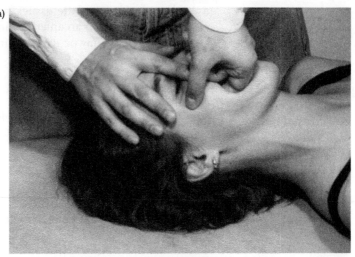

(a)

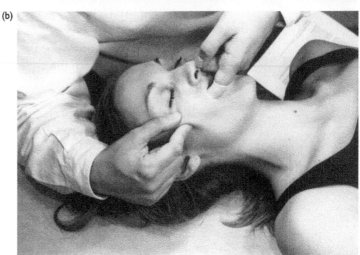

(b)

Median palatine suture *(Figs 7.23a,b)*

Therapist: Take up a position beside the patient's head.
Hand position: Cranial hand:

> ➤ Span the greater wings with your thumb and middle finger or index finger.

Caudal hand:

> ➤ Position your index finger and middle finger intraorally, on the two palatine processes of the maxillae anterior to the transverse palatine suture.

Method: ➤ Hold the greater wings firmly in the neutral position.
➤ At the same time, spread the index finger and middle finger of your caudal hand.

Figure 7.23 (a,b) Median palatine suture

(a)

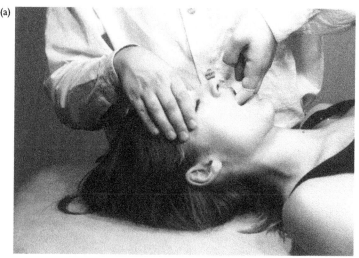

(b)

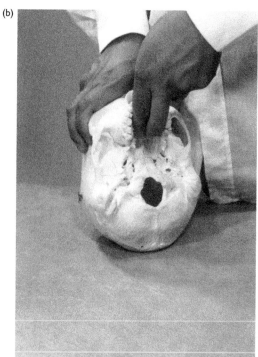

➤ Permit all movements/unwindings of the maxillae without reducing the gentle disengagement.
➤ With each release of the tissues, seek the new limit of motion of the maxillae laterally.
➤ Establish the PBMT and PBFT.
➤ A fluid impulse may be used to direct energy from the inion.
➤ At the end of the technique, the motion of the maxilla should be re-synchronized with the sphenoid motion in harmony with the PRM rhythm.

During the inspiration phase, go with the sphenoid and the maxillae into flexion and ER; during the expiration phase, go with the sphenoid and the maxillae into extension and IR.

References

1 Rohen JW. Morphologie des menschlichen Organismus, 2. Aufl. Stuttgart: Verlag freies Geistesleben; 2002:366.
2 Stone R. Polaritqätstherapie, 2. Auflage: Hugendubel; 1994:207.

8 The palatine bones

LOCATION, CAUSES AND CLINICAL PRESENTATION OF PALATINE DYSFUNCTIONS

Osseous dysfunction

a) Sphenopalatine suture:
All four constituent parts of this suture may become subject to dysfunction, but Sutherland mentions one in particular: the pterygoid notches of the sphenoid articulate with the pyramidal processes of the palatine bones, moving in grooves on the latter. The pterygoid processes converge anteriorly and separate posteriorly, so that the sphenoid spreads the small palatines in the inspiration phase and moves them into external rotation. According to Sutherland, this slight pendulum motion between the pterygoid processes of the sphenoid and these grooves on the palatines is particularly important for the effective transmission of motion to the palatine and maxillary bones, and also for its function as a 'speed reducer'. This mechanism is frequently disturbed, for example in SBS dysfunctions or in traumatic injuries to the face. The consequence is a restriction of the maxillary complex.

b) Other sphenopalatine sutures

c) The orbital process enters into the formation of the orbit.
Clinical presentation: Eye problems

d) Transverse palatine suture

e) Palatomaxillary suture

f) Vomeropalatine suture

g) Palatoethmoidal suture

h) Median palatine suture

Muscular dysfunction

Dysfunctions between the pyramidal and pterygoid processes and restriction of palatine bone motion can arise in cases of severe hypertonus of the lateral/medial pterygoid muscles.

a) Lateral pterygoid muscle on the external surface of the pyramidal process.

b) Medial pterygoid muscle on the posterior external margin of the pyramidal process.

c) Tensor veli palati muscle on the lower posterior region of the horizontal plate.

Nervous disturbances

a) Pterygopalatine ganglion

Cause: Blows, falling on to the frontal bone or a zygomatic bone, or falling on to the upper jaw may push the small palatine bone into the ganglion, leaving less space for the ganglion and impairing its function.

Clinical presentation: Functional disturbances of the lacrimal gland, and of the small glands of the nasopharyngeal space and palate, olfactory disturbance due to dryness of the nasal mucosae.

b) Maxillary nerve

The maxillary nerve extends into the orbit from the foramen rotundum via the pterygopalatine fossa and inferior orbital fissure. There it detours the small orbital process of the palatine bone, and then first passes into the maxillary canal before arriving at the surface. This small appendage to the palatine bone acts like a tension regulator for this nerve, so that it is not subjected to excessive tensile forces during the slight movements of the primary respiratory rhythm.

Clinical presentation: Paresthesias of the mid-facial region, etc.

c) Major and minor palatine nerves

Causes: Blows or falling onto the upper jaw, resulting in a dysfunction of the transverse palatine suture and palatomaxillary suture.

Clinical presentation: Disturbances of sensitivity and pain in the mucosa of the hard and soft palate.

d) Pharyngeal branch of maxillary nerve dysfunction in the sphenopalatine suture, particularly in the palatovaginal canal.

Sensory disturbance of the pharyngeal mucosa

Vascular disturbances

Symptoms in the vessels listed below are only rarely induced solely by palatine dysfunction.

a) Descending palatine artery (branch of the middle meningeal artery): in the greater palatine canal.

b) Sphenopalatine artery (branch of maxillary artery): in the sphenopalatine foramen.

c) Ascending pharyngeal artery (branch of maxillary artery): in the palatovaginal canal.

Causes of dysfunctions of the palatines

Primary dysfunction

- Intraosseous
- Traumatic injury: blows, dental extractions, poor masticatory habits, or other examples of force affecting the upper jaw can lead to restrictions of maxillary and palatine motion, and of the motion of the pterygopalatine ganglion.

Secondary dysfunction

- Due to dysfunction of the sphenoid (e.g. in association with SBS dysfunctions) and of the maxilla.
- Developmental disturbances of the cranial base at the embryonic stage lead to developmental disturbances of the palatine bone.
- In combination with dysfunction of the temporomandibular joint (see Muscular dysfunction).

Examination and techniques

- History-taking
- Visual assessment
- Palpation of the position
- Palpation of the PRM rhythm
- Motion testing
- General mobilization of the palatine
- Sphenopalatine (pterygopalatine) suture
- Pterygopalatine ganglion
- Transverse palatine and palatomaxillary suture, see The Maxillae
- Median palatine suture

DIAGNOSIS

History-taking

Nasal symptoms (rhinitis, sinusitis, hayfever), oral or pharyngeal symptoms, ocular symptoms, asthma.

Visual assessment

- Palate: lowered/flat (ER of maxilla and palatine)
- Palate: elevated (IR of maxilla and palatine)
- Unilaterally lowered or elevated palate: torsion or lateroflexion-rotation of SBS.

Palpation of the position

Horizontal plate: lowered (ER) or elevated (IR).

Palpation of primary respiration *(Figs 8.1a,b)*

- Biomechanical/biodynamic palpation, motion testing as required.
- If palpation reveals a restriction, the therapist may induce an impulse in the direction of the restriction. This will emphasize it, making it easier to sense from which structure it originates.

Figure 8.1 (a,b) Palpation of primary respiration of the palatine bones

(a)
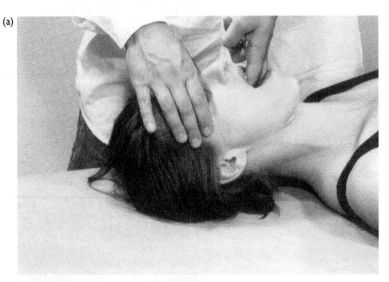

(b)
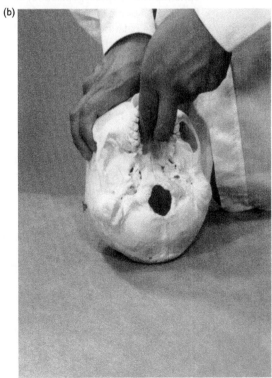

Therapist: Take up a position beside the patient's head.
Hand position: Cranial hand:

> ➤ Span the greater wings with your thumb and your middle or index finger.

Caudal hand:

> ➤ Place your index and middle fingers intraorally, one on either horizontal plate of the palatine bone laterally to the median palatine suture.
> ➤ To position them exactly, slide the fingers along the medial margin of the upper molars. Just behind the last molars, position them slightly medially on the hard palate.
> ➤ For the unilateral test, only the index finger of the caudal hand is positioned intraorally on the horizontal plate of one palatine bone (see Fig. 8.4).

Biomechanical approach
- An external rotation of the palatine bone occurs during the inspiration phase.
- The horizontal plate moves down; the median palatine suture moves downward and posterior. The transverse diameter increases.
- The orbital process and sphenoid process move inferior, following the body of the sphenoid.
- The pyramidal process moves outward and in a downward and posterior direction, following the pterygoid process of the sphenoid.
- The sphenoid lowers the palatine bone via the pterygoid process and the vomer.
> ➤ With your cranial hand, passively follow the motion of the SBS into extension and flexion.
> ➤ With your caudal hand, you will be able to sense whether the palatine bone moves in harmony with the motion of the SBS.

Inspiration phase, normal finding (Fig. 8.2):

> ➤ The horizontal plate moves inferior (and somewhat laterally).

Expiration phase, normal finding:

> ➤ The horizontal plate moves superior (and somewhat medially).

Biodynamic/embryological approach
Inspiration phase, normal finding (Fig. 8.3):

> ➤ The hands may perceive a force on the palatines in an anterior, inferior direction.

Expiration phase, normal finding:

> ➤ The hands may perceive a force on the palatines in a posterior, superior direction.
> ➤ Compare the amplitude, strength, ease and symmetry of the motion of the palatines.

Figure 8.2 PR inspiration phase/biomechanical approach

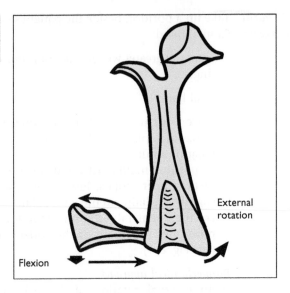

Flexion

External rotation

Figure 8.3 PR inspiration phase/biodynamic approach

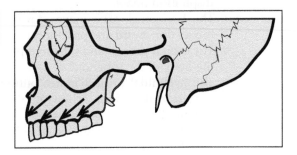

➤ Other types of motion of the palatine bones may sometimes occur during external and internal rotation. These provide an indication as to further dysfunctions of the particular palatine involved.
➤ Palatine dysfunctions may be unilateral or bilateral, symmetrical or asymmetrical.

Motion testing

Hand position: As above.
Method: Testing of ER and IR.
During the inspiration phase:

➤ With your middle finger and thumb, deliver an impulse caudad to the greater wings (motion into flexion).
➤ With the index and middle fingers that are on the horizontal plates, you will perceive a minute inferior motion in response to this pressure.

During the expiration phase:

➤ With your middle finger and thumb, deliver an impulse in a cephalad direction (motion into extension).

➤ With the index and middle fingers that are on the horizontal plates, you will perceive a minute superior motion in response to this pressure.
➤ Compare the amplitude and the ease of motion of the palatine under consideration, or the force needed to bring about motion.

TREATMENT OF THE PALATINE BONES

The sphenoid and the maxilla not infrequently need to be corrected before treating the palatine.

General mobilization of the palatine bones *(Fig. 8.4)*

Therapist: Stand beside the patient's head.
Hand position: Cranial hand:

➤ Span the greater wings with your thumb and your middle or index finger.

Caudal hand:

➤ Place your index finger intraorally on the horizontal plate of the palatine, laterally to the median palatine suture.
➤ To position it exactly, slide the index finger along the medial margin of the upper molars. Just behind the last molar, position the finger slightly medially on the hard palate.

Method: Cranial hand:

➤ Establish the PBMT of the sphenoid. Hold the sphenoid in PBMT.

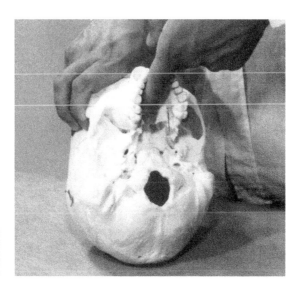

Figure 8.4 General mobilization of the palatine bone

Caudal hand:

➤ With your index finger, apply pressure in a superior direction (release from the maxilla).

➤ Then, using your index finger, administer traction in a lateral direction (release from the opposite palatine).

➤ Now administer gentle traction medially using your index finger.

➤ Finally, lower your index finger and administer a degree of traction in an inferior direction.

At the end of the technique, the motion of the palatine bone should be re-synchronized with the motion of the sphenoid in harmony with the PRM rhythm.

➤ During the inspiration phase, go with the sphenoid and palatine into flexion and ER (greater wing of the sphenoid inferior, horizontal plate inferior).

➤ During the expiration phase, go with the sphenoid and the palatine into extension and IR (greater wing of the sphenoid superior, horizontal plate superior).

Note: Proceed only very gently, especially in the case of a cranially directed impulse, as there is otherwise a risk of restricting the palate.

Alternative hand position: (Fig. 8.5)

Therapist: Stand at the head of the patient.

Hand position: Bilateral.

➤ Position the index fingers of both hands intraorally one on either side, on the horizontal plates of the palatines laterally to the median palatine suture.

Method: As above, except that the sphenoid is not involved and the two palatines are mobilized simultaneously.

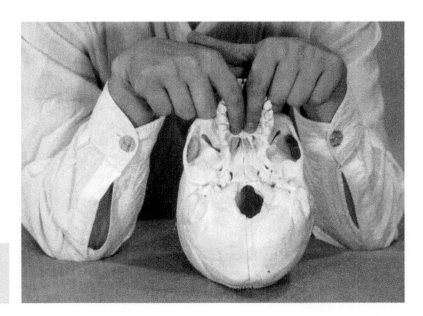

Figure 8.5 General mobilization of the palatine bone. Alternative hand position

Sphenopalatine suture *(Fig. 8.6)*

Suture margin:
- The lower lateral surface of the body of the sphenoid articulates with the sphenoid process of the palatine bone.
- The bottom anterior corner of the sphenoid body articulates with the orbital process of the palatine.
- The anterior margin of the medial plate of the sphenoid pterygoid process articulates with the posterior margin of the palatine perpendicular plate.
- The pterygoid notch articulates with the pyramidal process of the palatine.

Suture type: (All four joints):
Plane suture. (The technique releases in particular the pterygoid notch of the sphenoid from the pyramidal process of the palatine.)

Patient: Supine.

Therapist: Stand beside the patient's head, on the opposite side to the dysfunction.

Hand position: Cranial hand:

➤ Span the greater wings with your thumb and your middle or index finger.

Caudal hand:

➤ Position the index finger intraorally on the horizontal plate of the palatine (at the height of the last molar) on the dysfunctional side.

Method: Disengagement:

➤ Move the palatine anterolaterally, to release the pyramidal process from the pterygoid notch.
➤ At the same time, guide the greater wings caudad (flexion).

Establishing the PBMT:

➤ Maintain the disengagement, while at the same time establishing the PBMT between the sphenoid and the palatine.

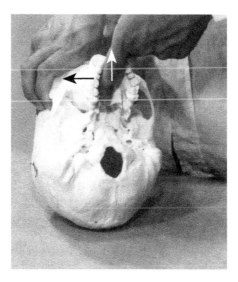

Figure 8.6 Sphenopalatine suture

➤ Follow the sphenoid in the direction of greater motion (in the motion axes of flexion/extension, torsion and side bending-rotation, etc.).
➤ Move it just far enough in these directions for the membrane tensions (between flexion and extension, torsion right and left, etc.) to be in the best possible reciprocal balance.
➤ Follow the palatine in the directions of greater motion (of ease).
➤ Follow it just far enough in these directions for the tensions on the sphenopalatine suture to be in the best possible reciprocal balance.
➤ This makes it possible for a new tension equilibrium to be established between palatine and sphenoid.
➤ Establish the PBFT.
➤ Maintain the PBT until the abnormal tension has corrected itself and the inherent homeostatic forces (PRM rhythm etc.) have stabilized.
➤ Breathing assistance: The patient can assist as follows: at the end of an in-breath, hold the inhalation for as long as possible, while performing a plantar flexing of both feet. Repeat for several breathing cycles.
➤ A fluid impulse may be used to direct energy from the opposite parietal tuber.

Median palatine suture *(Fig. 8.7)*

Therapist: Stand beside the patient's head.
Hand position: Cranial hand:

➤ Span the greater wings with your thumb and your middle or index finger.

Caudal hand:

➤ Position your index and middle fingers intraorally one on either side, on the horizontal plates of the palatines.

Method: Disengagement:

➤ Immobilize the greater wings in the neutral position.
➤ Spread the index and middle fingers of your caudal hand to gently disengage the suture.
➤ Permit all palatine motions/tissue unwinding without reducing the gentle disengagement.
➤ With each release of the tissues, seek the new limit of motion of the palatines laterally.

Establishing the PBT:

➤ Maintain the disengagement while establishing the PBMT between the sphenoid and the palatine – the position in which the abnormal tensions in the joints are in the best possible reciprocal balance – and the PBFT.
➤ Breathing assistance: The patient can assist as follows: at the end of an in-breath, hold the inhalation for as long as possible, while

Figure 8.7 Median palatine suture

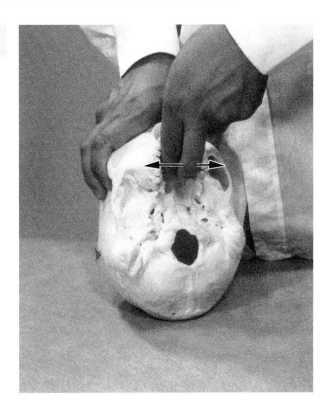

performing a plantar flexing of both feet. Repeat for several breathing cycles.

➤ A fluid impulse may be used to direct energy from the mid-line.

➤ At the end of the technique, the motion of the palatine should be re-synchronized with the motion of the sphenoid in harmony with primary respiration.

➤ During the inspiration phase, go with the sphenoid and the palatines into flexion and ER; during the expiration phase, go with the sphenoid and the palatines into extension and IR.

9 The zygomatic bones

THE MORPHOLOGY OF THE ZYGOMATIC BONE ACCORDING TO ROHEN[1]

In its motion dynamics, the zygomatic bone corresponds to the clavicle. The relationship between the maxilla and the neurocranium, with interposition of the zygomatic bone, is analogous to the separation of the upper limb and thorax by the clavicle. By connecting the maxilla to the frontal and temporal bones, the zygoma links the expressivity of the three bones and thus plays a crucial role in physiognomic expression. It serves to integrate the viscerocranium and neurocranium or, to be more precise, the viscerocranium, skull-cap and cranial base. Binocular vision, the means by which we receive an accurate image of our environment, is possible only as a result of the evolutionary forward migration of the eyes; laterally, the zygomatic bone forms a border between the orbit and the temporal sinus.

LOCATION, CAUSES AND CLINICAL PRESENTATION OF DYSFUNCTIONS OF THE ZYGOMATIC BONE

Osseous dysfunction

The zygomatic bone links the bones of the face to the temporal bone via the intermediary of the sphenoid and under the influence of the occiput. Its relationship with the four bones which surround it, is thus one of integration and balance.

a) Sphenozygomatic suture

Causes: Falling on or a blow to the cheek, and SBS dysfunctions.

b) Temporozygomatic suture

Causes: Falling on or a blow to the cheek, and SBS dysfunctions.

The sliding motion of the zygomatic and temporal processes at the temporozygomatic suture integrates the influences of the sphenoid and occiput. If the suture is compressed, the mobility relative to the temporal bone is restricted.

Sequelae: Impaired mobility of the temporal and zygomatic bones.

Blocking of the temporozygomatic suture could result in the zygomatic process of the temporal bone being unable to slide downward and outward with the temporal process of the zygomatic bone during the inspiration phase. This would obstruct the temporal bone in internal rotation during the inspiration phase. *Remember*: The zygomatic bone is largely influenced by the sphenoid, while the temporal bone is influenced by the occiput.

c) Frontozygomatic suture

Clinical presentation: Orbital disturbance, resulting in visual impairment.

d) Zygomaticomaxillary suture

Causes: Falling, or a blow to the face.

Clinical presentation: Orbital disturbance, disturbance of the maxillary sinus, resulting in sinusitis.

Muscular dysfunction

Masseter muscle

Sequelae: Restriction of the mobility of the zygomatic bone.

Fascial dysfunction

Masseteric fascia, temporal fascia.

Causes: Tension in the anterior cervicocranial fascias and dysfunction of visceral structures.

Sequelae: Restriction of the mobility of the zygomatic bone.

Causes of dysfunctions of the zygomatic bone

Primary dysfunction

- Intraosseous
- Traumatic injury: falling on and blows to the zygomatic bone

Secondary dysfunction

- Due to dysfunction of the frontal bone, temporal bone and maxilla, more rarely due to dysfunction of the sphenoid and occipital bone.

Examination and techniques

- History-taking
- Visual assessment
- Palpation of the position
- Palpation of primary respiration
- Motion testing
- Rotation dysfunction
- Decompression of the zygomatic bone
- Sphenozygomatic suture
- Frontozygomatic suture, see The Frontal bones
- Temporozygomatic suture, see The Temporal bones
- Zygomaticomaxillary suture, see The Maxillae

DIAGNOSIS

History-taking

Falling on or blows to the zygomatic bone; in rare cases very frequent supporting of the head on the hand at the zygomatic bone can lead to a dysfunction.

Visual assessment

- Zygomatic bone: prominent (ER) or recessive (IR)
- Orbital diameter: enlarged (ER) or reduced (IR)

Palpation of the position

- Zygomatic bone: prominent (ER) or recessive (IR)
- Eye margin: everted (ER) or inverted (IR)
- Temporozygomatic suture: downward, outward and slightly anterior (ER), or upward, inward and slightly posterior (IR)

Palpation of primary respiration *(Fig. 9.1)*

- Biomechanical/biodynamic palpation, motion testing as required.
- If palpation reveals a restriction, the therapist may induce an impulse in the direction of the restriction. This will emphasize it, making it easier to sense from which structure it originates.

Therapist: Take up a position at the head of the patient.

Hand position:
- Your two thumbs should touch one another and form a fulcrum.
- Position the index fingers, middle fingers and ring fingers of both hands on the two zygomatic bones. Place your index fingers on the maxillary processes, your middle fingers on the lower margins and your ring fingers on the posterior margins of the zygomatic bones.

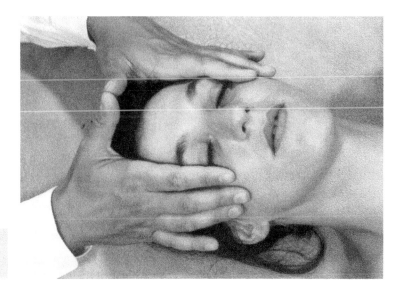

Figure 9.1 Palpation of primary respiration of the zygomatic bones

Figure 9.2 (a,b) Palpation of primary respiration of the zygomatic bones. Alternative hand position

(a)

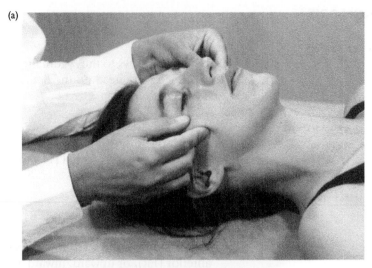

(b)

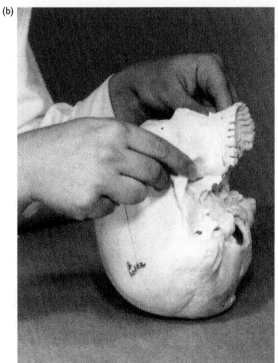

Alternative hand position: (Figs 9.2a,b)

➤ Place your thumbs anterior on the two frontal processes of the zygomatic bones (on the orbital margins).
➤ Place your index fingers on the posterior-inferior margins of the two zygomatic bones.
➤ Position your middle fingers posterior on the frontal processes of the two zygomatic bones (on the posterior-superior margins).

Biomechanical approach

- During the inspiration phase, an external rotation of the zygomatic bone occurs.
- The motion of the zygomatic bone is induced by the sphenoid via the sphenoidal greater wings. It is also dependent upon the movement of the frontal bone, maxilla and temporal bone.
- The orbital surface moves anterior, outward and slightly downward (influenced by the sphenoid).
- This results in enlargement of the orbit at the diameter running from an inside, upper position to an outside, lower position. The angle between zygomatic bone and frontal bone is also increased.
- The temporal process moves in an outward, downward and slightly anterior direction, while the zygomatic process of the temporal bone moves outward, downward and slightly posterior. The sliding motion of the two processes at the temporozygomatic suture integrates the influences of sphenoid and occipital bone.

Inspiration phase of the PR, normal finding (Fig. 9.3): ER

➤ The maxillary process moves in a lateral, anterior and slightly superior direction.
➤ The frontal process moves anterolaterally.
➤ The posterior-inferior margin moves inferiorly and medially.

Expiration phase of the PR, normal finding: IR

➤ The maxillary process moves in a medial, posterior and slightly inferior direction.
➤ The frontal process moves posteriorly and medially.
➤ The posterior-inferior margin moves superiorly and laterally.

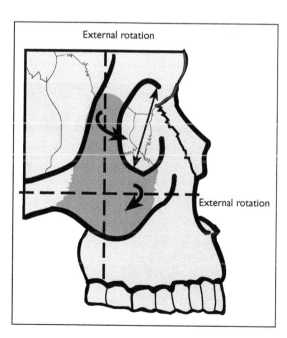

Figure 9.3 PR inspiration phase: biomechanical approach

Biodynamic/embryological approach

Inspiration phase of the PR, normal finding (Fig. 9.4):

➤ The zygomatic bone and maxilla move in an anterior, inferior direction.

Expiration phase of the PR, normal finding:

➤ The zygomatic bone and the maxilla move in a posterior, superior direction.
➤ Compare the amplitude, strength, ease and symmetry of the motion of the zygomatic bone.
➤ Other types of zygomatic bone motion may sometimes occur during external and internal rotation. These provide an indication as to further dysfunctions of the particular zygomatic bone involved.
➤ Zygomatic-bone dysfunctions may be unilateral or bilateral, symmetrical or asymmetrical.

Alternative hand position, unilateral: (Fig. 9.5)

Therapist: Take up a position at the head of the patient on the side to be tested.

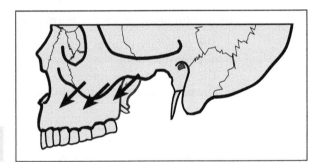

Figure 9.4 PR inspiration phase: biodynamic approach

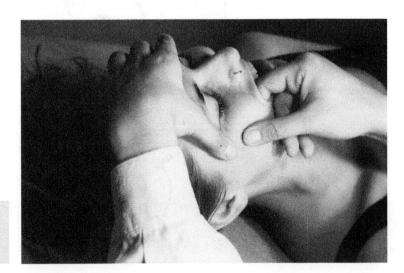

Figure 9.5 Palpation of primary respiration of the zygomatic bones. Alternative hand position, unilateral

Hand position: Cranial hand:

> ➤ Span the greater wings with your thumb and your middle or index finger.

Caudal hand:

> ➤ Position your index finger intraorally on the inner surface of the zygomatic bone.
> ➤ Place your thumb on the outer surface of the zygomatic bone.

Method: ➤ With your cranial hand, passively follow the motion of the SBS into extension and flexion.
> ➤ With your caudal hand, you will be able to sense whether the zygomatic bone moves in harmony with the motion of the SBS.

Inspiration phase, normal finding: ER

> ➤ The maxillary process moves in an anterolateral and slightly superior direction.
> ➤ The frontal process moves anterolaterally.

Expiration phase, normal finding: IR

> ➤ The maxillary process moves in a medial, posterior and slightly inferior direction.
> ➤ The frontal process moves in a medial, posterior direction.

Motion testing

Hand position: As above.
Method: Testing of ER and IR.
During the inspiration phase: ➤ On the frontal processes and maxillary processes, direct an impulse in an anterolateral direction.
> ➤ On the lower margin of the zygomatic bone, direct an impulse medially and superior.

During the expiration phase:

> ➤ On the frontal processes and maxillary processes, direct an impulse medially and posterior.
> ➤ On the lower margin of the zygomatic bone, direct an impulse laterally and inferior.
> ➤ Compare the amplitude and the ease of motion, or the force needed to bring about motion at the zygomatic bones.

TREATMENT OF THE ZYGOMATIC BONES

Rotation dysfunction *(Fig. 9.6)*

Therapist: Take up a position at the head of the patient, somewhat away from the side of the dysfunction.

Figure 9.6 Rotation dysfunction

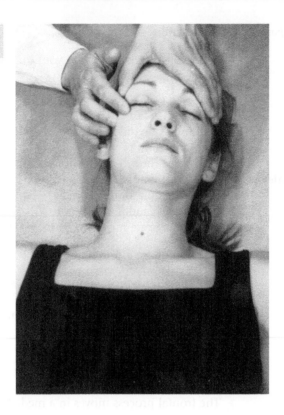

Hand position: Hand on the frontal bone:

> Span the frontal bone with your thumb and middle finger (and/or index finger), by hooking them firmly around the outside of the zygomatic processes of the frontal bone.

Hand on the dysfunctional side on the zygomatic bone:

> Position your index finger on the orbital margin.
> Place your middle finger on the posterior-inferior margin of the zygomatic bone.

Method: Establishing the PBMT:

> With the hand that is on the frontal bone, passively follow the motion of the frontal bone into extension and flexion.

During the inspiration phase, follow the ER of the zygomatic bone.

> The index finger on the frontal process and maxillary process follows anteriorly and laterally.
> The middle finger on the lower margin follows inferiorly and medially.

During the expiration phase, follow the IR of the zygomatic bone.

> The index finger on the maxillary process follows in a medial, posterior and slightly inferior direction.

➤ The middle finger on the frontal process follows posteriorly and medially.

➤ The PBMT is the position between ER and IR in which the abnormal tensions on the joints are in the best possible reciprocal balance. Establish the PBFT.

➤ Maintain the PBT until a correction of the abnormal tension has been achieved and the inherent homeostatic forces (PRM rhythm, etc.) have stabilized.

➤ At the end of the technique, the motion of the zygomatic bone should be re-synchronized with the sphenoid motion in harmony with the PRM rhythm.

➤ During the inspiration phase, go with the sphenoid and the palatine bones into flexion and ER; during the expiration phase, go with the sphenoid and the palatine bones into extension and IR.

Biodynamic approach

Encourage the spontaneous occurrence of a still point or corrective inspiration phase, external rotation and expansion or expiration phase, internal rotation and retraction of the zygomatic bone, by means of palpation, carried out in a state of relaxed, non-invasive attention and empathy. Synchronize this treatment with the inherent homeodynamic forces and rhythmic patterns. This approach requires no encounter or confrontation with tissue resistances and no inhibition of any phase of primary respiration.

Alternative hand position: (Fig. 9.7)

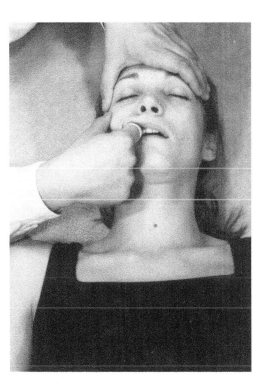

Figure 9.7 Rotation dysfunction. Alternative hand position

Therapist: Take up a position at the head of the patient somewhat away from the side of the dysfunction.

Hand position: Hand on the frontal bone:

> Span the frontal bone with your thumb and middle finger (and/or index finger), by hooking them firmly around the outside of the zygomatic processes of the frontal bone.

Hand on the zygomatic bone on the dysfunctional side:

> Position your index finger intraorally on the lower margin of the zygomatic bone.
> Place your thumb outside, on the zygomatic bone. Grasp the zygomatic bone with your two fingers.

Method: As above.

Decompression of the zygomatic bone *(Fig. 9.8)*

Therapist: Take up a position beside the patient's head, on the same side as the dysfunction.

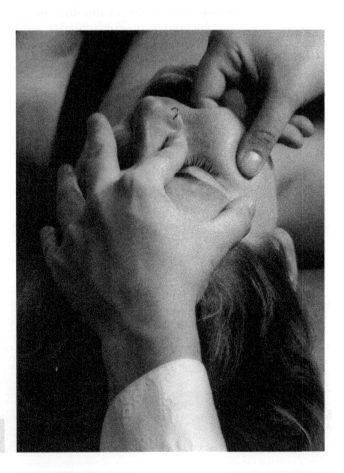

Figure 9.8 Decompression of the zygomatic bone

Hand position: Cranial hand:

> ➤ Span the frontal bone with your thumb and ring finger.
> ➤ Also position your thumb on the greater wing on the affected side.
> ➤ Place your index finger on the frontal process of the maxilla on the affected side.

Caudal hand:

> ➤ Place your index finger intraorally, on the lower margin of the zygomatic bone.
> ➤ Place your thumb outside, on the zygomatic bone. Grasp the zygomatic bone with your two fingers.

Method: ➤ Hold the frontal bone and sphenoid and the maxillae firmly in the neutral position. While doing this, administer laterally-directed traction on the zygomatic bone.
> ➤ Permit all motions/tissue unwinding without reducing the traction.
> ➤ Establish the PBMT, PBFT.

Sphenozygomatic suture *(Fig. 9.9)*

Suture margin: The anterior-directed zygomatic process joins the anterior margin of the greater wing.
Suture type: Serrated suture.
Therapist: Take up a position beside the patient's head, on the opposite side to the dysfunction.
Hand position: Cranial hand:

> ➤ Span the greater wings with your thumb and your middle finger.
> ➤ Place your index finger on the zygomatic process of the frontal bone.

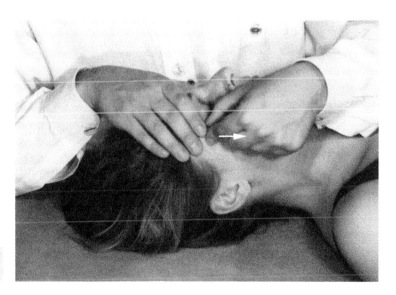

Figure 9.9
Sphenozygomatic suture

Caudal hand:

➤ Grasp the frontal process of the zygomatic bone with your thumb and index finger.

Method: *a)* Disengagement:

Cranial hand:

➤ Hold the sphenoid firmly in the neutral position. Similarly, hold the affected side of the zygomatic process of the frontal bone in position with your index fingers.

Caudal hand:

➤ At the same time, administer traction on the zygomatic bone caudad with your thumb and index finger.
➤ Permit all motions/tissue unwinding without reducing the traction.

b) Direct technique

➤ A dysfunction in ER is treated by going with the sphenoid into the extension position during the expiration phase and holding it there.
➤ A dysfunction in IR is treated by going with the sphenoid into flexion during the inspiration phase and holding it there.

c) Establishing the PBT

➤ Maintain the gentle disengagement while you establish the PBMT of the zygomatic bone – the position between ER and IR in which the abnormal tensions on the joints are in the best possible reciprocal balance – and the PBFT.
➤ Maintain the PBT until a correction of the abnormal tension has been achieved and the inherent homeostatic forces (primary respiration, etc.) have stabilized.
➤ A fluid impulse may be used to direct energy from the opposite lambdoid suture or caudad of it.

Note: An exaggeration technique may be indicated, rather than a direct technique.

➤ If the dysfunction is in ER, go with the sphenoid into flexion during the inspiration phase and hold it there.
➤ In the case of a dysfunction in IR, go with the sphenoid into extension during the expiration phase and hold it there.

Alternative hand position: (see Fig. 9.5)
Patient: The patient's head is turned toward the opposite side from the dysfunction.
Therapist: Take up a position beside the patient's head, on the same side as the dysfunction.
Hand position: Cranial hand:

➤ Span the greater wings with your thumb and middle finger.

Caudal hand:

> ➤ Grasp the zygomatic bone, by placing your thumb outside on the zygomatic bone and your index finger on the zygomatic bone from inside (intraorally).

Temporozygomatic suture *(Fig. 9.10)*

Suture margin: The posterior-directed temporal process of the zygomatic bone joins the zygomatic process of the temporal bone.

Suture type: Serrated suture.

Patient: The patient's head is turned toward the opposite side from the dysfunction.

Therapist: Take up a position beside the patient's head, on the opposite side from the dysfunction.

Hand position: Cranial hand on the temporal bone:

> ➤ Grasp the zygomatic process with your thumb and index finger.
> ➤ Position your middle finger in the external acoustic meatus.
> ➤ Place your ring finger on the mastoid process.
> ➤ Place your little finger on the mastoid portion.

Caudal hand on the zygomatic bone:

> ➤ Grasp the temporal process of the zygomatic bone with your index finger and thumb.

Method: Disengagement:

> ➤ Administer traction posterior with the index finger and thumb that are on the temporal bone.
> ➤ Administer traction anterior with the index finger and thumb that are on the zygomatic bone.

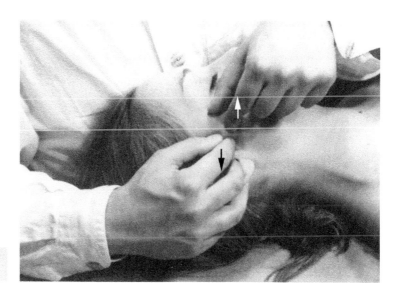

Figure 9.10
Temporozygomatic suture

➤ Permit all motions/tissue unwinding that occur.

➤ Hold this position until you sense a release of the tension at the suture.

Direct technique

➤ Hold the zygomatic bone gently in position. During the inspiration phase, go with the temporal bone into an external rotation and hold it there.

➤ Establish the PBMT, PBFT.

At the end of the technique, the motion of the zygomatic bone should be re-synchronized with the temporal-bone motion in harmony with the PRM rhythm.

➤ During the inspiration phase, go with the temporal bone and zygomatic bone into ER; during the expiration phase, go with the temporal bone and zygomatic bone into IR.

➤ A fluid impulse may be used to direct energy from the opposite lambdoid suture or caudad of it.

Reference

1 Rohen JW. Morphologie des menschlichen Organismus, 2. Aufl. Stuttgart: Verlag freies Geistesleben; 2002:367.

10 The nasal bones, lacrimal bones and inferior nasal conchae

THE NASAL BONES

> ### Causes of dysfunctions of the nasal bones
>
> #### Primary dysfunction
> - The primary cause as a rule is traumatic injury due to blows, falls or a tightly-fitting glasses frame.
>
> #### Secondary dysfunction
> - Secondarily due to dysfunction of the maxilla and frontal bone.
>
> #### Examination and techniques
> - History-taking
> - Visual assessment and palpation of the position
> - Palpation of primary respiration
> - Motion testing
> - Global technique of the nasal bone
> - Frontonasal suture
> - Nasomaxillary suture, see The Maxillae (lift and spread technique)
> - Internasal suture

DIAGNOSIS

History-taking

Disturbance of nasal secretion and nasal breathing, prior traumatic injuries

Visual assessment and palpation of the position

➤ Asymmetric nasal bones
➤ Painful nasal-bone cranial sutures

Palpation of primary respiration *(Fig. 10.1)*

Therapist: Take up a position at the head of the patient.

Hand position: ➤ Position your index fingers on both sides of the nose, one on each nasal bone.

➤ Rest the other fingers passively on the cranium.

Figure 10.1 Palpation of primary respiration of the nasal bones

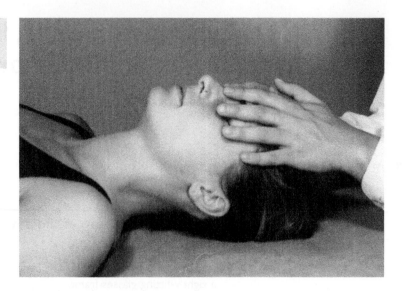

Alternative hand position: (see Fig. 10.3)

Therapist: Take up a position beside the patient's head.

Hand position: Cranial hand:

➤ Place your cranial hand on the frontal bone with your middle finger on the metopic suture, immediately above the frontonasal suture.
➤ Position your index and ring fingers next to the middle finger.

Caudal hand:

➤ Place your thumb and index finger one on either nasal bone.

Biomechanical approach
● During the inspiration phase, an external rotation of the nasal bone occurs.
● The nasal bone is influenced by the frontal bone and maxilla and, via them, by the sphenoid.

Inspiration phase of the PR, normal finding (Fig. 10.2): ER

➤ The internasal suture moves posterior.

Expiration phase of the PR, normal finding: IR

➤ The internasal suture moves anterior.
➤ Compare the amplitude, strength, ease and symmetry of the motion of the nasal bones.
➤ Other types of motion of the nasal bones may sometimes occur during external and internal rotation. These provide an indication as to further dysfunctions of the particular nasal bone involved.
➤ Nasal bone dysfunctions may be unilateral or bilateral, symmetrical or asymmetrical.

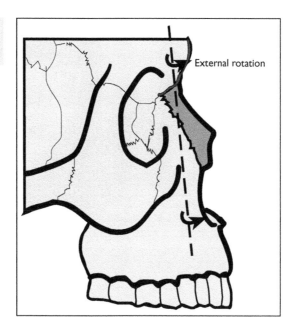

Figure 10.2 Inspiration phase of the PR/biomechanical approach

External rotation

Motion testing

This differs from palpation of primary respiration in one feature only: external and internal rotation of the nasal bone are now actively induced by the therapist in harmony with the PRM rhythm. Compare the amplitude and the ease of motion of the nasal bone under consideration, or the force needed to bring about motion.

TREATMENT OF THE NASAL BONES

When treating a nasal bone, it is usually necessary to treat the maxilla and frontal bone also.

Global technique to treat the nasal bones *(Fig. 10.3)*

Therapist: Take up a position beside the patient's head.

Hand position: Cranial hand:

> ➤ Place your cranial hand on the frontal bone with your middle finger on the metopic suture, immediately above the frontonasal suture.
> ➤ Place your index and ring fingers next to the middle finger.

Caudal hand:

> ➤ Place your thumb and index finger one on each nasal bone.

Method: ➤ Register the cranial movements of the frontal bone with your hand resting passively on the frontal bone.
> ➤ During the inspiration phase, deliver an impulse into ER with the thumb and index finger that are on the nasal bones.

Figure 10.3 Global technique to treat the nasal bones

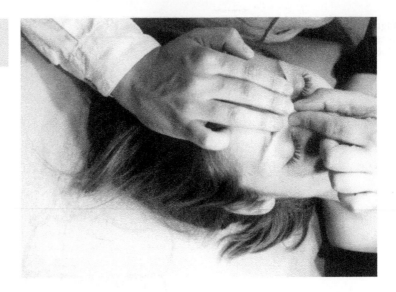

> During the expiration phase, deliver an impulse into IR with the thumb and index finger that are on the nasal bones.

Biodynamic approach

Encourage the spontaneous occurrence of a still point or corrective inspiration phase, external rotation and expansion or expiration phase, internal rotation and retraction of the nasal bone, by means of palpation, carried out in a state of relaxed, non-invasive attention and empathy. Synchronize this treatment with the inherent homeodynamic forces and rhythmic patterns. This approach requires no encounter or confrontation with tissue resistances and no inhibition of any phase of primary respiration.

Frontonasal suture

Suture margin:
> The upper margin of the nasal bone articulates with the medial portion of the nasal part of the frontal bone (serrated suture).
> The bony ridge of the nasal bone (nasal crest) articulates with the medial pointed projection (nasal spine) of the frontal bone (plane suture).

Therapist: Take up a position beside the patient's head.
Hand position: (Fig. 10.4)
Cranial hand:

> Place your cranial hand on the frontal bone. Position your index and middle fingers immediately above the frontonasal suture.

Caudal hand:

> Place your thumb and index finger one on each nasal bone.

Figure 10.4 Frontonasal suture

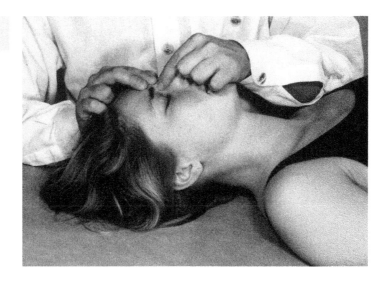

Figure 10.5 Frontonasal suture. Alternative hand position

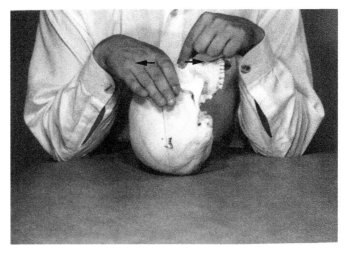

Alternative position of the cranial hand I: (Fig. 10.5)

➤ Grasp the frontal bone at the zygomatic processes with your thumb and index finger. Position the basal joint of your index finger against the glabella.

Alternative position of the cranial hand II, according to Magoun: *(Fig. 10.6)*

➤ Position your middle finger on the glabella.
➤ Place your index and ring fingers alongside the metopic suture.

Method: Disengagement:

➤ Administer gentle traction cephalad on the frontal bone.
➤ At the same time administer traction caudad on the nasal bones.
➤ Permit all motions/tissue unwinding that occur.

Figure 10.6 Frontonasal suture. Magoun's alternative hand position

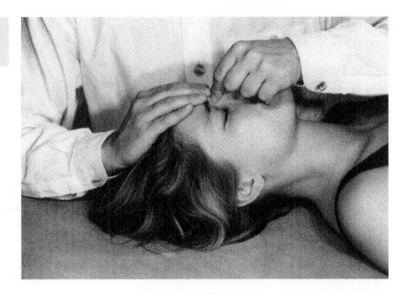

Figure 10.7 Internasal suture.

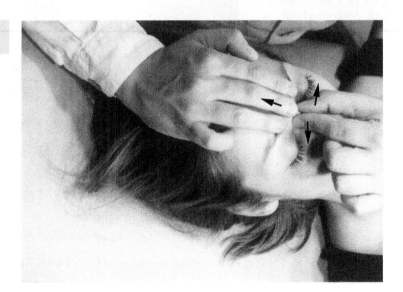

Internasal suture *(Fig. 10.7)*

Therapist: Take up a position beside the patient's head.

Hand position: Cranial hand:

> ➤ Place your cranial hand on the frontal bone with your middle finger on the metopic suture, immediately above the frontonasal suture.
> ➤ Position your index and ring fingers next to the middle finger.

Caudal hand:

> ➤ Place your thumb and index finger one on each nasal bone.

Method: Disengagement:

> ➤ Administer gentle traction cephalad on the frontal bone.
> ➤ Maintain this traction while spreading the nasal bones away from one another.
> ➤ Permit all motions/tissue unwinding that occur.

LACRIMAL BONES

Causes of dysfunctions of the lacrimal bones

Primary dysfunction

● Primary traumatic injury due to blows or falling.

Secondary dysfunction

● Secondarily due to dysfunction of the maxilla, frontal bone or ethmoid.

Examination and techniques

● History-taking
● Palpation of primary respiration
● Motion testing
● Global technique to treat the lacrimal bones
● Frontolacrimal suture
● Ethmoidolacrimal and lacrimomaxillary sutures, see The Ethmoid bone and The Maxillae

DIAGNOSIS

History-taking

Disturbance of lacrimation (nasolacrimal duct), possibly also disturbances of motion at the orbit, or disturbances of the ethmoid air cells.

Palpation of primary respiration *(Fig. 10.8)*

Therapist: Take up a position beside the patient's head on the side to be tested.

Hand position: ➤ Place your cranial hand on the frontal bone.
➤ Place the index finger of your caudal hand on the lacrimal bone.

Biomechanical approach

The lacrimal bone is influenced by the maxilla, frontal bone and ethmoid and, via these bones, by the sphenoid. During the inspiration phase it rotates slightly outward relative to the frontal process of the maxilla. The nasolacrimal duct enlarges.

Fig.10.8 Palpation of primary respiration of the lacrimal bones

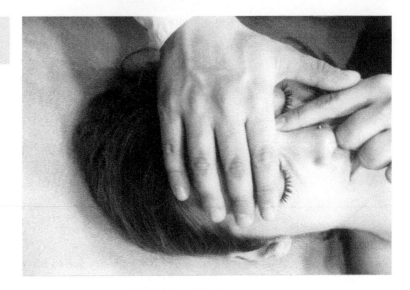

Figure 10.9 Inspiration phase of PR/biomechanical approach

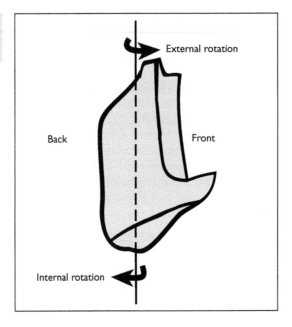

Inspiration phase, normal finding (Fig. 10.9): ER

➤ The lateral margins move anterolaterally.

Expiration phase, normal finding: IR

➤ The lateral margins move in a medial, posterior direction.

Biodynamic/embryological approach
Inspiration phase, normal finding (Fig. 10.10):

➤ Rotation of the lacrimal bone, during which its inferior portion moves in a lateral direction.

Figure 10.10 Inspiration phase of the PR/biodynamic approach

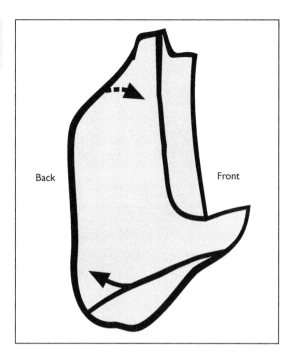

Expiration phase, normal finding:

> ➤ Rotation of the lacrimal bone, during which its inferior portion moves in a medial direction.

Motion test

This differs from palpation of primary respiration only in one feature: the external and internal rotation of the lacrimal bone are now actively induced by the therapist in harmony with primary respiration.

TREATMENT OF THE LACRIMAL BONES

When treating a lacrimal bone it is usually necessary to treat the maxilla and the frontal bone also.

Global technique to treat the lacrimal bones *(Fig. 10.11)*

Therapist: Take up a position beside the patient's head, on the side to be tested.

Hand position:
> ➤ Place your cranial hand across the frontal bone.
> ➤ Position the index and middle fingers of your cranial hand on the upper orbital margins, as close as possible to the frontolacrimal suture.
> ➤ Place the index finger of your caudal hand on the lacrimal bone.

Method:
> ➤ Register the cranial motion of the frontal bone with your hand resting passively on it.
> ➤ During the inspiration phase, with your index finger direct an impulse into ER on the lacrimal bone.

Figure 10.11 Global technique to treat the lacrimal bones

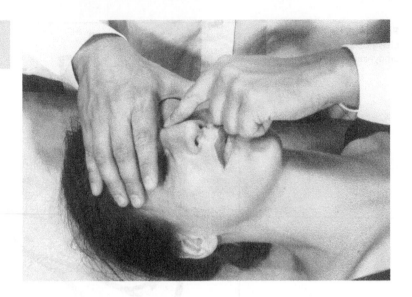

➤ During the expiration phase, with your index finger direct an impulse into IR on the lacrimal bone.

Alternative method: ➤ During the inspiration phase, with your index and middle fingers begin to tilt the frontal bone (flexion), while applying pressure on the glabella in a posterior and superior direction with the basal joint of your index finger (ER).

➤ Hold the frontal bone in flexion and ER, while directing impulses into ER and IR on the lacrimal bone in harmony with the PRM rhythm.

Biodynamic approach

Encourage the spontaneous occurrence of a still point or corrective inspiration phase, external rotation and expansion or expiration phase, internal rotation and retraction of the lacrimal bone, by means of palpation, carried out in a state of relaxed, non-invasive attention and empathy. Synchronize this treatment with the inherent homeodynamic forces and rhythmic patterns. This approach requires no encounter or confrontation with tissue resistances and no inhibition of any phase of primary respiration.

Frontolacrimal suture *(Fig. 10.12)*

Suture margin: The upper part of the lacrimal bone articulates with the anterior quadrant of the ethmoidal notch.

Suture type: Squamous suture.

Hand position: As above.

Method: ➤ During the inspiration phase, with your index and middle fingers begin to tilt the frontal bone (flexion), while applying pressure on the glabella in a posterior and superior direction with the basal joint of your index finger (ER).

➤ Hold the frontal bone in flexion and ER.

Figure 10.12
Frontolacrimal suture

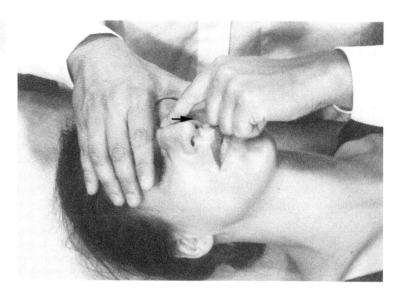

> At the same time move the lacrimal bone caudad (disengagement).
> Permit all motions/tissue unwinding of the lacrimal bone that occur.
> With each release of the suture, seek the new limit of motion of the frontal bone in the direction of external rotation and flexion.
> Establish the PBMT and PBFT.
> A fluid impulse may be used to direct energy from the occipital bone.

INFERIOR NASAL CONCHAE

Causes of dysfunctions of the inferior nasal conchae

Primary dysfunction

● Traumatic injury due to blows, operations on the nose.

Secondary dysfunction

● Secondarily, due to dysfunction of the maxilla, palatine bone and ethmoid bone, deviation of the nasal septum.

History-taking

Disturbance of nasal breathing.

TREATMENT OF THE INFERIOR NASAL CONCHAE

Dysfunctions of the inferior nasal conchae are corrected by treating the maxilla, ethmoid bone, palatine bone, and sometimes the vomer.

11

The mandible and temporomandibular joint

The temporomandibular joint (TMJ), viewed as part of the body as a whole, was the subject of attention from the beginning of osteopathy. To mention just a few examples, Still[1] and Sutherland[2] both mention techniques for the treatment of temporomandibular joint dysfunctions, while Magoun[3], Fryette[4] and Frymann[5,6] describe possible causes, and diagnostic and therapeutic methods for problems of the temporomandibular joint.

In osteopathy – in contrast to the accepted treatments of traditional medicine – considerable importance is also assigned to the temporal bones in the development of temporomandibular dysfunctions.[7,8]

Smith, Hruby and Blood[9–11] all speak of a close association between dysfunctions of the temporomandibular joint and multiple disturbances affecting the whole body.

ANATOMY OF THE TEMPOROMANDIBULAR JOINT (TMJ) *(Figs 11.1, 11.2)*

The temporomandibular joint (TMJ) plays a direct or indirect role in a number of functions, such as chewing, swallowing and sucking, articulation of sounds, breathing and facial expression. The joint is composed of the head of the mandible, which is cylindrical in shape, and the mandibular fossa and articular tubercle of the temporal bone. Between these lies the articular disk, which divides the joint into an upper and a lower compartment, the meniscotemporal and meniscocondylar joint spaces.

- Head of the mandible (condylar process of the mandible)
- Mandibular fossa and articular tubercle (temporal bone)
- Articular disk
- Articular capsule
- Ligaments
- Muscles
- Nerves

The head of the mandible *(Fig. 11.3)*

- The head of the mandible forms the cranial end of the condylar process (of the ramus of the mandible). It protrudes medially, and its surface is convex, being cylindrical or ellipsoid in shape.[12] The cartilaginous layer is highly vascularized in newborns, a feature

291

Figure 11.1 The temporomandibular joint

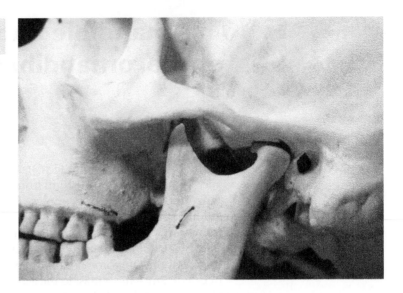

Figure 11.2 Histological section through the central region of the TMJ (preparation and photograph: Priv-Doz. Dr C. Schmolke, Anatomisches Institut, University of Bonn). From: Tillmann B. Farbatlas der Anatomie. Zahnmedizin-Humanmedizin. New York/Stuttgart: Thieme; 1997:63, Figure 150

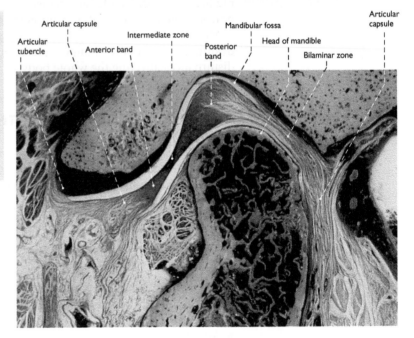

that decreases with age. There is a reduction in thickness of the cartilage at the articular head during the life of the individual.

- The anterior portion of the mandibular head is oriented anteriorly and superiorly. It is covered with fibrocartilage, and it articulates with the articular tubercle of the temporal bone. Between the two lies a disk.

- The transverse axis of the mandibular head runs from anterolateral to posteromedial, and obliquely downward. The extended axes normally intersect at the anterior border of the foramen magnum.[13]

- In its frontal and sagittal aspects the head of the mandible is convex. The two mandibular heads are seldom symmetrical. They

Figure 11.3 Right condylar process (anterior view)

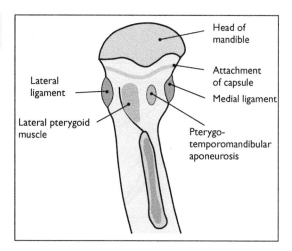

are flat at birth, and only become hemispherical when the child begins to chew and the deciduous molars appear. The head of the mandible attains its final cylindrical form when the permanent dentition is complete.[14]

● The anterior surface of the mandibular head is the main articular surface. It is covered with fibrocartilage.

● The posterior, smooth portion of the mandibular head is oriented posterosuperiorly. Although it is enclosed in the articular capsule, it does not act as part of the joint. It is covered in taut connective tissue.

● The attachment of the articular capsule runs around the condylar process.

● Below this the bone is narrower and forms the neck of the mandible.

● Immediately below the head of the mandible, on the anterior surface of the condyle, is a small depression, the fovea, for the insertion of the lateral pterygoid muscle.

The mandibular fossa and articular tubercle *(Fig. 11.4)*

● The mandibular fossa is situated on the inferior surface of the temporal squama. It is two to three times the size of the articular surface of the head of the mandible.

● Only the anterior portion of the mandibular fossa, belonging to the squamous part, forms part of the joint. It runs from the articular tubercle dorsally to the petrosquamous fissure, and measures about 19 mm in the anteroposterior direction by about 25 mm wide.

   The posterior portion does not form part of the joint. It belongs to the tympanic part, and lies outside the articular capsule. It is covered in taut connective tissue. The chorda tympani emerges at the petrotympanic fissure.[15]

● The axis of the mandibular fossa, like that of the mandibular head, runs posteromedially. In its frontal and sagittal aspects the fossa is concave.

Figure 11.4 Mandibular fossa and articular tubercle of the temporal bone

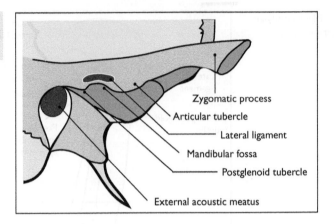

Zygomatic process
Articular tubercle
Lateral ligament
Mandibular fossa
Postglenoid tubercle
External acoustic meatus

- Anteriorly the fossa gives way to the saddle-shaped articular tubercle, which has a slanting articular surface, oriented posteriorly and inferiorly.
- The anterior part of the fossa and the tubercle are covered in fibrocartilage. The fibers are mainly collagenous and run both obliquely and parallel, from the petrotympanic fissure and the superior anterior portion of the posterior zygomatic (postglenoid) tubercle to the articular tubercle. The intermediate zone is capable of proliferation and so of initiating repair processes throughout life.
- In sagittal section the fossa and the tubercle describe an S-shaped course.

The bone architecture of the masticatory system[16–18]

The structure of the cranium makes it highly resistant to the effects of force. A number of factors contribute to this resistance: the elasticity of the bone, the buttressed structure, the tensile restraint of the dural system, the absorption of vibration by the paranasal sinuses, and the way in which the viscerocranium articulates with the skull.

The enormous forces generated by the muscles during mastication affect the anterior and middle cranial fossae in particular. The masticatory muscles exert a downward tension on the middle cranial fossa, while the pressure generated by chewing is transmitted upward by buttresses of the maxilla and mandible.

In the case of the maxilla, these are the buttress of the canine, the zygomaticomaxillary buttress and the less robust pterygomaxillary buttress. The buttress of the canine transmits the forces from the alveoli of the canine teeth around the piriform aperture to the frontal process of the maxilla and medial orbital margin. The zygomatico-maxillary buttress distributes the forces from the alveoli of the molars to the zygomatic bone. From there, they are transmitted to the frontal bone via the frontal processes of the zygomatic bones, then onward to the inferior temporal line and forward to the lateral superior roof of the orbit. A second route leads from the zygomatic bone to the zygomatic arch and articular tubercle. The pterygomaxillary buttress, which is less robust, transmits the pressure from the rear molars to the middle of the cranial base.

In the mandible, the forces are transmitted to the basal arch, which comprises the base of the mandible, the central part of the ramus and the condylar process. The bone fibers in the condylar process run in an oblique vertical direction from posterior cranial to anterior caudal. In addition to the basal arch, the mandible includes the apophysis for the insertion of the temporalis muscle, the masticatory muscle extending from the coronoid process to the body of the mandible, and the angular apophysis, on the angle of the jaw.

The course of the fibers in the temporal region of the joint is complex. In the horizontal plane the fibers are oriented along the course of the zygomatic arch. They divide at the roots of the zygomatic processes of the temporal bone. Transverse fibers continue into the infratemporal crest of the greater wings of the sphenoid, and combine with the pterygo-sphenoidal-frontal buttress. Other, longitudinally oriented fibers continue into the squamous part of the temporal bone.

In the frontal plane, the fibers run vertically and link the tabulae of the temporal bone.

The articular disk *(Figs 11.5, 11.6)*

The articular disk divides the TMJ into an upper and a lower compartment and forms the effective joint socket. The disk is biconcave and made of fibrocartilage.

There are individual variations in shape, since the disk adapts to the adjacent components of the joint.[19-22]

The central portion is shallow (1–2 mm). At the time of birth, however, it is of even thickness throughout.[23-26]

The disk consists of an anterior, central (intermediate) and posterior parts or bands. The posterior part splits into two layers to create the bilaminar zone; however, there are differences in the structure of the bands.

The peripheral parts are firmer than the central parts of the disk.[27]

- Anterior: taut connective tissue and cartilage.
- Middle: taut connective tissue.
- Posterior, superior layer: elastic connective tissue (collagen and many elastic fibers).
- Posterior, inferior layer: taut, non-elastic connective tissue.

Adjacent structures

- Anteriorly, medially and laterally the disk is connected to the articular capsule.
- Anteriorly the disk connects with the lateral pterygoid muscle.

Figure 11.5
Temporomandibular joint, sagittal section

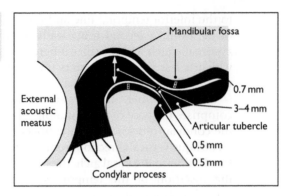

Figure 11.6 Lateral view of the right TMJ

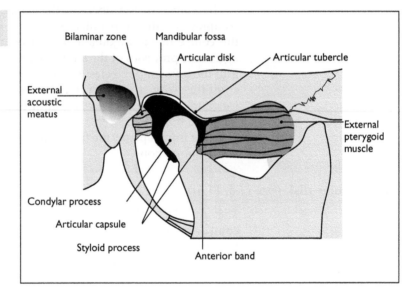

- The posterior superior layer is attached to the border of the tympanosquamous and petrosquamous fissures (discotemporal ligament).
- The posterior, inferior layer is attached to the rear aspect of the neck of the mandible (discocondylar ligament).
- Posteriorly, the bilaminar (retrodiscal) zone gives way to loose, fat-rich connective tissue through which run blood vessels including a venous plexus (the retrodiscal pad).
- This pad of tissue provides protection from pressure to the chorda tympani, which exits at the petrotympanic fissure. It also has an effect on motion in the TMJ.[28]

Embryonic development

The articular disk develops in the 7½ week *in utero*.[29]

During embryonic development it extends to penetrate the tendons of the pterygoid muscle. Posteriorly, the superior lamina is attached in the region of the petrosquamous fissure, the medial lamina moves through the fissure to the malleus and the anterior ligament of the malleus in the middle ear and the inferior lamina of the disk attaches to the condyle.

Function: The disk serves the function of evening out the difference in size and shape between the head of the mandible and the joint cavity. It improves the distribution of pressure in the joint by enlarging the effective surface, so reducing the forces on the TMJ from masticatory pressure.[30] It also serves as a movable joint cavity that changes its position with the movements of the condyle. The disk divides the joint compartment into an upper joint (gliding motion) and a lower joint (combined rotation and gliding motion). The taut discocondylar ligament maintains the disk in its location on the head of the mandible. This makes it highly important for the coordination between the disk and the condyle during movement of the jaw.

Biomechanics of the disk[31]

Physiological closing of the mouth: the disk lies centrally in the mandibular fossa. During mouth closure, a physiological position exists between the condylar process and the joint surface of the temporal bone. The retrodiscal pad is folded and the discotemporal ligament relaxes. Increased load has the effect of making the disk tend to glide posteriorly. The lateral pterygoid muscle (superior belly) opposes this motion.

● Opening of the mouth: the discotemporal ligament is stretched, preventing further opening of the mouth.
● Middle stage of mouth opening: The disk glides anteriorly in absolute terms, but posteriorly in relation to the condyle.
● Maximum opening of the mouth: The disk glides posteriorly in relation to the condyle.

The articular capsule *(Fig. 11.7)*

The articular capsule extends from the condyle to the disk and from the disk to the temporal bone, so that it is possible to distinguish an upper and a lower joint space. Only on the lateral side do true capsule

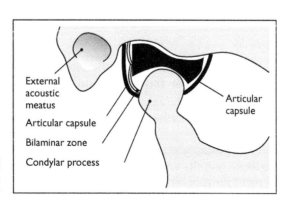

External acoustic meatus

Articular capsule

Articular capsule

Bilaminar zone

Condylar process

Figure 11.7 The capsule and disk of the TMJ

fibers run directly from the condyle to the temporal bone. The joint capsule is fairly wide, looser above and tauter below the disk.[15,32] It can be seen as a peripheral, fibrous and synovial continuation of the disk.[21]

The anterior attachment of the capsule allows plenty of room for motion to the articular head, especially in the anterior direction, and is usually able to prevent tearing of the capsule in the case of luxation.[33,34]

Attachment to the temporal bone: circular

- Anteriorly: to the tubercle. A layer of collagenous fibers runs medially. This layer can be described as a continuation of the disk or a thickening of the fascia of the lateral pterygoid muscle.
- Laterally the fibers of the disk and capsule connect with the lateral ligament of the temporomandibular joint and approach the masseter and temporalis muscles.[35]
- Medially and laterally: to the bone-cartilage boundary.
- Posteriorly: to the bone, immediately anterior to the petrotympanic fissure.

Attachment to the mandible

- Anteriorly, medially and laterally: to the bone-cartilage boundary.
- Posteriorly: to the transition between the head and the condyle.
- The posterior attachment of the joint capsule is approximately 5 mm deeper than anterior.
- Posteriorly there is transition of the capsule into the retrodiscal pad.[33]
- Fibers of the superior head of the lateral pterygoid muscle attach to the anterior side of the capsule.[33]

Note: There is no vascularization or innervation of the joint surfaces of the mandible and temporal bone, or of the disk. The articular capsule and the posterior bilaminar (retrodiscal) tissue, in contrast, are highly vascularized and richly supplied with nerves, especially nociceptors; they are therefore extremely pain-sensitive and susceptible to inflammatory processes. The anterior attachment of the disk is also vascularized and innervated, but less so than the posterior attachment.[31,33]

Ligaments *(Figs 11.8, 11.9)*

Lateral ligament of the temporomandibular joint (lateral or temporomandibular ligament)[33]

Origin: Root of the zygomatic arch of the temporal bone.

Anterior part: Surrounds the articular tubercle and runs from anterior to the tubercle on the zygomatic process of the temporal bone in an obliquely posterior direction.

Insertion: Laterally and posteriorly on the neck of the mandible.

Posterior part: Runs behind the articular tubercle on the zygomatic process.

Figure 11.8 Ligaments of the TMJ

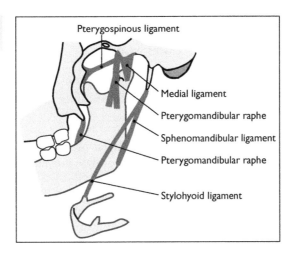

Figure 11.9 Lateral view of the right TMJ

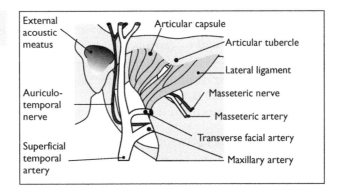

Insertion: Posteriorly and slightly inferiorly on the condyle, together with the middle and posterior part of the capsule.

Posteriorly the ligament is firmly interlinked with the articular capsule.

Function: ● Strengthens the temporomandibular joint capsule.
● Limits extreme protrusion and retrusion of the mandible.
● Resists inferior movement of the mandible as the mouth begins to open.
● Gives support during the transition from rotation to gliding movement and the reverse.
● Stabilizes the mandibular head on the operative side during molar grinding movements.

Lateral collateral ligament

The lateral collateral ligament has been distinguished from the lateral ligament of the temporomandibular joint.[36]

This ligament is fairly thin and weak. The superior part is wider than the inferior part.

Origin: Disk.
Insertion: Condyle.
Function: Controls jaw movement.

Medial (collateral) ligament

This ligament is significantly thicker than the lateral collateral ligament.

Origin: Disk.
Insertion: Medially on the condylar process.
Function: Supports and limits condyle movement.

Stylomandibular ligament

Origin: Styloid process of the temporal bone.
Insertion: Posterior border of the angle of the mandible; fascia of medial pterygoid muscle.
Function: ● Limits protrusion.
● Reinforces the parotid fascia and masseteric fascia.

Sphenomandibular ligament: thin, broad ligament, medial to capsule

Origin: Spine of the sphenoid.
Insertion: Lingula of the mandible, mandibular foramen on the medial surface of the ramus.
Function: Limits inferior movement and protrusion of the mandible.

Pterygomandibular raphe

Origin: Pterygoid hamulus of the sphenoid.
Insertion: Internal surface of the body of the mandible, above the mylohyoid line.
Function: Limits extreme movements of the mandible.

Tanaka ligament[33]

Origin: Medial ligament.
Insertion: Wall of the middle fossa, immediately posterior to the attachment of the superior part of the lateral pterygoid muscle to the disk.
Course: Medially and slightly anteriorly.
Function: Provides medial reinforcement; holding function during the anterior and posterior movement of the disk.

Anterior ligament of the malleus

Origin: Anterior process of the malleus in the middle ear.
Insertion: ● Petrotympanic fissure; a few fibers run to the spine of the sphenoid and onward with the sphenomandibular ligament to the ramus of the mandible.
● Continuity of connective tissue through to the tympanic membrane has been found to exist.[33]

Pintus ligament: occurrence not regular

Origin: The malleus, in the middle ear.
Insertion: Passes through the petrotympanic fissure to the head of the mandible.

Muscles (Fig. 11.10)

Temporalis muscle (Fig. 11.11)

Origin:
- Temporal fossa (temporal, sphenoid, parietal and frontal bones)
- Fan-shaped origin
- Deep layer: inferior temporal line.
- Superficial layer: temporal fascia.
- Further origins: temporal fascia of the sphenoid bone and posterior of the zygomatic bone.

Insertion: Coronoid process. Further fibrous attachments to the middle part of the anterior capsule (not directly to the disk).[35]

Course of fibers:
- Anterior part: vertically, from inferior to superior.
- Medial part: from anterior and inferior to posterior and superior.
- Posterior part: from anterior and inferior to posterior and superior or horizontally.

Function:
- Elevation of the mandible. Active in posteriorly directed biting force (anterior and posterior parts).[37]
- Adduction of the mandible.
- Positioning of the mandible to ensure optimum bite using masseter and pterygoid muscles.
- Tensing of capsule.[21]
- Pars posterior: Retrusion.
- Innervation: mandibular nerve (CN V3).
- (Each of the three parts of the muscle has its own nerve branch.)

Masseter muscle (Fig. 11.12)

Innervation: mandibular nerve (CN V3).

Deep part

Origin: Posterior third of the zygomatic arch.

Insertion:
- Almost perpendicular at the masseteric tuberosity of the ramus of the mandible.
- Deep part: lateral part of the anterior articular capsule (not directly to the disk).[35]

Course of fibers: Vertical.

Function:
- Elevation of the mandible, especially in the case of anteriorly directed biting force; laterotrusion; tensing of capsule.[38]
- Active in laterally directed biting force on the ipsilateral side.[37]

Superficial part

Origin: Anterior two-thirds of the zygomatic arch.

Insertion: Obliquely at the angle of the mandible.

Course of fibers: From superior and anterior to posterior and inferior.

Function: Elevation of the mandible and protrusion.

Medial pterygoid muscle (Fig. 11.13)

Covered by the deep (muscular) fascia of the masseter muscle; forms a muscle sling together with the masseter muscle.

Origin: Pterygoid fossa (inner surface of the lateral plate of the pterygoid process).

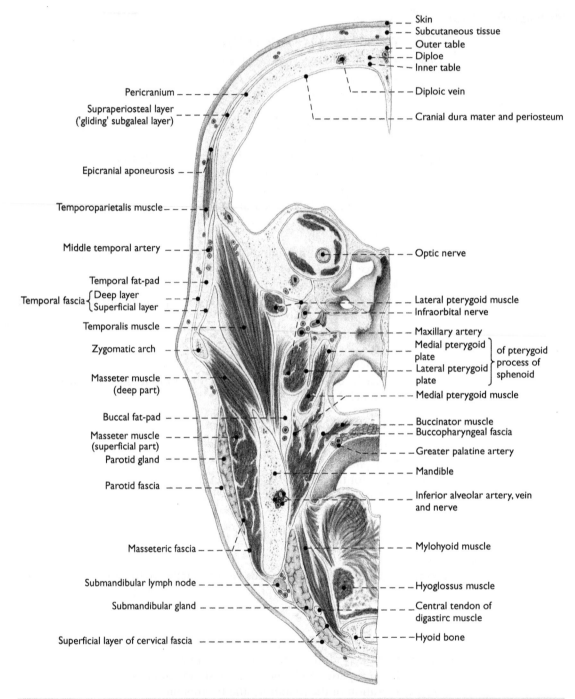

Figure 11.10 Frontal section through the right half of the face, level with the ramus of the mandible. From: Tillmann B. Farbatlas der Anatomie. Zahnmedizin-Humanmedizin. New York – Stuttgart: Thieme; 1997

Figure 11.11 Temporalis
muscle

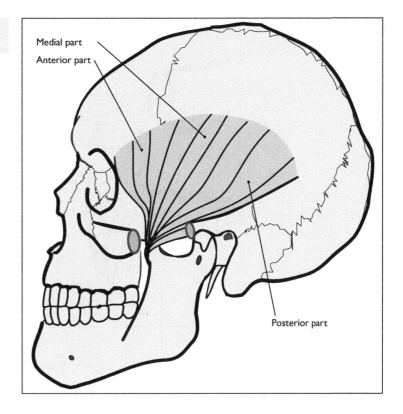

Medial part

Anterior part

Posterior part

Figure 11.12 Masseter
muscle

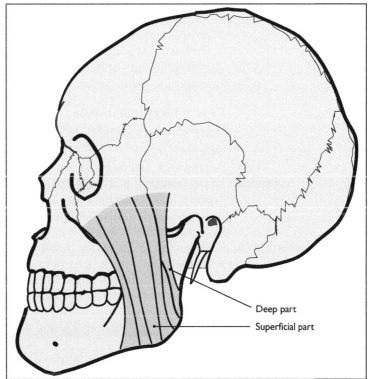

Deep part

Superficial part

Figure 11.13 Medial and lateral pterygoid muscles

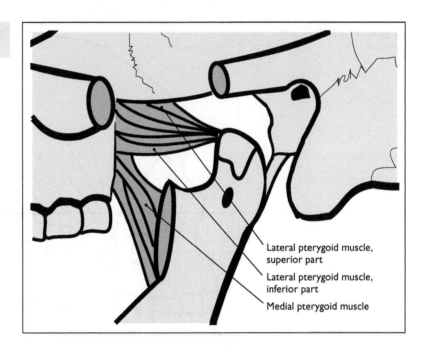

Lateral pterygoid muscle, superior part

Lateral pterygoid muscle, inferior part

Medial pterygoid muscle

Insertion: Inner aspect of the angle of the mandible (pterygoid tuberosity); may form raphe with the tendon of insertion of the masseter muscle.

Course of fibers: Nearly vertical, obliquely to inferior and posterior; outward.

Function:
- Elevation of the mandible (together with masseter).
- Protrusion when teeth occluded (opposing retrusion by temporalis muscle, posterior part).
- Unilateral: Medial movement of the mandible.[39]
- Innervation: mandibular nerve (CN V3).

Note: Excessive medial movement leads to hypertrophy of the muscle.

Lateral pterygoid muscle (see *Fig. 11.13*)

Innervation: mandibular nerve (CN V3).

Superior part:

Origin: Infratemporal surface and infratemporal crest of the sphenoid.

Insertion: Upper border of pterygoid fovea, anterior and medial to the articular capsule; disk. (Attachment to the disk is a matter of some debate: is the attachment functionally effective, not functionally effective, or non-existent?)[35,40]

Course of fibers: Slightly oblique, from inside, anterior and superior, running outward and posterior.

Function:
- Elevation of the mandible (mouth closure).
- Anterior movement of the disk and condyle and unilateral medial movement.
- Stabilization of the capsule and disk at the terminal stage of mouth opening.
- Positioning and stabilization of the condylar head and disk during mouth closure.[41]

● Stabilization of the resting condyle on the operative side during molar grinding movement.

Inferior part

Origin: Outer aspect of the lateral pterygoid plate.

Insertion: Anterior of condyle in the pterygoid fovea.

Course of fibers: Horizontally oriented, from inside, inferior, running outward and superior.

Function: ● Protrusion with or without mouth opening.

● Unilateral: molar grinding (medial movement).

● Works in synergy with the suprahyoid muscles in movements of mouth opening.

● Gives support in the translation of the condylar head caudad, anteriorly and contralaterally during the opening of the mouth.[41]

Sphenomandibular muscle[40]

Innervation: mandibular nerve (CN V3).

Origin: Greater wing of the sphenoid.

Insertion: Coronoid process or adjacent area.

Function: Stabilization of the mandible if required.

Indirectly involved muscles

Muscles of the floor of the mouth (mylohyoid, digastric, geniohyoid muscles).

Function: Opening of the mouth (rotation movement); provide foundation for movements of the tongue.

Suprahyoid muscles

● Mylohyoid muscle: from the mylohyoid line of the mandible to the body of the hyoid bone and median raphe (CN V3).

The left and right portions of the mylohyoid muscle form a mobile diaphragm in the floor of the mouth. When the mouth is closed, the fibers run in a superior, lateral and slightly anterior direction from the hyoid to the raphe of the mandible. The course of the muscle fibers between their bony attachments is not straight, as is often stated, but curved. This is caused by the connection between the muscle and the geniohyoid above and the anterior belly of the digastric below.[42]

● Geniohyoid muscle: from the mental spine of the mandible to the body of the hyoid bone (CN XII, C I).

● Digastric muscle: from the mastoid notch of the temporal bone, via a tendinous loop at the hyoid bone, to the digastric fossa of the mandible (CN V3, CN VII).

● Stylohyoid muscle: from the styloid process of the temporal bone to the lesser horn of the hyoid (CN VII).

● Hyoglossus muscle: from the body and greater horn of the hyoid bone to the side of the tongue (CN XII).

● Chondroglossus muscle: from the lesser horn of the hyoid bone to the side of the tongue (CN XII).

Infrahyoid muscles
- Omohyoid muscle: from the upper border of the scapula to the body of the hyoid bone (C I–C III).
- Sternohyoid muscle: from the upper sternum and the sterno-clavicular joint to the body of the hyoid bone (C I–C III).
- Thyrohyoid muscle: from the thyroid cartilage to the greater horn and body of the hyoid bone (C I carried by CN XII).
- Sternothyroid muscle: from the sternum and first rib to the thyroid cartilage (C I–C III).

Muscles located behind the hyoid bone
- Middle constrictor of pharynx: from the greater and lesser horns of the hyoid bone (CN IX, CN X, cervical sympathetic trunk).
- Stylohyoid muscle: from the styloid process to the lesser horn (CN VII).
- Digastric muscle (posterior belly) (CN VII).

Muscles of the tongue
- Genioglossus muscle: from the mental spine of the inner surface of the mandible into the tongue; fan-shaped (CN XII).
- Hyoglossus muscle: see above.
- Chondroglossus muscle: see above.
- Styloglossus muscle: from the styloid process into the side of the tongue.
- Myloglossus (inconsistent): posterior of the mylohyoid line to the base of the tongue.
- Palatoglossus: from the palatine aponeurosis into the side of the tongue.
- Superior and inferior longitudinal muscles, transverse muscle of the tongue, vertical muscle of the tongue.
- The facial muscles (facial expression; muscle system of the lips and cheeks) (CN VII) (Fig. 11.14).

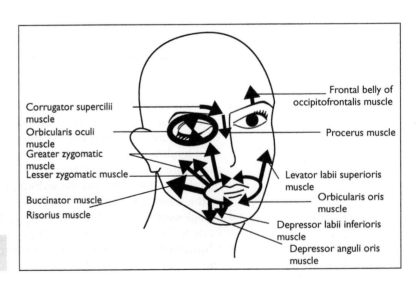

Figure 11.14 Function of the facial muscles

e.g. buccinator muscle: from the pterygomandibular raphe and the maxilla and mandible to the angle of the mouth, and orbicularis oris muscle (assists movement of food in the mouth; also sucking and blowing).

- Pharyngeal muscles (swallowing) (CN IX, CN X).
- Muscles of the palatopharyngeal arches: the palatine muscles and pharyngeal muscles (CN V, CN IX, CN X).
- Muscles of the larynx (formation of sounds) (CN X).
- Nuchal muscles (indirect opening of the jaw, by drawing the head/nape of neck backward) (cervical nerves).
- Sternocleidomastoid muscle (indirect opening of the jaw by extension of the head on bilateral contraction)[43] (CN XI, cervical plexus).

Fasciae

- Investing layer of cervical fascia: especially the temporal fascia and also the masseteric, parotid, and buccopharyngeal fasciae.
- Pterygo-temporo-mandibular aponeurosis: at the anterior edge of the neck of the condylar process (Fig. 11.15).
- There are also functional links with the falx cerebri and cerebelli and the tentorium cerebelli, and the nuchal muscles. The intracranial structures transmit the balance of forces between the viscerocranium and the compensating tonus of the nuchal muscles. The function of the temporomandibular joint and the occlusion patterns of the upper and lower jaw are dependent on this balance (Fig. 11.16).

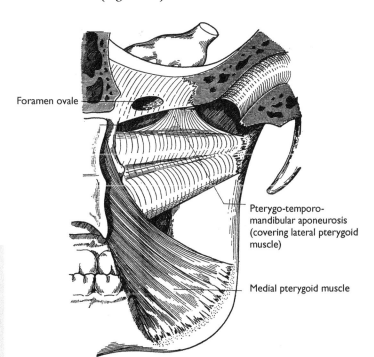

Foramen ovale

Pterygo-temporo-mandibular aponeurosis (covering lateral pterygoid muscle)

Medial pterygoid muscle

Figure 11.15
Interpterygoid region, pterygo-temporo-mandibular aponeurosis. From: Perlemuter L, Waligora J. Cahiers d'anatomie 1, système nerveux central. Paris; Masson: 1980

Figure 11.16 Diagrammatic representation of the balance between the neurocranium and viscerocranium and the cervical spine. The weight of the viscerocranium is compensated by means of the tonus of the nuchal muscles. The effect of these extends into the interior of the cranium via the falx cerebri and cerebelli and tentorium cerebelli. From: Delaire J. L'analyse architecturale et structurale cranio-faciale (de profil). Rev Stomatol 1978; 79:8

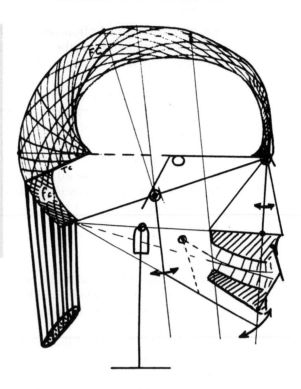

Innervation of the temporomandibular joint[44] *(Figs 11.17, 11.18)*

- Auriculotemporal nerve (branch of the mandibular nerve, CN V3): The articular branches of the auriculotemporal nerve run from outside inward and posteriorly to enter the articular capsule.
- Masseteric nerve and deep temporal nerve (both branches of the mandibular nerve, CN V3): their articular branches run from anterior to enter the articular capsule.
- Facial nerve (CN VII): A twig of this nerve sometimes enters the joint from outside.
- Autonomic innervation via the otic ganglion: Preganglionic parasympathetic fibers begin in the lesser petrosal nerve (CN IX), are reoriented in the otic ganglion and pass into the articular capsule from medially. These are concerned with the production of synovial fluid. Sympathetic innervation is supplied from the carotid plexus without reorientation in the otic ganglion.
- The lateral ligament of the TMJ and surrounding fatty tissue are also richly innervated.

Additional nerves of the mandible
- Buccal nerve (from CN V3) (entirely sensory branch).
- Nerve to the medial pterygoid muscle (from CN V3).
- Inferior alveolar nerve (from CN V3): in the mandibular canal.
- Mental nerve (branch of inferior alveolar nerve) (from CN V3): at the mental foramen.

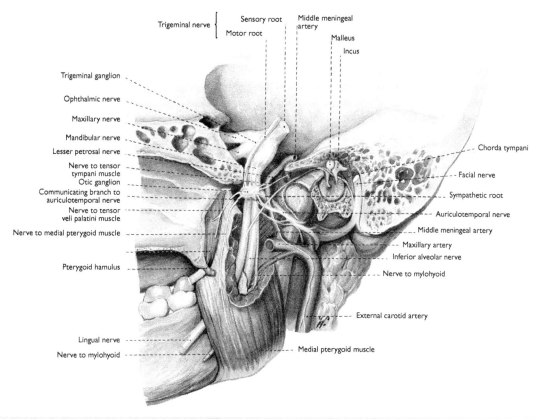

Figure 11.17 Retrocondylar structures: medial view of the right half of the head (paramedian section). From: Tillmann B. Farbatlas der Anatomie. Zahnmedizin-Humanmedizin. Stuttgart – New York: Thieme; 1997

- Nerve to mylohyoid (branch of inferior alveolar nerve): in the mylohyoid groove.
- Masseteric nerve (from CN V3): at the mandibular notch.
- Otic ganglion and submandibular ganglion supply innervation to the salivary glands.

Mechanoreceptors[45-52]

Four different types of mechanoreceptor are found in proximity to the joint:

- Ruffini corpuscles (endings): information relating to present position of the joint and its movement (direction, speed, amplitude of condylar movement).
- Lamellated (pacinian) corpuscles: dynamic receptors in the articular capsule register acceleration of TMJ movements.
- Golgi tendon organs: isolated corpuscles in the lateral articular capsule reinforcement; maximum forces cause these corpuscles to produce reflex relaxation of the masticatory muscles. The condyles can then glide freely sideways.

Figure 11.18 Sensory innervation of the TMJ: auriculotemporal nerve (4 articular branches), deep temporal nerve (1 articular branch) and masseteric nerve (4 articular branches). From: Tillmann B. Farbatlas der Anatomie. Zahnmedizin-Humanmedizin. Stuttgart – New York: Thieme; 1997

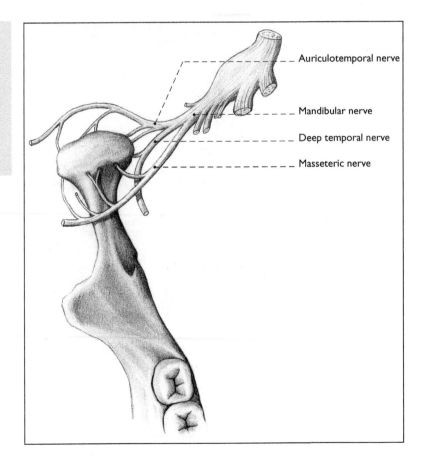

- Numerous free nerve endings: depolarization occurs in sudden pronounced translation movements in the TMJ.

The proprioceptive impulses produced by these structures, which derive from the first branchial arch, are mainly transmitted to the nucleus of the trigeminal nerve. The proprioceptive information processed includes that from the TMJ, together with the capsule-disk-muscle complex, the mallei anterius and sphenomandibular ligaments. This connection means that any disturbance of the masticatory system may also affect the proprioceptive system of the entire first branchial arch.

Of the three, the lateral pterygoid, masseter and temporalis muscles, it is the temporalis that possesses the greatest number of neuromuscular spindles. 1A and 1B fibers continue to the posterior horn of the spinal cord. These react to stretching of the muscles and to the speed of stretch.

Blood vessels (Figs 11.19a,b; see also Figs 11.9, 14.18)

- The maxillary artery (branch of the external carotid artery) has branches to the mandible and masticatory muscles.

Figure 11.19 (a) Arterial supply to the teeth and gums of the maxilla. From: Tillmann B. Farbatlas der Anatomie. Zahnmedizin-Humanmedizin. Stuttgart – New York: Thieme; 1997 (b) Arterial supply to the teeth and gums of the mandible by the inferior alveolar artery and branches of the buccal artery. From: Tillmann B. Farbatlas der Anatomie. Zahnmedizin-Humanmedizin. Stuttgart – New York: Thieme; 1997

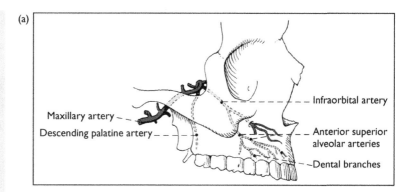

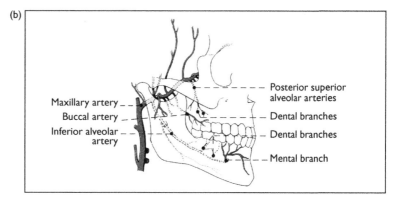

- The inferior alveolar artery (branch of the maxillary artery): in the mandibular canal.
- The mental branch of the inferior alveolar artery: at the mental foramen.
- Artery to the mylohyoid (branch of the inferior alveolar artery): in the mylohyoid groove.
- The masseteric artery (branch of the maxillary artery): at the mandibular notch.
- The superficial temporal artery (branch of the facial artery): structures supplied include the TMJ.

Lymph drainage
- The retropharyngeal, sub- and preauricular, and submandibular lymph nodes.
- The occipital lymph nodes.
- Also: the cervical lymph nodes.

Connections with other structures

Parotid gland: (Fig. 11.20) at and behind the ramus of the mandible.

Figure 11.20 The interpterygoid region. Location and connections of the parotid gland. From: Perlemuter L, Waligora J. Cahiers d'anatomie 1, système nerveux central. Paris; Masson: 1980

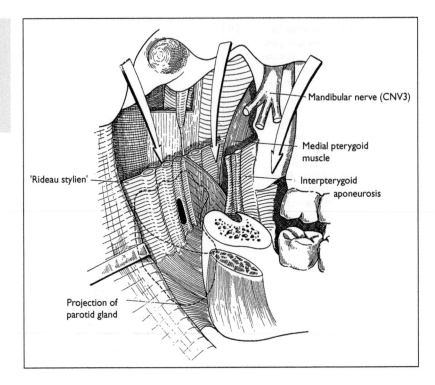

Mandibular nerve (CNV3)

Medial pterygoid muscle

Interpterygoid aponeurosis

'Rideau stylien'

Projection of parotid gland

BIOMECHANICS OF THE MANDIBLE

The articular surfaces of the TMJ are highly incongruent, and the articular capsule is very lax. As a result the joint has considerable mobility, with a large range of motion.[53,54] Joint movement options include opening and closing, laterotrusion and mediotrusion.[55-58]

The temporomandibular joints enable movement around three axes.[59,60] Rohen[34] and others have described the temporomandibular joint as a turning and sliding joint. There is no fixed centralized position of the condyles in the mandibular fossa.[61]

Movements of the jaw are always a combination of movements, making it impossible to define fixed axes of jaw movement. On the contrary, according to Koolstra and van Eijden 1997, the patterns of muscle contraction determine the helical axis of motion at any moment for the open-close movement.[55,62,63] This means that not only does the muscle function of the TMJ depend on the immediate helical axis of motion, but conversely the axis depends on the muscle function.[54]

Opening of the jaw, for example, begins with movement around an axis of rotation about 1 cm posterior and inferior to the condyle. At the end of mouth opening, the axis of rotation lies below the coronoid process, approximately at the transition from the ramus to the body of the mandible. Many of the movements of the human TMJ are not symmetrical.

An example of this is lateral movement of the TMJ. Here, the contralateral condyle moves anteriorly, to the articular tubercle, while the ipsilateral condyle remains in the mandibular fossa and moves only slightly toward the ipsilateral side.[55,58,64]

Koolstra and van Eijden (1995–97, 1999) developed a biomechanical model of the human masticatory system which does not limit its movements to fixed, immutable axes. Their model combines effects of the joint surfaces, the force of active and passive muscles, dynamic properties of the muscles and the mass of the structures moved. However, the primary factor for the movements of the TMJ is the direction of movement of the involved muscles in relation to the center of gravity.[54,63,65,66]

All movements of the mandible involve both the superior and the inferior joint compartment. In the superior joint compartment, mainly sagittal gliding movements take place, and in the inferior compartment, mainly rotation movements.

Certain main movements can be distinguished:

- Opening and closing of the mouth (abduction and adduction).
- Protrusion and retrusion of the mandible.
- Laterotrusion.

In the rest position there is no contact between the teeth. The mandibular head is located at the posterior slope of the articular tubercle. The posterior part of the disk fills the fossa.[67]

Biomechanical demands on the temporomandibular joint[52]

The act of chewing imposes loads on the TMJ.[68-73]

These underlie overloading of the joint, as in parafunctional activities.[74-77] However, loading of the TMJ is highly variable according to individual and habit,[78-80] since the mandible operates like a balance beam together with the adjacent muscles of the TMJ[81-88] and the muscles of the floor of the mouth and other hyoid muscles, and numerous other regulatory mechanisms, and so is integrated into a supraordinate regulatory system. The smooth functioning of all the components in the regulatory equation, which are being constantly adjusted to current requirements by processes of feedback and adaptation, is essential for normal TMJ function.

Various muscle forces can be activated to produce a particular masticatory pressure. The physiological contact forces can vary between 0% and 50% of total masticatory force. With a contact force of 0% and when the condyle is supported on the articular tubercle while biting onto a solid piece of food, the load on the joint is almost zero.[89-91] The positioning of the condyle on the articular tubercle is in turn dependent on the angle of opening of the TMJ.

Simulation of static load with jaw closed indicates that the transmission of stress and tension mainly affects the intermediate zone of the disk (especially the lateral parts). Even relatively minor joint loading is stated to produce distinct deformations, and relatively large differences in the direction of the loads on the joint are stated to have little influence on the distribution of the deformations.

The smooth functioning of the virtual neuromuscular axis that governs the masticatory apparatus is essential for normal TMJ function. Without it, overloading of the system and damage to the temporomandibular joint occur.[91]

Opening and closing of the mouth

Combined rotation and gliding movements are involved in the opening and closing of the mouth (Fig. 11.21).[92]

When the mouth is opened, the first movement is a rotation of the condylar process (inferior discomandibular joint). This produces an opening of about 12° (Fig. 11.22).[93]

The next step is a protrusion movement. The condylar process and disk are drawn anteriorly, under the articular tubercle (superior discomandibular joint). The lateral pterygoid muscle, aided by the digastric muscle, produces protrusion of the disk and condylar process.

Closing of the mouth involves retrusion and posterior rotation of the condylar process. Mouth closure is controlled by the lateral pterygoid muscle (superior part) (Fig. 11.23).[93]

A more detailed analysis of mouth opening and closing is given below.

Mouth opening

Initiation of mouth opening:

● The superior part of the lateral pterygoid muscle relaxes.
● Forward rotation of the condylar process.

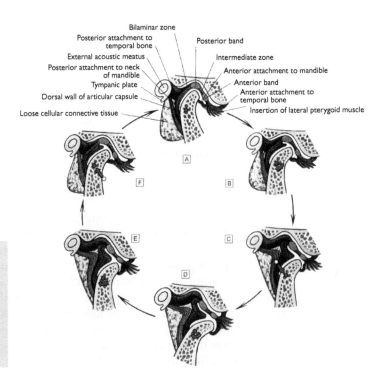

Figure 11.21 Diagrammatic illustration of the effects in the TMJ of opening and closing of the mouth, according to Rees. From: Williams PL, et al. Gray's Anatomy. 38th edn. New York: Churchill Livingstone; 1995

Figure 11.22 Opening of the mouth according to Amiguez. 1. Superior part of the lateral pterygoid muscle relaxes. 2. Inferior part of the lateral pterygoid muscle contracts. 3. Digastric muscle (anterior belly) contracts

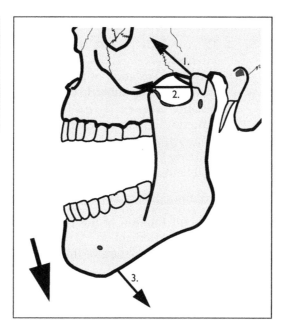

Figure 11.23 Closure of the mouth according to Amiguez. 1. Suprahyoid muscles relax. 2. Temporalis muscle contracts. 3. (a) Medial pterygoid muscle contracts. (b) Masseter muscle contracts

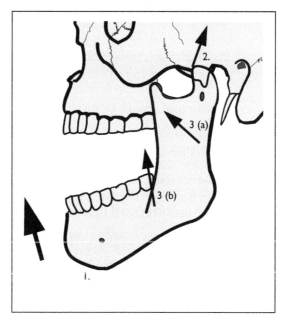

● Posterior translation of the disk relative to the gliding movement of the condyle.
● The digastric muscle (in particular the anterior belly) contracts to initiate mouth opening, assisted by the mylohyoid and geniohyoid muscles. The hyoid bone acts as a fixed point, stabilized by the infrahyoid muscles.

Middle stage of mouth opening:

- The condylar process rotates forward and glides anteriorly and inferiorly.
- Forward translation of the disk (along the oblique course created by the articular tubercle of the temporal bone and condyle). The distance traveled is less than that of the condyle, resulting in posterior movement relative to the condyle.[67]
- Contraction of the lateral pterygoid (inferior part) and digastric muscles, assisted by the mylohyoid and geniohyoid muscles, enable the middle stage of mouth opening.[94]

Maximum opening of the mouth:

- Forward rotation of the condylar process; this transmutes into a gliding movement.
- Posterior translation of the disk relative to the gliding movement of the condyle.
- Contraction of the digastric muscle (assisted by the mylohyoid and geniohyoid muscles) produces the final stage in mouth opening.
- Opening of the mouth is limited by the lateral ligament of the temporomandibular joint, the retrodiscal connective tissue (disco-temporal ligament) and the temporalis muscle (posterior fibers).

If tensing of the masseter and temporalis muscles restricts the opening of the mouth, a change in the fixed point leads to flexion of the head and cervical spine.

Mouth closing

Initiation of mouth closure:

- The condylar process rotates backward.
- Anterior translation of the disk in absolute terms.
- Anterior translation of the disk relative to the gliding movement of the condyle.
- Relaxation of the suprahyoid muscles begins closure of the mouth.
- The discotemporal ligament is fully tensed.

Middle stage of mouth closure:

- The condylar process rotates backward and glides posteriorly and superiorly.
- Posterior translation of the disk. The distance traveled is less than that of the condyle, resulting in anterior movement relative to the condyle.
- Contraction of the temporalis muscle enables the mouth-closing movement.
- The discotemporal ligament increasingly relaxes.

Final position:

- Closing rotation of the condylar process.
- Relative anterior translation of the disk.

- The final position is produced by contraction of the temporalis and masseter muscles, the lateral pterygoid (superior part) and medial pterygoid muscles.
- The movement is limited by the lateral ligament of the TMJ and discocondylar ligament.
- The vascular retrodiscal pad empties.

Note: The disk glides more slowly than the condyle when the mouth is opened or closed, in order to maintain the balance of form and function.[95]

Protrusion and retrusion *(Fig. 11.24)*[96]

- The movement involved in protrusion of the mandible is relatively slight.
- An anterior and inferior gliding movement of the condylar processes occurs (in the superior discomandibular joint). The angle of inclination is between 5° and 55°.
- A slight turning around a transverse axis also occurs in the TMJ, so that the lower incisors can slide downward on reaching the upper incisors.
- The lower incisors are raised again once they have passed the upper front teeth.
- Retrusion is the reverse of the protrusion process.

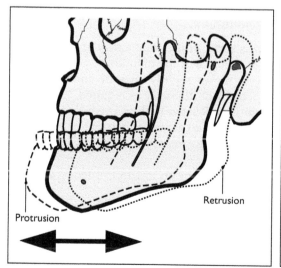
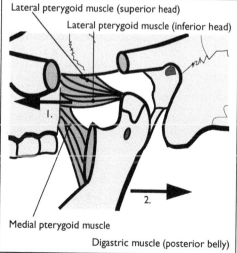

Figure 11.24 Protrusion and retrusion, according to Amiguez. 1. Protrusion: Contraction of the lateral pterygoid (inferior part), medial pterygoid, and masseter muscles and anterior part of the temporal muscle. 2. Retrusion: Contraction of the lateral pterygoid (superior part), medial pterygoid, and masseter muscles (deep part), the posterior part of the temporalis muscle and posterior belly of the digastric muscle

Protrusion

- Anterior translation of the condylar process, together with slight rotation.
- The disk glides anteriorly. The distance traveled is less than that of the condyle, resulting in posterior movement relative to the condyle.
- Protrusion is enabled mainly by contraction of the lateral pterygoid muscle (inferior part), assisted by the medial pterygoid and masseter muscles and the anterior fibers of the temporalis muscle.
- Protrusion is limited by the discocondylar, sphenomandibular and stylomandibular ligaments.

Retrusion

- Posterior translation of the condylar process occurs, together with slight rotation.
- The disk glides posteriorly. The distance traveled is less than that of the condyle, resulting in anterior movement relative to the condyle
- Retrusion is enabled mainly by contraction of the lateral pterygoid muscle (superior part), medial pterygoid and masseter muscles (deep part), assisted by the posterior fibers of the temporalis muscle and the posterior belly of the digastric muscle.
- Retrusion is limited by the discocondylar ligament and lateral ligament of the TMJ.
- The vascular retrodiscal pad empties.

Laterotrusion *(Fig. 11.25)*[93]

On the side of the laterotrusion:

- The condylar process turns in the joint cavity, rotating around a vertical axis through the neck of the mandible.
- The condylar process moves slightly laterally and posteriorly or anteriorly; also superiorly or inferiorly as required.
- Lateral rotation of the disk. Relative to the movement of the condyle the disk moves in a medial and anterior direction.

On the side of the mediotrusion:

- The condylar process moves in an anterior, inferior and slightly medial direction.
- There is anterior and medial translation of the disk in absolute terms, but in relation to the movement of the condyle its movement is posterior and lateral.
- On the side of the laterotrusion: contraction of the lateral pterygoid muscle (superior part), the posterior fibers of the temporalis muscle, the masseter and digastric muscles.
- On the side of the mediotrusion: contraction of the lateral pterygoid muscle (inferior part), the medial pterygoid and masseter muscles and the anterior fibers of the temporalis muscle.

Figure 11.25 Laterotrusion according to Amiguez. (a) Side of mediotrusion: condylar process moves antero-inferiorly and slightly medially. Contraction of lateral pterygoid (inferior part), medial pterygoid, masseter and anterior part of temporalis. (b) Side of laterotrusion: condylar process moves laterally and posteriorly. Contraction of lateral pterygoid (superior part), posterior part of temporalis, and masseter and digastric muscles

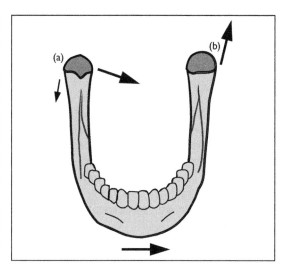

- Laterotrusion is limited by the lateral ligament of the TMJ and discocondylar ligament on the side of laterotrusion.
- Laterotrusion is limited by the sphenomandibular and stylomandibular ligaments on the side of mediotrusion.

CONTROL OF THE ACT OF CHEWING

A biological system of feedback control governs the operation of the TMJ and integrates its many functions (chewing, swallowing, sucking, speaking, facial expression, etc.).[52] The biomechanical parameters governed by this control system are not limited to the joint itself, but have to include all neighboring structures (muscles of mastication, the tongue, the hyoid, and of facial expression, the teeth and dental ligamentous apparatus, and the mucous membranes of the cheeks and mouth); all of these must be registered and processed.

The extrapyramidal system is mainly responsible for nervous control, which means that chewing and swallowing do not take place under voluntary control, although this can be achieved via the cerebral cortex.

Afferent information is conveyed by means of mechanoreceptors, chemoreceptors and thermoreceptors.

Mechanoreceptors are present in muscles, in the articular capsule, in the mucosa of the mouth, and in the parodontal region. Thermoreceptors are located in the mucosa of the mouth and dentinal canals, and chemoreceptors in the taste buds.

The afferent information is transmitted to the cranial nerve centers and so to the CNS by the trigeminal (CN V), facial (CN VII), glossopharyngeal (CN IX) and vagus (CN X) nerves.

On reaching the CNS this information is passed to the thalamus in the diencephalon or to the masticatory center (probably in the pons).

In the thalamus impulses are directed as appropriate to the extrapyramidal system, basal ganglia, or cerebral cortex on the basis of the afferent information from the sensory organs.

From the basal ganglia, stimuli pass via the red nucleus to the origins of cranial nerves V, VII, IX, X and XII and spinal nuclei of the first three cervical nerves, which regulate and control the act of chewing and swallowing.

The process of mastication can be governed consciously in the cerebral cortex. The information passes from the primary somatosensory cortex to the primary motor cortex. From there the stimulus can be transmitted by way of the corticospinal tract to the origins of the cranial nerves already mentioned, and of the cervical nerves, and on to the structures involved in mastication.

PHYLOGENETIC AND ONTOGENETIC INFLUENCES ON THE DEVELOPMENT OF THE JAW

Phylogenesis

Phylogenesis throws a particularly clear light on the supreme importance of the human temporomandibular joint. In fish, the tracts of ingestion and respiration run parallel. In land-living vertebrates, however, the nasal cavity forms dorsally and the respiratory organ ventrally, with the respiratory tract crossing at the pharynx.

The reshaping of the buccal cavity in humans to create a universal, closed and adaptable hollow space was the prerequisite for the development of differentiated speech.

Portmann,[97] referring back to Reichert (1838), describes certain homologous features in the phylogenesis of the temporomandibular joint in vertebrates, focusing on the joint between the articular and quadrate bones and the mammalian joint between the malleus and incus (Table 11.1).

Two phylogenetic processes are discussed in relation to the emergence of the temporomandibular joint in mammals.[97] One assumption is that the dentary of the dermal bones expanded laterally so that it eventually covered the articular bone. That enabled a new joint

Table 11.1 Homologous features in the phylogenesis of the TMJ in vertebrates		
Stapes	Hyomandibular in fish Columella auris of amphibians, reptiles and birds
Incus	Quadrate
Malleus	Articular
Anterior process of malleus	Prearticular
Tympanic ring	Angular

to take shape on the same axis as the primary temporomandibular joint and laterally to it. Another, less likely hypothesis assumes that the new mammalian joint (the squamosal/dentary joint) formed rostrally from the primary articular/quadrate bone joint. Whatever the case, the existence of these two joints, located one behind the other, has been demonstrated in some vertebrates.

The development toward upright gait produced certain structural changes in the body, including the development of the clavicle, the use of the upper limbs in place of the jaw for grasping objects, and the development of the mouth and laryngeal region to become a highly specialized organ of speech.

For Delattre and Fenart,[98] the most important change in the skull in the development of human beings was the posterior rotation of the occiput. This completely alters the intracranial volume and leads to further changes, for example those to the masticatory apparatus:

- The extension of the pterygoid processes.
- The increase in height of the maxillae and rami of the mandible, combined with a lowering of the hard palate and horizontal body of the mandible.
- The reinforcement of the nasal spine of the maxilla and the mandibular symphysis, with a retreat of the alveolar process relative to the maxilla, and of the alveolar part in relation to the mandible.
- The outward and downward rotation of the external petrous (mastoid) part.[98]
- The gliding hinge movement is only found in humans.

Embryology of the mandible and temporomandibular joint

The temporomandibular joint in human beings is a recent development in their history.[52] In this they are unlike primitive vertebrates, in which the posterior and anterior parts of the first branchial arch connect in the primary jaw (differentiating to form the malleus-incus joint). In humans, however, the mandible connects with the temporal bone.[99]

The mandible develops from mesenchymal tissue, around Meckel's cartilage (cartilage of the first branchial arch), by membranous ossification. The maxilla, zygomatic bone and squama of the temporal bone develop by membranous ossification from the mesenchymal maxillary process of the first branchial arch. Movements of the jaw can be detected in the embryo at 2 months *in utero*.

- Until the 7th week the face is confined between the growing brain and the bulge of the early heart, leading to the broad embryonic face with its widely spaced eyes and nose and crooked mouth opening.

    When the embryonic heart and viscera migrate progressively downward with the diaphragm and the brain ascends as it continues to grow, there is at last room for the face to elongate (Fig. 11.26).

Figure 11.26 Influences on the growth of the skull: effect on the growth of the maxillary complex of the downward and anteriorly directed force associated with growth of the nasal septum

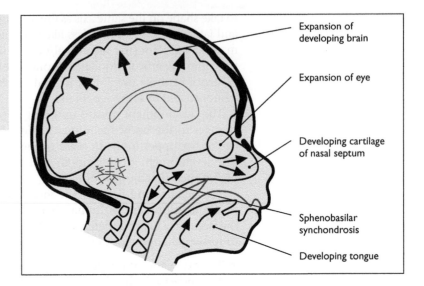

Expansion of developing brain

Expansion of eye

Developing cartilage of nasal septum

Sphenobasilar synchondrosis

Developing tongue

Figure 11.27 Growth movement of the mandible

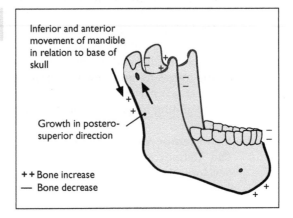

Inferior and anterior movement of mandible in relation to base of skull

Growth in postero-superior direction

++ Bone increase
— Bone decrease

Growth movements and factors affecting the growth of the lower third of the face

● Growth of the ramus posteriorly and superiorly (Fig. 11.27).

Explanation: Bone formation in the condyles of the mandible.

● Overall downward and anterior repositioning of the mandible.

Explanation: Growth of the ramus in a posterior and superior direction in relation to the cranial base.

● Posterior separation of the two halves of the body of the mandible. (Fig. 11.28).

Explanation: Posterior growth of the condylar heads.

Further factors involved in the growth of the mandible
(see also Fig. 11.29)

● The mandibular nerve is the first structure to form in the mandibular region. It probably induces the formation of the early mandible from a membranous thickening of the mesectoderm. In the 6th

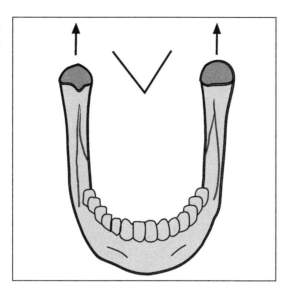

Figure 11.28 Lateral expansion of the ramus of the mandible

week an ossification center for each half of the mandible is formed (near the bifurcation of the inferior alveolar nerve and artery). Ossification proceeds along the alveolar nerve and its branches, and the cartilage of the branchial arch almost completely disappears.

- The transformation of woven bone into lamellated bone takes place at an earlier stage in the mandible than in other bones in response to the fetus's early swallowing and sucking activity (fifth month *in utero*).
- In the 12th week *in utero* secondary cartilage appears, independently of the pharyngeal arch cartilage, as precursors to part of the condylar process, for the head of the mandible and the mental protuberance. The secondary cartilage of the condyle is replaced by bone, but the upper part remains as articular cartilage and as a growth center. This growth center is of particular importance for the further shaping of the mandible.
- The activity of the lateral pterygoid muscle regulates the development of the condylar process.[100]
- The activity of the temporalis muscle influences the development of the coronoid process.
- The activity of the masseter and pterygoid muscles influences the development of the angle and ramus of the mandible.
- The primordial teeth form the basis for the development of the alveolar part.
- The vertical movement of the teeth.
- The growth and movement of the tongue also affect the development of the maxillae.

Cartilaginous growth of the mandibular head

The type of growth undergone by this cartilage is unlike normal cartilaginous growth by interstitial cartilage cell division. Cartilage

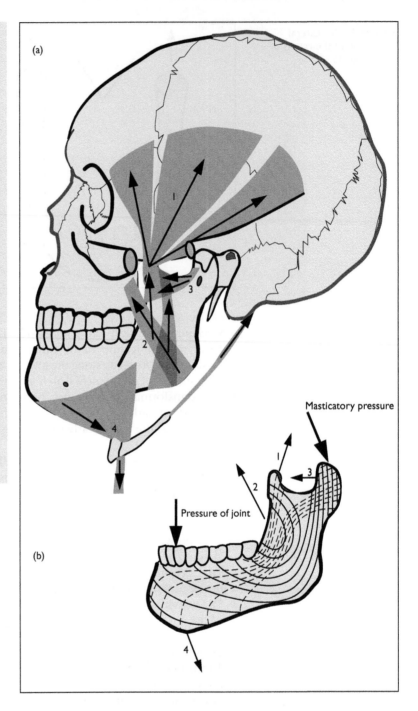

Figure 11.29 Effects of forces on mandibular growth and course of trajectories. (a) Effects of forces on mandibular growth:
1. Posterosuperior pull of the temporalis muscle.
2. Anterosuperiorly directed force of the masseter and medial pterygoid muscles.
3. Anteroinferior pull of the lateral pterygoid muscle in interaction with the temporalis muscle (posterior part). 4. Direction of force of the suprahyoid and infrahyoid muscles. (b) Effect of forces on course of trajectories: 1. Posterosuperior pull of the temporalis muscle.
2. Anterosuperior direction of force of the masseter and medial pterygoid muscles.
3. Anteroinferior pull of the lateral pterygoid muscle in interaction with the temporalis muscle (posterior part). 4. Directions of force of the suprahyoid and infrahyoid muscles. Dotted lines, trajectories of pull; Solid lines, pressure trajectories

cells are present, which divide very little but do produce important ground substance and fibers. The secondary cartilage develops from the mesenchyme, as does the secondary mandible. Like the mandible, it is covered with a layer of connective tissue. Cartilage cells differentiate from this connective tissue layer, subsequently leaving the layer and forming the cartilage of the mandibular head. In a sense this process corresponds to the growth of bone that occurs on the surface, the periosteum (appositional bone growth), rather than by interstitial cell division. Consequently the head of the mandible reacts like any cartilage and yet also has properties of bone.

Growth of the temporal joint components

The ossification center of the squamous part (with the zygomatic process) appears in the neurocranium when the embryo is 30 mm long. Membranous ossification begins when it reaches a length of 35 mm. The zygomatic process of the temporal bone appears and extends anteriorly. The mandibular fossa is formed medially.

Synchronicity of ossification[101-104]

When an embryo reaches a length of 28 mm (vertex-coccyx) the ossification centers of the zygomatic bone, squamous part and ramus of the mandible appear, along with the masseter muscle.

The tooth-bearing parts of the bone, the alveolar process of the maxilla and alveolar part of the mandible, begin membranous ossification at the same stage of embryonic growth (around the 40th day *in utero*). The premaxilla appears around the 45th day.

The ossification centers of what will become the greater wing, pterygoid process of the sphenoid, condylar process, and pyramidal process of the palatine bone appear when the embryo reaches 40 mm, along with the temporalis and the medial and lateral pterygoid muscles.

Although the origin and ossification of the condylar process and the temporal joint surface differ, ossification of both begins around the same time and same place. This synchronous ossification also reflects the functional destiny and design of these structures.[101]

The capsule, disk and muscle complex[105-108]

In the course of ontogenesis the tissue of the first branchial arch – that is to become the capsule, disk and muscle complex – develop between the ossification centers of the mandible and the temporal bone. The unity of tissue is apparent during the embryonic stage, during childhood and adulthood.

Ontologically, the masticatory muscles form anteriorly on the blastema. Fibers of the lateral pterygoid, temporalis and masseter muscles attach to capsule and disk.

In the newborn the masticatory apparatus is sufficiently mature to enable sucking. In the adult the complex of capsule, disk and muscle has adapted to the mechanical demands of the form of nutrition.

Histologically the disk corresponds to the surface of the TMJ. The connective tissue fibers of the capsule run parallel and in continuity with the fibers of the disk, and with the tissue covering the articular surfaces.

An understanding of the functional, structural and dynamic unity of the capsule, disk and muscle complex and the bony parts is of key importance when treating disturbances of the masticatory system.

The influence of mandibular growth on disturbances of the TMJ, of facial growth, and of craniocervical balance

As described above, the growth of the mandible plays an important role in the development of the face. Both genetic and epigenetic factors govern the growth of the mandibular head. Biomechanical factors play a large role.

Dibbets showed that in objectively established symptoms of a craniomandibular dysfunction (CMD) (see below), no morphological changes or disorders of growth of the jaw are found. However, subjective symptoms of CMD are often associated with changes in the shape of the jaw: with a blunter shape for the angle of the mandible or a deeper location of the TMJ.[109]

The head of the mandible normally grows quickly, but if this is retarded, compensation immediately takes place in the form of heightened appositional bone growth activity, which is normally slower. Dibbets demonstrated that this process is not sufficient to compensate completely, resulting in disorders. The mandible is no longer able to perform its functions of support for the adjacent tissues at the right time. These include support to the teeth, the functional relationship of the upper and lower teeth, as a relay point for the masticatory and hyoid muscles, holding open the digestive and respiratory tracts. The consequence is that the adjacent parts adapt more than normally to the mandible, leading to altered growth of the middle part of the face, altered craniocervical balance (muscular and in terms of growth), and the emergence of CMD.

Displacement of the respiratory tract alters the growth of the face, and produces an elongated profile, open mouth and retruding mandible.[109, 110]

To this is added an anteverted posture of the head and neck and extension of the head to ease breathing.[111]

A prominent chin leads to backward tilting of the head (the process is the reverse of the retruding chin). It has been shown that the backwardly tilted head position was associated with altered growth of the head and mandible.[112]

THE MANDIBLE AS METAMORPHIC REFLECTION OF THE LOWER LIMB[113]

The two evident design principles in the function of the lower limbs are the use of arches as a means of support to the upright body, and of angled levers for locomotion. Rohen sees these functions of the lower limbs as having their metamorphic equivalents in the dynamics of the mandible.

In the case of the lower limbs, it is only for dynamic reasons that both sides are required to work functionally together (in this the legs and arms differ). In the case of the mandible, this cooperation is complete in that both halves fuse to form a single bone during embryonic development.

The architecture of the mandible, the arch with its alveolar and coronoid (muscular) processes is metaphorically equivalent to the supporting and load-bearing arch structures of the lower limbs.

These mandibular structures are, however, mainly responsible for the work of mastication. Rohen sees this work as the beginning of the digestive process, expressing the 'dissolution of an object in space' in contrast to the function of the lower limbs, which is characterized more by the act of 'integration into three-dimensional space'.

The principle of the angled lever, too, which is important for locomotion, can be seen in the mandible on account of its unmistakable angled shape and the condylar process that connects it to the TMJ. Here the relationships are reversed, according to Rohen, in that the human TMJ is largely relieved of mechanical stress during chewing by the extended length of the angled lever. This gives us a relatively freely movable temporomandibular joint, combined with a kind of physiological luxation on wide opening of the mouth, while further movement combinations of the joint are made possible by the disk.

The remarkable angled construction of the mandible therefore releases it from three-dimensional space, quite unlike the lower limbs. The movable joint of the human jaw, relieved as it is of stress, in combination with the development of an arched palate, continuous row of teeth, mobile tongue and lowered position of the larynx, also provides the basis for the development of language. These dynamics can be seen as a kind of anti-movement, in which the development of language serves as a new framing of the powers with which we shape physical space.

CRANIOMANDIBULAR DYSFUNCTION (CMD)

Antczak-Boukoms' (1995) review of the literature between 1980 and 1992 finds more than 400 instances of temporomandibular disorder.[114] There is no agreed single definition of this concept in the literature.

In 1934 a set of symptoms was described by Costen which he linked with malfunction of the TMJ (Costen syndrome: loss of hearing, dizziness, tinnitus, restriction of the jaw, preauricular pain, burning sensation of the tongue and globus hystericus).[115] In 1968, Schwarz grouped together the involvement of all the structures of the masticatory system and of psychological factors in the development of increased muscular tension, in the concept of temporomandibular joint pain dysfunction syndrome.[116]

Laskin introduced the concept of myofascial pain dysfunction syndrome, which he used to denote unilateral TMJ symptoms with painless palpation of the TMJ and after excluding radiological changes.[117] The present book combines the definition of TMJ dysfunction given by Solberg (1982) and De Boever and van Steenberghe (1988) and the definition given by Dibbets (1991)[118] of craniomandibular dysfunction (CMD).[119]

Craniomandibular dysfunction (CMD) is said to exist if one or more of the following symptoms are present:

- Subjective symptoms (reported by the patient): pain and sensitivity in the region of the masticatory muscles and TMJ, clicking, crepitation, restriction of movement of the TMJ.
- Objective signs (observed by the examiner): palpation of clicking and crepitation and observation of movement restriction[120-125] and abnormal movement patterns of the TMJ.
- Abnormal shape and position of the mandibular head on a radiograph performed for the purpose.

This definition provides no information on the affected structures (myogenous, arthrogenous, occlusal, neurogenous, ligamentous etc.) and causes. These are described further later (see also Ch. 12).

THE TEMPOROMANDIBULAR JOINT AND BODY POSTURE *(See also Fig. 11.50)*

There is a close interrelationship between body posture and the function and structure of the temporomandibular joint.[126] The effect of body posture on the masticatory system in the course of human development, with the development of upright posture and of the cerebrum, has already been described.

Littlejohn described a gravity line linking the symphysis of the mandible with the pubic symphysis (Fig. 11.30).[127] He also identified functional triangles in the body that establish an interrelationship between the TMJ and other body structures (Fig. 11.31).

Robert Samoian produced a model to demonstrate the integration of the TMJ in vertical body posture (Fig. 11.32):

- Functional links also exist with the falx cerebri and cerebelli and tentorium cerebelli, the nuchal muscles and spine[128] (see also Fig. 11.33). Delaire[129] states that the intracranial structures serve to transmit the balance of forces between the weight of the viscerocranium and the compensating tonus of the nuchal muscles, although this hypothesis is the subject of controversy.[130] The function of the temporomandibular joint and the occlusional patterns of the upper and lower jaw are dependent on this balance (Fig. 11.33; see also Fig. 11.16). Incorrect posture should be redressed in order to ensure the long-term success of treatment.[131] Crooked pelvic posture and unequal leg length affect occlusion to an electromyographically measurable degree.[132] Bahnemann[128] indeed sees the overwhelming majority of cases of dysgnathia

Figure 11.30 Descending anteroposterior gravity line: Course, from the anterior border of the foramen magnum through the body of T11 and T12 and the articulations of L4/L5 to the tip of the coccyx. Function, unites the spine into a single functional joint system, centered on T11 and T12. **Ascending posteroanterior gravity line:** Course, begins bilaterally at the hip joint, as a result of the pressure of the head of the femur in its articulation with the acetabulum. These lines run anterior to L3 and anterior to T4 to end at the posterior border of the foramen magnum. Function, reinforces support for the organs of the pelvis and abdomen; directs the forces at the atlanto-occipital joint to T2 and the second rib. The double line removes stress from L3 by directing tensions toward the head of the femur. **Ascending anterior gravity line:** Course, parallel to the descending gravity line. Function, links the symphysis of the mandible with the symphysis pubis. **Descending central gravity line:** Course, from the vertex, passing posterior to the clinoid processes, posterior third of the foramen magnum, transverse processes of C3–C6, anterior to T3 and T4, past the lower border of the third rib, body of L1–L4, and inside of the knee, to the feet. Function, L3 is the center of gravity of the body

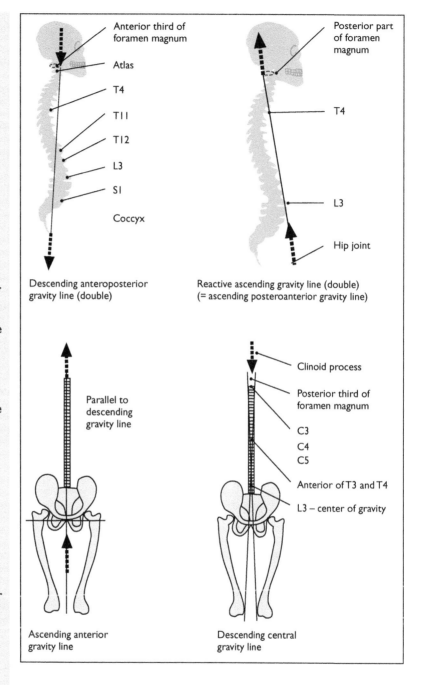

Anterior third of foramen magnum

Atlas

T4

T11

T12

L3

S1

Coccyx

Descending anteroposterior gravity line (double)

Posterior part of foramen magnum

T4

L3

Hip joint

Reactive ascending gravity line (double) (= ascending posteroanterior gravity line)

Parallel to descending gravity line

Ascending anterior gravity line

Clinoid process

Posterior third of foramen magnum

C3
C4
C5

Anterior of T3 and T4

L3 – center of gravity

Descending central gravity line

as due to a spinal syndrome, termed a gnatho-vertebral syndrome.

According to Schöttl and Broich, the following associations can be found between functional units, on the basis of studies by Haberfellner, Bahnemann, Rocabado and Treuenfels:[133–137]

- Retrusive occlusion (prognathism) and anteflexion of the head (70% of cases according to Rocabado).
- Temporomandibular joint and occipito-atlanto-axial joints: cross-bite and raised shoulder.
- Open bite (side) and crooked pelvic posture.
- Head and neck posture and speech.
- Mouth breathing/open bite and lymphatic reaction and digestive tract disturbances.
- Motor function of the tongue and skeletal muscles/total body posture.
- Ear, eye and occlusal planes and spine.
- Temporomandibular joint and hyoid.

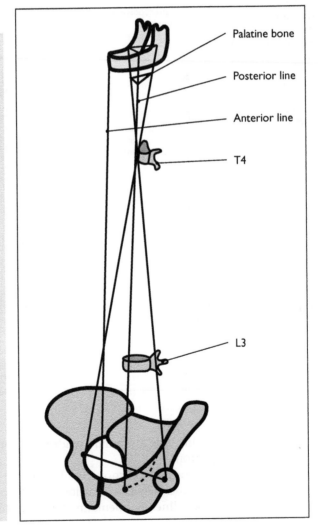

Figure 11.31 Polygon of forces acting on the spine, according to Littlejohn. One line runs from the anterior border of the foramen magnum to the coccyx. This is balanced by two lines running from the posterior border of the foramen magnum to the acetabulum, crossing these at the level of T4 to create a triangle above and another below the third rib and T4 (center of gravity). A functional line connects the symphysis of the mandible and pubic symphysis. Function: The triangles support the spine and organs. The upper triangle contains the joint structures with links to the foramen magnum, providing a base for the skull, which is balanced on T4. Effects of rotation of the skull are felt down as far as T4. Any imbalance in the palatine bone and its muscles affects the function of the upper triangle. The lower triangle helps maintain abdominal function by transmitting the rhythmic activity of the thorax. Normal posture of the pelvis (base of triangle) is necessary for support of abdominal tension

Figure 11.32 Model by Robert Samoian; modified by Torsten Liem. 1. (a) Nuchal muscles. (b) Back muscles. 2. Prevertebral muscles. 3. Omohyoid muscle. 4. Temporalis, masseter, and medial pterygoid muscles. 5. Lateral pterygoid muscle. 6. Suprahyoid muscles. 7. Infrahyoid muscles. 8. Muscles of the tongue (styloglossus m.) that move tongue posteriorly and superiorly. 9. Hyoglossus and chondroglossus muscles: lower and retract tongue. 10. Genioglossus muscle

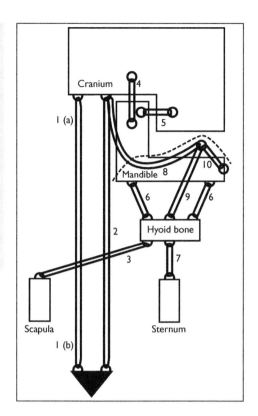

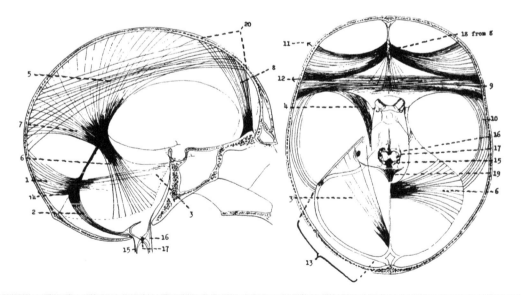

Figure 11.33 Stress fibers of the dura mater. From: Arbuckle BE. The selected writings of Beryl E. Arbuckle DO, FACOP. Indianapolis: American Academy of Osteopathy; 1994. Horizontal: 1. Falx cerebri inferior. 2. Falx cerebelli. 3. Tentorium cerebelli. 4. Sphenoidal. 5. Falx cerebri superior. Vertical: 6. Tentorium. 7. Falx cerebri posterior. 8. Falx cerebri anterior. 9. Transverse. Circular: 10. Squamosal. 11. Cranial vault anterior. 12. Cranial vault medial. 13. Cranial vault posterior. 14. Cranial fossa posterior. 15–17. Spinal

The relationship between the functional triangles and the temporomandibular joint

Posterior *(Fig. 11.34)*

1) Posterior-superior triangle

The trapezius muscle (descending part) and the more deeply located cervical muscles link the occiput with the scapula and account for the mobility of the cervical spine.

2) Posterior-inferior triangle

The trapezius muscle (ascending part) and the deeper-lying pectoral muscles continue to the lumbosacral transition and coccyx. Lateral support is given by the latissimus dorsi muscle.

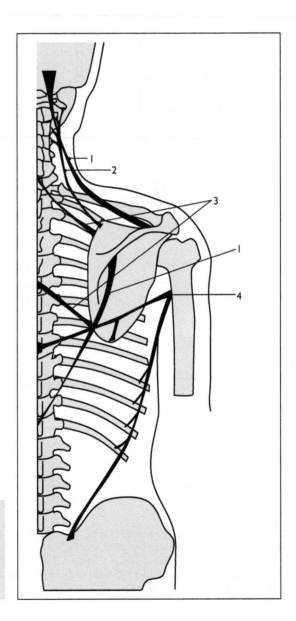

Figure 11.34 Muscles of the posterior functional triangle. 1. trapezius muscle. 2. levator scapulae muscle. 3. rhomboid major and minor muscles. 4. latissimus dorsi muscle

Anterior *(Fig. 11.35)*

1) Superior inframandibular triangle

- The digastric muscle (anterior belly), mylohyoid and geniohyoid muscles link the mandible with the hyoid.
- The triangle also incorporates the muscles of the tongue.

2) Inferior inframandibular triangle

The sternocleidomastoid, thyrohyoid, sternohyoid and sternothyroid muscles link the hyoid and the thyroid cartilage with the sternoclavicular and sternocostal joints.

Lateral triangle *(Fig. 11.36)*

- The digastric muscle links the mastoid with the hyoid and the mandible.
- The sternocleidomastoid muscle links the occiput and the mastoid with the sternum and clavicle.
- The stylohyoid muscle links the temporal bone with the hyoid.

Myers describes the TMJ as part of the deep frontal line,[139] whose function is the balancing of the head and nape of the neck on the body, the stabilization of the thorax, support of the lumbar spine, stabilization of the leg segments and raising of the medial arch of the foot. Course of the deep frontal line in the superior region: cranium → masticatory muscles → mandible → suprahyoid muscles → hyoid → infrahyoid muscles → pretracheal layer of cervical fascia

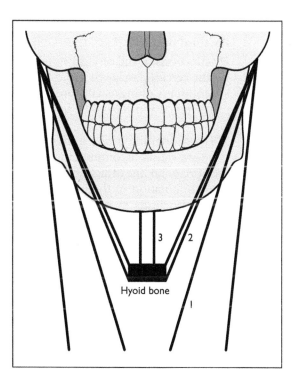

Figure 11.35 Anterior functional triangles (model by Landouzy[138]). 1. sternocleidomastoid muscle. 2. stylohyoid muscle. 3. digastric muscle

Hyoid bone

Figure 11.36 Lateral functional triangle (model by Landouzy[138]). 1. Digastric muscle (anterior belly). 2. Digastric muscle (posterior belly). 3. Sternocleidomastoid muscle. 4. Stylohyoid muscle. 5. Suprahyoid muscles. 6. Infrahyoid muscles. 7. Omohyoid muscle. 8. Temporalis muscle. 9. Muscles of the back

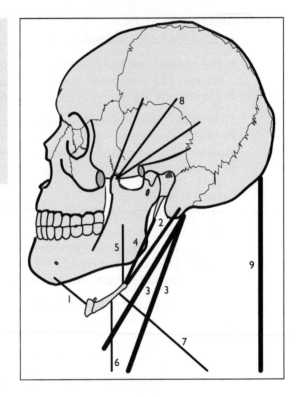

→ posterior border of subcostal cartilage, xiphoid process → anterior diaphragm, crura of diaphragm → body of the lumbar vertebrae.

Postural patterns *(Figs 11.37–11.39, Table 11.2)*[140,141]

Dysfunctions of the cervical vertebrae can have an effect on the TMJ via the cervical fasciae or hyoid bone.

Mouth breathing usually produces extension of the head according to Lawrence and Razook,[142] to ensure the best airway in the mouth area.

The shortening of the nuchal muscles and resulting extension of the head causes accommodative protrusion of the head to maintain the horizontal line of sight. Hypertonus of the nuchal muscles results. The combination of the inclination of the head, neck and pectoral girdle also leads to backward and downward displacement of the mandible, through the tension of the hyoid muscles. This leads to compression of the condylar process into the joint cavity of the TMJ, and increased tonus of the masticatory muscles.

Sidebending with contralateral rotation of the head causes the mandible to shift contralaterally to the sidebending, as in congenital torticollis.[143,144]

Dysfunction of the pectoral girdle can affect the TMJ via the omohyoid muscle to the hyoid bone and via the suprahyoid muscles. Further possible effects of pectoral girdle dysfunctions are to the temporal bone via the sternocleidomastoid muscle and so to the TMJ.[143]

Figure 11.37 Postural pattern, according to Hall T and Wernham J: normal gravity line. The gravity line runs from the dens axis via the sacral promontory, the middle of the hip and knee to the calcaneocuboid joint. The gravity line is derived from the combination of forces holding the body upright. The cranium is aligned with the center of the pelvis and the pectoral girdle is aligned with the pelvic girdle. The anterior line runs from the tip of the mental protuberance to the pubic symphysis. It runs parallel to the gravity line and perpendicular to the pubic line, and is the result of thoracic and abdominal tensions. Thoracic and abdominal pressure is normal

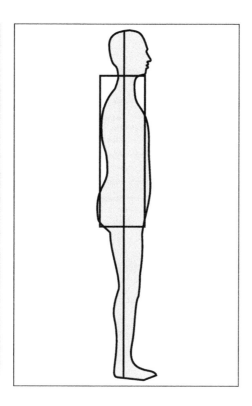

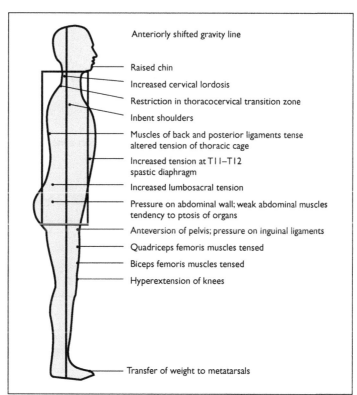

Anteriorly shifted gravity line

Raised chin

Increased cervical lordosis

Restriction in thoracocervical transition zone

Inbent shoulders

Muscles of back and posterior ligaments tense
altered tension of thoracic cage

Increased tension at T11–T12
spastic diaphragm

Increased lumbosacral tension

Pressure on abdominal wall; weak abdominal muscles
tendency to ptosis of organs

Anteversion of pelvis; pressure on inguinal ligaments

Quadriceps femoris muscles tensed

Biceps femoris muscles tensed

Hyperextension of knees

Transfer of weight to metatarsals

Figure 11.38 Postural pattern: anteriorly displaced gravity line. Tendency to crural hernia; inguinal hernia; visceral ptosis; bladder irritation

Figure 11.39 Postural pattern: posteriorly shifted gravity line. General enfeebled appearance; tendency to constipation, hemorrhoids and rectal prolapse

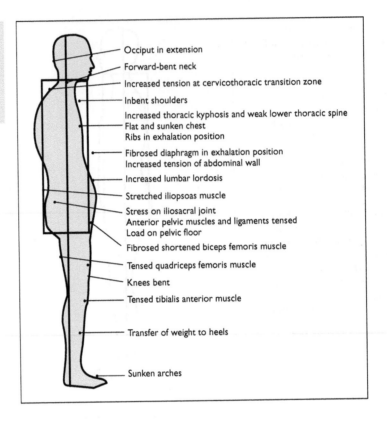

Occiput in extension
Forward-bent neck
Increased tension at cervicothoracic transition zone
Inbent shoulders
Increased thoracic kyphosis and weak lower thoracic spine
Flat and sunken chest
Ribs in exhalation position
Fibrosed diaphragm in exhalation position
Increased tension of abdominal wall
Increased lumbar lordosis
Stretched iliopsoas muscle
Stress on iliosacral joint
Anterior pelvic muscles and ligaments tensed
Load on pelvic floor
Fibrosed shortened biceps femoris muscle
Tensed quadriceps femoris muscle
Knees bent
Tensed tibialis anterior muscle
Transfer of weight to heels
Sunken arches

Table 11.2 Posture types according to Hall, Wernham and Littlejohn

Posture type	Ventral (anterior type)	Dorsal (posterior type)
Joint problems	Increased cervical lordosis Restriction in cervicothoracic transition zone Increased tension of posterior muscles and ligaments of the back Restriction and increased tension at T11 and T12 (T10-L1) Load on lumbosacral transition zone	Occiput in extension (and compression) Stress in cervicothoracic transition zone Increased thoracic kyphosis and weakened lower thoracic spine Compression of sternocostal joints Increased lumbar lordosis Load on iliosacral joints
Respiratory-circulatory	Tensions in diaphragm (often inspiratory) Weak overstretched abdominal muscles	Tensions in diaphragm (often in expiration) Disturbed pressure relationships between abdominal and thoracic cavities Increased tension of abdominal wall
Visceral	Tendency to ptosis of organs Reduced tension of parietal peritoneum Tendency to hernias and irritation in the lesser pelvis	Increased pressure on abdominal and pelvic organs Tendency to circulatory disorders Tendency to respiratory problems Tendency to obstipation

Source: Fossum C. Allgemeine Diagnostik. In: Liem T, Dobler T, eds. Leitfaden Osteopathie; Munich: Urban and Fischer; 2002.

Effects of craniomandibular dysfunction on body posture

Craniomandibular dysfunction (CMD) can of course affect body posture in its turn (Figs 11.40, 11.41, see Fig 11.42).

There is a close connection between the occipitocervical transition zone and the tonus of the muscles of the neck, and the position and function of the temporomandibular joint. The head is involuntarily held in the position that ensures the best occlusion of the teeth. Bahnemann[128] was almost always able to demonstrate changes in spinal posture in cases of malpositioning of the jaw. It is very important in this connection that not only the masticatory muscles in the wider sense, but also the specialized muscles of mastication can be used to stabilize the head[145] (see also dysfunction of the cervical spine).

In cases of prognathism where there is abnormal projection of the mandible, or of extreme open bite, inferior position of the atlas is found with a frequency of 30%. The proposed cause is the frequent inflammation of the nasopharyngeal region found with this dysfunction of the jaw, because of the proximity to the atlas.[136]

This corresponds to the extension position of the occiput (occipital condyles located anteriorly on the atlas). In this position the posterior arch of the atlas is approximated to the occiput.

- Ligamental strain between the anterior arch of the atlas and the dens can impinge on the subarachnoid space (and cerebrospinal fluid) at the second cervical vertebra.[136]
- The vertebral arteries (supplying the cerebellum and brainstem), the meninges of the brain and spinal cord, spinal cord, medulla oblongata and adjacent cranial nerve nuclei, the hypoglossal nerve (CN XII), superior cervical ganglion and vagus nerve (X) can be compromised.

Clinical presentation: Disturbances of speaking and swallowing, disturbance of tongue movement, dizziness, headache, and neurovegetative symptoms.[134]

Postural signs of craniomandibular dysfunction

Easily observed external signs may be: differently raised eyebrows, crooked posture of the head, and unilaterally raised clavicle.

1. Ipsilateral CMD: sidebending in the atlanto-occipital joint and secondary compensation of the atlanto-axial joint.
2. In the case of prognathism/retrusive occlusion: gravity line, especially at the head, cervicothoracic transition zone, and shoulders, is anteriorly displaced; extreme lordosis of the cervical spine and lumbar spine.[128]
3. In the case of protrusive occlusion: gravity line, especially at the head, cervicothoracic transition zone, and shoulders, is posteriorly displaced; cervical and lumbar spine extended.[128]
4. Restriction of the hyoid.
5. Cephalad and medial movement of the scapula.
6. In the case of ipsilateral CMD dysfunction: produces latent scoliosis.[146]

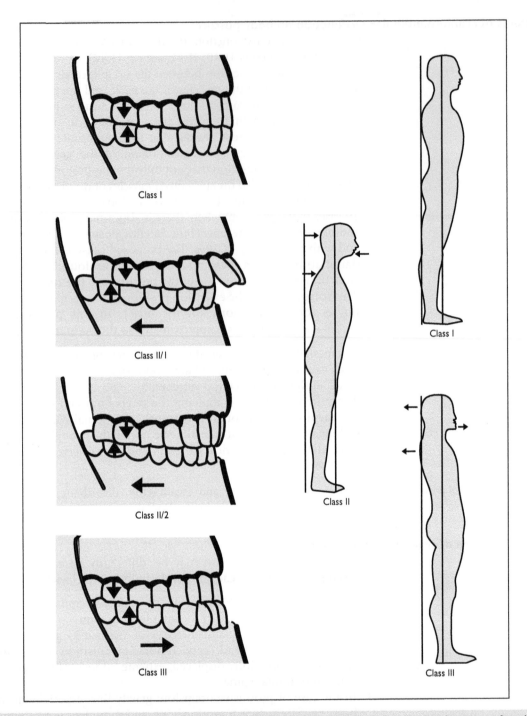

Figure 11.40 Effect of mandibular position on the cervicothoracic transition zone. Abnormal position of teeth with neutral occlusion: class I. Prognathism (retrusive/distal occlusion): class II with protruding upper front teeth ("buck teeth"): class II/1; with closed bite of upper front teeth: class II/2. Progenia (protrusion/mesial occlusion): class III

Figure 11.41 Myofascial interaction between TMJ and body. 1. Temporalis muscle. 2. Masseter muscle. 3. Suprahyoid muscles. 4. Stylohyoid muscles. Digastric muscle (posterior belly). 5. Infrahyoid muscles. 6. Sternocleidomastoid muscle. 7. Omohyoid muscle. 8. Cervical muscles (posterior and anterior). 9. Infraspinatus/supraspinatus muscles. 10. Biceps brachii muscle. 11. Thoracic back muscles. 12. Serratus anterior muscle. 13. External oblique muscle. 14. Diaphragm. 15. Iliopsoas muscle. 16. Lumbar back muscles. 17. Adductor muscles. 18. Biceps femoris muscle

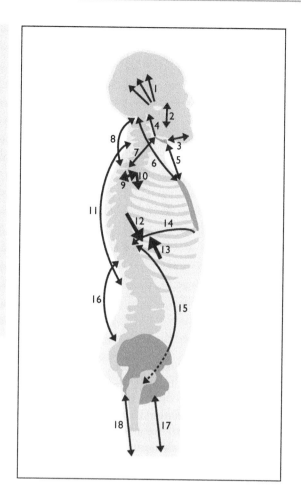

7. In the case of ipsilateral CMD dysfunction: imbalance of the pelvic girdle.[146]
8. In the case of cross-bite: asymmetry of the face and scoliosis.[128]
9. In the case of open bite: atlas-axis dysfunction.[128]

Barre's vertical alignment test *(Fig. 11.42)*[147]

1. Ascending dysfunction (pelvis deviates to the side): short leg, lumbar pain, dysfunction of the foot, knee, hip or pelvis.
2. Descending dysfunction (head/neck deviate to the side): cervical pain, dysfunction of the clavicle, shoulder, mandible, old craniocervical trauma, disturbance of the eyes or of vision.
3. Dysfunction ascending and descending (head/neck deviate to one side; pelvis to the opposite side).
4. Compensatory state: in this state any therapeutic intervention brings with it a risk of decompensation.
5. Unilateral hypertonus (head, upper body and pelvis deviate to the same side): central or vestibular disturbance.

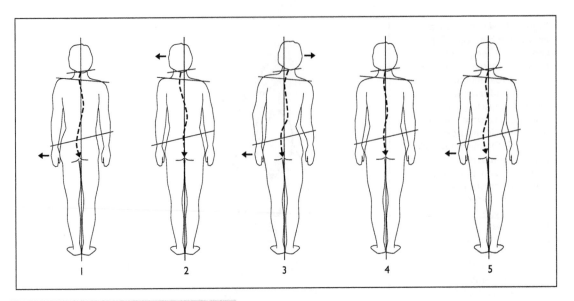

Figure 11.42 Barre's vertical alignment test

Dynamic signs of craniomandibular dysfunction

Motion or mobility restriction of body structures is far more important to the osteopath in diagnosis and treatment than static positional findings relating to individual body structures, or to the posture of the body. It is therefore essential to the success of osteopathic treatment to carry out dynamic local and global motion tests in addition to positionally based diagnosis.

1. Rotation restriction of the head on the side of the raised scapula.
2. The atlas and axis are usually rotated toward the side of the lowered scapula.
3. Lateral redistribution of weight leads to instability of the lower limb on the side of the lowered scapula.

Fascial organization according to Zink

Zink described the interaction between fascial patterns and postural organization. He ascribes particular importance to the transition zones – the craniocervical (O-A joint), cervicothoracic, thoracolumbar and lumbosacral regions – for diagnosis and therapy.

The ideal fascial organization would be a body without fascial motion restrictions, in which rotation in both directions is equally possible in all the above regions. The ideal is not found in practice; fascial organization in fact reflects not only trauma, but asymmetry of gait, organic disturbances, and a host of other factors in life.

Compensatory fascial organization *(Fig. 11.43a)*

Compensatory fascial organization is the most common situation in healthy individuals. The direction of fascial organization varies from one region to the next.

Figure 11.43
(a) Compensatory fascial organization
(b) Decompensatory fascial organization

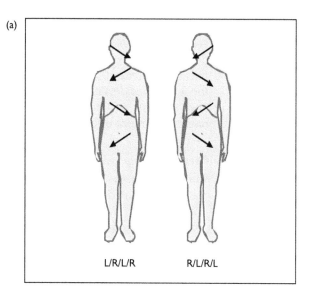

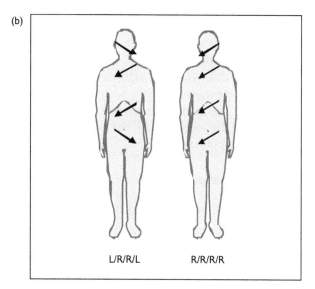

The one most frequently found (80% of cases) is expressed in greater ease of rotation in the left craniocervical, right cervicothoracic, left thoracolumbar and right lumbosacral (L/R/L/R) rotation. The compensatory pattern of fascial organization arranged R/L/R/L is less frequently found.

Decompensatory fascial organization *(Fig. 11.43b)*

This is characterized by the situation in which the direction of fascial mobility does not change from one region to the next. This may arise, for example, as the result of trauma.

Diagnostic procedure

- Test the regions described with the patient standing, and lying down.
- Locate the areas of compensatory fascial organization and identify the levels that deviate from this type of organization.
- The success of treatment is usually accompanied by the re-establishment of compensatory fascial organization.

Differential diagnosis

1. Standing/sitting: If the parameters remain unchanged when the patient has sat down, a descending dysfunction is more likely. Improvement in the parameters indicates that an ascending dysfunction is probable.
2. Paper test: Place a piece of paper between the teeth on the side of the raised scapula. An improvement in the parameters means that a dysfunction of the masticatory apparatus can be assumed as the origin of symptoms.
3. Meersseman test (differential diagnosis of ascending or descending dysfunction).

Patient standing

Posterior: Compare the height of the superior iliac crests, of the shoulders, and of the ears.

Lateral: Set against a body plumbline held laterally to the body and observe the position of the shoulder, the greater trochanter and lateral malleolus.

Patient supine

- Examine leg length and the position of the medial malleoli.
- Compare the abduction and internal rotation of the legs.
- Compare the active hip movement with legs extended.
- Compare the turning of the head.
- Establishment of contact between the teeth of the upper and lower jaw: With the patient supine, insert a separator of maximum thickness 3 mm between the teeth of the patient's upper and lower jaw, extending over the whole row of teeth (to prevent posterior displacement of the mandible) immediately posterior to the incisors.
- Ask the patient to take a few steps while biting gently together and swallowing the saliva.
- Then repeat the test.
- Evident improvement of the parameters: descending dysfunction (cranium; TMJ) (see Table 11.3).
- No change: ascending dysfunction.
- Partial improvement only: further general osteopathic examination is needed.

Table 11.3 Differentiation of ascending and descending dysfunctions associated with the TMJ

	Functional restriction and/or pain in masticatory apparatus	Positional or dynamic signs in TMJ	Tissue and motion changes of par./visc. structures	After treatment of identified dysfunction
Ascending dysfunction	Yes	No	Yes	Imp. of TMJ signs
Ascending dysfunction with CMD	Yes	No	Yes	Dynamic + positional TMJ signs → th. TMJ
Descending CMD	Yes + in par. system, e.g. pain in cervical spine	Yes		Imp. of par. system signs
Descending CMD with dysfunction of the par./visc. system	Yes + in par. system	Yes		Partial or no imp. of par. signs and posture → par. + visc. dysfunction

Imp., improvement; par., parietal; visc., visceral; th., therapy; → leads to par., parietal system, musculoskeletal fascial system of the body; visc., visceral system, internal organs and associated structures

LOCATION, CAUSES AND CLINICAL PRESENTATION OF CRANIOMANDIBULAR DYSFUNCTIONS

Osseous and diskal dysfunction

Clinical presentation: Pain, restrictions of the TMJ, joint sounds

a) Mandible
Powerful blows to the mandible, or falling and hitting the lower jaw may lead to fractures or subluxation. Less powerful blows or less serious falls usually cause an asymmetric displacement of the lower jaw, resulting in one side moving anterior and the other posterior. The consequence is one temporal bone in IR (on the side with the anteriorly displaced condyle) and one temporal bone in ER (on the side with the posteriorly displaced condyle), with disturbance of the tentorium cerebelli.

Other sequelae may be intraosseous dysfunction of the mandible, and disturbances of the intracranial membranes, SBS, hyoid bone and sacrum.

But many other causes may also lead to dysfunctions of the TMJ (see below).

Inflammatory or degenerative processes in the TMJ lead, via pain receptors and mechanoreceptors, to an alteration of muscular contraction, which causes a change in the position of the TMJ as a way of avoiding pain.

- Osteopathic dysfunction of the condyle process
- Traumatic injury, or chronic contraction of certain muscles of mastication can cause the condyles to become locked in a certain position. This phenomenon may be unilateral or bilateral.

Locking of the condyle in an anterior position (Fig. 11.44)
This dysfunction arises when the mouth is opened too wide, during tooth extractions, or as a result of a fall on to, or a blow on the tip of the chin, with spasm of the lateral pterygoid muscle.

Sequelae: 1. Temporal bone in external rotation.
2. Posteriorization of the hyoid bone, e.g. via the digastric muscle, stylohyoid muscle, etc.)

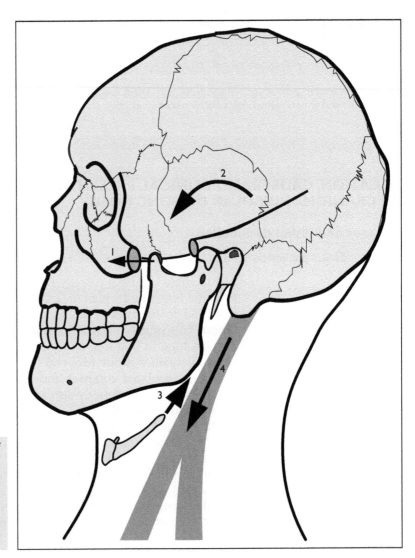

Figure 11.44 Restriction of a condyle in an anterior position. 1. Condyle in anterior position. 2. Temporal bone in external rotation. 3. Posteriorization of the hyoid bone. 4. Contraction of the sternocleidomastoid muscle

3. Dysfunction of the fourth thoracic vertebra; symptom: possible disturbances of cardiac rhythm.
4. Secondary contraction of the sternocleidomastoid muscle.

Symptoms: Venous stasis of the cranial vessels, or vagal problems and functional disturbance of the thyroid.

Restriction of the condyle in a posterior position[148–165] *(Fig. 11.45)*

This dysfunction usually arises in association with traumatic injury or a dysfunction of the atlanto-occipital joint, and is sustained by a spasm of the posterior fibers of the temporal muscle. For the role of the lateral pterygoid muscle.

Posterior displacement of the condyle is associated with an anterior displacement of the disk, during mouth-closure movement in the intercuspal position[158,166] (see also The Disk).

For Weinberg, posterior displacement of the condyle is an important factor in TMJ pain syndrome.[167]

Sequelae: 1. Temporal bone in internal rotation.
2. Diskal dysfunction: luxation or clicking. The clicking usually precedes locking of the jaw joint.

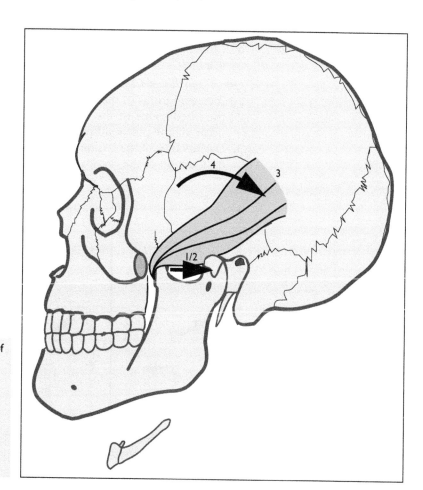

Figure 11.45 Restriction of a condyle in a posterior position. 1. Condyle in posterior position. 2. Contraction of the lateral pterygoid muscle. 3. Contraction of the temporal muscle (posterior part). 4. Temporal bone in internal rotation

Reciprocal clicking during mouth-opening is the result of a release of the TMJ. Reciprocal clicking during the closure movement is due to a displacement of the disk and condyle.

In cases of chronic reciprocal clicking and locking, the disk remains dislocated anterior during the normal extent of movement of the mandible.[166]

3. Strain of the petrosphenoidal ligament with disturbances of the sixth cranial nerve.
4. The pterygoid process of the sphenoid is shifted posterior (and in a lateral, inferior direction).
5. Disturbance of the hamulus in the middle ear, e.g. via the anterior ligament of the malleus: auditory disturbances.
6. Dysfunction of the carotid sympathetic plexus.
7. Dysphagia.

Restriction of the condyle in a lateral position (Fig. 11.46)
This dysfunction usually arises in association with traumatic injury.

Sequelae:
1. Asymmetric motion of the temporal bones.
2. Compression of the parietotemporal suture.
3. Torsion of the tentorium cerebelli.
4. Asymmetric opening and closure of the jaw.
5. Limited opening of the jaw.
6. Lateralization of the hyoid bone to the side of the laterally displaced condyle.

Other sequelae of CMD
1. Increased tonus of the orbicularis oris and buccinator.
2. Increased tonus of the constrictor muscles of the pharynx may occur via the pterygoid process of the sphenoid.
3. Dysfunction of the basilar part of the occipital bone can lead to a dysfunction of the cervical spine.

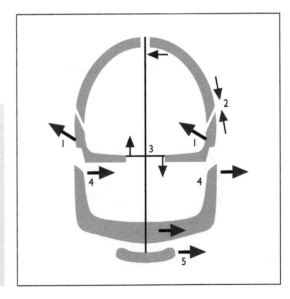

Figure 11.46 Restriction of a condyle in a lateral position. 1. Asymmetric motion of the temporal bones. 2. Compression of the parietotemporal suture. 3. Torsion of the tentorium cerebelli. 4. Lateralization of the mandible and asymmetric opening and closure of the jaw. 5. Lateralization of the hyoid bone to the side of the laterally displaced condyle

b) Temporal bone

Unlike conventional medical therapies, osteopathy also ascribes great importance to the temporal bones in the development of craniomandibular dysfunctions (CMD).[7,8] All disturbances of the temporal bones are capable of impairing the TMJ.

The most common dysfunction is IR of both temporal bones (associated with perinatal trauma).

In IR, displacement of the mandibular fossae in an antero-lateral direction occurs, resulting in anterior displacement of the mandible. In ER of both temporal bones, the mandible is displaced posterior.

(A dysfunction of the lower jaw can of course also lead to dysfunction of the temporal bone.)

However, secondary dysfunctions of the mandible are usually only manifested once the child begins to chew.

Mechanism of neuromuscular dysfunction
1. Dysfunction of temporal bone and sphenoid leads, via the facial nerve (CN VII), to abnormal contraction of the digastric muscle (posterior belly), resulting in CMD.
2. Dysfunction of the temporal bone and sphenoid leads, via the trigeminal ganglion and mandibular nerve (V3), to abnormal contraction of the temporal muscle, masseter muscle, pterygoid muscle, and digastric muscle (anterior belly), resulting in CMD.

c) SBS (Fig. 11.47)

The occipital bone governs the temporal bone, which in turn influences the mandible.

Example: An occipital bone in extension brings the temporal bones into IR; these in turn cause displacement of the mandible anterior.

The sphenoid governs the anterior facial bones (including the maxilla), but not the mandible.

Mechanism of neuromuscular dysfunction
1. Via the accessory nerve (CN IX) and the cervical plexus, dysfunction of the occipital bone causes abnormal contraction of the sternocleidomastoid muscle, leading to a restriction of the temporal bone with consequent CMD.
2. Via motor nuclei of the nerve V3, dysfunction of the occipital bone leads to abnormal contraction of the temporal muscle, masseter muscle, pterygoid muscles and digastric muscle (anterior belly), with consequent CMD.
3. Torsion of the SBS with compression of the oval foramen causes, via the mandibular nerve (V3), a spasm of the masticatory muscles with consequent CMD.

Mechanism of myofascial dysfunction

Torsion of the SBS leads, via the pterygoid process, to abnormal contraction or hypertonicity of the lateral pterygoid muscle, as a result of which the condyle process is restricted anterior.

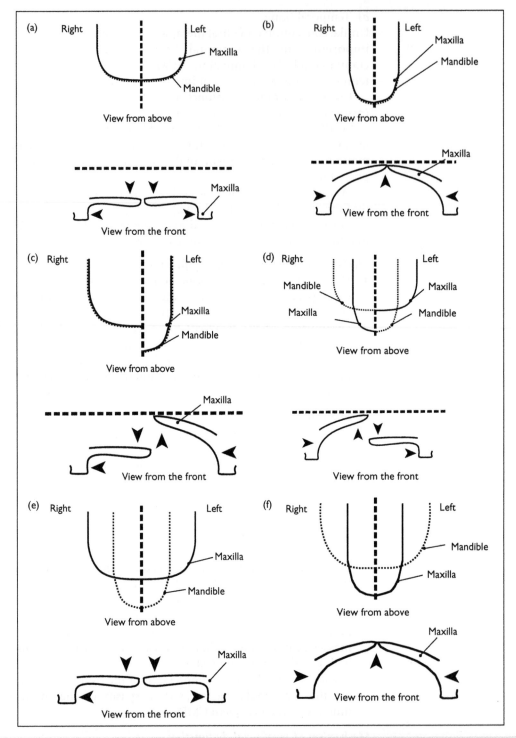

Figure 11.47 Influence of the SBS on the occlusion. (a) Flexion of the SBS (b) Extension of the SBS (c) Torsion right of the SBS (d) Side-bending/rotation right of the SBS (e) Superior vertical strain of the SBS (f) Inferior vertical strain of the SBS

d) Disk

The effects of stress and of the transmission of tension are produced primarily in the intermediate zone of the disk (especially in its lateral parts). Even relatively minor loading of the joint can induce distinct deformation.[168,169]

During a forceps delivery, the disk may be damaged by the pressure of the forceps on the pre-auricular region.[126] As a rule, however, the damaged tissues of the baby quickly regenerate.

Extreme mouth-opening movements, or holding the mouth fully open for long periods (e.g. during dental treatment, etc.) can lead to over-extension of the bilaminar structures. Traumatic injuries caused e.g. by falling or by blows, may lead to excessive posterior compression of the bilaminar (retrodiskal) structures, resulting in inflammation, pain and swelling which in some circumstances may cause anterior displacement of the disk.

As a result of a malocclusion, tooth extractions, muscle imbalances, and dysfunctions of the skeletal-muscle system etc., sustained asymmetric forces (extension or compression) may affect the disks, leading to increased diskal wear and problems with the bilaminar (retrodiskal) structures. Another notable cause of anterior dislocation of a disk is orthopedically-induced retrusion of the mandible, resulting in histological and microscopic changes in the disk and its attachments, e.g. flattening of the posterior diskal region.[170]

Anterior displacement of the disk may be induced by excessive contraction of the superior part of the lateral pterygoid muscle.[171,172] However, the associated posterior displacement of the condyle may also be caused by the temporal muscle (see restriction of the condyle in the posterior position).[173]

Changes in the position of the menisci are frequently encountered, but are usually symptomless.[172] Retrodiskal disturbances may exist with or without alteration of the disk-condyle relationship. However, investigations have confirmed that anterior dislocation of the disk in static occlusion represents the most common intra-articular symptomatic disturbance of the TMJ.[148-165,174-177] While an anterior dislocation of the disk does not necessarily co-exist with CMD, it is frequently associated with a convex disk shape and perforation of the posterior disk attachment, as well as with an increased susceptibility to the occurrence of CMD.[178-181]

More recently, it has been demonstrated that lateral or medial disk displacements, in contrast to the rare posterior displacements, are observed more frequently now than in the past.[148-165,182] An anteromedial position of the disk is more common than the anterolateral position.

Clinical presentation: Joint sounds (clicking, crepitation), subluxation and, especially in association with diskal dislocation, severe restriction and pain may occur.[183] In the anteromedial position of the disk, the head of the condyle is moved laterally somewhat and therefore appears to be more prominent.[184] In the anterolateral disk position, the head of the condyle is displaced medially and is less prominent. This is associated with severe trismus.[185]

Secondary abnormal contractions of the masseter and temporal muscles arise as an arthrokinetic protective reflex associated with an abnormal disk position.[186]

Analysis of mandibular-joint clicking (Fig. 11.48a)

e) Hyoid bone (Fig. 11.48b)

The hyoid bone may be dysfunctional owing to mandibular-joint disturbances (disturbances of swallowing or vocalization, etc.) and induce CMD via myofascial chains. However, it may also participate in the development of CMD.

f) Teeth[187]

Causes: Dental extractions, orthodontic surgery, traumatic injury, CMD, poorly fitting dental prostheses and dental fillings,[188] genetic factors, dietary factors, and birth trauma.[189] Laughlin mentions that, if certain conditions exist, some dental surgery and orthodontic operations are capable of inducing cranial dysfunctions.[190] These include, e.g. rigid dental bridges, especially ones which span the front teeth, solid metal or non-metal dental prostheses or partial prostheses, amalgam fillings, and rigid dental braces and dental crowns, static somatic dysfunctions, mental and physical stresses, etc.

Disturbances of occlusion in turn lead to disturbances of muscle function or muscle spasms, and may cause a CMD.[191]

An occlusal factor is very often implicated in the causation of a CMD. Patients who have had dental treatment, for example, suffer from CMD more frequently than patients with intact teeth.[188]

Just as there is a correlation between disturbances of occlusion and parafunctional habits, a positive correlation has also been demonstrated between the degree of TMJ dysfunction and the degree of malocclusion and parafunctional habits.[192] For example, it has been established that in TMJ patients by comparison with healthy volunteers, occlusion of the upper and lower teeth is less frequently simultaneous and less frequently symmetric.[193]

A clear correlation exists between a muscle imbalance of the anterior part of the temporal, and TMJ symptoms. In association with maximum voluntary bite, the anterior part of the temporal muscle has a more significant effect on tooth contact than the masseter muscle,[193] although the occurrence of TMJ dysfunctions cannot be explained on the basis of occlusal relationships alone.[194]

Crossbite appears to cause neither symptoms nor disease in the TMJ. Nor is there any evidence that an over-bite influences non-arthrotic disturbances of the TMJ in any way, whereas a clear association exists between an anterior open bite and osteoarthritis of the TMJ.[195]

Any premature contact of the teeth is communicated to the central nervous system via the nerve endings (mechanical stimuli, pain) in the periodontal ligament. In response to this, the jaw muscles contract. Abrasion of the impeding tooth surface or the exertion of force on the tooth are two ways of correcting the premature contact; alternatively the chewing surfaces involved are avoided by

(a)

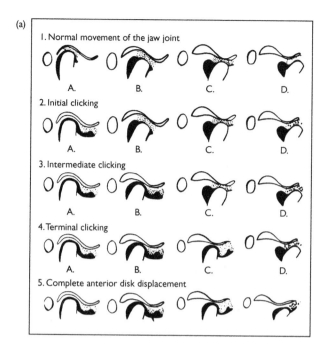

(b)

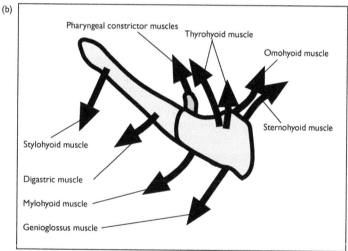

Figure 11.48 (a) Analysis of jaw-joint clicking. With thanks to WB Farrar and WL McCarty, Jnr, on whose work (A clinical outline of temporomandibular joint diagnosis and treatment. Normandie publications, Montgomery, 1982), the description below is very largely based. 1. Normal movement of the jaw joint. 2. Clicking begins immediately on opening the mouth (initial clicking): the bilaminar (retrodiskal) tissue has been displaced immediately in front of the condyle. The sound is due to backward displacement of the condyle into the disk. 3. Clicking during mouth opening (intermediate clicking): the bilaminar (retrodiskal) tissue has moved a greater distance in front of the condyle. The condyle must therefore travel further rearward to reach the disk. 4. Clicking during the end of mouth opening (terminal clicking): the disk has moved forward again beneath the articular tubercle of the temporal bone. The condyle regains contact with the disk only at the end of mouth opening. The sound is indicative of damage to the disk. 5. Complete anterior disk displacement: the disk is positioned in front of the articular tubercle of the temporal bone. The condyle can no longer move into the disk. At this stage, there is normally no clicking noise. This stage can progress to a true arthrosis. (b) Muscles which act upon the hyoid bone

hypertonicity of the muscles. Contraction of these muscles causes a displacement of the mandible (laterotrusion, protrusion).

Combination with other factors (emotional states, stress, dysfunction of the cervical spine, joint disease, cold or damp, metabolic disturbance and hormonal factors) leads to additional contraction of the muscles of mastication, and ultimately to a triggering or deterioration of symptoms. The consequences are bruxism (grinding of the teeth without a functional purpose), pain, tendinomyopathies, further compensation and degenerative processes (joint diseases) (Fig. 11.49).

Mechanism of myofascial dysfunction

Disturbance of occlusion → contraction of the neck muscles → dysfunction of the cervical or thoracic spine.

Disturbance of occlusion → contraction of the cervical flexors and suprahyoid muscles → reduction of lordosis of the cervical spine, displacement of the hyoid in a posterior, superior direction, lowering and posterior displacement of the tongue → the consequence may be bruxism, especially if conditions are favorable due to simultaneous contraction of the retrohyoid muscles and posterior part of the temporal muscle → the infrahyoid muscles follow the suprahyoid and, via their influence on the scapula and thorax, can impair breathing.

Laughlin's dysfunction mechanism[190]

Excessively narrow maxilla and mandible → extraction of the bicuspids to create more space → posterior displacements of the anterior teeth and pre-maxilla by orthodontic measures → possible compression of cranial sutures, flattening of the facial profile and lateral compression of the facial structures.[196–200]

Figure 11.49 Effect of premature contact on the TMJ. Compensatory contraction of the muscles of the jaw. (a) Premature contact: information is conducted via nerve endings in the periodontal ligament. The muscles of mastication contract. (b) In some circumstances, this contraction counterbalances the premature contact, and may cause a displacement of the mandible

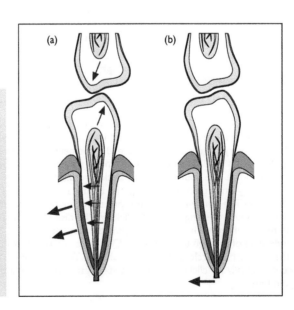

→ Possible compression of the sphenobasilar synchondrosis → posterior displacement of the mandible due to posterior displacement of the maxillary complex → TMJ syndrome with displacement of the disk, and cervical and sacral imbalance.[199,201]

The further back the position of the premature bite in the mouth, the greater the load or compressive force on the opposite TMJ. At the same time, the ipsilateral joint is subjected to a reduced load and increased tension.

Reduced posterior tooth contact, e.g. due to tooth extractions or dental treatment etc., leads to increased activity of the temporal muscle, masseter muscle, and the medial and lateral pterygoid muscles (superior part), and to increased compression of the TMJ.[202]

Note:
- However, opinions vary as to the importance of occlusal disharmonies in the occurrence of a CMD.[195]
- Myofascial adaptation in the example of premature contact of the first molar on the left (Fig. 11.50).

g) Maxilla

Cause:
- Traumatic injury (a fall or a blow).
- The fact that the maxilla is displaced posterior leads to ER of the zygomatic bone and compression of the complex of maxilla-palatine-pterygoid process. The consequence is an ipsilateral displacement of the condyle anterior.

Clinical presentation: Clicking sounds, reduced mouth opening, pain on chewing.

h) Cervical spine

Mechanism of neuromuscular dysfunction
1. Dysfunction of the upper cervical spine leads, via the nerves C1 to C3, to an abnormal contraction of the infrahyoid muscles. These restrict the hyoid bone and influence the suprahyoid muscles, resulting in a CMD (see also under dysfunction of the suprahyoid muscles).
2. Dysfunction of the upper cervical spine leads, via the accessory nerve (CN IX) and cervical plexus, to abnormal tension of the sternocleidomastoid muscle with restriction of the temporal bone, resulting in a CMD.
3. By means of mutual reinforcement of dysfunctions of the neck muscles and TMJ via the trigeminal nucleus.

Mechanism of myofascial dysfunction
- Dysfunction of the upper cervical spine leads to a CMD via the suprahyoid muscles or the deep cervical fascia and the investing layer of the cervical fascia.
- A dysfunction of the upper cervical spine may also give rise to stimulation of the auriculotemporal nerve, with consequent pain in the jaw joint, and earache.
- Hyperlordosis of the CS can give rise to distocclusion.[128]
- A hyperextended/kyphotic CS may lead to a prognathic occlusion.[128]
- Scoliosis may cause an ipsilateral CMD and a crossbite.
- An atlas-axis dysfunction can give rise to an open bite.

Figure 11.50 Myofascial adaptation in the example of premature contact of the first molar on the left

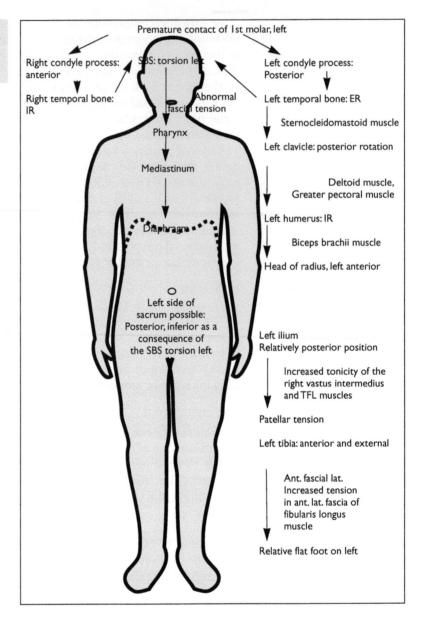

Premature contact of 1st molar, left

Right condyle process: anterior

SBS: torsion left

Left condyle process: Posterior

Right temporal bone: IR

Abnormal fascial tension

Left temporal bone: ER

Sternocleidomastoid muscle

Pharynx

Left clavicle: posterior rotation

Mediastinum

Deltoid muscle, Greater pectoral muscle

Left humerus: IR

Diaphragm

Biceps brachii muscle

Head of radius, left anterior

Left side of sacrum possible: Posterior, inferior as a consequence of the SBS torsion left

Left ilium Relatively posterior position

Increased tonicity of the right vastus intermedius and TFL muscles

Patellar tension

Left tibia: anterior and external

Ant. fascial lat. Increased tension in ant. lat. fascia of fibularis longus muscle

Relative flat foot on left

i) Shoulder girdle

Mechanism of myofascial dysfunction

1. Dysfunction of the scapula leads, via the omohyoid muscle, to a restriction of the hyoid bone and, via the suprahyoid muscles, to a CMD.
2. Via the sternocleidomastoid muscle, and owing to the continuity of the infrahyoid muscles with the digastric muscle (posterior belly) and stylohyoid muscle, dysfunction of the clavicle and sternum causes a restriction of the temporal bone, resulting in a CMD.
3. Drawing back the shoulders can cause protrusion.

Muscular dysfunction

A large number of investigations have concluded that most pain of the jaw joint is of muscular origin.[203,204] It is also possible that muscular imbalances give rise to pain and finally to masticatory disturbances[204] or inflammatory and degenerative changes in the joints.[205] However, there is no consensus as to whether muscular hyperactivity is of local (occlusal, articular) or central causation (stress, psychoemotional factors).[206]

The masseter, lateral pterygoid and temporals are the muscles of mastication most commonly involved in CMD.

Causes of muscular hypertonicity:

- Malocclusion, bruxism.
- Dysfunction of the cervical spine, as well as of the rest of the spinal column and the extremities.
- Poor posture.
- Stress and psychic factors (gnashing of the teeth and grinding of the teeth).
- Traumatic injury: falling on and hitting the lower jaw, or a blow to the mandible or head, and supporting one's head with the hand or arm under the lower jaw; this can result in acute muscle spasm.
- CMD.
- Degenerative and inflammatory diseases of the TMJ (pain leads to further muscular contraction).
- Neurovascular: associated with dysfunction of the sphenopetrosal synchondrosis or oval foramen. This leads to compression or edema of the mandibular nerve (V3) either directly or via a circulatory stasis.
- Hormonal influences: menopause, puberty, thyroid dysfunctions.
- Metabolic influences.
- Other effects: cold, damp and air-conditioning.
- Shaper[144] states that shortness of one leg is the commonest single cause of spasm of the masticatory muscles.

Clinical presentation: Pain, restrictions of motion.

a) Temporal muscle (Fig. 11.51)

Causes: Psychoemotional factors, dental dystopia, premature tooth contact, immobilization of the jaw, bruxism, gnashing of the teeth, cold or traumatic injury, secondarily in association with dysfunction of the upper trapezius muscle and sternocleidomastoid muscle.[207]

In hypertonicity, the muscle may compress the squamous suture and then the disk and articular surface of the temporomandibular joint.

Clinical presentation:
- Pain in the maxillary sinus and in the molars of the upper jaw.
- Pain in the temporal region.
- Hypersensitivity and pain in the upper teeth.[208,209]

Anterior part:
- Pain in the parietal bone (compression of the sphenoparietal and coronal sutures), malocclusion.[193]
- Grinding, central pressure.

Figure 11.51 Hypertonicity of the temporal muscle

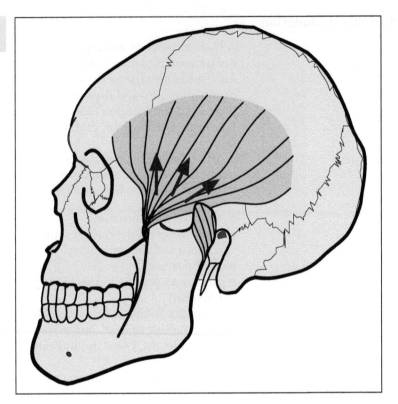

- Limited mouth opening.
- Muscle spasm draws the mandible cephalad.
- Possible compression in the TMJ, with diskal dysfunction.
- Temporal bone in anterior rotation.

Medial part:

- Temporal headache.
- Muscle spasm draws the mandible cephalad (with the anterior part).
- Pain radiating into the larynx.

Posterior part:

- Headache focused on the temporal bone or occipital bone (compression of the occipital mastoid suture).
- Disturbance of venous backflow of the cranial vessels.
- Muscle spasm draws the mandible posterior.
- Limited mouth opening.
- Temporal bone in external rotation (as the condyle is positioned posterior), while the parietal bone is in internal rotation.
- Pain radiating into the larynx.

b) Masseter muscle (Fig. 11.52)

Causes: Chronic muscle strain (bruxism, gum-chewing, dummy-sucking).[210]

Sudden strong contraction (cracking nuts), malocclusion, premature contact, mouth breathing, emotional trauma, CMD,

Figure 11.52 Hypertonicity of the masseter muscle. 1. Hypertonicity of the masseter muscle. 2. Temporal bone in external rotation. 3. Zygomatic bone in external rotation. 4. Compression of the TMJ.

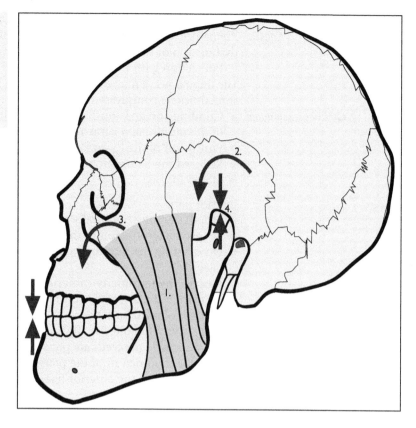

over-extended opening of the mouth during dental surgery, traumatic injury, secondarily in association with trigger points of the sternocleidomastoid muscle.[207]

Pain in the TMJ is very often associated with increased muscle activity (sometimes with simultaneous contraction of the neck muscles).[211]

Interaction with the contralateral gluteus medius (Rossaint and Thie).[212]

Clinical presentation:
- Increased tension in the masseter muscle,[211] grinding of the teeth (protrusive bruxism), pain in the upper jaw and lower molars, and in the mid-facial region (maxillary nerve (V2)) and maxillary sinus, and retro-ocular pain.[213]
- Limited mouth opening.
- In cases of unilateral hypertonicity, the mandible may deviate to the ipsilateral side.
- Compression of the TMJ.

Deep part:
- Unilateral tinnitus, frontal headache.
- Radiation into the TMJ and deep into the ear.

Superficial part:
- Radiation into the eyebrow region, maxilla, mandible and upper and lower molars.

c) Lateral pterygoid muscle (Fig. 11.53)

Causes: Premature contact, bruxism, excessive gum-chewing, secondary to dysfunction of the sternocleidomastoid muscle and neck muscles.[207]

Interaction with the adductor muscles (after Rossaint and Thie).[212] The lingual nerve may extend through the belly of the muscle, and so sometimes be compressed.[214]

Clinical presentation:
- Grinding and gnashing of the teeth, pain in the TMJ, maxilla, floor of the mouth, and earache.
- Protrusion of the lower jaw, with slightly reduced mouth opening.
- Reduced medial motion of the lower jaw.
- Malocclusion.

Inferior part:
- Mouth opening minimally reduced.
- Reduced laterotrusion to the contralateral side.
- On opening the mouth, the midline between the incisors deviates laterally.
- Muscle hypertonicity anteriorizes the condyle, resulting in premature contact of the contralateral front teeth and malocclusion of the ipsilateral back teeth.
- As a result, a full bite usually triggers pain on the ipsilateral side. The more strongly the teeth are pressed together, the greater the pain.
- Possible dysfunction of the pterygopalatine ganglion.
- Dysfunction of the anterior ligament of the malleus.

Superior part open:
- Muscle hypertonicity displaces the disk anterior, resulting in clicking of the joint.

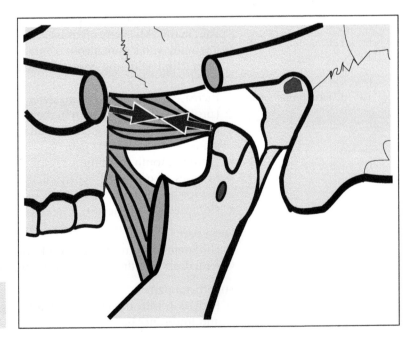

Figure 11.53 Hypertonicity of the lateral pterygoid muscle

d) Medial pterygoid muscle (Figs 11.54a,b)

Causes: Malocclusion, bruxism, excessive gum-chewing and post-childhood thumb-sucking, emotional stress and anxiety, rarely muscle spasm due to cellulitis in the pterygomandibular fossa; secondarily in association with dysfunction of the lateral pterygoid muscle or opposite medial pterygoid muscle.[207]

Interaction with the contralateral adductor muscles/psoas muscle (Rossaint and Thie).[212]

Clinical presentation:
- As for masseter muscle, pain in the TMJ and floor of the mouth.
- Mouth opening as a rule reduced and painful.
- Dysphagia.
- Radiation into the posterior region of the mouth and the pharynx, inferior and posterior of the TMJ, and deep into the ear.
- Displacement of the midline of the incisors.
- (A displacement of the mandible to the contralateral or ipsilateral side, or to neither side has been described).[215,216]
- Muscle spasm moves the condyle in an anterior and cranial direction, and the pterygoid process of the sphenoid in a posterior direction.
- Possible dysfunction of the pterygopalatine ganglion.

e) Sphenomandibular muscle

Causes: Muscle spasm, with compression of the maxillary nerve against the posterior wall of the maxillary sinus.[217]

Clinical presentation: Retro-orbital pain, possible involvement in the causation of cluster headache.

f) Mylohyoid muscle

Clinical presentation: Functional disturbances of the tongue,[218] dysphagia, tightness of the throat, or globus syndrome, sore throat, TMJ symptoms. Glossoptosis (pressure of the root of the tongue against the cervical spine, resulting in mouth breathing).

g) Digastric muscle

Causes: Bruxism (unilateral tenderness: anterior-posterior bruxism; bilateral tenderness: eccentric bruxism), mouth breathing, over-long styloid process; secondary to dysfunction of the masseter muscle.[207]

Clinical presentation:
- Grinding of the teeth, pain and functional disturbances of the mouth floor, tongue and pharynx, pain in the lower incisors (anterior belly), dysphagia, TMJ symptoms, possibly pseudopain in the sternocleidomastoid muscle (posterior belly).
- Hypertonicity of the muscle can restrict the hyoid bone in a cranial position, make it difficult to close the mouth, and cause an external rotation of the temporal bone.
- Hypertonicity of the posterior belly draws the mandible towards the ipsilateral side. This does not usually become manifest, however, as other muscles compensate for the effect (contralateral temporal muscle, posterior part, and masseter muscle, deep part).

h) Geniohyoid muscle

Clinical presentation: TMJ symptoms, similar symptoms to digastric muscle.

Figure 11.54 (a,b) Hypertonicity of the medial pterygoid muscle. 1. Muscle spasm moves the pterygoid process of the sphenoid in a posterior direction and therefore the greater wing in flexion position. 2. Muscle spasm moves the condyle in an anterior and cranial direction

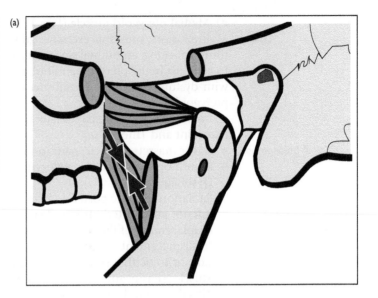

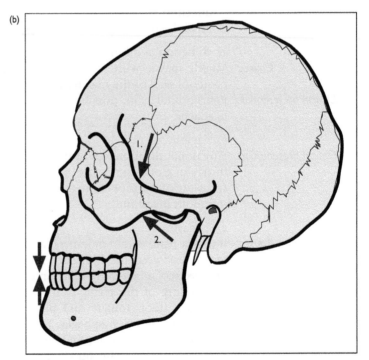

i) Stylohyoid muscle

Causes: Bruxism (unilateral tenderness: anterior-posterior bruxism; bilateral tenderness: eccentric bruxism).

Clinical presentation:
- Associated with muscle spasm: cranial motion of the hyoid bone and difficulties closing the mouth.
- Radiation of the pain into the tongue, floor of the mouth, pharynx and larynx.

- Hypertonic suprahyoid muscles may draw the mandible posterior. During the growth phase, this leads to reduced sagittal growth by comparison with the bones of the upper jaw, resulting in a distocclusion and withdrawal of the tongue from the palate due to the loss of its opposing member.
- A hypertonic suprahyoid musculature may also compress the articular surfaces and disk of the jaw joint, as well as the vessel-conducting retrodiskal pad, while moving the articular processes of the mandible into the posterior part of the TMJ groove. The infrahyoid muscles and the pharyngeal constrictor must then produce a counterforce in order to hold the hyoid bone in position in response to contraction of the suprahyoid muscles. This reactive contraction may in turn produce symptoms in the infrahyoid muscles. A reactive chronic hypertonicity of the pharyngeal constrictor may, via its connections with the neck, lead to strain in this region.
- The suprahyoid muscles also interact with the opposite psoas muscle (Rossaint and Thie).[212]

j) Superior pharyngeal constrictor

Clinical presentation:
- Pain and functional disturbance of the mouth floor and pharynx.
- In association with hypertonicity: via the pharyngeal raphe, dysfunctions of flexion and extension of the SBS.

k) Genioglossus muscle

Clinical presentation: Functional disturbance of the tongue.

l) Sternohyoid, thyrohyoid, omohyoid muscles (Fig. 11.55)

Clinical presentation: Associated with muscle spasm: cranial motion of the hyoid bone and difficulties closing the mouth, possibly thyroid disturbances.

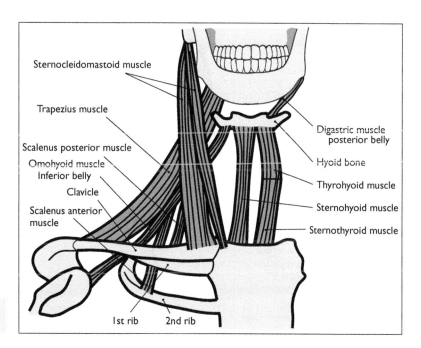

Figure 11.55 Hyoid muscles

m) Tongue

Clinical presentation: Dysphagia.

n) Sternocleidomastoid muscle (Fig. 11.56)

Causes: Postural imbalance due to a difference in leg length and shoulder-girdle dysfunction, disturbances of breathing (asthma), a sequela from CSF puncture, chronic sinusitis, dental abscess, herpes simplex in the mouth region.[207]

Clinical presentation:
- Soreness of the neck (patient lies in bed, usually on the dysfunctional side).
- Tension headache, sweating of the forehead on the ipsilateral side, conjunctival redness, lacrimation, rhinitis, blurred vision.

Sternal part:
- Pain at the temple, cheek and orbit.

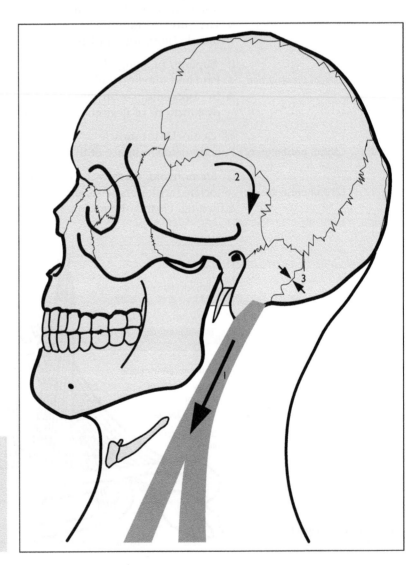

Figure 11.56 Hypertonicity of the sternocleidomastoid muscle. 1. Contraction of the sternocleidomastoid muscle. 2. Internal rotation of the temporal bone. 3. Compression of the occipitomastoid suture

Clavicular part:
- Frontal headache, disturbance of balance, postural dizziness, seasickness or travel sickness, possibly with nausea.
- Associated with hypertonicity: internal rotation of the temporal bone with secondary TMJ disturbance and compression of the occipitomastoid suture.

Dysfunction of the ligaments

Clinical presentation: Pain, restriction (joint sounds, possibly associated with dysfunctions of the articular capsule).

a) Stylomandibular ligament
Dysfunctions due to dental extractions associated with anterolateral displacement of the disk.
 Symptoms: neuralgic pain, dysphonia, earache, dysphagia and carotodynia,[29] as well as possibly sensitivity to pain over the styloid process.

b) Sphenomandibular ligament
Dysfunctions due to dental extractions: immobilization of the head, and the act of opening the mouth wide result in restriction of the temporal bones in internal rotation.
 Extraction of a tooth in the lower jaw leads to traction on the sphenomandibular ligament on the opposite side.
 Since the ligament is attached to the sphenoid posterior to the transverse flexion/extension axis, the traction on the ligament causes a cranial movement of the greater wing on this side (= the side opposite the dental extraction).
 Extraction of a molar from the lower jaw: cranial motion of the greater wing on the opposite side (torsion).
 Extraction of a molar from the upper jaw: cranial motion of the greater wing on the same side (torsion).
 This results in stretching of the petrosphenoidal ligament on the side of the cranial greater wing.

Clinical presentation: Visual disturbances (CN VI), facial pain (CN V, trigeminal ganglion), disturbances of blood outflow in this region, tinnitus.

c) Articular capsule and lateral ligament
On account of the good nerve supply in particular of the articular capsule and lateral ligament, but also of the other structures, inflammation and subluxations of the jaw joint can cause severe pain. This massive sensory input is transmitted into the trigeminal ganglion, which therefore in turn acts as a type of facilitated segment in the maintenance of the CMD.

d) Anterior ligament of the malleus and Pintus ligament
Clinical presentation: Hearing difficulties, tinnitus.

e) Sphenopetrosal ligament at the sphenopetrosal synchondrosis

Fascial dysfunction

All fascial structures are capable of transmitting tensions caused by a CMD or, conversely, of conducting dysfunctions from other regions of the body to the TMJ (see also: the jaw joint and body posture).

Dural dysfunction

Because dural innervation is provided via the trigeminal nerve (CN V), a CMD may also result in headache. Dural dysfunctions and CMD may lead to facilitation of the trigeminal ganglion.

Evidence has been produced that the tentorium cerebelli plays a role in disk dislocation. In post-mortem investigations, for example, a correlation has been reported between disk dislocation, the degree of ossification of the petrotympanic fissure, and fibrosis of the tentorium cerebelli.[220]

Disturbances of the nerves

Dysfunction of the joints, sutures, dura mater and fascias may directly impair the nervous structures and facilitate motor innervation in such a way as to give rise to a CMD. However, such disturbances may also be caused indirectly by venous stasis, e.g. in the cavernous sinus, or by stimulation of the periarterial sympathetic nerves. This leads, either directly or via a circulatory stasis, to edema or compression of the nerve. The consequence could be a change in the pH at the nerve, and altered stimulus conduction.

In association with dysfunction: due to the many nerve connections in the TMJ, the lateral ligament and the surrounding adipose tissue, dysfunctions or inflammation of the jaw joint may be associated with severe pain.

a) Trigeminal ganglion
Pain in the TMJ and dental structures may spread throughout the entire region innervated by the trigeminal nerve. For example, information may be conducted via the trigeminal nerve (CN V) to the trigeminal nucleus, which extends to the height of the second or third segment of cervical spinal cord, and may even reach the upper thorax via intermediate neurons. The nerve receptors in the mouth region are furthermore much more sensitive than in other regions of the body. The trigeminal nucleus in the mid-brain simultaneously receives afferent proprioceptive information from the periodontal ligaments and the muscle spindles. The stimuli may be mutually reinforcing in this trigeminal nucleus. The ganglion too may facilitate, and give rise to a vicious circle.

In close proximity to the trigeminal ganglion, the trigeminal nerve may be impaired by high-pressure within the internal carotid artery or by venous congestion at the level of the cavernous sinus.

The branches of the trigeminal nerve may furthermore be impaired by dysfunctions of the temporal bones and sphenoid, by abnormal dural tensions and venous congestion of the sinus, as well as by disturbances of cranial outflow.

- Mechanism of neuromuscular dysfunction: dysfunction of the temporal bone and sphenoid leads, via the trigeminal ganglion and CN V3, to abnormal tensions of the temporal muscle, masseter, pterygoid muscles and digastric muscle (anterior belly), resulting in a CMD.

b) Mandibular nerve (CN V3)

Masseteric nerve, the deep temporal nerves, and the lateral pterygoid, lingual and inferior alveolar nerves:

Causes: The causes include hypertonicity of the lateral pterygoid muscle, dysfunction at the oval foramen (sphenopetrosal synchondrosis), abnormal dural tensions, dysfunction of the pterygospinous ligament, and CMD. The lingual nerve may course through the belly of the lateral pterygoid muscle, and so be compressed in some circumstances.[214]

The inferior alveolar nerve may become compressed within the mandibular canal.[221,222]

Accelerated demyelination of the mandibular nerve (generation of abnormal impulses).

- Mechanism of neuromuscular dysfunction: Via motor nuclei of the nerve CN V3, dysfunction of the occipital bone leads to abnormal tension of the temporal, masseter, pterygoid and digastric (anterior belly) muscles, with consequent CMD.

Clinical presentation: Pain in the TMJ and pain referral, abnormal tension in the muscles of mastication (sequelae: CMD, malocclusion), pain in the teeth of the lower jaw, disturbances of salivation, sensory disturbances and pain in the skin of the lower facial region, headache (innervation of the dura of the middle cranial fossa).

c) Auriculotemporal nerve (V3)

This nerve runs between the neck of the mandible and the sphenomandibular ligament, winds around the neck in a lateral direction, and courses upward beneath the parotid between the TMJ and the external acoustic meatus.

Clinical presentation: Pain in the side of the face and temporal regions, and earache.

d) Maxillary nerve (V2)

The maxillary nerve passes through the foramen rotundum into the pterygopalatine fossa, where it subdivides further into the infraorbital nerve, zygomatic nerve and sensory root of the pterygopalatine ganglion.

Causes: Congestion within the cavernous sinus, dysfunction of the foramen rotundum and pterygopalatine suture, spasm of the sphenomandibular muscle with compression of the maxillary nerve against the posterior wall of the maxillary sinus.[217]

Clinical presentation: Disturbances of lacrimation, disturbances of secretion into the nasal and paranasal sinuses, aching of the upper teeth, disturbances of sensitivity and pain in the skin of the mid-facial region, mucosa and upper teeth, retro-orbital pain.

e) Infraorbital nerve (V2)
Through the inferior orbital fissure into the infraorbital canal, and on through the infraorbital foramen into the soft tissue of the face.
Clinical presentation: Disturbances of sensitivity and pain in the skin of the mid-facial region, mucosa and upper teeth.

f) Superior alveolar nerves (V2)
In the alveolar canals on the back of the infratemporal surface. The branches which supply the teeth and gums of the upper jaw branch off from the infraorbital nerve in the pterygopalatine fossa.
Clinical presentation: Toothache and painful gums.

g) Major palatine nerve
Clinical presentation: Disturbances of sensitivity and pain in the mucosa of the hard palate.

h) Sympathetic fibers of the deep petrosal nerve, via the pterygopalatine ganglion, sensory root of the pterygopalatine ganglion, maxillary nerve and zygomatic nerve to the lacrimal nerve (lacrimal gland)
Clinical presentation: Disturbance of the lacrimal gland.

i) Chorda tympani (VII)
Causes: Dysfunction of the temporal bone, CMD, in association with its course from the petrotympanic fissure, infratemporal fossa, and beneath the lateral pterygoid muscle.
Clinical presentation: Disturbance of taste (anterior two thirds of the tongue) and of salivation (sub-mandibular ganglion) affecting the submandibular and sublingual glands.

j) Zygomatic nerve
Clinical presentation: Disturbances of sensitivity and pain in the skin in the region around the temporal and zygomatic bones.

k) Otic ganglion
Clinical presentation: Disturbance of secretion of the parotid salivary glands, and pain referral.

Vascular disturbances

Although the arteries are not as susceptible to dysfunctions as the veins on account of their stronger walls, they nevertheless also merit consideration.

a) Superficial temporal artery
This vessel is important for the TMJ.

b) Infraorbital artery and vein
Clinical presentation: Functional disturbance of the front teeth, bones and gums of the upper jaw.

c) Anterior superior alveolar arteries
Clinical presentation: Functional disturbance of the front teeth.

d) Posterior superior alveolar artery

Clinical presentation: Functional disturbance of the maxillary sinus, and of the molars, bones and gums of the upper jaw.

e) Descending palatine artery: in the greater palatine canal

Clinical presentation: Functional disturbance of the pharyngeal mucosa, gingivae of the front teeth, and soft palate.

f) Inferior alveolar artery (branch of the maxillary artery): in the mandibular canal.

g) Mental artery (branch of the inferior alveolar artery): on the mental foramen.

h) Mylohyoid branch (branch of the inferior alveolar artery): in the mylohyoid groove.

i) Masseteric artery (branch of the maxillary artery): on the mandibular notch.

j) According to Wittlinger,[223] the body has somewhat over 600 lymph nodes, more than 160 of which are located in the neck region. The outflow of lymph from the masticatory organ is impaired, inter alia, by elevated myofascial tensions within the neck region and cervicothoracic transition, and by the masticatory muscles.

Disturbances of the salivary glands

Those affected are the parotid gland, sublingual gland and submandibular gland.

Disturbances of the endocrine glands

Thyroid and parathyroid glands: e.g. via the thyrohyoid muscle.

Psyche, stress

Causes: Mental and physical over-exertion, chronic emotional stress and conflict situations, suppressed aggression or anxiety, frustration.

Expressions such as 'to grit one's teeth,' 'to get one's teeth into something,' 'to show one's teeth,' as well as the fact that primates use baring of the teeth to threaten an opponent are all evidence that the biting apparatus is also used to assuage aggressive confrontations, and as a kind of release valve for excessive emotional tension.[224] Huter sees the mandible as an expression of impulsiveness, power, stamina, dignity, pride and stability (Fig. 11.57).[225,226]

The limbic system in particular appears to play a key role in muscle hypertonicity caused by stress and psychological factors. Elevated muscle tonus has been induced e.g. by stimulating the reticular formation, thalamus, hypothalamus and amygdaloid body.

Figure 11.57 Diagram of the mandible

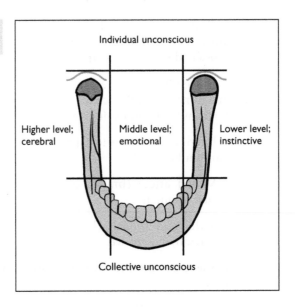

Chronic stress and psychic overload lead to muscle hypertonicity, which can in turn trigger bruxism, with the possible consequence of tendinomyopathies and joint disease.

Clinical presentation: Mental symptoms, hypertonicity of the masseter, pain in the TMJ, spasmophilic signs, grinding surfaces on teeth.

Important: True mental disorders such as depression may also lead to the development of symptoms in the region of the teeth and jaw. If mental illness is suspected, the patient should be referred to a specialist for further investigation. The treatment of the TMJ is contraindicated in such cases.[227]

On the other hand, continuous stimulation of the nociceptive system at the peripheral and central levels leads to changes in the processing of stimuli, and thus to altered pain perception.[211,228,229] Chronic pain will also impair other brain functions; there is, for example, a close relationship between pain and anxiety and pain and depression.[230,231] Pain and depression in turn impair tolerance to pain.[232-234]

Causes of craniomandibular dysfunctions

The occurrence of CMD (Table 11.4) is usually multi-factorial. Dysbalances, compensation within the structures of the TMJ or dysfunctions of the jaw may in time lead to structural TMJ changes (due, for example, to altered muscular activity) (Fig. 11.58). Pain states of the jaw joint may also induce reactions (neurological, muscular) that can give rise to a vicious circle or produce mental changes.

- Factors affecting the relative positions of the upper and lower jaw.
- Hypotonicity of the neck muscles, visual disturbances → abnormal head posture, reclination of the head → anterior displacement of the mandible.

Table 11.4 Causes of craniomandibular dysfunctions

Primary dysfunction	Congenital: the treatment of choice is usually orthodontic surgery
	Traumatic:
	Perinatal trauma, affecting the whole cranium; intraembryonic or postnatal causes are also possible, however; these may involve dysfunctions of the TMJ or intraosseous dysfunctions (the mandible originally consisted of two parts). Due to falling or blows to the face, with the possible consequence of one TMJ moving in an anterolateral direction and the other posteriorly and medially; a blow centrally on the tip of the chin usually moves both temporal bones into IR. Other sequelae could be muscular dys-balances and damage to the capsule or disk.
	Tooth extractions, or other forceful interventions on the lower jaw.[235]
	Extreme mouth-opening movements, e.g. during dental surgery, intubation etc.
	Blows to, or falling on to the pelvis may also cause restrictions of the lower jaw.
	This may lead both to intra-articular and to intraosseous dysfunctions.
Secondary dysfunction	Dysfunctions of the bones of the cranium and the cranial sutures, in particular of the temporal bone and occipital bone; this results in restriction of the TMJ and changes its position.
	Generalized hypermobility may occur in some circumstances.[236,237]
	Abnormal tensions in the masticatory muscles, hyoid muscles and ligaments of the TMJ.
	Poor chewing and swallowing habits, or a dysfunction of the tongue, especially the anterior position of the tongue: this may lead to dental misalignment and malocclusion.
	Disturbances of the teeth: malocclusions (premature contact etc.), orthodontic appliances,[238] dental prostheses, etc.
	Bottle-fed babies which have not been breast-fed: breast-feeding is an important stimulus to the growth of the as yet relatively underdeveloped mandible, and encourages closure of the mouth; it also stimulates the development of all organs involved in sucking, insalivation, chewing and swallowing.[239]
	Disturbance of nasal breathing or of the diaphragm: consequences are an alteration of lip position, possibly an alteration of tongue position, a lower jaw that is drawn down slightly and, sometimes, altered growth of the lower and middle thirds of the face.[240]
	Dysfunction of the upper cervical spine and of the atlanto-occipital joint: the cervical spine has a major influence on the TMJ, e.g. hypertonus of the muscles of the cervical spine can lead to hypertonus of the masticatory muscles.
	Dysfunction of the shoulder girdle (scapula, clavicle, 1st rib, e.g. via the omohyoid muscle, etc).
	Static dysfunctions: poor posture, poor working position, scolioses and dysfunctions of the pelvis, sacrum and lower extremities (e.g. a difference in leg length)[144] may lead to CMD via myofascial links.
	Visceral dysfunctions, via their fascial connection with the cranium, via the influence on the statics of the human body or on the meridian system.
	Disposition of the tissues: hyperlaxity of the capsular/ligamentous apparatus, deficiency of the connective tissue (opinions vary).[241,242]
	Psychological-emotional factors: stress, or emotional damage may lead directly or indirectly to increased muscle tonicity (e.g. in association with nocturnal grinding or gnashing of the teeth, nailbiting).
	Psychosocial factors
	Neurological disturbances, e.g. overactivity of the trigeminal ganglion, or reticular formation.

Table continued

Table continued

Imbalance of the meridian system: especially the gallbladder, sanjiao, small-intestine and stomach meridians.

Foci/disturbance fields: scars, dental foci, septic tonsils, and diseases of the stomach and small intestine can have a remotely-acting influence on the TMJ.[243]

Degenerative and inflammatory rheumatic disorders: osteoarthritis (the commonest rheumatic disorder), rheumatoid arthritis, psoriatic arthropathy, Chauffard syndrome, soft-tissue rheumatism, Bechterew disease.

Vitamin and mineral deficiencies: C, D, E, F, Ca, Mg, phosphorus.[243]

Elevated sugar consumption.[244]

Other causes: infectious osteitis, osteopathies (toxic, endocrine, cancerous), endocrine disturbances, foci and allergies.[243]

- Laxity of the TMJ ligaments → hypotonus of the temporal and masseter muscles → dropping of the jaw.
- Smallness of the nasal sinuses, polyps, tonsilar hypertrophy → narrowing of the upper airways, mouth breathing → extension and forward inclination of the head → dropping and anterior displacement of the mandible.
- Smallness of the oral cavity, large and/or thick tongue → prolapse of the tongue, tongue presses against the lower lip → anterior displacement of the mandible.
- Birth trauma, falling, blows, tooth extractions → dysfunction of the SBS (LFR, vertical strain).
- Difference in leg length, pelvic obliquity → transmission via the muscle chains to the TMJ.

Sequelae: Atypical deglutition and disturbances of articulation, craniomandibular dysfunction.

DIAGNOSIS

No joint, especially not the TMJ, may be regarded as an individual joint in isolation; rather it must be understood in the context of the structure and function of the body as a whole. Moreover, for treatment to be successful, it is especially important to be aware of the occurrence of a CMD as a multi-factorial phenomenon. For successful therapy that is not simply directed at the symptoms, it is therefore essential to study the whole body and to recognize the links and interactions between the body's structures and functions. The therapist must try to evaluate the importance and weighting of the various causal factors with reference to the TMJ problem if he or she is to be equal to their task. Examination of the jaw joint always comprises history-taking with the aid of standardized questionnaires, visual assessment, palpatory diagnosis, auscultation and X-ray examination. Other diagnostic methods are: nuclear spin resonance tomography,[245] computed tomography, arthrography, psychometric testing, bioelectronic testing, liquid-crystal thermography, EMG etc.

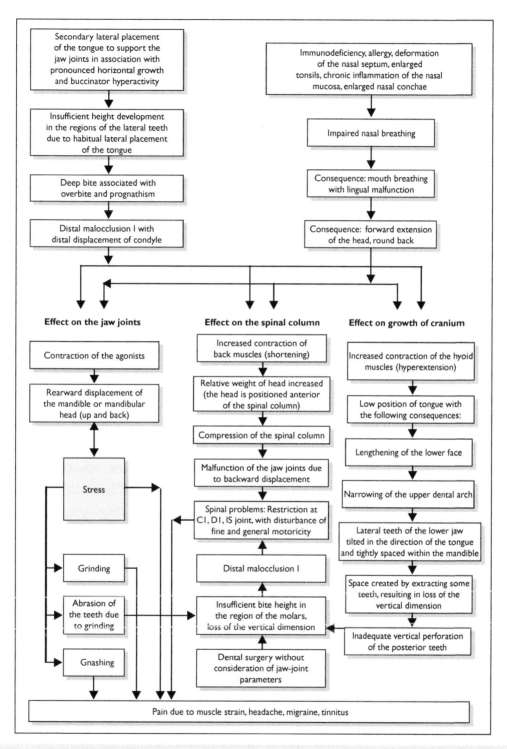

Figure 11.58 Causes of jaw joint-cervical spine dysfunction (Garry, Yerkes and Bowbeer, modified by Wolz)

A reliable diagnosis of the observed signs is only possible with a combination of various diagnostic parameters (Fig. 11.59).

History-taking

General:

Start of the symptoms, identification of possible causes of the symptoms, dental surgery or orthodontic surgery, deformation of the cranium.

- Family history.
- Disturbances of the jaw-joint structures (joint surfaces, articular capsules, articular ligaments, retrodiskal pad):
  - Pain in the TMJ or retrodiskal zone, associated with trismus, pain on opening the mouth or when biting into solid food, specific pattern of pain.
  - Restriction of the TMJ: restriction after waking up is an indication of nocturnal teeth-grinding, or similar; if the mouth can be opened further after clicking of the jaw joint, this is evidence of a disk problem.
  - Joint sounds (although no joint sounds occur in association with disturbances of the retrodiskal pad):

    Clicking while opening or closing the mouth is indicative of a disk problem, rarely of alterations of the joint surfaces. Loud clicking audible to those standing nearby, usually gives rise to social difficulties, but rarely to pain.

    Quiet clicking perceptible only to the patient by bone conduction, very often arises in conjunction with pain and functional disturbance of the TMJ. Crepitation is an indication of perforation of the disk and/or of the retrodiskal tissue, and possibly of arthrotic changes in the joint.
  - Malocclusions.
- Grinding.
- Disturbances of the temporomandibular joint muscles: pain in the muscles of mastication and restriction of the TMJ; in particular radiating pain in the lateral pterygoid muscle, masseter muscle (deep part), sternocleidomastoid muscle or medial pterygoid muscle may induce pain in the TMJ.
- Speech disturbances and dysphagia.
- Aural symptoms (otalgia, tinnitus, hearing impairment) may accompany a CMD.[197]
- Disturbances of the immune system.[246]
- Triggering factors: for example, orthodontic surgery (e.g. extraction of molars), alterations of bite, stress, accidents, falling on or blows to the head, face, back, pelvis and lower extremities.[167]
- Headache.[247,248]
- Radiating pain, e.g. in the head, back of the neck and shoulder, and lower lumbar spine.[197,247]
- Static-dynamic changes in the spinal column.[197]
- Neurovegetative symptoms.

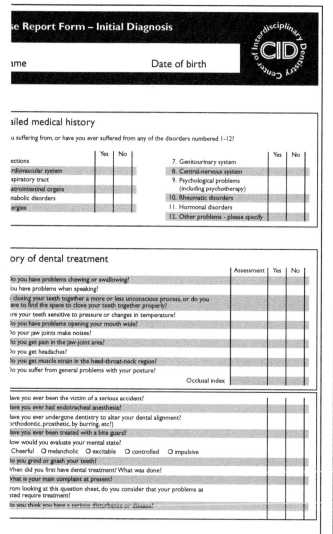

CID Center of Interdisciplinary Dentistry

ame Date of birth

ailed medical history

u suffering from, or have you ever suffered from any of the disorders numbered 1-12?

	Yes	No			Yes	No
ections			7. Genitourinary system			
rdiovascular system			8. Central-nervous system			
spiratory tract			9. Psychological problems (including psychotherapy)			
strointestinal organs			10. Rheumatic disorders			
:tabolic disorders			11. Hormonal disorders			
ergies			12. Other problems - please specify			

ory of dental treatment

	Assessment	Yes	No
)o you have problems chewing or swallowing?			
'ou have problems when speaking?			
: closing your teeth together a more or less unconscious process, or do you ave to find the space to close your teeth together properly?			
ire your teeth sensitive to pressure or changes in temperature?			
)o you have problems opening your mouth wide?			
)o your jaw joints make noises?			
)o you get pain in the jaw-joint area?			
)o you get headaches?			
)o you get muscle strain in the head-throat-neck region?			
)o you suffer from general problems with your posture?			
	Occlusal index		
lave you ever been the victim of a serious accident?			
lave you ever had endotracheal anesthesia?			
lave you ever undergone dentistry to alter your dental alignment? orthodontic, prosthetic, by burring, etc?)			
lave you ever been treated with a bite guard?			
low would you evaluate your mental state? Cheerful ○ melancholic ○ excitable ○ controlled ○ impulsive			
)o you grind or gnash your teeth?			
Vhen did you first have dental treatment? What was done?			
Vhat is your main complaint at present?			
rom looking at this question sheet, do you consider that your problems as sted require treatment?			
)o you think you have a serious disturbance or disease?			

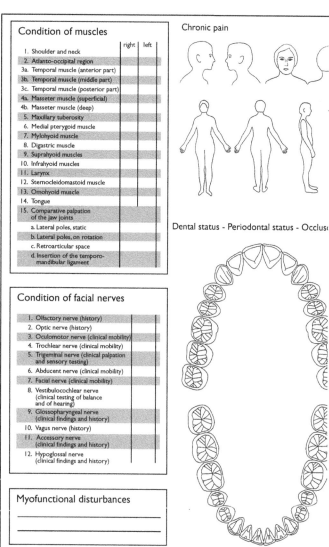

Condition of muscles

	right	left
1. Shoulder and neck		
2. Atlanto-occipital region		
3a. Temporal muscle (anterior part)		
3b. Temporal muscle (middle part)		
3c. Temporal muscle (posterior part)		
4a. Masseter muscle (superficial)		
4b. Masseter muscle (deep)		
5. Maxillary tuberosity		
6. Medial pterygoid muscle		
7. Mylohyoid muscle		
8. Digastric muscle		
9. Suprahyoid muscles		
10. Infrahyoid muscles		
11. Larynx		
12. Sternocleidomastoid muscle		
13. Omohyoid muscle		
14. Tongue		
15. Comparative palpation of the jaw joints		
a. Lateral poles, static		
b. Lateral poles, on rotation		
c. Retroarticular space		
d. Insertion of the temporo-mandibular ligament		

Condition of facial nerves

1. Olfactory nerve (history)		
2. Optic nerve (history)		
3. Oculomotor nerve (clinical mobility)		
4. Trochlear nerve (clinical mobility)		
5. Trigeminal nerve (clinical palpation and sensory testing)		
6. Abducent nerve (clinical mobility)		
7. Facial nerve (clinical mobility)		
8. Vestibulocochlear nerve (clinical testing of balance and of hearing)		
9. Glossopharyngeal nerve (clinical findings and history)		
10. Vagus nerve (history)		
11. Accessory nerve (clinical findings and history)		
12. Hypoglossal nerve (clinical findings and history)		

Myofunctional disturbances

_____

_____

Chronic pain

Dental status - Periodontal status - Occlus

1.59 Case report form – initial diagnosis, after Prof. R. Slavicek

- Clarification of other symptoms: dysphagia, disturbances of sucking, sensory impairment (taste, hearing, touch, etc.), dizziness, paresthesias, nausea, motor function. Possibly nasopharyngeal symptoms (disturbance of breathing, polyps, adenoid vegetations, sinusitis etc.); important differential diagnosis to TMJ pain.
- Current and previous diseases (e.g. cardiac disorders, gastrointestinal or rheumatic diseases). A number of authors point out that TMJ patients frequently show other somatic symptoms in addition to their TMJ symptoms.[211,220]

Summary of possible TMJ symptoms: pain in and around the TMJ, and in the muscles thereof, restriction of the TMJ, joint sounds, prominent condyle, pain in the head and face, back of the neck and shoulders, paresthesias in the facial and mouth region, aural symptoms, dizziness, presence of triggering factors, other somatic symptoms.

The following disorders must be excluded in the differential diagnosis

Tension headache, migraine, temporal arteritis, spondylarthrosis or Bechterew disease of the cervical spine, sinusitis, otitis media, trigeminal neuralgia, tumors, the rheumatic disorders (acute articular rheumatism, chronic rheumatism, primary chronic polyarthritis, gout, psoriasis), infection (infectious osteitis), true mental illnesses.

Visual assessment

Visual assessment of the face, oral cavity, teeth, tongue etc.

- To give an example, the following constitute evidence of non-specific hyperactivity: generalized hyperkinesia in the facial region, wear of chewing surfaces, indentations in soft tissues, fingernails, nail beds, pencil-chewing etc.; bruxism: evidence of grinding or gnashing.
- Teeth ground down, and indentations in soft tissues.
- Grinders: distinct faceting of the teeth, and wear of chewing surfaces.
- Low premolars, with canine 'drop-off'.
- Gnashers: teeth unfaceted, and little wear of chewing surfaces.
- Visible hypertrophy of the masseter.

Visual assessment of the position of the chin tip (Fig. 11.60)

- Deviation to the side of the CMD, or to the side on which the temporal bone is in IR.

Visual assessment of the position of the midline between the incisors (Fig. 11.61)

- ➤ Ask the patient to open the lips with the teeth parted.
- ➤ Compare the midline between the upper incisors with the midline between the lower incisors. The test is positive when the midlines do not coincide.

Figure 11.60 Visual assessment of position of chin tip

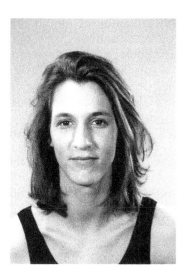

Figure 11.61 Visual assessment of position of midline between the incisors

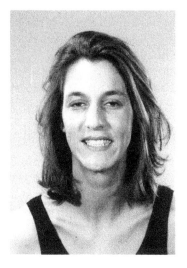

➤ The midline of the lower incisors is displaced towards the dysfunctional side of the TMJ.

➤ If no asymmetric movement can be perceived when the mouth is opened, the deviation may be caused by a maxillary dysfunction.

Mouth opening and mouth closure:

➤ Perceive the width and symmetry of mouth opening and mouth closure, as well as any associated sounds and pain.

➤ Enlargement of the mouth opening may occur in association with a hypermobile joint, or over-rotation, hyperextension and subluxation of the retrodiskal ligament.

Cardonnet and Clauzade's interpretation of reduced mouth opening (and laterotrusion):[249]

➤ A reduced mouth opening (44–35 mm) indicates muscular and diskal dysfunction.

➤ A distinct limitation of mouth opening (3–21 mm) indicates a relatively acute luxation.

➤ A severe limitation of mouth opening (<21 mm) is usually present if there is ankylosis or acute muscle spasm (often with underlying luxation).

➤ The ratio of the amplitude of the mouth opening to the minimum possible laterotrusion should be 4:1. A deviation of more than 2 mm is a clear sign of disk dislocation.

Interpretation of the deviation of the incisor midline during the opening and closure movement according to Sebald and Kopp:[250]

Discoordination: Deviations from the midline occur during the opening and closure movement. At the end of mouth opening, the lower jaw is once again in the midline position.

Interpretation: ● Usually myogenic dysfunction.
● The greater the deviation, the greater the dysfunction.

Prognosis: Very good.

According to Landeweer, a greater or lesser degree of incapacity during active movements and isometric contractions is an indication of discoordination.[251]

Active movement: inability to perform isolated protrusion, mouth opening from maximum protrusion, closure in maximum protrusion, or sideways movement of the mandible (lateral pterygoid muscle).

The degree of incapacity is evaluated as follows:

➤ Much activity in the auxiliary muscles without movement of the mandible.

➤ Much activity in the auxiliary muscles with movement of the mandible, but jerky, abrupt, atactic, etc.

➤ Little activity in the auxiliary muscles and relatively free mandibular movement.

➤ Little activity in the auxiliary muscles and smooth, free movement of the mandible.

Isometric contraction of the lateral pterygoid muscle[251]

➤ Evaluate the muscular response.

➤ The best result is obtained when the mandible remains in a stable position in response to the application of variable pressure.

➤ A dysfunction is indicated if the mandible is not capable of maintaining its position in response to variable pressure.

Note: Discoordination never occurs in the absence of muscle hypertonus or hyperactivity. Conversely, hypertonus and hyperactivity can occur without discoordination.

Deviation: During the opening and closure movement, a unilateral distinct deviation from the midline occurs. At the end of mouth opening, the mandible is once again in the midline position.

Interpretation: ● Possible disturbance of the joint surfaces (e.g. cartilaginous obstruction in the joint surfaces, intermediate clicking).

    ● Deviation to the side of the TMJ disturbance.

Prognosis: Moderately good.

Deflection: During the opening movement, a unilateral distinct deviation from the midline occurs. At the end of mouth opening, the mandible has deviated most distinctly from the midline.

Interpretation: ● Diskopathy, ankylosis (e.g. terminal clicking).

    ● Deviation to the side of the TMJ disturbance.

Prognosis: ● Acute diskopathy: very good.

    ● Chronic diskopathy: uncertain.

    ● Ankylosis: indication for surgery.

If a deviation of the midline of the incisors occurs during mouth opening, a test may be performed to ascertain whether the lateral pterygoid muscle is the cause of this deviation (this muscle is very often involved in a CMD).

➤ Ask the patient to move the tongue against the posterior part of the roof of the palate.

➤ If mouth opening is now symmetric, the lateral pterygoid muscle is very probably the cause.

➤ If the mouth opening movement remains asymmetric, the deviation is caused by something else.

Note: This tongue position prevents translation of the condyle over the articular tubercle.

    ● Joint sounds during mouth opening and mouth closure may be indicative of a hypermobile joint, as well as disturbance of the disk, lateral ligament or motion pathway of the joint.

    ● Clicking at the end of mouth opening and at the beginning of mouth closure indicates a hypermobile joint.

The three-finger metacarpal-joint test according to Dorrance (Fig. 11.62):

➤ Ask the patient to open the mouth sufficiently wide to accommodate the metacarpal joints of the index finger, middle finger and ring finger between the upper and lower incisors. The test is positive when this is not achieved, and indicates a CMD of articular or myogenic origin.

Watt's test:[252]

➤ Ask the patient to close the teeth together quickly several times.

Interpretation: ● Sharp, clear sound (teeth come together at high speed): high-quality occlusion or high-quality regulating function (proprioceptive integration).

Figure 11.62 3-finger metacarpal joint test according to Dorrance

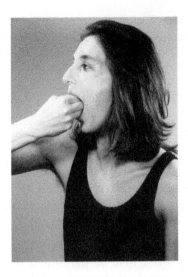

- Soft sound (teeth come together at low speed): poor-quality occlusion or poor-quality regulating function (proprioceptive integration).
- A sharp sound indicates only that, when the teeth come together, the same, large number of points (40–50) always meet simultaneously. It does not necessarily say anything about the condition of the occlusion, as a poor-condition occlusion can be compensated for by a high regulation function.
- We know that, in the case of a soft sound, the occlusal points do not come together simultaneously. This suggests a malocclusion, an impairment of centering or over-exertion of the proprioceptive mechanisms.

Palpation

Test of the position of the TMJ *(Fig. 11.63)*

Therapist: Place your index or middle fingers on the two temporomandibular joints, and note the position of the condyles.

Differential diagnosis of tenderness of the TMJ *(Table 11.5)*

Palpation or application of pressure is always bilateral.

The pressure should be applied not only statically, but also during mouth opening and mouth closure. If pressure induces pain, the test is positive.

Palpation of the PRM rhythm at the mandible *(Fig. 11.64)*

The lower jaw is influenced by the occiput via the temporal bones. If there is a flexion dysfunction of the occiput or of the SBS, the temporal bones are in external rotation. This places the mandibular

Figure 11.63 Testing the position and movement of the temporomandibular joints

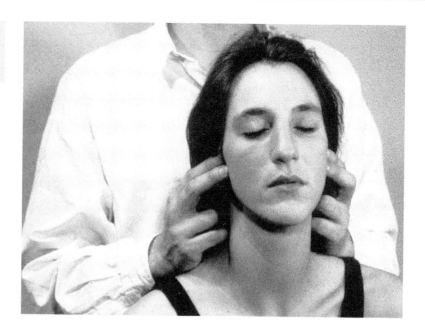

Table 11.5 Differential diagnosis of tenderness of the TMJ

Palpation	Finger position	If tenderness is present
From the side	MF[a] 1.5 cm anterior of the margin of the tragus	Minor arthrogenic disturbance, disturbance of the lateral ligament, diskal ligaments, or lateral displacement of the mandible
From a posterolateral direction	Mouth slightly opened; MF posterior of the condyle at several points	Disturbance of the bilaminar zone, posterior capsular inflammation, acute luxation with traction on the bilaminar zone
From a dorsal direction	LF[b] in the external acoustic meatus, pressure applied in an anterior direction	Severe arthrogenic disturbance, posterior inflammation of the disk
From a dorsal direction with the mouth open	LF in the external acoustic meatus, pressure applied in an anterior direction	Retrodiskal disturbance, muscular disturbance
From a dorsal direction with the mouth closed	LF in the external acoustic meatus, pressure applied in an anterior direction	Capsulitis, subluxation

[a]MF, middle finger; [b]LF, little finger

fossae of the temporal bones in a posterior, medial position, with the result that the mandible shifts backward.

In association with an extension dysfunction of the occiput or SBS, the temporal bones are in internal rotation. This places the mandibular fossae of the temporal bones in an anterolateral position, with the result that the mandible shifts forward.

Figure 11.64 Palpation of primary respiration at the mandible

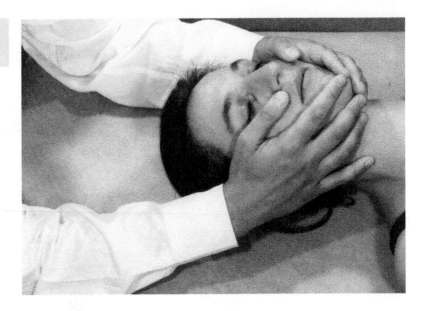

In a unilateral IR of the temporal bones, the TMJ on the same side tends to be positioned anterolaterally.

In a unilateral ER of the temporal bones, the TMJ on the same side tends to be positioned posterior and medially.

It is also possible for one temporal bone to be in IR and the other in ER, and for the one TMJ to be displaced anterolaterally and the other posteriorly and medially, with resulting disturbances of bite.

Therapist: Take up a position at the head of the patient.

Hand position:
➤ Place the palms of the hands on the mandible on both sides so that they cover the TMJ.
➤ The index fingers meet at the gnathion (the lowest median point of the lower jaw) and span the chin.
➤ Place the other fingers alongside, with the little fingers on the angles of the mandible.

a) Biomechanical approach
Inspiration phase, normal finding (Fig. 11.65): ER

➤ With your index fingers, sense a movement of the chin tip posterior.
➤ With your other fingers you will be able to perceive the angle of the mandible moving outward (forward and down).
➤ The articular processes (condyle processes) move inward, back and down. (They follow the mandibular fossae of the temporal bones. Owing to the flexibility of bone, the angles of the mandible move outward, while the articular processes are moving inward.)

Expiration phase, normal finding: IR

➤ With your index fingers, sense a movement of the chin tip anterior.
➤ With your other fingers you will be able to perceive the angle of the mandible moving inward (back and up).

Figure 11.65 PR inspiration phase/biomechanical approach

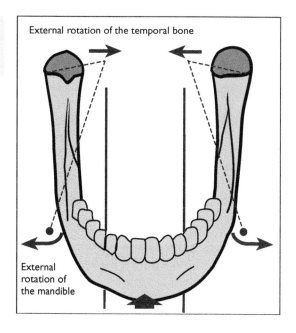

> External rotation of the temporal bone

> External rotation of the mandible

> ➤ The articular processes (condyle processes) move outward, forward and up.

b) Biodynamic/embryological approach
Inspiration phase, normal finding (see Figs 11.26, 11.27):

> ➤ The mandible moves downward and forward.
> ➤ The two halves of the body of the mandible move away from one another in the posterior region.

Expiration phase, normal finding:

> ➤ The mandible moves upward and back.
> ➤ The two halves of the body of the mandible move toward one another in the posterior region.
> ➤ Compare the amplitude, strength, ease and symmetry of the motion of the mandible.
> ➤ Other types of motion of the mandible may sometimes occur during external and internal rotation. These provide an indication as to further dysfunctions of the mandible.
> ➤ Mandibular dysfunctions may be unilateral or bilateral, symmetric or asymmetric.

Palpation of primary respiration and mobility of the temporal bone, SBS, occipital, atlantoaxial joint, and of the occiput/sacrum link

Motion testing

> ● This differs from palpation of primary respiration only in one feature: the external and internal rotation of the mandible is now actively induced by the therapist.
> ● Compare the amplitude, symmetry and ease of the movements, or the force needed to bring about motion.

Testing the motion of the TMJ *(Fig. 11.66)*

Patient: Seated.

Therapist: Take up a position behind the patient.

Hand position: Place your middle fingers in the ears, or your index and middle fingers immediately in front of the ears on the temporomandibular joints.

Method:
- ➤ Ask the patient to open and close the mouth slowly.
- ➤ Palpate the rolling and gliding motion in the temporomandibular joints.
- ➤ Any asymmetry, and any palpable or audible noise (grinding or clicking, etc.) is an indication of a CMD.
- ➤ Other movements of the mouth may also be palpated (protrusion, retrusion, laterotrusion).

Testing the passive motion of the TMJ *(Fig. 11.67)*

If mouth opening is limited, the mobility should be tested passively.

Patient: The patient is supine.

Therapist: Take up a position beside the patient at the level of the shoulder.

Hand position:
- ➤ Position your thumbs inside the mouth on the lower teeth, one on each side.

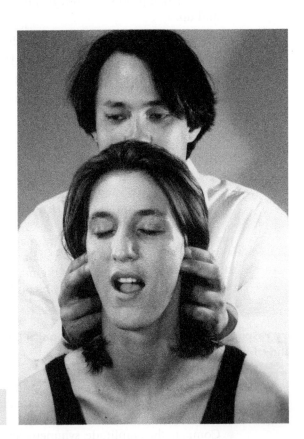

Figure 11.66 Mouth-opening palpation test

Figure 11.67 Testing the passive motion of the TMJ

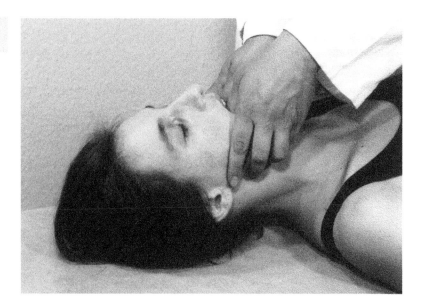

➤ Position the other fingers on the body of the mandible. With your middle fingers, grasp the angle of the mandible on both sides.

Method: Testing of mouth opening
Testing of cranial-caudal mobility:

➤ Administer pressure cephalad and traction caudad.

Testing of anterior-posterior mobility:

➤ Administer traction posterior and anterior.

Testing of rotation:

➤ Induce rotation to the right and to the left.

Testing of lateral displaceability:

➤ Induce a lateral displacement to the right and to the left.
➤ Compare the ease, amplitude, end sensation and symmetry of the movements of the mandible. A normal terminal sensation is perceivable as a hard ligamentous resistance (Table 11.6).

Interpretation:
● A light, resilient resistance at the end of mouth opening: disk.
● A solid resistance at the end of mouth opening: muscle cramp.
● Limited lateral displaceability to the right: CMD on the left (arthrogenic, muscular, etc.).
● A positive test result (= limitation of mobility), but a negative result in the isometric test: arthrogenic dysfunction.
● A negative test result: probably myogenic dysfunction.

Table 11.6 Differential diagnosis of the terminal sensation

Terminal sensation	+ Pain	+ Reduced amplitude	+ Normal amplitude
Sudden resistance	Sudden muscular contraction	Muscle cramp	
Softer resistance*	Slow muscular contraction, poss. shortening of the muscle	Muscle inhibition	Muscle inhibition
Harder resistance*		Connective-tissue obstruction, possibly shrinkage of the capsule	Connective-tissue obstruction
Osseous resistance		Osseous obstruction	
Elastic resistance		Dislocation of the disk without reduction	

*compared with the terminal sensation of ligamentous resistance

Other indications:
- Arthrogenic disturbance
  - If lateral mobility is severely limited (unilaterally or bilaterally), with reduced or almost normal mouth opening.
  - When an existing pain changes as a result of passive motion, in contrast with isometric testing.
- Probably no arthrogenic dysfunction:
  - If mouth opening is reduced, with normal or almost normal lateral mobility.
  - When an existing pain does not change as a result of passive motion.
  - When an existing restriction does not change as a result of passive testing (possible disturbance of muscle innervation).
- Myogenic dysfunction:
  - When an existing pain changes as a result of passive motion, in accordance with isometric testing.
  - Passive mouth opening with cranially-directed compression of the TMJ (Sebald and Kopp):[253]
  - This test is indicated if clicking occurs during active movement of the jaw. It is used for further differentiation of the clicking (Table 11.7).

Hand position:
- Position your thumbs inside the mouth on the lower teeth, one on each side.
- Position the other fingers on the body of the mandible. With your middle fingers, grasp the angle of the mandible on both sides.

Method:
- Induce passive opening of the mouth.
- At the same time, administer cranially-directed compression on the TMJ.

Table 11.7 Differential diagnosis of joint clicking

Clicking	Diagnosis
Later in the course of mouth opening*	Dislocation of the disk
Later in the course of mouth opening, but no clicking on closing the mouth or in association with repeated opening	Good prognosis
At the same point during mouth opening as without compression cephalad, but duller	Disturbance of the cartilage or bone of the articular surface
No clicking during compression cephalad	Disturbance of the lateral ligament

*compared with mouth opening without compression cephalad

Test of the motion of the retrodiskal tissue[31] *(Fig. 11.68)*

Palpation of the masticatory muscles *(Fig. 11.69)*

The degree of sensitivity or pain on palpation of the TMJ muscles provides an indication of the severity of the TMJ disturbance, and of hyperactivity or hypoactivity of the neuromuscular system. Apart from searching for the underlying cause, if the TMJ muscles are hypoactive they should be toned, and if they are hyperactive they should be relaxed. Further investigation of the interrelationship with the occlusion is essential.

Masseter muscle:

➤ Between the zygomatic arch and the angle of the mandible.

Temporal muscle:

➤ Posterior part: above the ears and behind the ears.
➤ Medial part: above the ears.
➤ Anterior part: above and in front of the ears.
➤ Point of attachment on the coronoid process: intraoral, between the cheek and the maxillary tuber toward the back in the direction of the coronoid process, at the height of the first molar on the buccal side.

Lateral pterygoid muscle:

➤ Intraoral, between the maxillary tuber and the ascending mandibular ramus, in the direction of the external acoustic meatus. Position your finger in the first instance so that the palmar surface faces medially, toward the gingivae, and turns to the side on the mandibular ramus.
➤ Move the finger in a posterior, cranial direction until the tip of the finger meets the tissue directly anterior of the muscle. This muscle cannot be palpated directly.

Medial pterygoid muscle:

➤ Intraorally, medially on the mandibular ramus, extending from the maxillary tuber to the angle of the mandible.

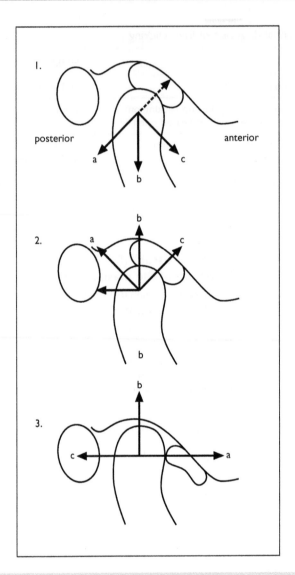

Figure 11.68 Testing the motion of the retrodiskal tissue; from J. Langendoen-Sertel and M. Hamouda: Die Bedeutung des retrodiskalen Gewebes bei temporo-mandibulären Arthropathien (The significance of the retrodiskal tissue in temporomandibular arthropathies). Manuelle Therapie 1998; 1:11. 1. Extension of the posterior, upper band (diskotemporal ligament): caudally-angled traction is exerted on the mandible, with a simultaneous posterior-anteriorly directed sliding motion of the mandible (from a to c). 2. Compression on the posterior lower and upper bands (discocondylar ligament and discotemporal ligament): angled cephalad, with simultaneous anterior-posteriorly directed sliding motion of the mandible (from c to a). 3. Diagnosis of an anterior displacement of the disk in static occlusion: (a) A posterior-anterior sliding motion of the mandible causes stretching of the retro-articular tissue, with pain. (b) An anterior-posterior sliding motion of the mandible leads to compression of the lower band (discocondylar ligament). (c) A purely cranial movement of the mandible will compress both the upper and the lower bands (discocondylar and discotemporal ligaments)

➤ (See also palpation of the mouth floor).
➤ Ask the patient to open the mouth wide.
➤ Extraorally: Position the finger medially on the angle of the mandible, and apply pressure in a superior direction.

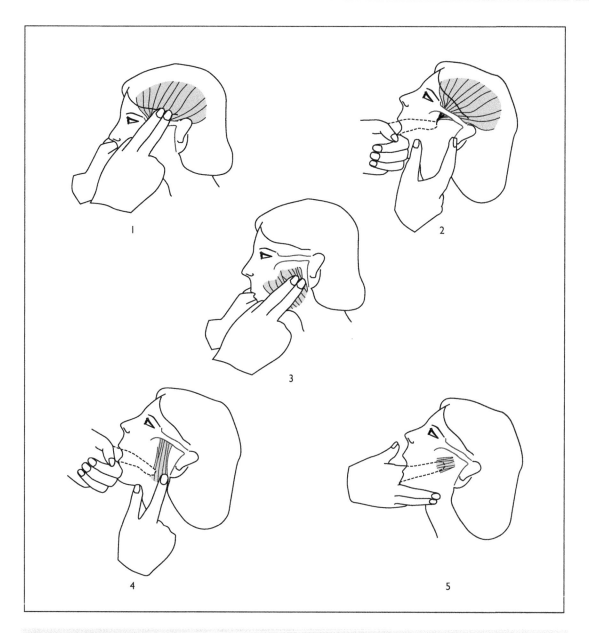

Figure 11.69 Palpation of the muscles of mastication. 1. Temporal muscle; 2. Temporal muscle, intraoral; 3. Masseter muscle; 4. Medial pterygoid muscle, intraoral; 5. Lateral pterygoid muscle, intraoral

Digastric muscle: with head extension.

➤ Posterior belly: posterior of the angle of the mandible, in front of the sternocleidomastoid muscle, in the direction of the ear; meanwhile, press inwards with the finger.

➤ Anterior belly: beneath the tip of the chin, extending along the floor of the mouth on both sides of the midline.

Further palpation

➤ Palpation of the hyoid muscles
➤ Palpation of the muscles of the neck and shoulder
➤ Palpation of the craniocervical fascias.

Trigger points (TP) *(Figs 11.70–11.79, Table 11.8)*
A trigger point is a hypersensitized/hyperstimulated region in a tissue (myofascial, cutaneous, ligamentous, fascial, periosteal). When pressure is applied, the effect is localized sensitivity to touch. Referred pain and referred contact sensitivity are encountered in some circumstances. Autonomous symptoms or proprioceptive disturbances may also occur.

Isometric muscle test according to Sebald and Kopp[254], after Winkel[255]

● The force and the duration of the contraction are tested.
● Isometric contraction should normally be strong and pain-free.

Patient: The patient is seated.
Hand position: ➤ Take up a position in front of the patient and grasp the jaw with your thumbs and thenar eminences outside on the alveolar part of the mandible and your index fingers on the angle of the mandible, whilst positioning the middle fingers on the underside of the mandible.
➤ For isometric contraction of the muscles responsible for mediotrusion, the thumb and thenar eminence are positioned on the opposite side from the mediotrusion on the outside of the mandible (as described above). Place the other hand on the temple on the mediotrusion side.
➤ For isometric contraction of the muscles which close the mouth, the palmar surface of the thumbs placed intraorally on the chewing surface of the lower teeth.

Alternative hand position for all tests: ➤ V-grip. Grasp the chin from the front with your thumb and index finger. The middle finger is bent under the chin.

Method: ➤ Ask the patient to relax the jaw joints, with the tongue lying relaxed in the mouth and the mouth slightly opened.
➤ Apply pressure in a given direction, while the patient resists this pressure.
➤ No movement should occur in the TMJ (isometric muscle contraction, Table 11.9).
➤ Increase the pressure slowly (over about 10 s).
➤ Then hold the pressure for about 10 s.

Note: If only one muscle is being tested, less force should be inserted than when testing muscle groups (Table 11.10).
Interpretation: (Tables 11.11, 11.12)
The test is negative if normal force is exerted and there is no pain: no myogenic dysfunction.
    The test is positive if the force is reduced and if pain is triggered: myogenic or arthrogenic dysfunction.

Figure 11.70 Trigger point of the temporal muscle (anterior and medial parts)

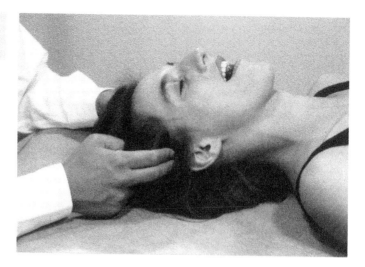

Figure 11.71 Trigger point of the temporal muscle (posterior part)

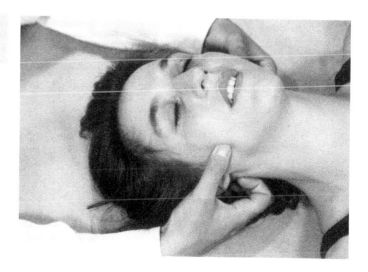

Figure 11.72 Trigger point of the masseter muscle (superficial part)

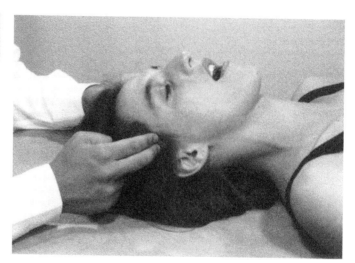

Figure 11.73 Trigger point of the masseter muscle (deep part)

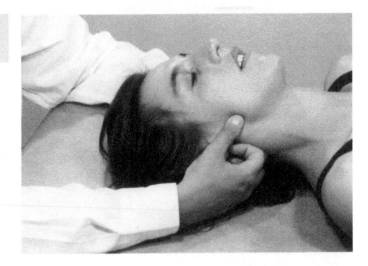

Figure 11.74 Trigger point of the lateral pterygoid muscle (anterior inferior part)

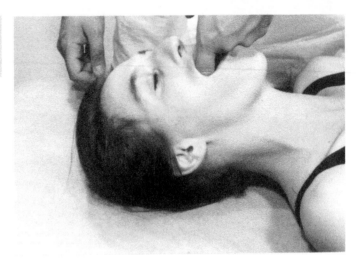

Figure 11.75 Trigger point of the lateral pterygoid muscle (posterior inferior part, and superior part)

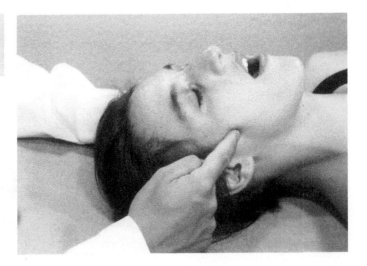

Figure 11.76 Trigger point of the medial pterygoid muscle (extraoral)

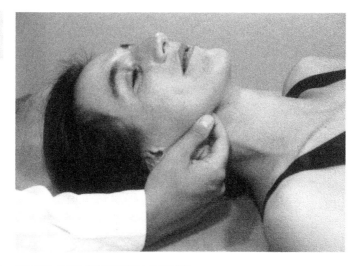

Figure 11.77 Trigger point of the medial pterygoid muscle (intraoral)

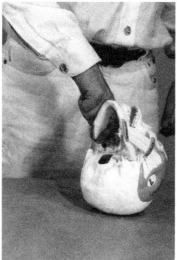

Figure 11.78 Trigger point of the digastric muscle, posterior belly

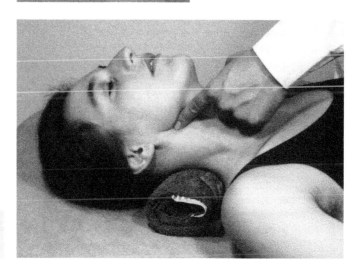

Figure 11.79 Trigger point of the digastric muscle, anterior belly

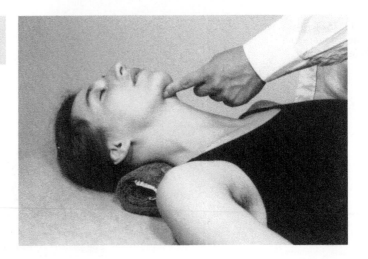

Table 11.8 Trigger points[207]

Muscle	Location + palpation	Referral	Trigger
Temporal muscle	Mouth opened 2–3 cm. Move one finger in a horizontal line from the zygomatic arch on each of the anterior, and middle and posterior portions of the muscle	Temporal region, eyebrow, upper teeth, more rarely maxilla and TMJ	Immobilization of the TMJ, grinding of the teeth, disturbance of occlusion, effect of cold or injury on the muscle, whiplash injury
Masseter muscle	With the mouth slightly opened for preliminary muscle stretch Superficial part: Press the muscle against the ramus of the mandible, or squeeze the muscle together with two fingers. Deep part: Press the muscle against the posterior part of the ramus and along the lower margin of the zygomatic bone (pressure in a posterior, upper position on the TP may possibly trigger tinnitus)	Superficial part: eyebrow, maxilla, mandible, upper + lower molars Deep part: TMJ and deep into the ear	Traumatic injury, grinding of the teeth, over-exertion, malocclusion, disturbance of occlusion
Lateral pterygoid muscle	Anterior part of the inferior muscle: Mouth opened 2 cm + mandible laterally displaced towards the test side. Finger intraorally between maxilla and coronoid process, pressure on the pterygoid process (lateral lamina) Posterior part of the inferior muscle + superior muscle: Mouth opened 3 cm: extraorally, via the masseter muscle beneath the zygomatic bone in the mandibular notch	TMJ, maxilla	Disturbance of occlusion

Table continued

Table continued

Muscle	Location + palpation	Referral	Trigger
Medial pterygoid muscle	Mouth wide open Extraorally: finger medially on the angle of the mandible, upward pressure Intraorally: slide the finger along the molars to the ramus of the mandible; the muscle is immediately posterior to the anterior border of the ramus	Back of the mouth + pharynx, beneath + behind the TMJ, deep into the ear	Usually secondary to dysfunction of the lateral pterygoid muscle or disturbance of occlusion
Digastric muscle	Extension of the head Posterior belly: Finger posterior of the angle of the mandible; slide it in front of the sternocleidomastoid muscle in the direction of the ear while pressing inwards with the finger Anterior belly: Fingers on the tissue beneath the chin tip, on both sides of the midline	Posterior belly: upper part of the sternocleidomastoid muscle (pseudo-pain in the sternocleidomastoid muscle) Anterior belly: Lower incisors *Note*: Pain becomes distinct when the sternocleidomastoid muscle is relaxed	Secondary to dysfunction of the masseter muscle, over-exertion of the muscle while grinding the teeth, retrusion of the mandible (associated with mouth breathing)
Sternocleido-mastoid muscle	On the sternal and clavicular portion	Sternal part: vertex, occiput, cheek, eye (atypical facial neuralgia), pharynx, sternum Clavicular part: Forehead, ear with dizziness, disturbance of balance	Over-exertion of the muscle due to structural somatic dysfunctions, problems with breathing

A reduction in force is an indication of a disturbance of innervation (neurogenic origin).

Pain localization:

- Pain in the muscles probably indicates a myogenic disturbance.
- Pain in the joint probably indicates an arthrogenic disturbance.
- Pain in various positions of the joint probably indicates a myogenic disturbance.
- Pain in only one position of the joint probably indicates an arthrogenic disturbance (further differentiation by passive motion testing, see above).

Palpation of the trigeminal nerve exits

A comparison of the pressure on the nerve exits of the trigeminal branches on both sides; the test is positive if there is tenderness and disturbances of sensitivity stop.

Table 11.9 Isometric testing

Isometric test	Initial position of the patient	Direction of pressure applied by the therapist
Muscles which open the mouth in centric relation	Mouth opened slightly	Cephalad
Muscles which open the mouth in protrusion	Protrusion of the mandible 3–4 mm when the mouth is slightly open	Cephalad
Muscles which open the mouth in mediotrusion	Mediotrusion of the mandible until the tips of the canines are opposite one another, with the mouth slightly open	Cephalad
Protractor muscles	Slight protrusion with the mouth slightly open	In a posterior direction
Muscles which produce mediotrusion, e.g. to the right	Mandible to the left, until the tips of the canines on the left are opposite one another, with the mouth slightly open	To the right
Muscles which close the mouth in centric relation	Mouth slightly open	Caudad
Muscles which close the mouth in protrusion	Protrusion of the mandible 3–4 mm when the mouth is slightly open	Caudad
Muscles which close the mouth in mediotrusion	Mediotrusion of the mandible until the tips of the canines are opposite one another, with the mouth slightly open	Caudad

Table 11.10 Muscle involvement

Isometric test	Muscles tested
Muscles which open the mouth	Digastric muscle, mylohyoid muscle, geniohyoid muscle, stylohyoid muscle, suprahyoid muscles, lateral pterygoid muscle
Protractor muscles	Lateral pterygoid muscle, masseter muscle (superficial part)
Muscles which produce mediotrusion	Lateral pterygoid muscle, medial pterygoid muscle
Muscles which close the mouth	Temporal muscle, masseter muscle, medial pterygoid muscle

Heat and warmth at the trigeminal nerve exits of the nerve.

Paradoxical sensations are possible in cases of bruxism. Total absence of sensation is an indication of neurological or neoplastic disease.

Further neurological investigation and examination of the paranasal sinuses are indicated.

Table 11.11 Interpretation of isometric testing according to Sebald and Kopp[254]

Isometric test	Possible disturbance in cases where the pain or pain-trigger changes	Follow-on investigation
Muscles which open the mouth in CR	DF of muscles which open the mouth	IT of mouth openers in protrusion
Muscles which open the mouth in protrusion	DF of muscles which open the mouth	IT of mouth openers in mediotrusion
Muscles which open the mouth in mediotrusion	Joint effusion, osteoarthritis, anterior dislocation of the disk	IT of muscles which produce mediotrusion. Test for arthrogenic disturbance
Protractor muscles	DF of protractor muscles	IT of muscles which produce mediotrusion
Muscles which produce mediotrusion	Muscles of mouth floor	Passive motion testing
Muscles which close the mouth in CR	Muscles which close the mouth	IT of mouth-closing muscles in protrusion
Muscles which close the mouth in protrusion	Muscles which close the mouth	IT of mouth-closing muscles in mediotrusion
Muscles which close the mouth in mediotrusion	Joint effusion, osteoarthritis, anterior dislocation of the disk	Passive motion testing. Test for arthrogenic disturbance

CR, centric relation; DF, dysfunction; IT, isometric test

Note: The interpretation of isometric testing serves merely as a diagnostic guide, and must be confirmed by further investigations.

Table 11.12 Interpretation of isometric testing according to Sebald and Kopp[254]

Isometric test	No change in pain or pain-trigger	Follow-on investigation
Muscles which open the mouth in CR	Mouth openers not involved	IT of the muscles which close the mouth at rest
Muscles which open the mouth in protrusion	Mouth openers not involved	IT of the muscles which close the mouth at rest. IT of protractors
Muscles which open the mouth in mediotrusion	Mouth openers not involved	IT of the muscles which close the mouth at rest
Protractor muscles	Protractors not involved	IT of the muscles which close the mouth at rest
Muscles which produce mediotrusion	DF of lat. + med. pterygoid muscle	Passive motion testing
Muscles which close the mouth in CR	Muscles which close the mouth not involved	Passive motion testing
Muscles which close the mouth in protrusion	Muscles which close the mouth not involved	Passive motion testing
Muscles which close the mouth in mediotrusion	Muscles which close the mouth not involved	Passive motion testing

CR, centric relation; DF, dysfunction; IT, isometric test

Note: The interpretation of isometric testing serves merely as a diagnostic guide, and must be confirmed by further investigations.

Masseteric reflex

This reflex involves the masseter (and the temporal muscle). The mandibular nerve (V3) innervates these muscles and is thus part of the monosynaptic reflex arc.

Method:
- ➤ Ask the patient to open the mouth slightly.
- ➤ Place your index finger on the patient's chin. Tap your finger with the reflex hammer.
- ➤ A slight tap is followed by closure of the mouth.
- ➤ The reflex is weaker if there is disease along the course of the trigeminal nerve (V), or bulbar paralysis.
- ➤ The reflex is stronger if there is a lesion of the first motor neuron, or pseudobulbar paralysis.

Auscultation

A double stethoscope is very useful for diagnosing jaw sounds (Table 11.13).

What to do next

- If the findings are arthrogenic, an imaging technique is indicated.
- For investigation of static and primary dysfunction in other regions of the body.

Other investigations

Function analysis, radiography, nuclear spin resonance tomography (more rarely computed tomography), functional investigation by magnetic resonance imaging, etc.

Table 11.13 Diagnosis of joint sounds

Sound	Diagnosis
Rubbing sounds	Maybe due to cartilaginous and osseous structures
Rubbing sounds without radiographic findings	Disturbance of occlusion
Clicking, general	Diskopathy
Reciprocal clicking	Diskopathy
Terminal clicks on closure, intensified when pressure applied cephalad on the angle of the jaw	Luxation in centric position
Terminal clicks on opening, and initial clicks on closure	Hypermobility, subluxation
Intermediate clicks	Localized thickening of the cartilage
Clear, loud clicking	Ligamentous, when the disk slides along the lateral and medial ligament

Reciprocal clicking, initial clicks on opening and terminal clicks on closure

Neurodynamic testing of the mandibular nerve (right), according to von Pieckartz.[256]

Patient: The patient is supine, with the head projecting beyond the table and touching the therapist's abdomen.

Therapist: Take up a position at the head of the patient.

Hand position: ➤ First, cup your hands under the occiput with your thumbs on the angles of the mandible.

Method: ➤ Bending of the head, with flexion of the CS about an imaginary transverse axis passing between the first and second cervical vertebrae (Fig. 11.80).

➤ Contralateral side-bending (= to the left) of the upper CS about an imaginary sagittal axis between the first and second cervical vertebrae (see Fig. 11.80).

➤ Flexion and side-bending are performed for as long as possible without triggering pain.

➤ While maintaining the position, carry out a contralateral sliding movement of the mandible (= to the left). To do this, place your right index and middle fingers parallel to the mandible, pointing anterior (Fig. 11.81).

➤ Ask the patient to relax the masticatory muscles and tongue, with the mouth opened about 1 cm.

➤ The test is positive if intraoral and craniocervical symptoms, deafness, burning, tingling, or extreme pressure and severe pain arise in the jaw region.

➤ A feeling of tension in the jaw region and slight sensory reactions in the facial region may be normal.

Interpretation: All structures capable of compressing the mandibular nerve and its branches or subjecting them to tensile stress may be causally involved. (Tables 11.14, 11.15)

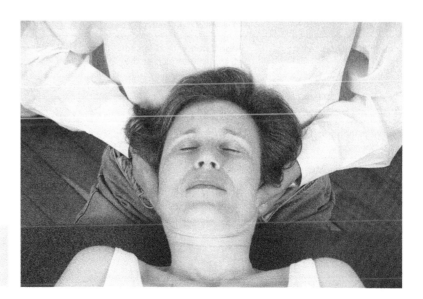

Figure 11.80
Neurodynamic testing of the mandibular nerve (von Pieckartz)

Table 11.14 Differential diagnosis of a CMD

	Myogenic	Arthrogenic	Occlusal
History-taking	First indication of presence of CMD		
Visual assessment Teeth Soft tissues Deviation of chin tip	Bruxism: (grinding, gnashing) Indication of the side of the dysfunction		Bruxism: (grinding, gnashing)
Active mouth opening and closure Dyscoordination Deviation Deflection	Indication of the side of the dysfunction and prognosis Probably myogenic	 Unilateral DF Unilateral DF, diskopathy, ankylosis	
3-finger test	Indication of a CMD		
Palpation of the TMJ: position and tenderness		Arthrogenic or bilaminar zone	
Palpation of the PRM rhythm	Indication of dysfunctions of widely varying origins, e.g. mandible, temporal bone, suture, membrane, ligament, etc.		
Test of TMJ movement	Indication of the side of the dysfunction and prognosis		
Test of passive mobility of the TMJ: Positive, but IT findings negative Negative	 Probably myogenic	 Arthrogenic	
DD of the jaw clicks with TMJ compression cephalad		Disk, joint surface, ligament	
Motion testing for the retrodiskal tissue		Retrodiskal + dislocation of the disk	
Palpation of the masticatory and hyoid muscles	Myogenic		
Trigger points	Myogenic; pain referral zones		
Isometric muscle testing	Associated with reduced strength* and pain in the muscles and while the joint is in various positions	Associated with reduced strength and pain in the joint, and only in one position of the joint	
Auscultation		Arthrogenic	Occlusal
Nerve palpation/reflex:	Neurogenic; disease of the paranasal sinuses		
Inconsistent findings with psychic signs	Possibly psychosomatic		
Radiographic investigation		Arthrogenic	

DF, dysfunction; DD, differential diagnosis

*Reduced strength without pain indicates a disturbance of innervation (neurogenic genesis)

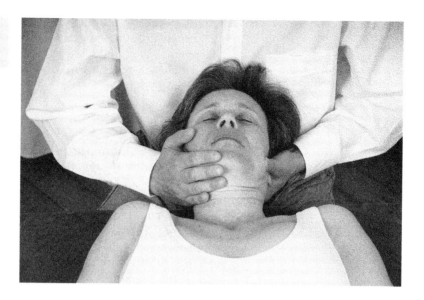

Figure 11.81 Contralateral sliding movement of the mandible

Table 11.15 Differential diagnosis of ascending and descending dysfunctions

	Interpretation
Palpation of the muscles of the neck and shoulder	Parietal involvement

Investigation of statics, positional:
   Static signs of a CMD
   Vertical test according to Barré
	DD of ascending and descending dysfunction

Investigation of statics, dynamic:
   Parameters: standing and sitting
   Paper test
   Meersseman test
   Table
	DD of ascending and descending dysfunction

Contradictory findings with psychic signs	Possibly psychosomatic

TREATMENT OF THE TEMPOROMANDIBULAR JOINT

Method of treatment

1. Treatment of all underlying muscular, fascial, osseous and visceral dysfunctions in the body that impair the function of the jaw joint and the postural patterns.
2. Treatment of the occipital bone and temporal bone.
3. Treatment of the masticatory muscles.
4. Treatment of the hyoid muscles.
5. Treatment of the neck muscles, see atlanto-occipital joint and Th4 (according to Littlejohn).
6. Treatment of the craniocervical fascias.
7. Treatment of the condyles and disks. A reduction in the intensity of pain in the facilitated segment should normally be achieved, before the alignment of the TMJ is normalized locally.

8. Auditory-tube technique II.
9. Treatment of the mandibular ligaments: sphenomandibular ligament, stylomandibular ligament.
10. Treatment of sphenopetrosal ligament at the sphenopetrosal synchondrosis.
11. Improvement of nasal breathing: treatment of the paranasal sinuses and tonsils.

Note: Osteopathic treatment of patients with symptoms of the masticatory apparatus should always be conducted in consultation and cooperation with an orthodontic or dental specialist. In addition to osteopathic treatment, orthotic therapy, dental hygiene treatment or, under certain conditions, drug treatment may also be indicated.

Underlying psychic components should also be clarified. Psychotherapy may be indicated in some cases.

A change of diet, focal therapy, etc. may also be necessary for the success of the therapy. A holistically-oriented treatment of the jaw ultimately involves the underlying causes.

Please also note: If inflammatory changes of the TMJ are present, extreme mouth opening should be avoided.

Other methods of treatment: Orthodontic techniques, arthroscopy of the TMJ,[257] discectomy, condylectomy, arthrotomy, sclerotherapy, pain-response training, psychosomatic therapy, repair of a disk perforation, arthrocentesis, soft splints, and transcutaneous nerve stimulation.

No influence of orthodontic treatment in adolescence on TMJ disturbances in later life have been identified in long-term studies.[258]

Of 300 TMJ disturbances with displacement of the disk (usually anteromedially to the condyle), 270 cases could be successfully treated with the aid of splints.[259]

Treatment of the masticatory muscles

Temporal muscle *(Fig. 11.82)*

Therapist: Take up a position at the head of the patient.
Hand position:
➤ For the posterior muscle fibers, position your hands on the muscles, above and posterior to the ears.
➤ For the medial muscle fibers, position your hands above the ears.
➤ For the anterior muscle fibers, position your hands above and anterior to the ears, approximately 1 cm posterior to the lateral ocular margins.
Method: ➤ At each position, administer gentle traction in a cranial direction to relax the muscle.

Masseter muscle *(Figs 11.83–11.85)*

Therapist: Take up a position at the head of the patient.
Hand position: ➤ Position your hands one on each masseter muscle, in the region between the zygomatic arch of the temporal bones and zygomatic bones and the muscle attachments at the angles of the mandible.

Figure 11.82 Temporal
muscle technique

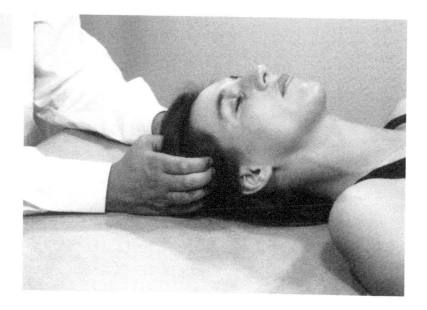

Figure 11.83 Masseter
muscle technique (fascia)

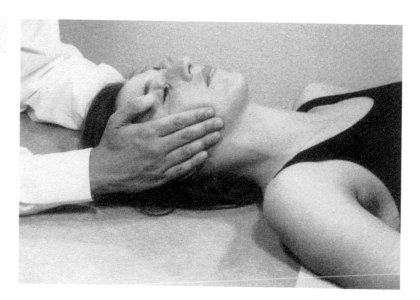

Method: ➤ (a) For the fascias of the muscle, administer very gentle pressure
and follow the fascial tensions of the muscle until the tension
is balanced.

➤ (b) For the superficial muscle portion, smooth the muscle on one
side slowly from the anterior two-thirds of the zygomatic arch
obliquely to the angle of the mandible with somewhat greater
pressure.

While you are doing this, grasp the chin with the other
hand while the patient opens the mouth slightly against the
gentle resistance (stretching the muscle).

Figure 11.84 Masseter muscle technique (superficial part)

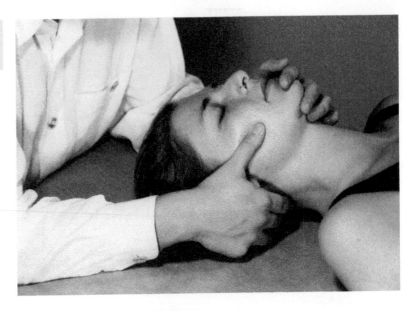

Figure 11.85 Masseter muscle technique (deep part)

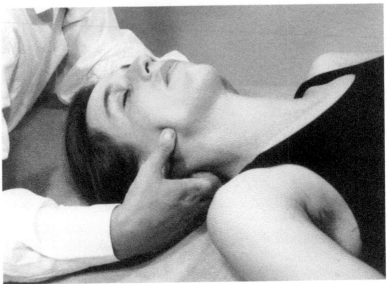

➤ (c) For the deep portion of the muscle, smooth the masseter muscle with stronger pressure from the posterior third of the zygomatic arch almost vertically towards the masseteric tuberosity of the ramus. The tensions in the muscle are then released point by point with small rotatory movements.

Lateral pterygoid muscle *(Figs 11.86a,b)*

Therapist: Take up a position beside the patient's head, on the opposite side to the dysfunction.

Hand position: ➤ Place the index finger or little finger of your caudal hand intraorally, and guide it along the outside margin of the alveolar process of the maxilla, in the direction of the external acoustic meatus. The palmar surface of the finger faces medially towards the gums (see Fig. 11.86a).

➤ When the finger comes into contact with the ascending ramus of the mandible, rotate it so that its palmar surface touches the cheek (Fig. 11.86b).

➤ It may be necessary to ask the patient to move the mandible slightly toward the ipsilateral side for you to be able to move your finger through medially to the ramus of the mandible.

➤ Move your finger posterior and cephalad sufficiently far for the tip to meet the tissue situated anterior of the muscle. Grasp the greater wings with the middle finger and thumb of your cranial hand.

(a)

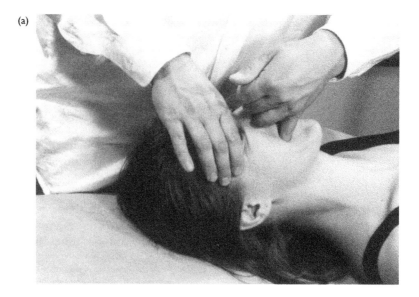

(b)

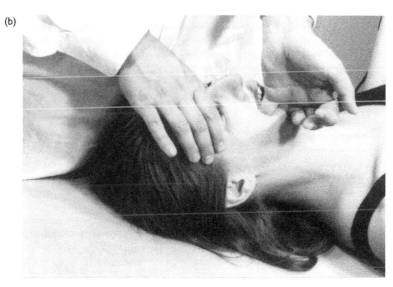

Figure 11.86 (a,b)
Technique for the lateral
pterygoid muscle

Method: ➤ With your cranial hand you are stabilizing the sphenoid without blocking the primary respiratory mechanism.

Caudal hand:

➤ With the tip of your index finger or little finger, apply gentle pressure on the muscle in the direction of the external acoustic meatus. The pressure should be maintained until a release of the muscle tone can be felt.

➤ The pressure should induce no pain.

➤ With each release of the tissue, seek the new limit of motion.

➤ At the end of the technique, administer somewhat greater pressure on the muscle 3 to 4 times to stimulate the tendon-receptor activity.

Medial pterygoid muscle *(Fig. 11.87)*

Therapist: Take up a position beside the patient's head, on the side to be treated.

Hand position: ➤ Position the index finger of your caudal hand intraorally.

➤ Inside the mouth, guide it along the row of teeth as far as the angle of the mandible, where its meets the medial pterygoid muscle.

Method: ➤ If possible, hook it round the muscle cord from posterior. If this induces retching, it is also possible to apply the gentle pressure to the muscle with the tip of the index finger without hooking it round. The pressure should be maintained until a release of the muscle tone can be felt.

➤ The pressure should induce no pain.

➤ With each release of the tissue, seek the new limit of motion.

➤ At the end of the technique, administer somewhat greater pressure on the muscle 3 to 4 times to stimulate the tendon-receptor activity.

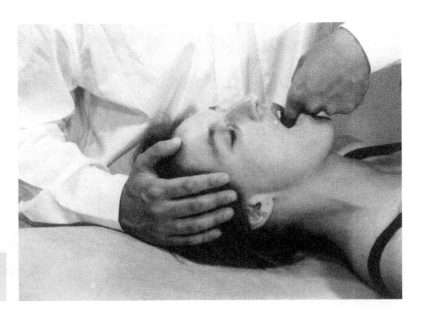

Figure 11.87 Technique for the medial pterygoid muscle

Isometric muscle contraction *(Figs 11.88–11.92)*

Indication: In cases of joint sounds, muscle spasm with limitation of mouth opening, and in association with asymmetric mouth-opening motion and muscle activity.

Hand position: ➤ Place your hands on the mandible in such a way that they can resist the particular motion of the jaw.

Method: For example, opening of the jaw.

➤ The patient relaxes the jaw joints, with the tongue lying relaxed in the mouth and the mouth slightly opened.

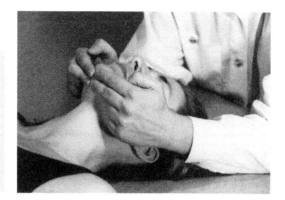

Figure 11.88 Isometric contraction of muscles which open the mouth. Hand position: Position your index and middle fingers against the base of the mouth, enclosing the chin. Method: Contraction in the mouth-opening direction against resistance

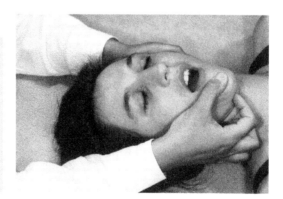

Figure 11.89 Isometric contraction of muscles which close the mouth. Hand position: Place the thumb of one hand anterior on the mandibular symphysis, while the other fingers grasp the lower jaw. The other hand is passive. Method: Contraction in the direction of mouth closure against resistance

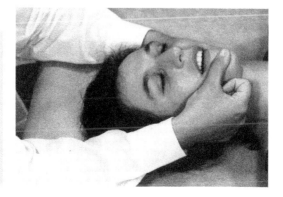

Figure 11.90 Isometric contraction of the protractor muscles. Hand position: Place the thumb of one hand anterior on the mandibular symphysis above the mental protuberance. The other hand is passive. Method: Contraction in the direction of protrusion against resistance

Figure 11.91 Isometric contraction of the retractor muscles. Hand position: Position your index and middle fingers against the base of the mouth, posterior to the mental protuberance. Method: Contraction in the direction of retrusion against resistance.

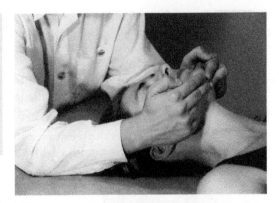

Figure 11.92 Isometric contraction of the laterally-contracting muscles. Hand position: Position the hand on the laterotrusion side against the mandible, while the other hand is placed on the opposite temple. Method: Contraction in the laterotrusion direction against resistance

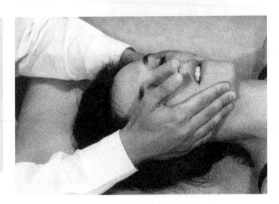

➤ Ask the patient to exert gentle contraction of the masticatory muscles in the direction of jaw opening. With your fingers, resist the muscular contraction so that no movement can take place in the TMJ (isometric muscular contraction).

➤ The force of muscle contraction should be only minimal and be exerted for about 6 s.

➤ Follow each contraction phase with a short relaxation phase.

➤ Each contraction/pause sequence should be repeated about three times.

➤ The technique is then performed accordingly for the mouth-closure, protrusion, retrusion and laterotrusion movements.

Treatment of the condyles

Compression and decompression of the temporomandibular joint (Figs 11.93–11.96)

The technique described below produces both the release of restrictions at the TMJ and squamous suture, and the release of tension of the intracranial membrane.

Therapist: Stand at the head of the patient.

Hand position: ➤ Position your arms on the table beside the patient's head.

➤ Hook your middle fingers beneath the angles of the mandible.

➤ The basal joints of the fingers cover the joints of the jaw, while the palms of the hands cover the ears and temporal regions.

Figure 11.93
Compression and decompression of the TMJ

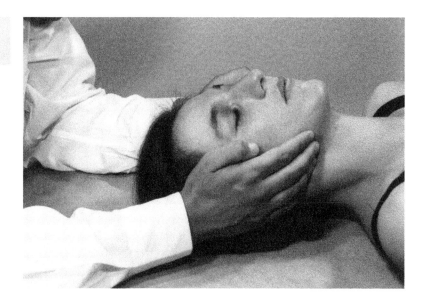

Figure 11.94
Compression of the TMJ

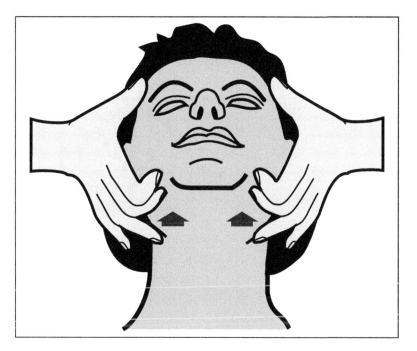

Method:

➤ Ask the patient to relax the TMJ, while not allowing the teeth to touch.

a) Compression (See Fig. 11.94):

➤ With your hands, apply cranially directed pressure on the mandible.

Figure 11.95
Decompression of the TMJ

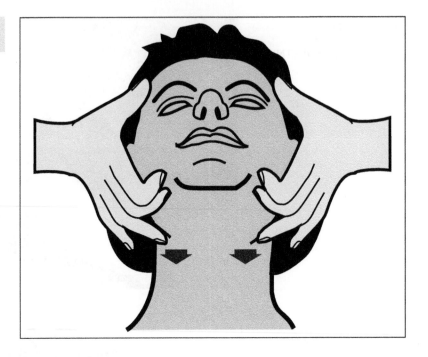

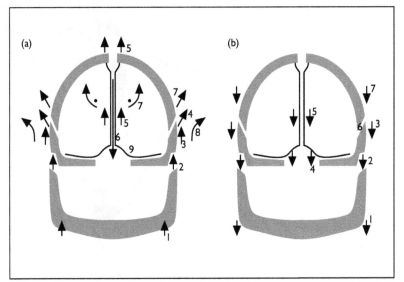

Figure 11.96 Schematic representation of the effect of the technique according to JE Upledger and JD Vreedevoogd. Lehrbuch der Kraniosakrale Therapie. 2nd edn. Heidelberg: Haug Verlag; 1994. (a) Compression of the TMJ. 1. Administration of cranially-directed pressure. 2. Minimal compression occurs at the TMJ. 3. Temporal bones: move in the cranial direction. 4. Shearing force at the squamous suture; on release of the suture, the upper margin of the temporal bone moves laterally. 5. Parietal bones: move in the cranial direction, taking the falx with them. 6. At a specific point, the falx prevents further motion of the parietals cephalad. 7. External rotation of the parietal bones. 8. External rotation of the temporal bones. 9. Consequent stretching of the tentorium cerebelli. (b) Decompression of the TMJ. 1. Administration of caudally-directed traction. 2. Release of the TMJ. 3. Temporal bones move caudally. 4. Consequence: tentorium cerebelli is drawn caudad. 5. Displacement of the straight sinus and falx cerebri. 6. Freeing of squamous suture. 7. Parietal bones move caudad

> Permit any movements of the mandible, without releasing the pressure cephalad.
> As soon as the restrictions of the mandible have been freed, the temporal bones too will execute a see-saw motion.
> The temporal bones move in a cranial direction, and at the same time exert a cranially-directed traction on the tentorium. When the squamous suture is released, the upper margin of the temporal bone tends to move laterally.
> The parietal bones also move in a cranial direction, drawing the falx cerebri with them.
> The falx prevents any further cranial movement of the parietal and temporal bones, thus causing these bones to rotate externally.
> Due to the external rotation of the temporal bones, the tentorium cerebelli is stretched between the two superior borders of the petrous part.
> During the ensuing release of the intracranial membrane, you will be able to perceive membrane tensions at the foramen magnum and in the dural sheath, right down to the sacrum.
> Note all motions of the bones and membranes without preventing them and without relaxing the gentle pressure cephalad.
> When no further relaxation can be perceived, gently reduce the pressure on the mandible and begin decompression by administering traction in a caudal direction.

b) Decompression (See Fig. 11.95):

Method: ➤ Now administer a caudally-directed traction on the mandible.
> The TMJ is freed, and the temporal bones move in a caudal direction.
> This draws the tentorium cerebelli caudad, resulting in a caudal displacement of the straight sinus and falx cerebri.
> The parietosquamous suture is released from restrictions, and the parietal bone also moves caudad.
> With increasing relaxation of the sutures, the tiny movements of the bones and membrane involved come to a standstill, so that the traction can be gently reduced.

c) Establish the PBMT, PBLT:

> Hold this position until a release at the joints and an improvement in the mobility occur.

Global treatment of the temporomandibular joint *(Fig. 11.97)*

Therapist: Stand at the head of the patient.
Hand position: ➤ Support your elbows on the treatment table.
> Position your middle or index fingers on the angle of the mandible.
> Rest your hands on the treatment table.

Method: Ask the patient to relax the TMJ, while not allowing the teeth to touch.

> Balance the angle of the mandible via the middle or index finger.
> Establish a PBLT, PBFT at the TMJ.

Figure 11.97 Global treatment of the TMJ

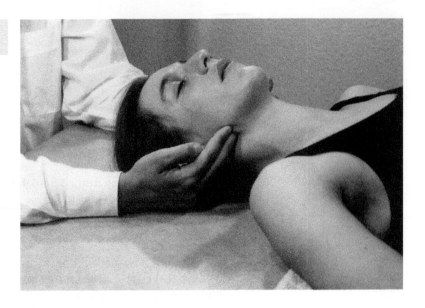

➤ Hold this position, until a relaxation at the joints and an improvement in the mobility occur.

Global treatment of the temporomandibular joint, intraoral (Fig. 11.98)

Therapist: Take up a position beside the patient at the level of the shoulder.

Hand position: ➤ Position your thumbs intraorally on the chewing surfaces of the lower teeth, one on each side.
➤ Hook the middle and index fingers behind the angles of the mandible.
➤ For the torsion and lateral movement, position your index fingers on the two maxillae.

a) Posterior/anterior release

Method: ➤ With your hands, apply a posteriorly-directed pressure on the mandible.
➤ Permit any movements of the mandible, without ceasing the posteriorly-directed pressure.
➤ When you can sense no further release, gently reduce the pressure on the mandible and administer traction anterior.

b) Torsion movement

➤ With your hands, apply a torsion movement to the mandible, while your index fingers stabilize the cranium via the maxillae.
➤ The mandible is first of all rotated in the direction of the dysfunction, i.e. in the direction of greater motion (of ease).
➤ Permit any movements of the mandible, without ceasing the rotation.
➤ When you can sense no further release, rotate the mandible in the direction of the restriction.

Figure 11.98 Global treatment of the TMJ, intraoral

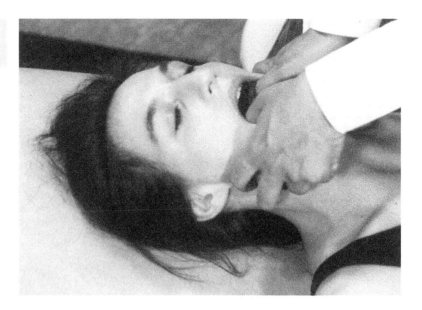

c) Lateral movement

➤ With your hands, apply a lateral movement to the mandible, while your index fingers stabilize the cranium via the maxillae.
➤ First, induce a lateral movement of the mandible in the direction of the dysfunction, i.e. in the direction of greater motion (of ease).
➤ Permit any movements of the mandible, without ceasing induction of the lateral movement.
➤ When you can sense no further release, induce a lateral movement of the mandible in the direction of the restriction.

d) Compression/decompression

➤ With your hands, apply cranially-directed pressure to the mandible.
➤ Permit any movements of the mandible, without ceasing the pressure cranially.
➤ When you can sense no further release, gently reduce the pressure on the mandible whilst administering a traction caudally and anterior (at an angle of 45°). Once again, permit all movements that occur.

Note: It is also possible to establish a PBLT, PBFT of all restrictions on the mandible.

Treatment of the TMJ according to Blagrave[260]

Dysfunction of the right temporomandibular joint I (Fig. 11.99).

Indication: Impairment of protrusion and/or left laterotrusion of the right TMJ.
Patient: The patient is supine, with a cushion under the upper TS to bring the CS into slight extension. Ask the patient to rotate the head to the left.
Therapist: Take up a position at the head of the patient.

Figure 11.99 Treatment of a right TMJ with impairment of protrusion and/or left laterotrusion (Blagrave)

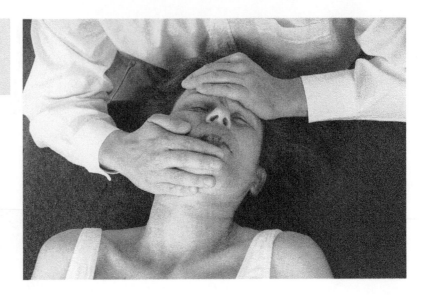

Hand position: Right hand:

> ➤ Place your index and middle fingers on the body of the mandible, with the fingers pointing anterior. Position the ring finger and little finger on the lower margin of the mandible.

Left hand:

> ➤ The left hand is on the forehead, with the fingers pointing in the direction of the ear.

Method:
> ➤ Ask the patient to open the mouth slightly.
> ➤ At the same time, move your hands in parallel but opposite directions. The right hand on the mandible is moved in an anterior, inferior direction and the left hand on the forehead is moved posterior and superior.

Dysfunction of the right temporomandibular joint II (Fig. 11.100)

Indication: Impairment of protrusion or opening of the right TMJ.
Patient: The patient is supine, with the head rotated slightly to the left.
Therapist: Take up a position beside the patient's head, on the opposite side to the dysfunction.
Hand position: Cranial hand:

> ➤ Place your cranial hand on the forehead to hold the head firmly in position.

Caudal hand:
> ➤ Position your thumb intraorally on the posterior lower molars.
> ➤ With your other fingers, grip the mandible from the outside.

Method: Ask the patient to close the mouth sufficiently for the posterior part of the thumb to come into contact with the upper molars.

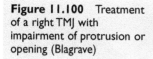

Figure 11.100 Treatment of a right TMJ with impairment of protrusion or opening (Blagrave)

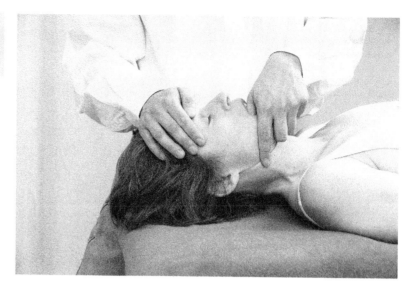

Flex the terminal joint of your thumb, so that the TMJ is passively mobilized against the upper molars by a lifting movement of the thumb.

In addition, with your caudal hand you may administer traction anterior in order to strengthen the movement.

Repositioning an anteromedial disk displacement according to a modification of the method of Kaluza/Goering[261] *(Fig. 11.101)*

Technique: Articulation.

Important: Before performing the technique, a reduction in the facilitation intensity of the affected segment should be achieved by myofascial and strain/counterstrain techniques.

Patient: The patient should be supine.

Therapist: Take up a position at the head of the patient.

Hand position:
- ➤ Place one hand on the side of the head to stabilize it.
- ➤ Position your other hand on the opposite angle and ramus of the mandible.

Method: Ask the patient to open the mouth as wide as possible.

- ➤ If maximal opening is achieved, with the hand that is on the mandible apply a continuous, lateral translation force. This should be directed towards the opposite TMJ.
- ➤ The hand positioned on the side of the head acts as a stabilizer and counterbalances the force from the other hand, so that no head movements occur.
- ➤ Maintain the forces exerted by the hands, while the patient slowly closes the mouth again.
- ➤ The aim is to achieve an opening between the mandibular condyle and the cranium.

Figure 11.101
Repositioning of an anteromedial disk displacement (modification of the method of Kaluza/Goering)

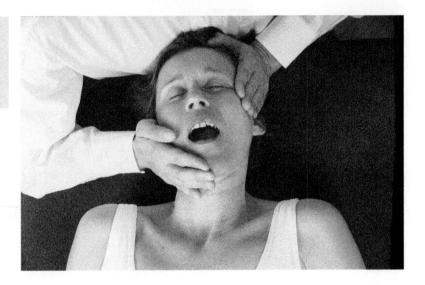

➤ When the treatment is successful, a palpable and sometimes audible change in the joint can usually be heard.
➤ The technique is then repeated on the other side.

● The number of repetitions is variable, but as a rule 4 to 8 repetitions are performed per side. The applied force may be increased as required.
● The signs of successful normalization are: normalization of the disk position, increased radius of movement, and pain and associated symptoms are reduced or disappear altogether.

Note: ● The repetitions are intended to reset the stretch receptors in the superior part of the lateral pterygoid muscle.
● If there is no clear improvement, the treatment may be repeated at weekly or fortnightly intervals.

Repositioning an anterolateral disk displacement according to Kaluza

This largely corresponds to unilateral treatment of the condyles, since the trismus associated with anterolateral disk displacement does not allow opening of the mouth sufficiently wide to use an articulatory technique. In some cases, however, the use of greater force is necessary than in the technique mentioned above.

Repositioning an anteromedially displaced disk according to Farrar[150,151,166] *(Fig. 11.102)*

A locked TMJ of no longer than 3–4 weeks' duration is usually relatively easy to release.

Hand position: ➤ With both hands, grasp the mandible firmly by positioning your thumbs on the posterior region of the lower teeth, one on each

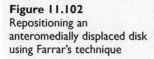

Figure 11.102
Repositioning an anteromedially displaced disk using Farrar's technique

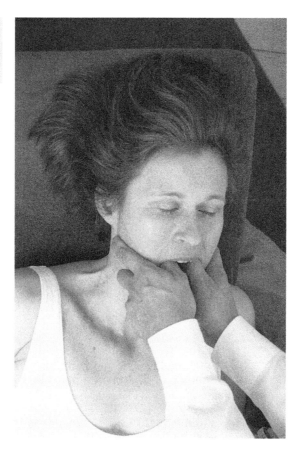

side, while the other fingers enclose the lower margin of the anterior mandible from the outside.

Method: ➤ On the side of the displaced disk, apply pressure caudad on the condyle while administering cranially-directed pressure with your fingers.

➤ The condyle on the affected side is then moved in an anterior, medial direction.

Unilateral treatment of the condyles *(Fig. 11.103)*

Therapist: Stand beside the patient's head on the opposite side to the dysfunction.

a) Decompression

Hand position: Cranial hand:

➤ Grip the angle of the mandible on the affected side with your thumb and index finger.

Caudal hand:

➤ Position the thumb intraorally, on the chewing surfaces of the lower teeth on the affected side. Place it on the last molars.

Figure 11.103 Unilateral treatment of the condyles

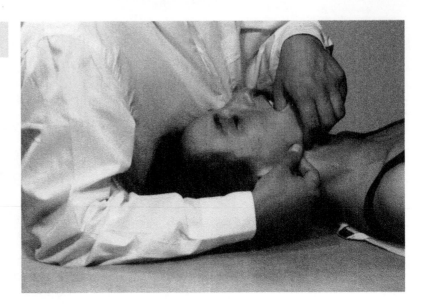

➤ Place the index finger outside on the lower margin of the horizontal part of the mandible.
➤ With your thumb and index finger, grip the horizontal part of the mandible.

Method: ➤ Administer traction in a caudal and anterior direction (at an angle of 45°) with the thumb and index finger of the caudal hand.
➤ Support this traction with your cranial hand.
➤ The cranial hand may additionally perform a gentle translation of the condyle anterior.
➤ Note all movements of the mandible that arise, without preventing them and without relaxing the gentle traction caudad and anterior.
➤ When no further release of the tissue (capsule, ligaments, muscles) can be sensed, the traction on the mandible can be stopped.
➤ Establish the PBLT, PBFT.
➤ A fluid impulse may be used to direct energy from the opposite occipitomastoid suture.

b) Harmonization of the temporal bone (Fig. 11.104)
Hand position: Caudal hand:
➤ With your thumb and index finger, maintain a grip on the angle of the mandible on the affected side.

Cranial hand:
➤ With your cranial hand, grasp the temporal bone with the '5-finger temporal-bone technique' palpation.
➤ The thumb and index finger grasp the zygomatic process.
➤ Position the middle finger in the external acoustic meatus.
➤ Place the ring finger on the tip of the mastoid process.
➤ The little finger will be on the mastoid part.

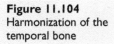

Figure 11.104
Harmonization of the temporal bone

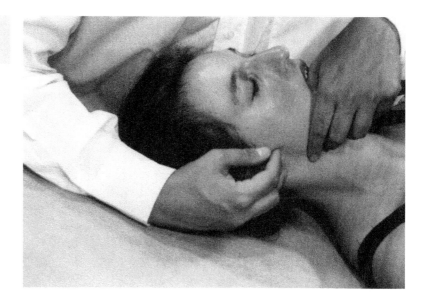

Method: ➤ After the TMJ has been decompressed, establish the PBMT, PBFT of the temporal bone.

Auditory-tube technique according to Magoun and Galbreath

Indication and effect: Release of the jaw joint, medial pterygoid muscle and myofascial structures of the nasopharyngeal space, etc.

'Multiple-hand technique' *(Fig. 11.105)*

Therapist 1 stands at the head of the patient.
Therapist 2 stands beside the patient's head.

Hand position: Therapist 1:
➤ Position your thenar eminences on the mastoid parts, one on each side.
➤ Position your thumbs on the anterior points of the mastoid process.
➤ Place the palms of your hands on the occiput.
➤ Clasp the fingers of the two hands.
➤ Position the elbows of both arms on the table.

Therapist 2:
➤ Position the thumbs intraorally, on the chewing surfaces of the lower teeth.
➤ Hook the middle fingers behind the angles of the mandible.

Method: ➤ Therapist 1 holds the occiput and temporal bones firmly in position.
➤ Therapist 2 administers caudally and anteriorly-directed traction (at an angle of 45°) on the mandible.

Figure 11.105 Multiple hand technique for the TMJ

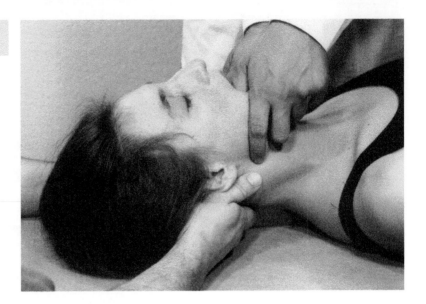

➤ Permit any movements of the mandible without terminating the traction caudad.
➤ When you can sense no further release, gently reduce the pressure on the mandible.
➤ Then, via the hand contact, establish a PBT between the mandible and the cranium.

TREATMENT OF THE MANDIBULAR LIGAMENTS

Sphenomandibular ligament according to Viola Frymann *(Fig. 11.106)*

Sphenomandibular ligament test

Therapist: Take up a position beside the patient's head, opposite the side to be tested.

Hand position: Cranial hand:
➤ Grasp the greater wings with your thumb and middle or index finger.

Caudal hand:
➤ Position the thumb on the biting surface of the last molar on the opposite side. With your fingers, grip the angle of the mandible.

Method: ➤ With your thumb, moved the mandible caudad.
➤ With your other hand, register the movements at the greater wings.

If there is an abnormal increase in tension of the sphenomandibular ligament, the greater wing on the tested side will move superior.

Note: The sphenomandibular ligament attaches on the spine of the sphenoid, which is located posterior of the flexion/extension axis of

Figure II.106 Treatment of the sphenomandibular ligament using Viola Frymann's technique

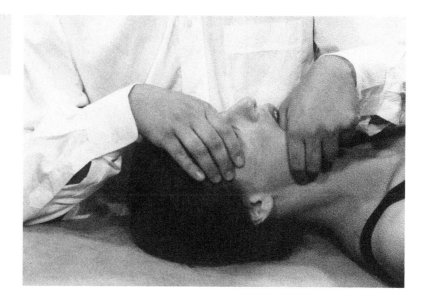

the SBS. For this reason, an increase in tension or fibrosis of the ligament causes caudal traction on the base of the sphenoid with a movement of the ipsilateral greater wing superior.

Treatment of the sphenomandibular ligament

Hand position: As above.
Method:
> ➤ With your thumb, move the mandible caudad.
> ➤ At the same time, administer a gentle traction caudad on the greater wings.
> ➤ Continue doing this until you sense a release of the sphenomandibular ligament.

Stylomandibular ligament according to Viola Frymann *(Fig. II.107)*

Stylomandibular ligament test

Therapist: Take up a position beside the patient's head, opposite the side to be tested.
Hand position: Cranial hand:
> ➤ '5-finger temporal-bone technique'
> ➤ Grip the zygomatic process with your thumb and index finger.
> ➤ Position the middle finger in the external acoustic meatus.
> ➤ The ring finger is positioned in front of the mastoid process.

Caudal hand:
> ➤ Position the thumb on the biting surface of the last molar on the opposite side. With your fingers, grip the angle of the mandible.

Method:
> ➤ With your thumb, move the mandible obliquely in a caudal, anterior and lateral direction (following the course of the ligament).
> ➤ With your other hand, register the movement at the temporal bone.

Figure 11.107 Treatment of the stylomandibular ligament using Viola Frymann's technique

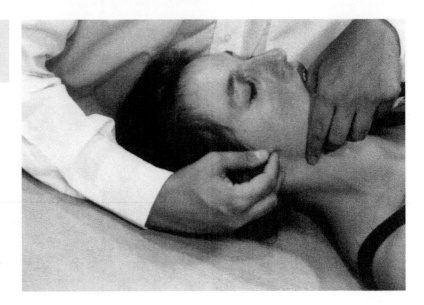

If there is an abnormal increase in tension of the stylomandibular ligament, the temporal bone on the tested side will move inferior.

Treatment of the stylomandibular ligament

Hand position: As above.

Method: ➤ With your thumb, move the mandible in a caudal, anterior and lateral direction.

➤ At the same time, hold the temporal bone in position.

➤ Continue doing this until you sense a release of the stylomandibular ligament.

Note: The sphenomandibular and stylomandibular ligaments may also be treated using the V-spread technique.

Self-help techniques

Decompression of the TMJ *(Fig. 11.108a)*

Indication: To release the tension in the joint in cases of muscular hypertonicity, inflammation of the joint, hardening of the tissue, pain, etc.

Patient: Seated.

Hand position: ➤ The two hands cover the angles and the ascending rami of the mandible. Do not support the elbows.

Method: ➤ Relax the joints of the jaw and the mouth as much as possible, allow the tongue to lie relaxed in the mouth, and open the mouth slightly.

➤ A slight decompression is exerted on the jaw joints simply by the weight of the arms.

Alternative technique *(Fig. 11.108b)*

Patient: Seated, with a roll of cotton wool between the posterior molars on each side.

Figure 11.108 (a) Self-help technique. Decompression of the TMJ **(b)** Decompression of the TMJ. Alternative technique

(a)

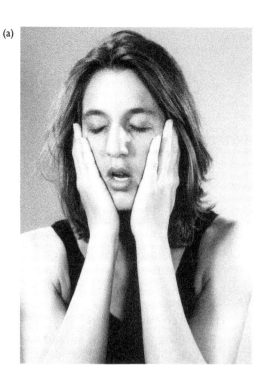

(b)

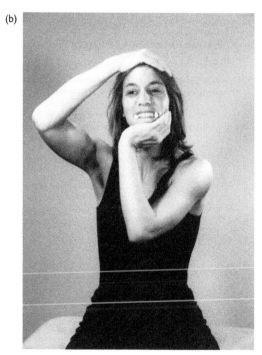

Hand position: ➤ Place one hand on the cranium and the other under the chin on the mandible.

Method: ➤ Relax the jaw joints and masticatory muscles as much as possible.
➤ With the hand that is on the chin, administer gentle pressure superior. The other hand on the cranium simultaneously stabilizes the head.

> A decompression in the TMJ occurs through the fulcrum of the cotton wool roll.

Release of the masticatory muscles

The techniques described below should be performed gently and should never cause pain.

Patient: Seated.

Temporal muscle *(Fig. 11.109)*

> Position your fingers on the muscles above the ears. Relax the mouth and jaw joints as best you can.
> Release the anterior, middle and posterior parts of the muscle by gentle traction in a cranial direction.

Masseter muscle *(Fig. 11.110)*

> Position your index and middle fingers on both masseter muscles. Relax the mouth and jaw joints as best you can.
> With your fingers, administer gentle pressure on the muscles, particularly on the hard areas in the muscles.

Lateral pterygoid muscle *(Fig. 11.111)*

> Guide your index finger or little finger intraorally along the outer margin of the alveolar process of the maxilla in the direction of the external acoustic meatus. The palmar surface of the finger must be turned laterally toward the cheek.
> Move the finger sufficiently far in a posterior and cranial direction for the tip to come up against the muscle.
> Apply gentle pressure to the muscle with your finger.

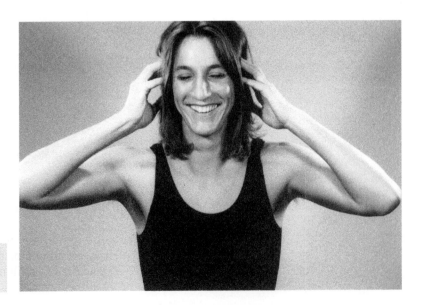

Figure 11.109 Self-help technique. Relaxation of the temporal muscle

Figure 11.110 Self-help technique. Relaxation of the masseter muscle

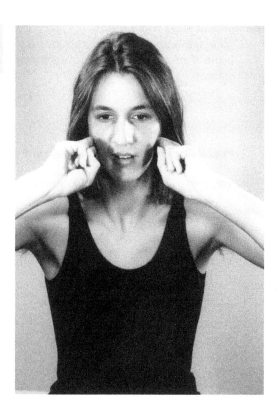

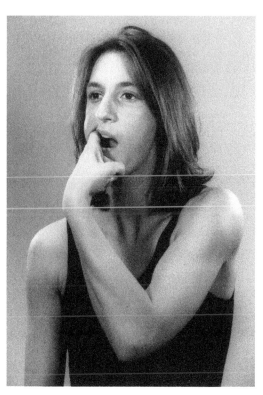

Figure 11.111 Self-help technique. Relaxation of the lateral pterygoid muscle

Improving the protrusion and sideways movement

This self-help technique can be used in cases of impairment of protrusion and sideways movement on account of elevated capsular tension.

It also teaches coordination and proprioceptive perception in the TMJ.

Patient: Seated or lying down.

Practicing the sideways movement *(Fig. 11.112)*

➤ Place your index finger that is on the opposite side from the dysfunction on the outside of the canine tooth of the upper jaw.
➤ Try to bite this finger.

Practicing the protrusion movement *(Fig. 11.113)*

➤ Position your index finger on the anterior incisors of the upper jaw.
➤ Try to bite this finger.

Isometric muscle contraction *(Fig. 11.114)*

Indication: Hypermobility of the TMJ, joints sounds, muscle spasm with restricted mouth opening, as well as in asymmetric mouth-opening motion and muscle activity.

Hand position: Place your two index fingers on the mandible, laterally of the tip of the chin.

Method: ➤ Relax the jaw joints, let the tongue lie relaxed in the mouth, and open the mouth slightly.
➤ Perform a gentle contraction of the masticatory muscles in the jaw-opening direction, against the resistance of the fingers. There should be no movement in the TMJ (isometric muscle contraction).

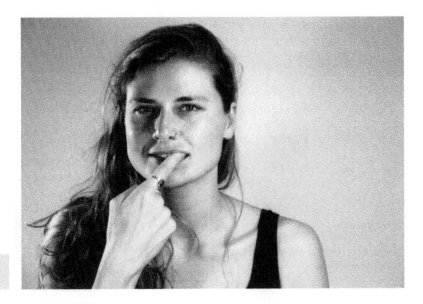

Figure 11.112 Practicing the sideways movement

Figure 11.113 Practicing the protrusive movement

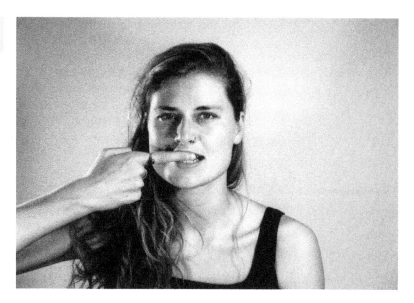

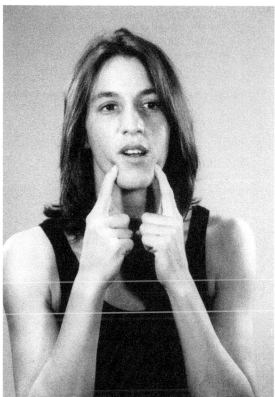

Figure 11.114 Isometric muscle contraction; mouth-opening movement. A gentle mouth-opening movement is executed against resistance of the fingers, without resulting in a movement of the jaw

➤ The force of the muscle contraction should be minimal, and be exerted for about 6 s.
➤ Each contraction phase should be followed by a brief relaxation phase.
➤ Each contraction/pause sequence should be repeated about three times.

➤ The technique is then performed in the same way for mouth closure, protrusion, retrusion and laterotrusion.

Alternative method: ➤ With your fingers, administer gentle pressure against the chin in the direction of mouth-closure. The muscles of the jaw should contract and counteract the gentle pressure of the fingers, with the result that no movement of the jaw takes place (isometric muscle contraction). The method continues as above.

This method has the advantage that the patient learns better control of his or her muscle activity.

References

1 Still AT. Osteopathy Research and Practice. Seattle: Estland Press; 1992:199–200.
2 Sutherland WG. The Cranial Bowl. Monkato, Minnesota: Free Press Company; 1939:99–100.
3 Magoun HI. Osteopathy in the Cranial Field. 3rd edn. Kirksville: Journal Printing Company; 1976:162–202.
4 Fryette HH. Principles of Osteopathic Technic. California: AAO; 1994:234–241.
5 Frymann VM. Cranial disorders and its role in disorders of the temporomandibular joint. Symposium on the temporomandibular joint dysfunction and treatment. Dent Clin N Am 1983:27.
6 Frymann VM. Why does the orthodontist need osteopathy in the cranial field. Cranial Lett 1988:41.
7 Magoun HI. Osteopathy in the Cranial Field, 3rd edn. Kirksville: Journal Printing Company 1976:162–202.
8 DiGiovanna EL, Schiowitz S. An Osteopathic Approach to Diagnosis and Treatment. Philadelphia: Lippincott-Raven; 1997:369.
9 Smith SD. (1981), Structural and facial influences on TMJ apparatus. JAOA 1981; 10.
10 Hruby RJ. (1985) The total body approach to the osteopathic management of temporo-mandibular joint dysfunction. JAOA 1985; 8.
11 Blood SD. (1986) The craniosacral mechanism and the temporomandibular joint. JAOA 1986; 8.
12 Lanz T, Wachsmuth W. Praktische Anatomie, Vol. 1. Part A. Berlin: Springer; 1985:215.
13 Benninghoff A. Anatomie des Menschen, Vol. 1, 14th edn. Munich: Urban & Schwarzenberg; 1985:525.
14 Schumacher GH. Anatomie für Zahnmediziner. Heidelberg: Hüthig; 1997:368.
15 Benninghoff A. Anatomie des Menschen, Vol. 1. 14th edn. Munich: Urban & Schwarzenberg; 1985:526.
16 Aumüller G. Gestaltungsfaktoren der schädelform. In: Staubesand J, Fleischhauer K, Zenker W, eds. Benninghoff, Anatomie. Makroskopische und Mikroskopische Anatomie des Menschen, Vol. 1. München: Urban und Schwarzenberg; 1985.
17 Sicher H, Dubral LE. Oral Anatomy, 5th edn. St Louis: Mosby; 1970.
18 Helluy L: Étude cinématique et dynamique du jeu mandibulaire dans l'abaissement et l'élévation simples. Actual Odonto-Stomat 1962; 58:147–180.
19 Hellsing G, Holmlund A. Development of anterior disk displacement in the temporomandibular joint: an autopsy study. J Prosthet Dent 1985; 53:397–401.
20 Choukas NC, Sicher H. The structure of the temporomandibular joint. Oral Surg 1960; 1203–1213.
21 Keith DA. Development of the human temporomandibular joint. Br J Oral Surg 1982; 20:217–224.
22 Marguelles-Bonnet R, Yung JP, Carpentier P, et al. Temporomandibular joint serial sections made with mandible in intercuspal position. J Craniomandib Pract 1989; 2:7.

23 Lanz T, Wachsmuth W. Praktische Anatomie, Part A. Berlin: Springer; 1985:126.

24 Carlsson GE, Oeberg T. Remodelling of the temporomandibular joint. Oral Sci Rev 1974; 6:53–86.

25 Strauss F, Christen A, Weber W. The architecture of the disc of the human temporomandibular joint. Helv Odontol Acta 1960; 4:1–4.

26 Moffett B. The prenatal development of the human temporomandibular joint. Contr Embryol 1957; 36:21–28.

27 Lai WF, Bowley J, Burch JG. Evaluation of shear stress of the human temporo-mandibular joint disc. J Orofac Pain 1998; 12(2):153–159.

28 Schumacher G-H. Anatomie für Zahnmediziner. Heidelberg: Hüthig; 1997:370.

29 Sperber GH. Embryologie des Kopfes. Berlin: Quintessenz; 1992:370.

30 Scapino RP, Canham PB, Finlay HM, et al. The behaviour of collagen fibers in stress relaxation and stress distribution in the jaw-joint disc of rabbits. Archives of Oral Biology 1996; 41:1039–1052.

31 Langedoen-Sertel J, Hamouda M. Die bedeutung des retrodiskalen gewebes beitemporo-mandibulären arthropathien. Manuelle Therapie 1998; 1:8–14.

32 Williams PL, Bannister LH, Berry MM, et al. Gray's Anatomy, 38th edn. New York: Churchill Livingstone; 1995:579.

33 Tanaka TT. TMJ Microanatomy: An Anatomy Approach to Current Controversies. An educational videotape. Chula Vista, CA: Clinical Research Foundation; 1992.

34 Rohen JW. Anatomie für Zahnmediziner. 2nd edn. Stuttgart: Schattauer; 1988:113–114.

35 Marguelles-Bonnet R, Yung JP, Carpentier P. Temporomandibular joint serial sections made with mandible in intercuspal position. J Craniomandib Pract 1989; 2(7):97–106.

36 Nell A, Niebauer W, Sperr W, et al. Special variations of the lateral ligament of the human. TMJ Clin Anat 1994; 7:267–270.

37 Kikuchi M, Watanabe M, Hattori Y. Three dimensional bite force and associated masticatory muscle activities.

38 Landeweer GG. Funktionelle anatomie der kaumuskeln. Update 2001; 2(2):20–24.

39 Schumacher G-H. Anatomie für Zahnmediziner. Heidelberg: Hüthig; 1997:388.

40 Hack GD, Dumm G, Toh MY. The anatomist's new tools. In: Encyclopaedia Britannica 1998 Medical and Health Annual. Chicago: NCMIC Insurance Co.; 1998:16–29.

41 McNamara J A. The independent functions of the two heads of the lateral pterygoid muscle. Am J Anat 1976; 138:197–206.

42 Van Eijden TMGJ, Koolstra JH. A model for mylohyoid muscle mechanics. J Biomechan 1998; 31:1017–1024.

43 Schumacher G-H. Anatomie für Zahnmediziner. Heidelberg: Hüthig; 1997:382.

44 Benner KU. Bau innervation und rezeptive strukturen des kiefergelenks. In: Benner K, Fanghänel J, Kowalewski R, et al., eds. Morphologie Funktion und Klinik des Kiefergelenks. Berlin: Quintessenz Verlag; 1993:43–60.

45 Baumann J. Contribution à l'étude de l'innervation de l'articulation temporomandibulaire. CRAA 1951; 2:120.

46 Boobennova MA. Innervation of the capsule of temporomandibular joint. Stomatolog 1950; 2:3–13.

47 Greenfield BE, Wyke B. Reflex innervation of the temporomandidular joint. Nature 1966; 211:940–941.

48 Klineberg IJ. Influences of temporomandidular articular mechanoreceptors on functional jaw movements. J Oral Rehabil 1980; 7:307–317.

49 Klineberg IJ, Greenfield BE, Wyke B. Afferent discharges from temporomandibular articular mechanoreceptors: An experimental study in the cat. Arch Oral Biol 1970; 15:935–952.

50 Klineberg IJ, Ash MM. Some temporomandibular articular reflex effects on jaw muscles. J Dent Res 1980; 57:130.

51 Zimny ML. Mechanoreceptors in articular tissues. Am J Anat 1988; 182:16–32.

52 Breul R. Bau und funktion des kiefergelenks. Osteopath Med 2002; 1:12–16.

53 Ostry DJ, Flanagan JR. Human jaw movement in mastication and speech. Arch Oral Biol 1989; 34:685–693.

54 Koolstra JH, Van Eijden TMGJ. Three-dimensional dynamical capabilities of the human masticatory muscles. J Biomechan 1999; 32:145–152.

55 Bennett NG. A contribution to the study of the movements of the mandible. J Prosthét Dent 1908, Reprinted 1958; 8:41–54.

56 Messerman T. A means for studying mandibular movements. J Prosthet Dent 1967; 17:36–43.

57 Gibbs CH, Messerman T, Reswick JB, et al. Functional movements of the mandible. J Prosthet Dent 1971; 26:604–620.

58 Goodson JM, Johansen E. Analysis of human mandibular movement. Monogr in Oral Sc 1975; 5:1–80.

59 Schumacher GH. Anatomie: Lehrbuch und Atlas. 1. Kopf, Orofaziales System, Auge, Ohr, Leitungsbahnen, 2nd edn. Leipzig: JA Barth; 1991.

60 Smith RD, Marcarian HQ. The neuromuscular spindles of the lateral pterygoid muscle. Anat Anz 1967; 120:47–53.

61 Slavicek R. La soi-disant relation centrée. Rev Orthop Dento Fac 1982; 16:413–415.

62 Gallo LM, Airoldi GB, Airoldi RL, et al. Description of mandibular finite helical axis pathways in asymptomatic subjects. J Dental Res 1997; 76:704–713.

63 Koolstra JH, van Eijden TMGJ. The jaw open–close movements predicted by biomechanical modelling. J Biomechan 1997; 30:943–950.

64 Lückerath W. Die bennettbewegung. Dtsch Zahnärztl Zeit 1991; 46:89–193.

65 Koolstra JH, van Eijden TMGJ. Biomechanical analysis of jaw closing movements. J Dent Res 1995; 74:1564–1570.

66 Koolstra JH, van Eijden TMGJ. Influence of the dynamical properties of the human masticatory muscles on jaw closing movements. Euro J Morphol 1996; 34:11–18.

67 Benninghoff A. Anatomie des Menschen, Vol. 1, 14th edn. Munich: Urban & Schwarzenberg; 1985:527.

68 Hatcher DC, Faulkner MG, Hay A. development of mechanical and mathematical models to study temporomandibular joint loading. J Prosth Dentistry 1986; 55:377–384.

69 Smith DM, McLachlan KR, McCall WD. A numerical model of temporomandibular joint loading. J Dent Res 1986; 65:1046–1052.

70 Faulkner MG, Hatcher DC, Hay A. A three-dimensional investigation of temporomandibular joint loading. J Biomechan 1987; 20:997–1002.

71 Koolstra JH, Van Eijden TMGJ, Weijs WA, et al. A three-dimensional mathematical model of the human masticatory system predicting maximum possible bite forces. J Biomechan 1988; 21:563–576.

72 Ferrario VF, Sforza C. Biomechanical model of the human mandible in unilateral clench: distribution of temporomandibular joint reaction forces between working and balancing sides. J Prosth Dentistry 1994; 72:169–176.

73 Throckmorton GS, Dechow PC. In vitro measurements in the condylar process of the human mandible. Arch Oral Biology 1994; 39:853–867.

74 O'Ryan F, Epker BN. Temporomandibular joint function and morphology: observations on the spectra of normalcy. Oral Surg 1984; 58:272–279.

75 Nickel JC, McLachlan KR, Smith DM. A theoretical model of loading and eminence development of the postnatal human temporomandibular joint. J Dent Res 1988; 67:903–910.

76 Newberry WN, Mackenzie CD, Haut RC. Blunt impact causes changes in bone and cartilage in a regularly exercised animal model. J Orthop Res 1998; 16:348–354.

77 McCormack T, Mansour JM. Reduction in tensile strength of cartilage precedes surface damage under repeated compressive loading *in vivo*. J Biomechan 1998; 31:55–61.

78 Hylander WI, Bays R. An *in vivo* strain-gauge analysis of the squamosal-dentary joint reaction force during mastication and incisal biting in macaca mulatta and macaca fasciculans. Arch Oral Biol 1979; 24:689–697.

79 Boyd RL, Gibbs CH, Mahan PE, et al. Temporomandibular forces measured at the condyle of macaca arctoides. Am J Orthod Dentofacial Orthop 1990; 97:472–474.

80 Brehnan K, Boyd RL, Laskin J, et al. Direct measurement of loads at the temporomandibular joint in macaca arctoides. J Dent Res 1981; 60:1820–1824.

81 Barbenel JC. The mechanics of the temporomandibular joint – a theoretical and electromyographical study. J Oral Rehabil 1974; 1:19–27.

82 Breul R. Die stellungsabhängige beanspruchung des kiefergelenks des menschen – eine biomechanische analyse. In: Benner K, Fanghänel J, Kowalewski R, et al., eds. Morphologie Funktion und Klinik des Kiefergelenks. Berlin: Quintessenz; 1993:111–119.

83 Breul R, Mall G, Landgraft, et al. Biomechanical analysis of stress distribution in the human temporomandibular joint. Ann Anat 1999; 181:55–60.

84 Freimann R. Untersuchungen über zahl und anordnung der muskelspindeln in den kaumuskeln des menschen. Anat Anz 1954; 100:258–264.

85 Gill HI. Neuromuscular spindles in human lateral pterygoid muscles. J Anat 1971; 109:157–167.

86 Honee GLJM. An investigation on the presence of muscle spindles in the human lateral pterygoid muscle. Ned Tijdschr Tandheilkd 1966; 73 (suppl 3):43–48.

87 Kummer B. Anatomie und biomechanik des unterkiefers. Fortschr Kieferorthop 1985; 46:335–342.

88 Molitor J. Untersuchungen über die beanspruchung des kiefergelenks. Z Anat Entw Gesch 1991; 129:109–140.

89 Kubein-Meesenburg D, Nägerl H, Fanghänel J. Elements of a general theory of joints. Anat Anz 1991; 172:309–321.

90 Nägerl H, Kubein-Meesenburg D, Fanghänel J, et al. Die posteriore Führung der Mandibula als neuromuskulär gegebene innere Gelenkkette. Dtsch Stomat 1991; 41:279–283.

91 Nägerl H, Kubein-Meesenburg D. Comparative examination of the determination of the individual contour-curve from the incisors and from the premolar region. Anat Anz 1990; 170:163–170.

92 Schumacher G-H. Anatomie für Zahnmediziner. Heidelberg: Hüthig; 1997:372.

93 Amiguez JP. L'ATM. Une Articulation Entre l'Osteopathe et le Dentiste. Aix en Provence: Verlaque; 1991:52.

94 Schumacher G-H. Anatomie für Zahnmediziner. Heidelberg: Hüthig; 1997:402.

95 Krogh-Poulsen W, Troest T. Form und funktion im stomatognathen System. In: Hupfauf L, ed. Funktionsstörungen des Kauorgans, 2nd edn. Munich: Urban & Schwarzenberg; 1989:15.

96 Amiguez JP. L'ATM. Une Articulation Entre l'Osteopathe et le Dentiste. Aix en Provence: Verlaque; 1991:54.

97 Portmann A. Einfuhrung in die vergleichende Morphologie der Wirbwltiere. 6. Aufl. Schwabe, Basel 1983; 105–108.

98 Delattre A, Fenart R. L'Hominisation du crâne. Paris: CNRS; 1954.

99 Starck D. Embryologie, 4th edn. Stuttgart: Thieme; 1978.

100 Petrovic A, Charlier JP. La synchondrose sphéno-occipitale de jeune rat en culture d'organes: mise en évidence d'un potentiel de creoissance indépendent. Paris: CRAcadSc; 1967;1511–1513.

101 Couly G. Articulations temporo-mandibulaires et interrelations fonctionnelles masticatrices. Actualités Odonto–Stomat 1976; 50:233–252.

102 Eschler J. L'influence des muscles masséter et ptérygoidien interne sur le développement et la croissance de la mandibule. Actualités Odonto-Stomat 1970; 89:7.

103 Maronneaud P. La constitution du squelette branchial méckelien primordial ses variations phylogénétiques les processus invoevolutifs observés à son niveau chez l'homme. Arch Anat Hist Embryo 1952; 34:285–295.

104 Oeconomos O. Le ménisque et les surfaces articulaires temporo-mandibulaires chez quelques animaux domestiques. CRAA; 1932:427.

105 Couly G, Brocheriou C, Vaillant J-M. Les ménisques temporo-mandibulaires. Rev Stomat. Paris; 1975:303–310.

106 Couly G, Guilbert F, Cernéa P, et al. The temporomandibular joint in the newborn infant. Oto-meniscal relations. Rev Stomatol Chir Maxillofac Jun 1976; 77(4):673–684.

107 Couly G, Hureau J, Vaillant J-M. The dynamic complex of the temporomandibular meniscus. Rev Stomatol Chir Maxillofac 1975; 76(8):597–605.

108 Delaire J, et al. Considération sur la physiologie du ménisque temporo-mandibulaire. Rev Stomat 1974; 2:447–454.

109 Dibbets JMH. Wachstum und kraniomandibuläre Dysfunktion. In: Steenks MH, Wijer A de, eds. Kiefergelenkfehlstellungen aus Physiotherapeutischer und Zahnmedizinischer Sicht: Diagnose und Therapie. Berlin: Quintessenz; 1991:104.

110 Linder-Aronson S. Adenoids, their effect on mode of breathing and nasal airflow and their relationship to characteristics of the facial skeleton and the dentition. Acta Otolaryngol 1970:265.

111 Schöttl W. Die Cranio-mandibuläre Regulation. Heidelberg: Hüthig; 1991:77.

112 Solow B, Siersbaek-Nielsen S. Growth changes in head posture related to craniofacial development. Am J Orthod 1986; 89:132–140.

113 Rohen JW. Morphologie des Menschlichen Organismus, 2nd edn. Stuttgart: Verlag Freies Geistesleben, 2002: p. 368.

114 Antczak-Boukoms A. Epidemiology of research for temporomandibular disorders. J Orofacial Pain 1995; 9:226–234.

115 Costen JB. A syndrome of ear and sinus symptoms dependent upon disturbed function of the temporomandibular joint. Ann Otol Rhinol and Laryngol 1934; 18:1–15.

116 Schwarz L. The pain-dysfunction syndrome In: Schwarz L, Chayes CM, eds. Facial Pain and Mandibular Dysfunction. Philadelphia: Saunders; 1968.

117 Laskin DM. Etiology of the pain dysfunction syndrome. J Am Dent Assoc 1969; 79:147.

118 Dibbets JMH. Wachstum und kraniomandibuläre dysfunktion. In: Steenks MH, Wijer A de, eds. Kiefergelenkfehlstellungen aus Physiotherapeutischer und Zahnmedizinischer Sicht: Diagnose und Therapie. Berlin: Quintessenz; 1991:99.

119 Winkel D. Nichtoperative Orthopädie, Part 4/2: Diagnostik und Therapie der Wirbelsäule. Stuttgart: Fischer; 1993:341.

120 Berrett A. Radiology of the temporomandibular joint. Den Clin N Am 1983; 27(3): July.

121 Hesse J, Hansson TL. Factors influencing joint mobility in general and in particular respect of the craniomandibular articulation: A literature review. J Craniomand Disord 1988; 1.

122 Clark GT, Seligman DA, Solberg WK, et al. Guidelines for the examination and diagnosis of temporomandibular disorders. J Craniomandib Disord 1989; 3:7–14.

123 De Wijer A, Lobbezzo-Scholte AM, Steenks MH, et al. Reliability of clinical findings in temporomandibular disorders. J Orofac Pain 1995; 9:2.

124 Augthun M, Müller-Leisse C, Bauer W, et al. Anteriore verlagerung des discus articularis des kiefergelenkes. J Orofac Orthop/Fortschr Kieferorthop 1998; 59:39–46.

125 Walker N, Bohannon RW, Cameron D. Discriminant validity of temporomandibular joint range of motion measurements obtained with a ruler. J Orthop Sports Phys Ther 2000; 30(8):484–492.

126 Garry JF. Frühe iatrogene Dysfunktionen von orofazialen Muskeln des Skeletts und des Kiefergelenks. In: Morgan D, House L, Hall W, et al., eds. Das Kiefergelenk und Seine Erkrankungen. Berlin: Quintessenz; 1985:96.

127 Wernham J. Lectures on Osteopathy. Maidstone College of Osteopathy.

128 Bahnemann F, ed. Der Bionator in der Kieferorthopädie. Grundlagen und Praxis. Heidelberg: Haug; 1993:28.

129 Delaire J. L'analyse architecturale et structurale cranio-faciale (de profil). Rev Stomatol 1978; 79:8.

130 Ferré JC, Chevalier C, Lumineau JP, et al. L'ostéopathie crânienne esseurreou réalité? Les Instantanés Médicaux, EMC 1990:36.

131 Kopp S. Die Bedeutung der oberen kopfgelenke bei der ätiologie von schmerzen im kopfHalsNackenbereich. Dtsch Zahnärztl Zeitschr 1989; 44(12):966–967.

132 Strachan F, Robinson MJ. Short leg linked to malocclusion. Osteopath News 1965; 4.

133 Schöttl W. Die Cranio-mandibuläre Regulation. Heidelberg: Hüthig; 1991:95.

134 Broich I. Kieferorthopädie und Orthopädie: fehlfunktionen im mund-kiefer-bereich ganzheitlich diagnostizieren und behandeln. Manuelle Therapie 1999; 3:32–96.

135 Haberfellner H. Wechselwirkung zwischen gesamtkörperhaltung und gesichtsbe-reich. Pädiatrie und Pädologie 1981; 16(2):203–225.

136 VonTreuenfels H. Kopfhaltung, Atlasposition und atemfunktion beim offenen biss. Fortschritte der Kieferorthopädie 1984; 45:111–121.

137 VonTreuenfels H: Orofaziale dyskinesien als ausdruck einer gestörten wechselbeziehung von atmung, verdauung und bewegung. Fortschritte der Kieferorthopädie 1985; 46:191–208.

138 Landouzy JM. Les A.T.M. Evaluation, traitements odontologiques et ostéopathies. Aix en Provence: Editions de Verlaque; 1993:107–108.

139 Myers TW. Anatomy Trains. Edinburgh: Churchill Livingstone; 2001.

140 Wernham J. Mechanics of the spine. Yearbook of Institute of Applied Osteopathy, Maidstone; 1956.

141 Wernham J. Mechanics of the spine. Yearbook of Maidstone College of Osteopathy, Maidstone; 1985.

142 Lawrence ES, Razook SJ. Nonsurgical management of mandibular disorders. In: Kraus LS, eds. Temporomandibular Disorders. 2nd edn. New York: Churchill Livingstone; 1994:130.

143 Solberg W, Clark G. Kieferfunktion – Diagnostik und Therapie Berlin: Quintessenz; 1985:152.

144 Shaper EP. Aspekte bei der behandlung von muskelspasmen. In: Morgan D, House L, Hall W, et al., eds. Das Kiefergelenk und Seine Erkrankungen. Berlin: Quintessenz; 1985:377–378.

145 Schöttl W. Die Cranio-mandibuläre Regulation. Heidelberg: Hüthig; 1991:106.

146 Kraus M, Lilienfein W, Reinhart E, et al. Das Kiefergelenk in der zahnärztlich-physiotherapeutischen Kombinationsbehandlung. Zeitschr Physioth 1998; 9:1545–1551.

147 Guillaume P. Vision et posture II. Paris: Agréssologie-Spei médical; 1988.

148 Bell W. Clinical diagnosis of the pain-dysfunction syndrome. J Am Dent Assoc 1969; 79:154.

149 Blackwood HJJ. Pathology of the temporomandibular joint. J Am Dent Assoc 1969; 79:118.

150 Farrar W. Diagnosis and treatment of anterior dislocation of the articular disc. J Dent 1971; 41:348.

151 Farrar W. Differentiation of temporomandibular joint dysfunction to simplify treatment. J Prosthet Dent 1972; 28:629.

152 Farrar W. Dysfunctional centric relation of the jaw associated with dislocation and displacement of the disc. Compendium Amer Equil Soc 1976; 13:272.

153 Graber T. Orthodontics – Principles and Practices, 2nd edn. Philadelphia: WB Saunders; 1967:481.

154 Kiehn CL. Meniscetomy for internal derangement of temporomandibular joint. Amer J Surg 1952; 83:364.

155 Posselt U. Physiology of Occlusion and Rehabilitation, 2nd edn. Oxford: Blackwell Scientific Publications; 1968.

156 Pringle J. Displacement of the mandibular meniscus and its treatment. Brit J Surg 1918; 6:385.

157 Ricketts R. Occlusion – the medium of dentistry. J Prostmet Dent 1969; 21:154.

158 Sarnat B. The Temporomandibular Joint. Springfield: Charles C Thomas; 1964:133–184.

159 Schwarz L, Chayes GM. Facial Pain and Mandibular Dysfunction. Philadelphia: Saunders; 1968.

160 Shore N. Occlusal Equilibration and Temporomandibular Joint Dysfunction. Philadelphia: JB Lippincott; 1959.

161 Silver CM, Simon SD. Meniscus injuries of the temporomandibular joint: Further experience. J Bone and Joint Surg 1963; 45:113.

162 Silver CM, Simon SD, Savastano AA. Meniscus injuries of the temporomandibular joint. J Bone Surg 1956; 38:54.

163 Thoma KH. Oral Surgery. St Louis: CV Mosby; 1958:705.

164 Wakeley C. The causation and treatment of displaced mandibular cartilage. Lancet 1929; 2:543.

165 Weinberg L. Posterior bilateral condylar displacement: its diagnosis and treatment. J Prosthet Dent 1976; 36:272.

166 Farrar WB. Characteristics of the condylar path in internal derangements of the TMJ. J Prosthet Dent 1978; 39(3):319–323.

167 Weinberg LA, Lager LA. Clinical report on the etiology and diagnosis of TMJ dysfunction-pain syndrome. J Prosthet Dent 1980; 44(6):642–653.

168 Beek M, Koolstra JH, van Ruijven LJ, et al. Three-dimensional finite element analysis of the human temporomandibular joint disc. J Biomechan 2000; 33:307–316.

169 Beek M, Koolstra JH, van Ruijven LJ, et al. Three-dimensional finite element analysis of the cartilaginous structures in the human temporomandibular joint. J Dent Res 2001; 80(10):1913–1918.

170 Isberg A, Isacsson G. TMJ tissue reactions following retrusive guidance of the mandible. J Dent Res 1985; 4:764.

171 Lafreniere CM. The role of the lateral pterygoid muscles in TMJ disorders during static conditions. J Craniomandib Pract 1997; 15:38–51.

172 Westesson PL. Posterior disc displacement in the temporomandibular joint. J Oral Maxillofacial Surg 1998; 56:1266–1273.

173 Hatala MP, Westesson PL, Tallents RH, et al. TMJ disc displacement in asymptomatic volunteers detected by MR imaging.

174 Paesani D, Westesson P-L, Hatala M, et al. Prevalence of temporomandibular joint internal derangement in patients with craniomandibular disorders. Am J Orthod Dentofac Orthop 1992; 101:41–47.

175 Weinberg LA. The etiology diagnosis and treatment of TMJ dysfunction-pain syndrome. J Prosth Dent 1980; 43:186–196.

176 Solberg WK, Clark GT. Keifergelenkdysfunktion. Diagnostik und Therapie. Berlin: Quintessenz; 1985.

177 Müller J, Schmid CH, Bruckner G, et al. Morphologisch nachweisbare formen von intraartikulären dysfunktionen der kiefergelenke. Deutsche Zahnärztl Zeitschr 1992; 47:416–423.

178 Louis TK, Douglas AO, Alexander SM, et al. Magnetic resonance imaging of the TMJ-disc in asymptomatic volunteers. J Oral Maxillofac Surg 1987; 852–854.

179 Solberg WK, Hansson TL, Nordstroem B. The temporomandibular joint in young adults at autopsy: a morphologic classification and evaluation. J Oral Rehab 1985; 12:303.

180 Äkerman S, Kopp S, Rohlin M. Histological changes in temporomandibular joints from elderly individuals. An autopsy study. Acta Odontol Scand 1986; 44:31–239.

181 Carlsson GE, Kopp S, Öberg T. Arthritis and allied diseases of the temporomandibular joint. In: Zarb GA, Carlsson GE, eds. Temporomandibular Joint Function and Dysfunction. Denmark: Munksgaard; 1979; 269–320.

182 Tasaki M, Westesson P-L, Isberg A, et al. Classification and prevalence of temporomandibular joint disk displacement in patients and symptom-free volunteers. Am J Orthod Dentofac Orthop 1996; 109(3):249–296.

183 Kurita K, Westesson P-L, Tasaki M, et al. Temporomandibular joint: diagnosis of medial and lateral disk displacement with anteroposterior arthography – correlation with cryosections. Oral Surg Oral Med Oral Pathol 1992; 73:364–368.

184 Kurita H. The relationship between the degree of disk displacement and ability to perform disk reduction. Oral Surg Oral Med Oral Pathol 2000; 90:16–20.

185 Williamson PC. Horizontal condylar angulation and condyle position associated with adolescent TMJ disk status. J Craniomandib Pract 1999; 17:101–107.

186 Isberg A, Widmalm SE, Ivarsson R. Clinical radiographical and electromyographical study of patients with internal derangement of the TMJ. J Dent Res 1985; 4:764.

187 Slavicek R. Les principes de l'occlusion. Rev Orthop Dento Faciale 1983; 17: 449–490.

188 Kampe T, Hannerz H. Five-year longitudinal study of adolescents with intact and restored dentitions: signs and symptoms of temporomandibular dysfunction and functional recordings. J Oral Rehabil 1991; 18:387–398.

189 Price WA. Nutrition and Physical Degeneration. Keats, Connecticut: Price-Pottenger Nutrition Foundation; 1997.

190 Laughlin JD. Bodywide Influences of Dental Procedures, Part I. J Bodywork and Movement Therapies. London: Churchill Livingstone; 2002; 1:9–16.

191 Huijbers AJM. Schienentherapie und okklusionskkorrekturen. In: Steenks MH, Wijer A de, eds. Kiefergelenkfehlstellungen aus physiotherapeutischer und zahnmedizinischer Sicht: Diagnose und Therapie. Berlin: Quintessenz; 1991:47.

192 Schiffman EL, Friction JR, Haley D. The relationship of occlusion, parafunctional habits and recent life events to mandibular dysfunction in a non-patient population. J Oral Rehabil 1992; 19(3):201–223.

193 Choi J-K. A study on the effects of maximal voluntary clenching on the tooth contact points and masticatory muscle activities in patients with temporomandibular disorders. J Craniomandib Disorders: Facial & Oral Pain 1992; 6:41–46.

194 De Laat A, van Steenberghe D, Sesaffre E. Occlusal relationships and temporomandibular joint dysfunction. Part II: Correlations between occlusal and articular parameters and symptoms of TMJ dysfunction by means of stepwise logistic regression. J Prosthet Dent 1986; 55:116–121.

195 Seligmann DA, Pullinger AG. The role of intercuspal occlusal relationships in temporomandibular disorders: A review. J Craniomandib Disorders: Facial & Oral Pain 1991; 5:96–106.

196 Bowbeer G, Facial Beauty and the TMJ, Part III. Isle of Wight: Cranio-View; 1993.

197 Fonder A. Dental Distress Syndrome. Rock Falls: Medical Dental Arts; 1990.

198 Escoto M, O'Shaughnessy T, Yerkes I. Functional forum. The Functional Orthodontist 2000; 17:32–34.

199 Gelb H, Goodheart G. Clinical Management of Head Neck and TMJ Pain and Dysfunction. Philadelphia: WB Saunders; 1977.

200 Witzig J, Spahl T. Clinical Management of Basic Maxiofacial Orthopedic Appliances. Littleton: Mosby; 1987.

201 Jecsmen J. Cranial Osteopathy-sidebend and Dentistry. Isle of Wight: Cranio-View; 1994.

202 De Boever JA, Functional disturbance of the temporomandibular joint. In: Zarb G, Carlsson G, eds. Temporomandibular Joint – Function and Dysfunction. Copenhagen: Munksgaard; 1979:194–195.

203 Bell WE. Management of masticatory pain. In: von Alling CC, Mahan PE, eds. Facial Pain. Philadelphia: Lea and Febiger; 1977:185.

204 Gelb H. Patient evaluation. In: Gelb H, ed. Clinical Management of Head Neck and TMJ Pain and Dysfunction. Philadelphia: Saunders; 1977:75.

205 Schwartz LL. Conclusions of the temporomandibular joint clinic at Columbia. J Peridontol 1958; 5:210–212.

206 Yermm R. Neurophysiological studies of temporomandibular joint dysfunction. Oral Sci Rev 1976; 7:31.

207 Travell JG, Simons DG. Myofascial Pain and Dysfunction, Vol. 1. Baltimore: Williams and Wilkins; 1983:240.

208 Shaper EP. Aspekte bei der behandlung von muskelspasmen. In: Morgan D, House L, Hall W, et al., eds. Das Kiefergelenk und seine Erkrankungen. Berlin: Quintessenz; 1985:392.

209 Kroening R. Die Leitungsanästhesie zur differenzierung von craniofacialem schmerz. In: Clark G, Solberg W, eds. Perspektiven der Kiefergelenkstörungen. Berlin: Quintessenz; 1988:137.

210 Bauer A, Gutowski A. Gnathologie. Einführung in Theorie und Praxis. Berlin: Quintessenz; 1975:83.

211 Schroeder H, Siegmund H, Santibánez H.: Causes and signs of temporomandibuar joint pain and dysfunction: an electromyographical investigation. J Oral Rehabilit 1991; 18:301–310.

212 Schöttl W. Die Cranio-mandibuläre Regulation. Heidelberg: Hüthig; 1991:63.

213 Kroening R. Die Leitungsanästhesie zur differenzierung von craniofacialem Schmerz. In: Clark G, Solberg W, eds. Perspektiven der Kiefergelenkstörungen. Berlin: Quintessenz; 1988:137.

214 Isberg AM, Isacsson G, Williams WN, et al. Lingual numbness and speech articulation deviation associated with temporomandibular joint disc displacement. Oral Surg Oral Medic Oral Pathol 1987; 1:9–14.

215 Bell WE. Nonsurgical management of the pain-dysfunction syndrome. J Am Dent Assoc 1969; 79:161–170.

216 Schwartz LL, Tausig DP. Temporomandibular joint pain-treatment with intramuscular infiltration of tetracaine hydrochloride: a preliminary report. NY State Dent J 1954; 20:219–223.

217 Hack GD, Dumm G, Toh MY. The anatomist's new tools. In: Encyclopaedia Britannica 1998 Medical and Health Annual. Chicago: NCMIC Insurance Co; 1998:16–29.

218 Garry JF. Frühe iatrogene Dysfunktionen von orofazialen Muskeln des Skeletts und des Kiefergelenks. In: Morgan D, House L, Hall W, et al., eds. Das Kiefergelenk und Seine Erkrankungen. Berlin: Quintessenz; 1985:94.

219 Lang J. Clinical Anatomy of the Masticatory Apparatus and Peripharyngeal Spaces. New York: Thieme; 1995.

220 Landeweer GG. Können spannungen im tentorium cerebelli einen einfluss auf die diskusposition im kiefergelenk haben? UpDate 2001; 2(1):21–23.

221 Williams PL, Warwick R, Dyson M, et al. Gray's Anatomy, 37th edn. New York: Churchill Livingstone; 1989.

222 Slegter R, Azouman M. Observation of the anterior loop of the inferior alveolar canal. International J Oral Maxillofac Implants 1993; 7:295–300.

223 Wittlinger H and G. Lehrbuch der Manuellen Lymphdrainage nach Dr Vodder, Vol. I, 10th edn. Heidelberg: Haug; 1992:51.

224 Graber G. Was leistet die funktionelle therapie und wo findet sie ihre Grenzen? Dtsch Zahnärztl Zeitschr 1985; 40:165.

225 Aerni F. Lehrbuch der Menschenkenntnis. Zürich: Kalos; 1988:363.

226 Lejoyeux J. Aspect comportemental morphologique et typologique du syndrôme algodysfonctioneel de appareil manducateur. Rev Orthop Dent Facial 1987; 21:561–578.

227 Graber G. Der Einfluss von Psyche und Stress bei dysfunktionsbedingten erkrankungen des stomatognathen systems. In: Hupfauf L, ed. Funktionsstörungen des Kauorgans, 2nd edn. Munich: Urban & Schwarzenberg; 1989:66.

228 Albe-Fessard D, Cordes-Lara M, Sanderson P, et al. Advances in pain research and therapy. In: Kruger L, Liebeskind JC, eds. Neural Mechanisms of Pain, Vol. 6. New York: Raven Press; 1984:167–182.

229 Perl ER. Advances in pain research and therapy. In: Kruger L, Liebeskind JC, eds. Neural Mechanisms of Pain, Vol. 6. New York: Raven Press; 1984:23–51.

230 Magni G. On the relationship between chronic pain and depression when there is no organic lesion. Pain 1987; 31:1.

231 Magni G, Merskey H. A simple examination of the relationships between pain organic lesions and psychiatric illness. Pain 1987; 29:295.

232 Benjamin S, Barness D, Berger S, et al. The relationship of chronic pain, mental illness and organic disorders. Pain 1988; 32:185.

233 France RD, Urban BJ, Pelton S, et al. CSF monoamine metabolites in chronic pain. Pain 1987; 31:189.

234 Kleinknecht RA, Mahoney ER, Alexander LD. Psychosocial and demographic correlates of temporomandibular disorders and related symptoms: an assessment of community and clinical findings. Pain 1987; 29:173.

235 Clark G, Solberg W, Monteiro AA. Kiefergelenkbeschwerden. Neue entwicklung in der klinischen behandlung in forschung und lehre. In: Clark G, Solberg W, eds. Perspektiven der Kiefergelenkstörungen. Berlin: Quintessenz; 1988:17.

236 Westling L. Craniomandibular disorders and general joint mobility. Acta Odontol Scand 1989; 47:293–299.

237 Greenwood L F. Is temporomandibular joint dysfunction associated with generalized joint hypermobility. J Prosthet Dent 1987; 58(6):701–703.

238 Seider R. Der Einfluss von kraniosakraler Therapie auf den Bewegungsumfang entfernt liegender grosser Gelenke, bei Zustand nach kieferorthopädischer Zahnstellungskorrektur mittels Zahnspange. Hamm: Diplomarbeit; 1999.

239 Bahnemann F. Anthropologische Grundlagen einer Ganzheitsmedizin aus kieferor-thopädischer Sicht. Heidelberg: Haug; 1992:84.

240 Bahnemann F., ed. Der Bionator in der Kieferorthopädie Grundlagen und Praxis. Heidelberg: Haug; 1993:3044.

241 Hupfauf L. Einführung in die problematik funktionsbedingter erkrankungen. In: Hupfauf L, ed. Funktionsstörungen des Kauorgans, 2nd edn. München: Urban & Schwarzenberg; 1989:6.

242 Chun DS, Koskinen-Moffett L. Distress jaw habits and connective tissue laxity as predisposing factors to TMJ sounds in adolescents. J Craniomandibular disorders: Facial Oral Pain 1990; 4:165–176.

243 Schöttl W. Die Cranio-mandibuläre Regulation. Heidelberg: Hüthig; 1991:30–35.

244 Garliner D. Myofunktionelle Diagnose und Therapie der Gestörten Gesichtsmuskulatur. München: Verlag Zahnärzte Schrifttum; 1980:83.

245 Kirk WS, Jr. Diagnostic disk dysfunction and tissue changes in the temporomandibular joint with magnetic resonance imaging. JADA 1989; 119:527.

246 Breiner M. Whole Body Dentistry. Fairfield: Quantum Health Press; 1999. Zeines V. Healthy Mouth, Healthy Body. New York: Kensington Books; 2002.

247 Fonder A. The Dental Physician. Blacksburg: University Publications; 1977.

248 Gelb H, Goodheart G. Clinical Management of Head, Neck and TMJ Pain and Dysfunction. Philadelphia: WB Saunders; 1977.

249 Cardonnet M, Clauzade M. Diagnosis différentiel des dysfonctions de l'ATM. Les Cahiers de Prothèse 1987; 58:125–169.

250 Sebald WG, Kopp S. Funktionsstörungen und Schmerzphänomene des Cranio-mandibulären Systems. Grundlagen und Basisdiagnostik. Jena; 1996:45–48.

251 Landeweer GG. Untersuchungsmethoden zur Beurteilung von Funktionsveränderungen im Kausystem. Update 2001; 2(2):25–29.

252 Schöttl W. Die Cranio-mandibuläre Regulation. Heidelberg: Hüthig; 1991:10–14.

253 Sebald WG, Kopp S. Funktionsstörungen und Schmerzphänomene des Cranio-mandibulären Systems. Grundlagen und Basisdiagnostik. Jena; 1996:39–41.

254 Sebald WG, Kopp S. Funktionsstörungen und Schmerzphänomene des Cranio-mandibulären-Systems. Grundlagen und Basisdiagnostik. Jena; 1996:117–132.

255 Winkel D. Nichtoperative Orthopädie, Part 4/2: Diagnostik und Therapie der Wirbelsäule. Stuttgart: Fischer; 1993:373.

256 Piekartz von HJM. Vorschlag für einen neurodynamischen Test des N mandibularis – Reliabilität und Referenzwerte. Manuelle Therapie 2001; 5:56–66.

257 Katzenberg RW, David AK, Ten Eick WR, et al. Internal derangements of the temporomandibular joint. An Assessment of Condylar Position in Centric Occlusion 1983; 49(2):250–254.

257 Steinfurth G. Einflusz osteopathischer dysfunktionen der ossa temporalia auf die maximale aktive mundöffnung. Diplom. SKOM. Düsseldorf: DAO; 2001.

258 Sadowski C. Temporomandibular disorders and functional occlusion after orthodontic treatment: Results of two long-term studies. Amer J Orthod 1984; 5(86):386.

259 Williamson EH, Sheffield JW. The non-surgical treatment of internal derangement of the temporomandibular joint: A survey of 300 cases. Facial Orthop Temporomandibular Arthrol 1985; 2(10):18–20.

260 Dobler T. Diagnostik und Behandlung der Art temporomandibularis. In: Liem T, Dobler T, eds. Leitfaden Osteopathie. München: Urban und Fischer; 2002.

261 Kaluza CL, Goering EK, Kaluza KN. Osteopathischer ansatz bei TMG-dysfunktion. Osteopath Med 2002; 1:4–7.

12

The orofacial structures, pterygopalatine ganglion and pharynx

The orofacial system comprises the following structures:

- Bones: the palatine bones, maxillae, mandible, and temporo-mandibular joints.
- The teeth and periodontal ligament.
- Muscles: the muscles controlling jaw opening and closure, the muscles of the tongue, oral cavity floor, and palatopharyngeal arch, and those governing facial expression.
- Soft tissues: the cheeks, lips, buccal and pharyngeal mucous membranes, salivary glands, tonsils, adenoids etc.
- Nerves and vessels supplying this region.
- Taste receptors.
- Pharynx: part of the digestive tube connecting the oral cavity, nasal cavity, and the esophagus.
- Larynx: this consists of an articulated cartilaginous framework, muscles, and a mucosal lining. Among other things, the larynx is involved in phonation.

Functions of the orofacial system: mastication, suckling, swallowing, respiration, phonation, sensory perception of taste, temperature, pain, and depth, expression of emotions etc.

THE ORAL CAVITY *(Figs 12.1, 12.2)*

The oral cavity is the central feature of the orofacial system. It is subdivided into the oral vestibule, which is the area outside the dental arch, and the oral cavity proper, which is the area inside the dental arch.

The oral cavity is bounded below by the suprahyoid muscles (floor of the mouth), above by the hard palate (maxillae and palatine bones) and soft palate, and laterally by the mandible and cheeks. It is bounded in front by the lips and behind by the oropharyngeal isthmus. The teeth and tongue are important organs in the oral cavity.

The tone of the soft posterior part of the palate depends in particular on the levator and tensor veli palatini muscles, the palatopharyngeus muscle, the tongue and the orientation of the pterygoid process of the sphenoid bone.

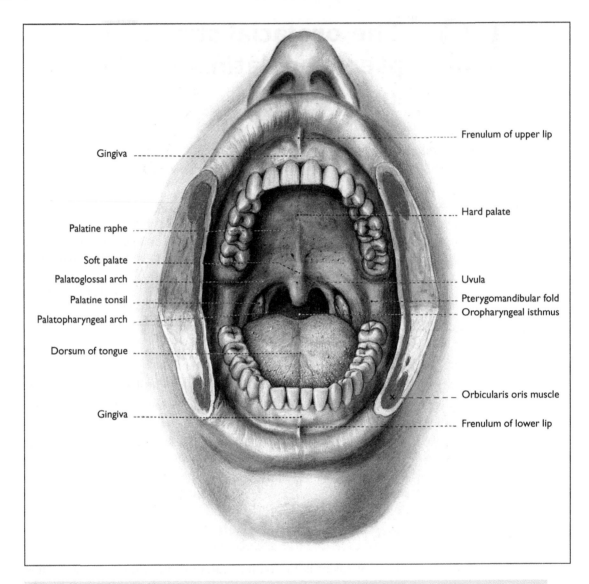

Figure 12.1 The oral vestibule and the oral cavity proper. The cheeks and lips are shown in cut-away view (From: Tillmann B. Farbatlas der Anatomie. Zahnmedizin – Humanmedizin. Stuttgart: Thieme; 1997)

Salivary gland innervation *(Fig. 12.3)*

In sensory terms the salivary glands are innervated by the mandibular nerve (CN V3). For secretory purposes, the parotid salivary gland is innervated by the glossopharyngeal nerve (CN IX) via the otic ganglion, and the submandibular and sublingual salivary glands are innervated by the intermedius nerve (CN VII) via the submandibular ganglion.

Figure 12.2 Sagittal section through the oral cavity. 3, Oral vestibule; 6, Upper lip; 9, Lower lip; 14, Oral cavity proper; 16, Hard palate; 17, Soft palate (From: Feneis H. Anatomisches Bildwörterbuch. 6th edn. Stuttgart: Thieme; 1988:109, Figure C)

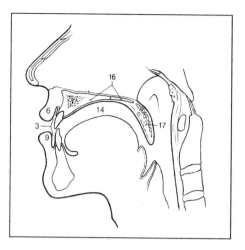

Figure 12.3 The innervation of the salivary glands (From: Tillmann B. Farbatlas der Anatomie. Zahnmedizin – Humanmedizin. Stuttgart: Thieme; 1997)

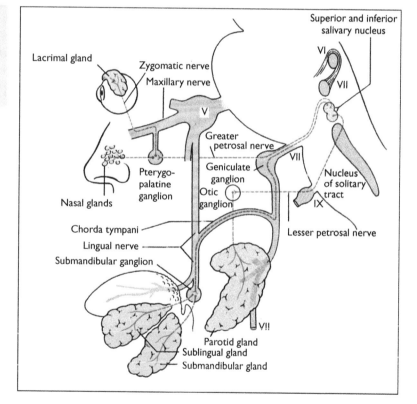

The otic ganglion: secretory innervation of the parotid gland *(Fig. 12.4)*

The parasympathetic ganglion is situated immediately below the foramen ovale, medial to the mandibular nerve (CN V3), and lateral to the tensor veli palatini muscle. It contains the perikarya of the postganglionic parasympathetic fibers. These fibers pass by communicating branches to the auriculotemporal nerve, by which they are conveyed to the parotid gland. The preganglionic fibers arrive at the ganglion from the glossopharyngeal nerve (CN IX) via the lesser petrosal nerve.

Figure 12.4 The otic ganglion

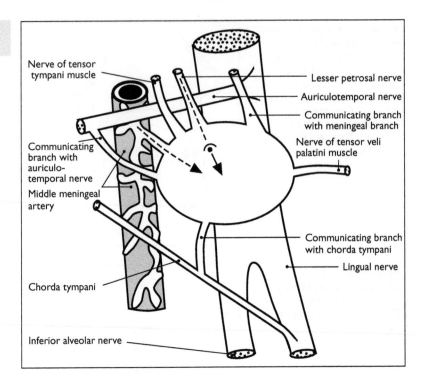

Nerve of tensor tympani muscle

Lesser petrosal nerve

Auriculotemporal nerve

Communicating branch with meningeal branch

Nerve of tensor veli palatini muscle

Communicating branch with auriculo-temporal nerve

Middle meningeal artery

Communicating branch with chorda tympani

Lingual nerve

Chorda tympani

Inferior alveolar nerve

However, the ganglion has non-synaptic connections with the:

- Tensor veli palatini nerve, which supplies the tensor veli palatini muscle.
- Tensor tympani nerve, which supplies the tensor tympani muscle.
- Meningeal branch of the mandibular nerve via the communicating branch of the same name.
- Sympathetic root: arising in the superior cervical ganglion, fibers from the external carotid plexus of the middle meningeal artery also pass through the otic ganglion without being interrupted.
- Chorda tympani nerve: via the communicating branch of the same name. Instead of relaying them via the chorda tympani nerve through the middle ear, this branch sometimes sends gustatory fibers from the anterior two-thirds of the tongue via the lesser petrosal nerve (CN IX) and the nerve of the pterygoid canal to the geniculate ganglion of the facial nerve.

The submandibular ganglion

Secretory innervation of the submandibular and sublingual salivary glands (Fig. 12.5).

The ganglion is located superior to the submandibular salivary gland and below the lingual nerve (CN V3) and contains the perikarya of the postganglionic parasympathetic fibers. The preganglionic fibers pass via the chorda tympani nerve from the intermedius nerve (CN VII) to enter the ganglion.

Figure 12.5 The submandibular ganglion

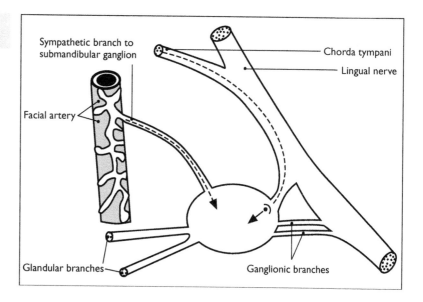

The submandibular ganglion has connections with:

- The sympathetic nervous system: commencing in the superior cervical ganglion, fibers from the sympathetic root on the facial artery pass through the ganglion without being interrupted. These supply the vascular smooth muscle in the submandibular and sublingual salivary glands.
- The submandibular and sublingual salivary glands: postganglionic parasympathetic and sympathetic as well as sensory fibers pass through the glandular branches to supply these glands.
- The lingual nerve: via ganglionic branches. As well as sensory fibers, postganglionic parasympathetic and sympathetic ganglionic fibers are carried in the lingual nerve to the glands of the oral mucosa.

Primary respiration

During the inspiration phase of primary respiration, the oral cavity widens transversely and its anteroposterior diameter is shortened.

Explanation: The mandible moves in a posterior direction as a result of ER of the temporal bones.

During the expiration phase of the PRM, the oral cavity shows transverse narrowing and its anteroposterior diameter is increased.

The teeth

Adults have a full complement of 32 permanent teeth. Each quadrant of the mouth contains 2 incisors, 1 canine, 2 premolars and 3 molars; (dental formula: 2-1-2-3). Deciduous teeth include no molars (dental formula: 2-1-2).

Adult dentition code

The first digit (1–4) identifies the quadrant of the mouth: 1 right upper, 2 left upper quadrant, 3 left lower and 4 right lower quadrant. The second digit (1–8) denotes the position of the tooth in the quadrant: incisors (1 and 2), canine (3), premolars (4 and 5) and molars (6 to 8).

18 17 16 15 14 13 12 11 | 21 22 23 24 25 26 27 28

48 47 46 45 44 43 42 41 | 31 32 33 34 35 36 37 38

Positional terms used in dental anatomy

- Buccal, labial: facing the cheek or lip
- Lingual, palatal: facing the tongue or palate
- Mesial: toward the midline of the dental arch
- Distal: away from the midline of the dental arch
- Occlusal: pertaining to the contact surfaces of the teeth

Dental structure

Teeth consist of three hard tissues: dentin, enamel and cement.

Dentin

Dentin forms the bulk of the tooth: it is harder than bone because it contains more inorganic substances. The odontoblasts are located only at the margin of the dentin and they send cellular processes into the interior of the tooth.

Enamel

The enamel forms an external layer coating the dentin. It is the hardest substance in the human body and is designed to protect the dentin. The enamel-forming cells are located at the outer surface of the enamel and are worn away rapidly after the teeth erupt. When the enamel is damaged (caries), it cannot regenerate itself.

Cement

The woven bone-like dentin in the alveolar bone is surrounded by cement instead of by enamel. The cement is perforated by fibers that are inserted into the alveolar bone, thus anchoring the tooth in the bone.

Other parts of the tooth

- Crown: coated with enamel.
- Root: coated with cement.
- Neck: the enamel-cement junction.
- Pulp cavity: the space within the dentin containing the blood vessels and nerves of the tooth; it extends from the root to the crown.
- Pulp: the tissue inside the pulp cavity (blood vessels, nerves, loose connective tissue etc.).

The periodontal ligament *(Fig. 12.6)*

The periodontal ligament (desmodontium) is a fibrous joint (syndesmosis) that suspends the root of each tooth in its alveolar bone socket. The periodontal ligament fibers are anchored in the cement layer of the tooth and in the alveolar bone. The periodontal ligament holds the teeth in sprung suspension, with the result that each tooth is capable of small movements in its alveolar bone socket. Blood vessels and nerves are also found at the junction between the dental root and alveolar bone. The nerves there transmit proprioceptive information via the periodontal ligaments, enabling the teeth to use the periodontal ligaments to adapt to the prevailing forces and to reposition themselves to a limited extent.

In this area, in particular, manual treatment can correct abnormal tensions in the ligamentous connections so as to positively influence the further transmission of proprioceptive information and the arterial blood supply to the teeth.[1] Influence can also be brought to bear on any reflex connections with other organ systems (Fig. 12.7).

Nerves and blood vessels *(Figs 12.8, 12.9)*

- The dental nerves in the mandible (inferior alveolar nerve) arise from the mandibular nerve (CN V3), and the dental nerves in the maxillae (superior alveolar nerves) arise from the maxillary nerve (CN V2). Dental pain may be felt as far down as the level of the second spinal cord segment due to the segmental interconnections of the trigeminal nerve.

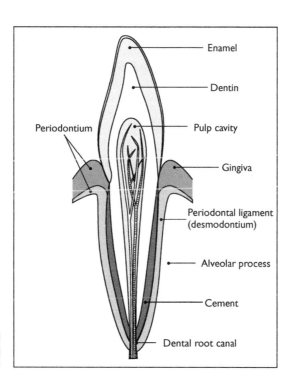

Figure 12.6 Sagittal section through a tooth

Enamel

Dentin

Periodontium

Pulp cavity

Gingiva

Periodontal ligament (desmodontium)

Alveolar process

Cement

Dental root canal

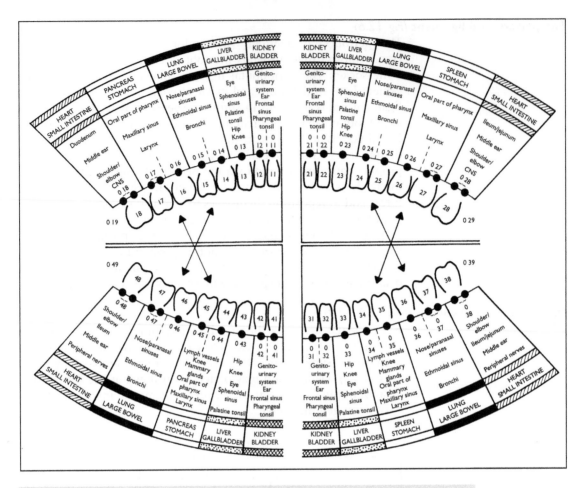

Figure 12.7 Interactions between teeth and organs (From: Pothmann VR, ed. Systematik der Schmerzakupunktur. Stuttgart: Hippokrates; 1996)

● The vascular supply of the teeth is provided by the inferior alveolar artery (mandible) and by the posterior superior alveolar artery and the anterior superior alveolar arteries (maxilla). These arise from the maxillary artery, a terminal branch of the external carotid artery. The nerves follow the same path as the blood vessels.

The influence of muscle forces on tooth development *(Fig. 12.10)*

The teeth are exposed to the outward pressure of the tongue and the inward pressure of the buccinator and orbicularis oris muscles. In normal circumstances, the pressure of the tongue during the processes of mastication, swallowing and phonation is compensated for by the peribuccal muscles. Any imbalance between the tongue and peribuccal muscles has repercussions for the positioning of the teeth.

Figure 12.8 The sensory innervation of the teeth and gingiva in the mandible (From: Tillmann B. Farbatlas der Anatomie. Zahnmedizin – Humanmedizin. Stuttgart: Thieme; 1997)

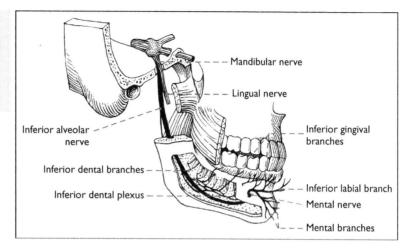

Figure 12.9 The sensory innervation of the teeth in the maxilla and of the maxillary sinus (From: Tillmann B. Farbatlas der Anatomie. Zahnmedizin – Humanmedizin. Stuttgart: Thieme; 1997)

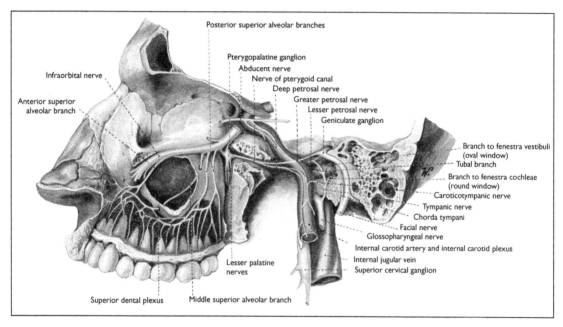

The tongue

The tongue is a muscular organ that is coated with highly differentiated mucosa. Its root rests on the floor of the mouth, with which it is fused.

Function: Bolus propulsion (initiation of the act of swallowing), food-grinding, receptor for tactile, thermal and gustatory stimuli, suckling, phonation, and organ of defense (lymphoid tissues at the root of the tongue). The tongue is also important for normal tooth development (see below).

Figure 12.10 The influence of muscle forces on tooth development

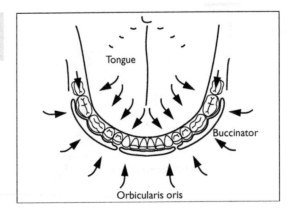

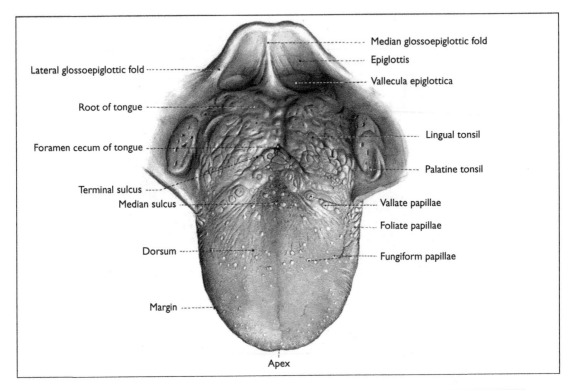

Figure 12.11 The muscles of the tongue and their anatomical relations (From: Tillmann B. Farbatlas der Anatomie. Zahnmedizin – Humanmedizin. Stuttgart: Thieme; 1997)

Anatomical relations of the tongue *(Fig. 12.11)*

While the tongue is suspended on the cranial base via muscles and ligaments, it has anterior and inferior attachments to the mandible and hyoid bone.

The cranial base (via the temporal bone), the mandible and the hyoid bone influence the tension balance of the tongue. The mandible represents a type of fulcrum for the tongue between the cranial base and the hyoid bone.

The muscles of the tongue *(Fig. 12.12)*

The tongue consists of extrinsic muscles that are attached to bony structures outside the tongue and of intrinsic muscles that are contained exclusively within the tongue.

Extrinsic muscles: The genioglossus muscle arises from the upper genial tubercle on the inner surface of the symphysis of the mandible and spreads out into the tongue in a fan-like form (CN XII).

This muscle is the most important muscle for tongue movement, for the resting position of the tongue in the oral cavity, and for drawing the tongue forward. It also moves the tongue upward.

Note: When the hypoglossal nerve is injured or diseased, the protruded tongue tends to be directed to the paralyzed side. The hyoglossus muscle arises from the body and greater horn of the hyoid bone and is inserted into the side of the tongue (CN XII).

The chondroglossus muscle arises from the lesser horn of the hyoid bone and is inserted into the side of the tongue (CN XII).

The styloglossus muscle arises from the styloid process and is inserted into the side of the tongue.

The palatoglossus muscle arises from the palatine aponeurosis and is inserted into the side of the tongue.

The myloglossus muscle (inconstant) runs from the posterior end of the mylohyoid line to the root of the tongue.

The nerves of the tongue *(Figs 12.13, 12.14, Table 12.1)*

Motor innervation: Glossopharyngeal nerve (CN IX): palatoglossus muscle.

Hypoglossal nerve (CN XII): intrinsic muscles of the tongue, genioglossus, hyoglossus, chondroglossus and styloglossus muscles.

General sensibility:

● Lingual branch of the mandibular nerve (CN V3): anterior two-thirds of the lingual mucosa.

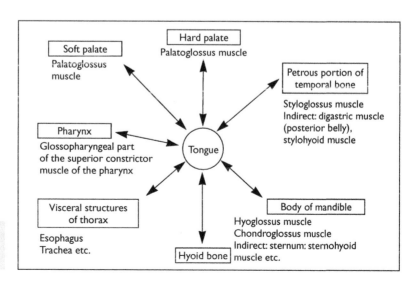

Figure 12.12 The relations of the tongue with muscles and other structures

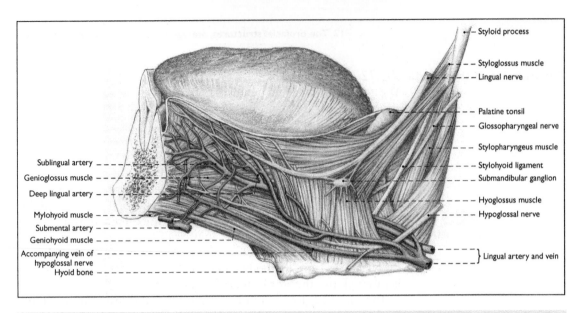

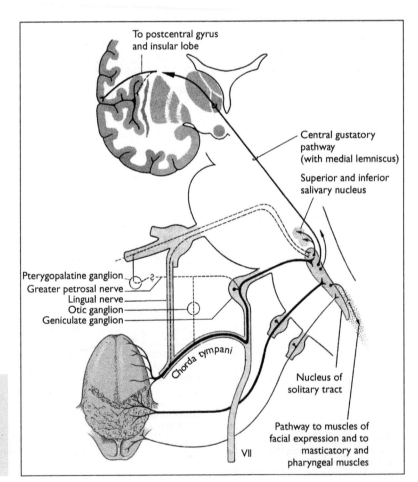

Figure 12.13 The hypoglossal nerve (From: Tillmann B. Farbatlas der Anatomie. Zahnmedizin – Humanmedizin. Stuttgart: Thieme; 1997)

Figure 12.14 Taste innervation of the tongue and the gustatory pathways (From: Tillmann B. Farbatlas der Anatomie. Zahnmedizin – Humanmedizin. Stuttgart: Thieme; 1997)

Table 12.1 Sensibility and sensory innervation of the tongue

Innervation	Anterior two thirds of tongue	Posterior third of tongue
Sensibility	CN V3	CN IX, (CN X in region of valleculae)
Sensory (taste)	CN VII	CN IX, (CN X at root of tongue)

- Glossopharyngeal nerve (CN IX): posterior third of the lingual mucosa.
- Vagus nerve (CN X): the area around the valleculae.

Sensory innervation (taste):

- Facial nerve (CN VII), chorda tympani: anterior two-thirds of the lingual mucosa.
- Glossopharyngeal nerve (CN IX): posterior third of the lingual mucosa.
- Vagus nerve (CN X): scattered taste cells at the root of the tongue.

THE CAUSES OF OROFACIAL STRUCTURE DYSFUNCTION

Because of the manifold functions of the orofacial system, interactions between a wide variety of factors may be involved in the causation of orofacial structure dysfunction.

Disturbances in early childhood

Through stimulation of the lips and tongue, the infant receives important impulses for the development of the nervous system, speech and personality. Hereditary reflexes form the basis for learned and practiced complex motor skills. If the tone of certain muscles is disturbed, reflexes are unable to develop properly, with the result that complex motor skills also cannot subsequently be learned as they should. If the chewing, suckling or swallowing reflex is disturbed, complex masticatory patterns, phonation, voluntary suckling and swallowing will later be impaired and may be executed with diminished coordination. For example, differentiated TMJ movement skills are necessary for the second babbling phase of language development at age 6 months. Abnormal structural development of the teeth or jaw leads in particular to disturbed phonation (apical, lingual, palatal and uvular sounds). Kinesthetic development is co-determined by early childhood experiences involving the oral region, for example, during breastfeeding. Somatopsychic interactions may occur in a wide range of ways. Limitation of masticatory function may also be reflected in personality development, for example, in the form of a diminished determination to see things through to completion (or to win through).

Structural factors

All the cranial bones may be involved in orofacial structure dysfunction and may require treatment in such cases. Dysfunction of the SBS (sphenobasilar synchondrosis) or temporal bone (peri or postnatally) may lead to disturbances in the oral cavity, via ligamentous, fascial and vascular connections, but also because of the influence of the cranial base on the growth of the middle and lower thirds of the face. Special attention should therefore be focused on the mandible and the maxillary complex. A maxillary complex in IR dysfunction may restrict the space available for the tongue, which is then displaced forward. The young child may then develop into a mouth breather with additional follow-on symptoms (e.g. problems with sleep and concentration etc.).[2] For Magoun,[3] diet is a more important factor than a traumatic etiology for the development of problems involving the jaws, oral cavity or pharynx.

The tongue

- Obstruction of nasal breathing leads to downward displacement of the tongue to allow increased mouth breathing. This results in narrowing of the maxillary arch.
- Enlargement of the lingual tonsils and, sometimes, of the adenoids may displace the tongue forward.
- A shortened frenulum will fix the tongue in a lowered position.
- Dysfunction of the cervical spine, especially hyperlordosis, may cause a functional disturbance of the tongue.
- An increase in styloglossus and palatoglossus muscle tone will cause the tongue to be drawn backward. Increased tone in the posterior fibers of the genioglossus muscle causes the tongue to protrude.
- A disturbance of the glossopharyngeal nerve (CN IX) and hypoglossal nerve (CN XII) or a flexion dysfunction of the SBS may disrupt the function of the styloglossus, palatoglossus and other lingual muscles, with subsequent swallowing disorders.

Note: The hypoglossal nerve (CN XII) may be disturbed, for example, in dysfunctions of the occipital bone and the upper cervical vertebrae (anastomosis of CN XII with the cervical nerve).

- According to Frymann, vertical strain dysfunction of the SBS in particular leads to increased fascial tension in the cervical region, with restriction of the hyoid bone and hence of the tongue. In superior vertical strain dysfunction there is flexion of the sphenoid bone and ER of the maxilla, with resultant maxillary widening and shortening. Furthermore, occiput extension produces IR of the temporal bone and mandible, causing the mandible to be moved posteriorly. As a result the tongue is displaced forward. In inferior vertical strain dysfunction there is narrowing of the maxilla and widening of the tongue, possibly causing the latter to push against the teeth.

Conversely, the tongue exerts an effect on the SBS

During the act of swallowing the tongue delivers a flexion impulse to the SBS.

When not engaged in mastication, swallowing, suckling, coughing and phonation, the tongue is usually located in a neutral position in the oral cavity. In this resting position the anterior upper part of the tip of the tongue is located immediately behind the upper incisors against the palate. The posterior part of the tongue is in contact with the soft palate, i.e. when the mouth is closed, it completely fills the oral cavity. In this position the tongue exerts an outward force on tooth development. It counterbalances the inward force exerted by the buccinator and other muscles of mastication. This is important for normal tooth development. When in the resting position, the tongue induces resting tone not only of the lingual muscles but also of the muscles controlling jaw closure.

An altered tongue position has an adverse effect on dental and mandibular-maxillary growth.

Glossoptosis is a special condition that is associated with strong pressure exerted by the root of the tongue against the cervical spine. Pressure on the glottis and blockage of the nasopharyngeal space lead to mouth breathing.

Consequences of an incorrect or fixed tongue position:

In backward displacement of the tongue (Fig. 12.15):[4]

- Swallowing disorder with impulse delivered to the cranium in the direction of the expiration phase of PRM.
- The mandible is drawn backward.
- Disturbance of phonation, auditory tube function, and pharyngeal drainage.

In forward displacement of the tongue (Fig. 12.16):[4]

- Swallowing disorder with impulse delivered to the cranium in the direction of the inspiration phase of PRM.

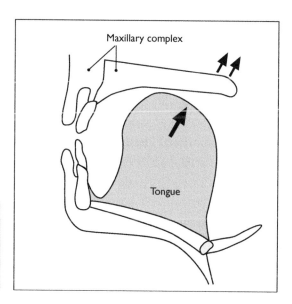

Figure 12.15 Incorrect tongue position and swallowing disturbance: backward displacement of the tongue (modified from Amiguez)

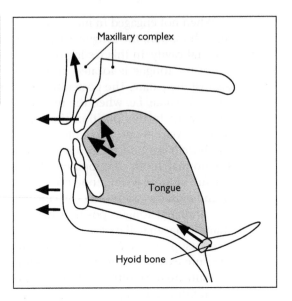

Figure 12.16 Incorrect tongue position and swallowing disturbance: forward displacement of the tongue (modified from Amiguez)

- The mandible is drawn forward.
- Phonation disturbance.
- Crooked teeth (especially front teeth) with subsequent jaw disturbance.
- The tongue may sometimes protrude between the teeth and lips.
- During the act of swallowing the orbicularis oris muscle is unable to contract in order to resist the pressure exerted by the tongue.
- Atonic lips.
- According to Knapp,[5] fixed forward displacement of the tongue exerts traction on the hyoid bone via the hyoglossus and genioglossus muscles. This tension is transmitted to the temporal bone (digastric muscle, posterior belly) and the cervico-occipital junction.

Possible symptoms:
- Nasal breathing disturbed when patient is supine.
- Common ENT symptoms.
- Swallowing disturbances.
- Speech disturbances.
- Delayed neuromotor development.
- Emotional instability.
- Dental problems, malocclusion and TMJ disturbances.

The teeth

The bones directly involved are the maxillae, the palatines (the incisive, intermaxillary, transverse palatine, and median palatine sutures), and the mandible. Dysfunctions involving the teeth may occur as a result of incorrect diet, disturbances of the bones of the jaw (with subsequent dental malocclusion), dental extractions, maxillofacial surgery, dental prostheses, nasal diseases, positional anomalies of the tongue, peribuccal muscle dysfunction, trauma or falls, and extreme overload due to gum-chewing etc. Correction of dental position using braces may produce functional limitations in the viscerocranium; as a result, manually measured restriction of mobility has been detected in remote large joints.[6] The sequelae of trauma to the teeth-bearing bones may in turn produce disturbances involving the eyes, nose, ears and throat. Moreover, an ascending dysfunction (e.g. postural curvature, scoliosis) may lead to dental malocclusion that in turn produces descending compensation. (The effect of our civilized diet is nowhere more apparent than on our teeth. Dental enamel, the hardest substance in the human body and usually sufficient to afford protection throughout life, commonly shows signs of wear after just a few years.)

Dental malocclusion, e.g. early contact, may result in grinding of the teeth, abnormal strain on the masticatory muscles, sinus formation, headache, and tinnitus.

According to Travell and Simons,[7] dental pain may occur as a result of pain referred from the temporal, masseter (superficial part) and digastric (anterior belly) muscles. Dental pain may be projected throughout the territory innervated by the trigeminal nerve, and dental, TMJ or neck pain may exacerbate each other or facilitate the trigeminal nerve and nucleus (see also Mandibular nerve dysfunction).

TREATMENT OF THE OROFACIAL STRUCTURES

Method of treating the orofacial structures (see also Pharynx)

According to Magoun,[3] all the cranial structures should be restored to normal.

- Treatment of the cranial base and the atlanto-occipital joint.
- Treatment of the maxilla and incisive suture.
- Treatment of the palatine bones.
- Treatment of the vomer.
- Treatment of the masticatory muscles.
- Treatment of the temporal bones, the mandible and the TMJ, including ligaments.
- Treatment of the teeth.
- Treatment of the muscles at the floor of the mouth, further hyoid muscles, as well as the hyoid bone and tongue.
- Treatment of the cervical spine, neck muscles and craniocervical fascia.
- Diet correction.[3]

Testing the teeth

Since the dental root is connected to alveolar bone via the periodontal ligaments, the fibrous joint (syndesmosis or gomphosis) between tooth and bone can also be released from abnormal tension, just like any other articulation.

Test *(Fig. 12.17)*

Therapist: Take up a position beside the patient's head.

Hand position: ➤ Place your index and middle fingers on the chewing surface of the teeth.

Method: ➤ Treat the tooth that appears to move in the direction of your fingers or generally appears to move more than the other teeth.

Alternative test *(Fig. 12.18)*

➤ Place one finger against the buccal surface of the row of teeth and ask the patient to chatter his/her teeth. Treat the tooth that presses outward against your finger.

Treatment of the teeth *(Fig. 12.19)*

Therapist: Take up a position beside the patient's head.

Hand position: ➤ Take hold of the affected tooth between your thumb and index finger.

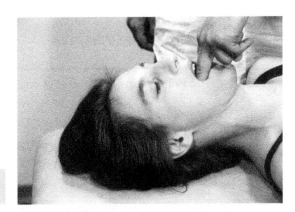

Figure 12.17 Testing the teeth

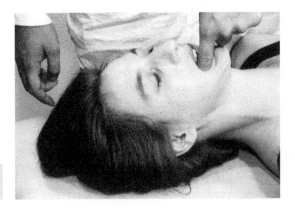

Figure 12.18 Alternative method of testing the teeth

Figure 12.19 Treatment of the teeth

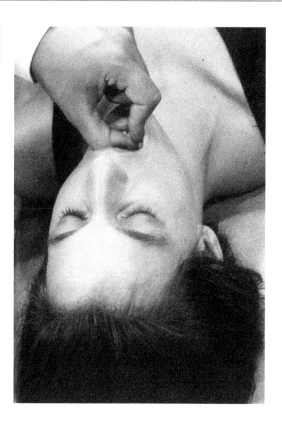

Method:
> Follow the intrinsic movements of the tooth. Unwind the tooth in its periodontal ligament.
> Then establish the PBLT in the periodontal ligament.

Alternative treatment:
> With your thumb and index finger, test each tooth in internal rotation and external rotation, and then treat using the exaggeration principle (indirect technique).

Treatment of the floor of the oral cavity

Palpation

Geniohyoid muscle:

- On intraoral palpation, a band of muscle running from the inferior mental spine on the inner surface of the mandible to the anterior surface of the hyoid.

Mylohyoid muscle:

- On intra- and extraoral palpation, a sheet of muscle attached to the whole length of the mylohyoid line of the mandible and extending to the body of the hyoid bone.

Digastric muscle:

- Posterior belly: posterior to the angle of the mandible (test for tenderness during jaw movement). Anterior belly: palpate from outside at the floor of the oral cavity.

Technique for the suprahyoid muscles *(Fig. 12.20)*

Therapist: Take up a position at the head of the patient.

Hand position: ➤ Place the index, middle and ring fingers of both hands on the midline at the floor of the oral cavity.

Method: ➤ With your index, middle and ring fingers, apply gentle cephalad pressure.
➤ While maintaining this pressure, stroke your fingers mediolaterally across the floor of the oral cavity.

Alternative technique I *(Fig. 12.21)*

Therapist: Take up a position at the head of the patient.

Hand position: ➤ Place your hands over both sides of the mandible.
➤ From below, direct the tips of the fingers of both hands upward toward the muscles of the floor of the oral cavity.

Method: ➤ With your fingers, apply cephalad and medial traction.
➤ Maintain traction until you sense release of tension.

Alternative technique II *(Fig. 12.22)*

Therapist: Take up a position beside the patient's head.

Hand position: ➤ Place the index finger of your cranial hand inside the patient's mouth at the floor of the oral cavity.
➤ Outside the patient's mouth, position the index finger of your caudal hand at the floor of the oral cavity opposite the location of your other index finger.

Method: ➤ With your index finger inside the patient's mouth, perform gentle circling movements on the muscles at the floor of the oral cavity, using the index finger outside as a fulcrum.

Note: Both methods should be comfortable for the patient. Stop the procedure if the patient experiences discomfort.

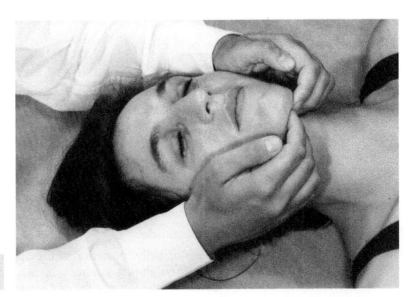

Figure 12.20 Technique for the suprahyoid muscles

Figure 12.21 Alternative technique I

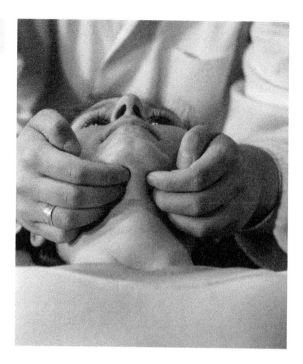

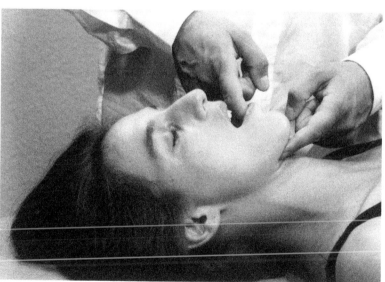

Figure 12.22 Alternative technique ii

Technique for the omohyoid muscle *(Fig. 12.23)*

Therapist: Take up a position at the head of the patient.

Hand position:
- ➤ Place the thumb of one hand at the posterior attachment of the omohyoid muscle to the scapula.
- ➤ Place your other hand on the underside of the mandible.

Method:
- ➤ The posterior inferior attachment of the omohyoid muscle cannot be treated directly. With your thumb, first push the trapezius in a posterior direction.

Figure 12.23 Technique for the omohyoid muscle

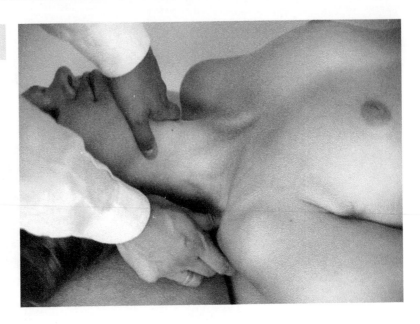

> Your thumb is now positioned along the course of the omohyoid muscle.
> By gentle contraction against resistance from the therapist, the muscles covering the posterior margin of this muscle can reduce the pressure on the jugular vein.

Technique for the hyoid bone *(Fig. 12.24)*

It is necessary to proceed with special care because of the sensitivity of the structures surrounding the hyoid bone. This caveat applies in particular to the use of direct techniques in this region.

Therapist: Take up a position beside the patient, on a level with the hyoid bone.

Hand position:
> Place one hand to provide dorsal support for the cervical spine.
> With your other hand, span the hyoid bone between index finger and thumb.

Method:
> Palpate the position of the hyoid bone (transverse or craniocaudal displacement).
> Gently test the lateral motion of the hyoid bone and then take it to its limit in the direction of ease (indirect technique).
> Once the tissues soften, seek the new limit of motion.
> Repeat this process until no further tissue softening can be detected.
> Then return the hyoid bone to the neutral position.
> To resolve any final asymmetries, a direct technique may now be used, i.e. move the hyoid bone in the direction of the restriction.
> Remove the hand supporting the cervical spine. Use it to fix the cranium laterally on the side of the restriction or barrier to motion.

➤ In all probability the amplitude of motion in this direction will already have increased markedly and have become balanced.

➤ A gentle procedure is extremely important. Never exceed the threshold at which the tissues display counter-contraction.

➤ In conclusion, place your hands above and below the patient's neck and perform tissue release as for the diaphragms described earlier.

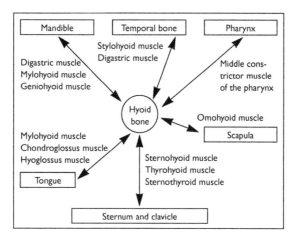

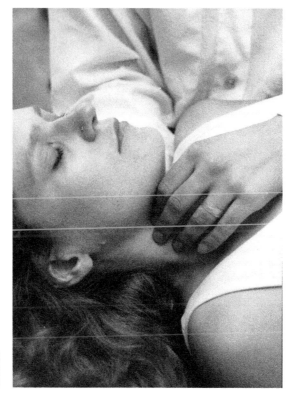

Figure 12.24 Technique for the hyoid bone

➤ A further way of releasing hyoid bone restrictions is to immobilize the hyoid bone in an inferior position while asking the patient to initiate the act of swallowing.

➤ The hyoid bone can also be treated in relation to the thyroid cartilage (thyrohyoid muscle). Take hold of the hyoid bone between the index finger and thumb of one hand, and the thyroid cartilage with your other hand. The method is the same as that described above, i.e. test the lateral motion of the hyoid compared with the thyroid cartilage. For correction, apply an indirect technique followed by a direct technique.

This exerts an effect on the hyoid bone and its muscles, ligaments and fascia, the first to 7th cervical vertebrae, the mechanics of swallowing, phonation, the thyroid, and psychological factors.

The cervical spine and the act of swallowing

a) Testing (Fig. 12.25)

Patient: Seated.

Therapist: Take up a position beside the patient.

Hand position: ➤ Place one hand on the neck muscles, as shown. With your other hand take the hyoid bone between the thumb and index finger.

Method: ➤ Ask the patient to swallow. Normally there should be no or only minimal discernible activity in the cervical spine and no

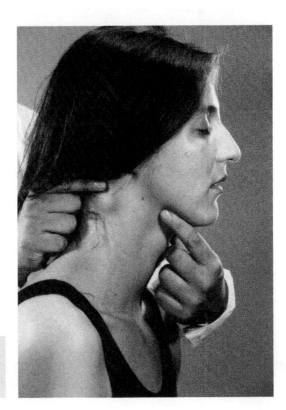

Figure 12.25 Testing the relationship between the cervical spine and the act of swallowing

head movement at all. A rapid craniocaudal movement at the hyoid should be detected. There should be minimal activity of the lips.

b) Treatment (see Fig. 12.24)

It is of course essential to implement all techniques required to eliminate dysfunctions involving the cervical spine and to conduct further tests of posture.

Hand position: The same as for testing, with the difference that treatment can also be performed with the patient supine.

Method: ➤ Establish a kind of PBT between the cervical spine and the hyoid bone.

Note: This component may also be integrated into the technique for the hyoid bone described above.

Treatment of the tongue

Chapman reflex points for the tongue

Anterior: On the second costal cartilage, 2 cm lateral to the sternum.

Posterior: Above and mid-way between the spinous process and the transverse process of the second cervical vertebra.

Chapman points are viscerosomatic reflexes that find expression through neurolymphatic reflex points in tissue. Local obstruction of lymphatic drainage occurs deep in the tissues of the reflex zone affected, presumably mediated by the orthosympathetic nervous system.

The points are palpated deep in the skin and subcutaneous tissues and, in particular, in the deep fascial layer or periosteum. Positive Chapman points are tender and tense to the touch, similar to a blister, with or without granular connective-tissue hardening.

Testing the tongue

With your index finger and thumb, take hold of the patient's lips, press them together and hold firmly, while instructing the patient to swallow.

The test is positive if the patient is unable to swallow while the lips are held firmly in this way. This is a physiological finding in early childhood but later it provides a pointer to a functional developmental disturbance of the tongue.

Alternative method: With your thumb and index finger, pull the patient's lower lip forward and hold it firmly in that position while the patient attempts to swallow.

Palpation of the PRM rhythm of the tongue

- In the inspiration phase of PRM the tongue shows transverse widening.
- In the expiration phase of PRM the tongue becomes longer.

Stretching the frenulum (Fig. 12.26)

> Place your index finger on the underside of the patient's tongue and stretch the frenulum laterally.

Unwinding the tongue *(Fig. 12.27)*

Therapist: Take up a position beside the patient's head.

Hand position: ➤ Take hold of the patient's tongue between your thumb, index finger and middle finger.

Method: ➤ Follow all the movements of the tongue (unwinding) until you sense that release has occurred.

THE PTERYGOPALATINE GANGLION

The pterygopalatine fossa *(Fig. 12.28)*

The pyramid-shaped pterygopalatine fossa is part of the infratemporal fossa. It contains the pterygopalatine ganglion.

It is bounded:
- In front: by the rounded eminence of the maxillary tuberosity.
- Behind: by the pterygoid process of the sphenoid bone.
- Above: by the under surface of the greater wing and body of the sphenoid bone.
- Medially: by the perpendicular plate of the palatine bone.
- Laterally: by the pterygomaxillary fissure (closed by connective tissue).
- Below: by the greater palatine canal.

It communicates with:
- The middle cranial fossa through the foramen rotundum (maxillary nerve, CN V2).
- The under surface of the cranial base through the pterygoid canal (nerve and artery of pterygoid canal, leading to the auditory tube).

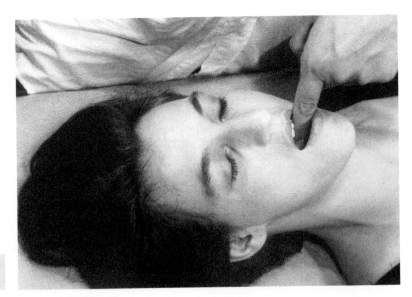

Figure 12.26 Stretching the frenulum

Figure 12.27 Unwinding the tongue

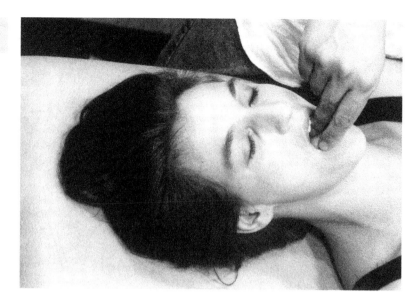

Figure 12.28 The pterygopalatine fossa

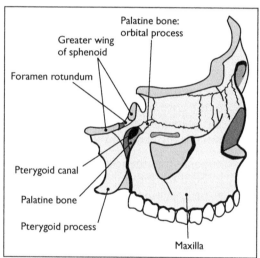

- The infratemporal fossa through the pterygomaxillary fissure (maxillary artery).
- The oral cavity through the greater palatine canal (greater palatine nerve and descending palatine artery).
- The nasal cavity through the sphenopalatine foramen (nasal branches from CN V2 and the sphenopalatine artery).
- The orbit through the inferior orbital fissure (infraorbital nerve, zygomatic nerve).

The pterygopalatine ganglion (*Fig. 12.29*)

Approximately 4 mm in diameter, the parasympathetic pterygopalatine ganglion, is one of the most important 'little things'

Figure 12.29 The pterygopalatine ganglion

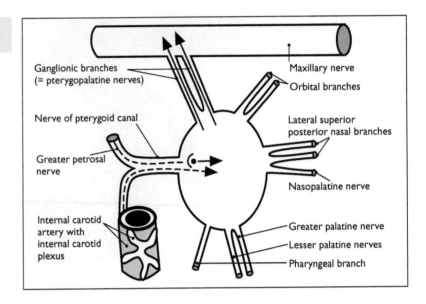

Ganglionic branches (= pterygopalatine nerves)

Maxillary nerve

Orbital branches

Nerve of pterygoid canal

Lateral superior posterior nasal branches

Greater petrosal nerve

Nasopalatine nerve

Internal carotid artery with internal carotid plexus

Greater palatine nerve

Lesser palatine nerves

Pharyngeal branch

in craniosacral osteopathy. This ganglion is attached above to two (ganglionic) branches of the maxillary nerve and is suspended in the pterygopalatine fossa like an overhead traffic light. It contains the perikarya of the postganglionic parasympathetic nerve fibers for the lacrimal gland and the small glands in the mucous membranes of the nose and palate. The preganglionic fibers run from the nerve of the pterygoid canal into the ganglion. The nerve of the pterygoid canal is formed from the:

- parasympathetic preganglionic greater petrosal nerve that issues from the intermedius nerve (CN VII), and the
- orthosympathetic deep petrosal nerve, which receives its postganglionic fibers from the internal carotid plexus, and these in turn derive from the superior cervical ganglion.

Parasympathetic and orthosympathetic nerve fibers emerge from the ganglion, as well as sensory elements from the maxillary nerve which, just like the orthosympathetic fibers, either pass through the ganglion without establishing synapses or else bypass it.

- The orbital branches enter the orbit through the inferior orbital fissure and sometimes continue into the mucous membrane of the posterior ethmoid air cells and the sphenoidal sinus.
- The lateral posterior superior nasal nerves (5–10 fine branches) pass through the sphenopalatine foramen to the superior and middle nasal conchae and to the mucous membrane of the posterior ethmoid air cells.
- The medial posterior superior nasal nerves also pass through the sphenopalatine foramen into the nasal cavity to supply the mucous membrane of the upper part of the nasal septum. The largest of these, the nasopalatine nerve, descends through the

incisive fossa to supply the mucous membrane of the anterior part of the palate and the gingiva behind the upper incisor teeth.

● The greater palatine nerve descends through the greater palatine canal to supply the mucous membrane of the hard palate. In addition, immediately before it traverses the greater palatine canal, it gives off branches that supply the mucous membrane of the inferior nasal concha and the inferior and middle nasal meatuses.

● The lesser palatine nerves pass through canals of the same name to innervate the mucous membrane of the soft palate and the palatine tonsils.

● The pharyngeal branch runs posteriorly and medially to supply the mucous membrane of the nasal part of the pharynx.

The causes of pterygopalatine ganglion dysfunction

Blows to or falls on the frontal or zygomatic bones and the maxilla may drive the small palatine bone into the ganglion, restrict the space available to the ganglion, and adversely affect its function. An extension dysfunction of the SBS may also compress and disturb the ganglion. Dysfunctions of the temporal and ethmoid bones and of the upper cervical vertebrae may also be involved.

Clinical signs: Disorders of tear secretion, asthma, dry or irritated nasal, nasopharyngeal and palatal mucosa, rhinitis, allergic rhinitis, sinusitis, eye disorders and ocular pain of nasal origin, as well as pain involving the temporal and auricular region and the auditory tube.

TREATMENT OF THE PTERYGOPALATINE GANGLION *(Figs 12.30a,b)*

In most cases it is necessary first to decompress the maxillary complex at the pterygopalatine suture (see The Maxilla). In addition, the sphenoid bone (extension of the SBS leads to narrowing of the pterygopalatine fossa), the maxilla, the palatine, ethmoid and temporal bones, the TMJ, and the upper cervical vertebrae in particular need to be examined, palpated and, where appropriate, treated.

Desired effect: To stimulate the pterygopalatine ganglion. The technique is indicated for the symptoms listed above.

Therapist: Take up a position beside the patient's head on the opposite side to the one being treated.

Hand position: ➤ Place your cranial hand as an 'observer' on one side of the cranial vault without applying pressure.

➤ Place the index finger or little finger of your caudal hand inside the patient's mouth.

➤ Move the finger along the outer edge of the alveolar process of the maxilla toward the ear. The palmar surface of the finger should face medially, toward the gingiva.

➤ It may be necessary to instruct the patient to perform slight sideways movements of the mandible to enable you to move your

Figure 12.30 (a,b)
Treatment of the
pterygopalatine ganglion

(a)

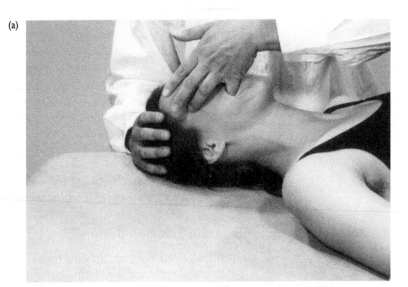

(b)

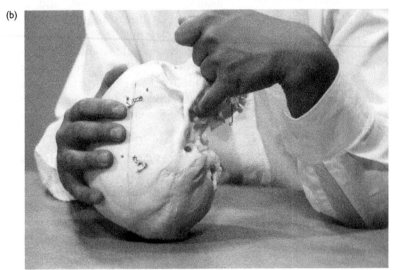

inserted finger through between the maxilla and the ramus of the
mandible.

➤ Advance your finger as far as the posterior end of the lateral aspect
of the maxilla and position it on the connective tissue in the
pterygomaxillary fissure. This is located between the maxillary
tuberosity and the pterygoid process.

Method: Caudal hand:

➤ With the tip of your index finger or little finger, administer gentle
pressure medially and slightly cephalad in the direction of the
pterygopalatine ganglion. In this process follow the tissue
movements with your finger.

➤ Maintain the pressure until you sense a release of tissue tone in the
fissure. In some circumstances this technique may be painful.

> Lacrimation will generally occur.
> With the cranial hand on the vault, deliver a fluid impulse toward the ganglion. Apply until you sense the release and physiological motion of the surrounding bones.

THE PHARYNX *(Fig. 12.31)*

The pharynx is a musculomembranous tube, some 12 to 15 cm in length and with openings into the nasal and oral cavities. It

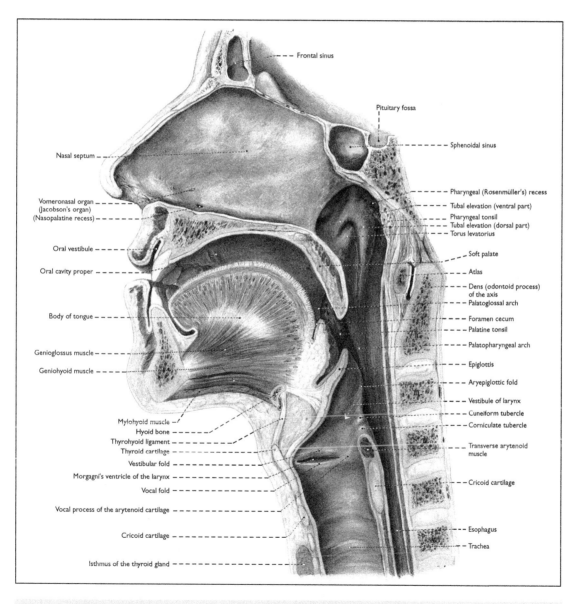

Figure 12.31 The pharynx. Sagittal section through the head and neck. Medial view (From: Tillmann B. Farbatlas der Anatomie. Zahnmedizin – Humanmedizin. Stuttgart: Thieme; 1997)

communicates laterally with the middle ear, and contributes to both the respiratory and the digestive tracts. It can be subdivided into a nasal, an oral, and a laryngeal part. However, the limits of these subdivisions are not rigidly defined.

The pharynx is suspended on the cranial base. Below, it is continuous with the esophagus at about the level of the 6th cervical vertebra. Behind, the pharyngeal wall lies against the cervical portion of the spinal column and the paravertebral muscles. In front, it opens into the respiratory and digestive tracts.

The pharynx communicates with the:

- Choanae: the paired openings between the nasopharynx and the nasal cavity.
- Pharyngeal openings of the auditory tube located in the lateral walls of the nasopharynx.
- Oropharyngeal isthmus: the constricted aperture between the oral part of the pharynx and the oral cavity.
- Mouth of the esophagus: the opening of the laryngeal part of the pharynx into the esophagus.
- Inlet of the larynx: the opening of the laryngeal part of the pharynx into the larynx.

The nasal part of the pharynx

The nasopharynx is located at the level of the nasal cavity.

It is bounded:
- Above, by the roof of the pharynx at the floor of the sphenoidal sinus where the pharyngeal tonsils are located.
- Behind, by the continuous downward slope of the posterior wall and the anterior arch of the atlas; a collection of lymphoid tissue lies in the mucous membrane here.
- In front, by the openings into the choanae.
- Laterally, by the pharyngeal openings of the auditory tubes, ~1–1.5 cm behind the inferior nasal concha; the lymphoid tissue present in the openings of the auditory tubes is known as the tubal tonsils. The pharyngeal opening of the tube is surrounded by the tubal elevation.
- Below, by the soft palate.

Pharyngobasilar fascia *(Fig. 12.32)*

The roof of the pharynx contains no muscle fibers and is formed by the pharyngobasilar fascia, by which it is attached to the cranial base.

The pharyngobasilar fascia originates at the upper margin of the superior constrictor muscles of the pharynx as a fusion of muscle fascia. Posterior to the pharyngeal tubercle of the occipital bone, the pharyngobasilar fascia forms a midline connective tissue seam – the pharyngeal raphe. This extends to the inferior end of the pharyngeal wall and provides attachment for the constrictor muscles of the pharynx.

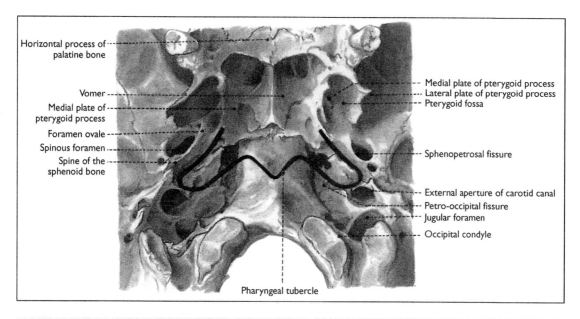

Horizontal process of
palatine bone

Vomer

Medial plate of
pterygoid process

Foramen ovale

Spinous foramen

Spine of the
sphenoid bone

Medial plate of pterygoid process
Lateral plate of pterygoid process
Pterygoid fossa

Sphenopetrosal fissure

External aperture of carotid canal
Petro-occipital fissure
Jugular foramen

Occipital condyle

Pharyngeal tubercle

Figure 12.32 Attachment of the pharyngobasilar fascia to the cranial base (From: Leonhardt H, Tillmann B, Töndbury G, Zilles K (eds). Rauber/Kopsch: Anatomie des Menschen. Volume I. Nervensystem. Stuttgart: Thieme; 1987)

Attachment of the pharyngobasilar fascia to the cranial base (posterior to anterior):

- Pharyngeal tubercle of the occipital bone.
- Bilaterally over the basilar portion of the occipital bone.
- Petrous part of the temporal bone medial to the carotid canal.
- Sweeps round ventrally.
- Passes medially to the tubal cartilage.
- Medial to the medial pterygoid plate of the sphenoid bone.
- Attaches to the lateral border of the choanae.
- Follows the pterygomandibular raphe.
- Mylohyoid line of the mandible.

The oral part of the pharynx

The oral part of the pharynx opens anteriorly into the oral cavity and is located approximately on a level with the second cervical vertebra. This portion of the pharynx is both respiratory and digestive in function.

It is bounded:
- In front: by the oropharyngeal isthmus; this consists of the root of the tongue, the soft palate with the uvula and the anterior (palatoglossal) and posterior (palatopharyngeal) palatal arches, and the muscles of the same name.
- Below: approximately on a level with the epiglottis.

The laryngeal part of the pharynx

The laryngeal part of the pharynx is continuous below with the esophagus and is on a level approximately with the 3rd to 6th cervical vertebrae.

It is bounded:
- Above: by the cranial border of the epiglottis.
- In front: by the inlet of the larynx and the larynx itself.
- Below: by the caudal border of the cricoid cartilage.

The transitional zone from the laryngeal part of the pharynx to the inlet of the larynx is bounded above by the epiglottis and laterally and below by the aryepiglottic folds. On each side of the laryngeal orifice, a mucosal recess, termed the piriform fossa, serves as a swallowing channel in which a large part of the bolus travels from the root of the tongue to the esophageal opening.

In neonates the nasal part of the pharynx is still relatively low and the laryngeal part of the pharynx has barely developed. Neonates are able to feed without closing the epiglottis because the larynx is still in a very high position in the neck.

The structure of the pharyngeal wall

The pharynx is composed of mucous membrane, submucosal connective tissue, glands, lymphoid tissue, muscle and an outermost adventitial coating. The mucous membrane does not possess a muscular layer.

While the epithelium of the nasal part of the pharynx is columnar and ciliated and is interspersed with goblet cells, the other parts of the pharynx are covered with non-keratinized stratified squamous epithelium.

In the upper part of the pharynx where muscle fibers are absent, the submucosal connective tissue thickens to become the pharyngobasilar fascia.

The submucosal layer is separated from the pharyngeal muscles by elastic connective tissue.

The nasal part of the pharynx contains seromucous glands, whereas the other parts of the pharynx possess only mucous glands.

The adventitia is connected to the spinal column by loose connective tissue and this enables the pharynx to glide in relation to the spinal column.

The muscles *(Figs. 12.33, 12.34)*

a) The constrictor muscles of the pharynx

Fiber pattern: The constrictor muscles of the pharynx are annular, being open anteriorly. Posteriorly at the pharyngeal wall, ascending, horizontal and descending fiber patterns are mingled.

Function: To constrict the pharynx; in some cases, because of their muscle fiber pattern, they may also elevate or lower the pharynx.

All the constrictor muscles of the pharynx have their attachment at the pharyngeal raphe. The pharynx is suspended from the cranial base by this strong fibrous band.

Figure 12.33 The muscles of the pharynx, posterior view. 15, Pharyngobasilar fascia; 20, Pharyngeal raphe; 22, Superior constrictor muscle of the pharynx; 27, Stylopharyngeus muscle; 29, Middle constrictor muscle of the pharynx; 32, Inferior constrictor muscle of the pharynx (From: Feneis H. Anatomisches Bildwörterbuch. 6th edn. Stuttgart: Thieme; 1988)

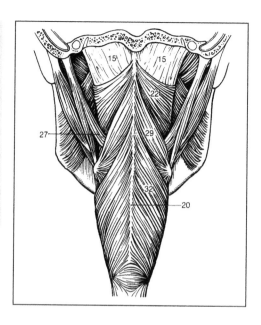

Figure 12.34 The muscles of the pharynx, lateral view. 15, Pharyngobasilar fascia; 21, Pterygomandibular raphe; 23–26, Superior constrictor muscle of the pharynx; 23, Pterygopharyngeal part; 24, Buccopharyngeal part; 25, Mylopharyngeal part; 26, Glossopharyngeal part; 30–31, Middle constrictor muscle of the pharynx; 30, Chondropharyngeal part; 31, Ceratopharyngeal part; 32, Inferior constrictor muscle of the pharynx; 33, Thyropharyngeal part; 34, Cricopharyngeal part (From: Feneis H. Anatomisches Bildwörterbuch. 6th edn. Stuttgart: Thieme; 1988)

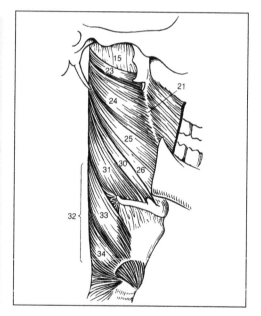

Innervation: The constrictor muscles of the pharynx are supplied by the pharyngeal plexus – in the upper pharynx more by the glossopharyngeal nerve (CN IX), and in the lower pharynx more by the vagus nerve (CN X).

The superior constrictor muscle of the pharynx (four parts)

Origin: ● Pterygopharyngeal part: the medial pterygoid plate and the pterygoid hamulus of the sphenoid bone.

- Buccopharyngeal part: pterygomandibular raphe.
- Mylopharyngeal part: the posterior end of the mylohyoid line.
- Glossopharyngeal part: intrinsic muscles of the tongue.

Dysfunction: The function of this muscle may be disturbed in dysfunctions involving the sphenoid, occipital, and palatine bones and as a result of abnormal tension in the cervical fascia.

On the other hand, according to Magoun, by drawing the mandible forward, the osteopath may reduce upper pharyngeal inflammation and lymph stasis.[8]

The middle constrictor muscle of the pharynx

Origin:
- Chondropharyngeal part: lesser cornu of the hyoid bone.
- Ceratopharyngeal part: greater cornu of the hyoid bone.

Dysfunction: The motion of the hyoid bone may be restricted by this muscle.

The inferior constrictor muscle of the pharynx

Origin:
- Thyropharyngeal part: oblique line of the lamina of the thyroid cartilage.
- Cricopharyngeal part: cricoid cartilage.

Dysfunction: Motion restriction of the thyroid and cricoid cartilage may impair vocal cord function.

Dysfunction of the constrictor muscles of the pharynx: Through the attachment of the pharyngeal raphe at the cranial base, a flexion dysfunction of the SBS may increase the tension in the fibers of the constrictor muscles of the pharynx. A torsion or side-bending – rotation dysfunction may cause deviation of the pharyngeal raphe and other fascial structures. The consequence may be reduced lymphatic drainage and swelling of the tubal mucosa with resultant auditory problems.

b) The elevator muscles of the pharynx
The elevator muscles of the pharynx descend from above (cranial base, palatine aponeurosis, auditory tube) down to the muscular wall of the pharynx.

The stylopharyngeus muscle

Origin: Styloid process of the temporal bone.
Insertion: Passes through the annular muscle layer between the superior and middle constrictor muscles of the pharynx, to the pharyngeal wall, thyroid cartilage and epiglottis.
Function: To elevate and broaden the pharynx.
Innervation: Glossopharyngeal nerve (CN IX).

The palatopharyngeus muscle (the most powerful elevator muscle of the pharynx, and the basis of the palatopharyngeal arch)

Origin: Palatine aponeurosis and pterygoid hamulus of the sphenoid bone.
Insertion: Lateral wall of the pharynx, thyroid cartilage.

Function: To elevate the pharynx, narrow the oropharyngeal isthmus, and lower the soft palate; according to Magoun, it also assists the opening of the auditory tube.[6]

Innervation: Pharyngeal plexus (glossopharyngeal nerve, CN IX, and vagus nerve, CN X).

The salpingopharyngeus muscle

Origin: Posterior medial part of the lip of the auditory tube cartilage; in some cases, the longitudinal muscles of the wall of the pharynx.

Insertion: Lateral wall of the pharynx.

Function: To elevate the pharynx, and prevent downward slippage of the levator veli palatini muscle.

Innervation: Pharyngeal plexus (glossopharyngeal nerve, CN IX).

c) The muscles of the soft palate and palatal arches

The tensor veli palatini muscle

Origin: The spine of the sphenoid bone on the under-surface of the greater wing, the scaphoid fossa, and the anterior lateral wall of the auditory tube.

Insertion: After turning medially round the pterygoid hamulus, it is inserted into the palatine aponeurosis.

Function: To tighten the soft palate (elevation to the level of the hamulus), widen the auditory tube, and seal off the nasal part of the pharynx during the acts of swallowing and speaking.

Innervation: Branch of the mandibular nerve (CN V3).

Dysfunction: If the pterygoid processes are out of balance, the result may be asymmetric tension in the right and left tensor veli palatini muscles. According to Magoun,[9] this may cause increased tension in the pharynx, associated with problems when swallowing or, in singers, with difficulty in reaching high notes.

The levator veli palatini muscle

Origin: Inferior surface of the petrous temporal bone, immediately in front of the carotid canal, cartilaginous inferior surface of the auditory tube.

Insertion: Palatine aponeurosis.

Function: To tighten and elevate the soft palate, widen the auditory tube, and seal off the nasal part of the pharynx during the acts of swallowing and speaking.

Innervation: Pharyngeal plexus (glossopharyngeal nerve, CN IX and vagus nerve, CN X, in some cases fibers from the facial nerve, CN VII).

Dysfunction: Asymmetric dysfunctions of the temporal bones (petrous parts) may contribute to asymmetric tension in the left and right levator veli palatini muscles.

The musculus uvulae

Origin: Palatine aponeurosis.

Insertion: Connective tissue at the tip of the uvula.

Function: To shorten and thicken the uvula, and seal off the nasal part of the pharynx.

Innervation: Pharyngeal plexus (vagus nerve, CN X).

The palatoglossus muscle (the basis of the palatoglossal arch)

Origin: Palatine aponeurosis.

Insertion: Transverse muscle of the tongue.

Function: To elevate the root of the tongue, lower the soft palate, and narrow the oropharyngeal isthmus.

The palatopharyngeus muscle (see Constrictor muscles of the pharynx)

The nerves of the pharynx *(Fig. 12.35)*

The glossopharyngeal nerve (CN IX), vagus nerve (CN X) and the sympathetic trunk together form the pharyngeal plexus in the wall of

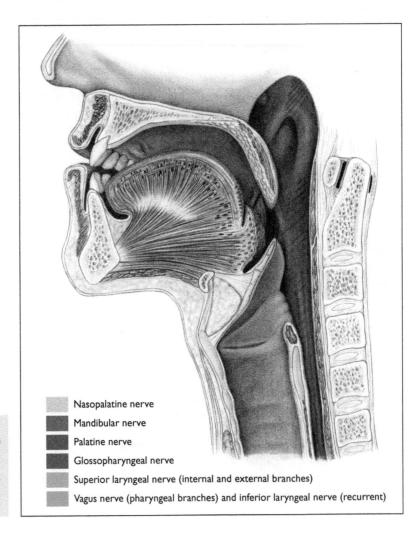

Figure 12.35 The sensory innervation of the oral cavity, pharynx, larynx and trachea (From: Tillmann B. Farbatlas der Anatomie. Zahnmedizin – Humanmedizin. Stuttgart: Thieme; 1997)

Nasopalatine nerve

Mandibular nerve

Palatine nerve

Glossopharyngeal nerve

Superior laryngeal nerve (internal and external branches)

Vagus nerve (pharyngeal branches) and inferior laryngeal nerve (recurrent)

the pharynx. This plexus sends motor fibers to muscles, and sensory and secretory fibers to mucous membrane.

Motor innervation:

See the sections on the respective muscles; the upper pharynx tends to be supplied by branches of the glossopharyngeal nerve, and the lower pharynx by branches of the vagus nerve.

Sensory innervation:

- Maxillary nerve (CN V2): roof of the pharynx and area around the opening of the auditory tube.
- Glossopharyngeal nerve (CN IX): root of tongue, lower nasal part of the pharynx, palatine tonsils, oral part of the pharynx.
- Vagus nerve (CN X): the laryngeal and sometimes the oral part of the pharynx.

The vessels of the pharynx

Arterial supply:

- Ascending pharyngeal artery (branch of the external carotid artery): most important artery, it ascends lateral to the wall of the pharynx as far as the cranial base.
- Ascending palatine artery (branch of the facial artery): wall of the pharynx.
- Superior laryngeal artery (branch of the superior thyroid artery).
- Sphenopalatine artery (terminal part of the maxillary artery): wall of the pharynx.
- Inferior thyroid artery (branch of the subclavian artery): inferior region of the pharynx.

Venous supply:

- The pharyngeal veins form a venous network (pharyngeal plexus) around the muscles of the pharynx. Close to the inlet to the esophagus the veins form a kind of cushion that lends the mucous membrane a degree of elasticity, confers protection against pressure forces, and may constrict the lumen in certain circumstances.
- The pharyngeal veins end in the internal jugular vein. They additionally open into the pterygoid venous plexus and the meningeal veins.
- The superior laryngeal vein, superior thyroid vein and the lingual vein are located on a level with the larynx.

Lymphatic supply:

- Retropharyngeal lymph nodes and deep cervical lymph nodes.

The act of swallowing (see also The Tongue)

- Contraction of the muscles at the floor of the mouth produces cranial and anterior movement of the hyoid bone, causing the tongue to be pressed against the bony palate. The tongue (hyoglossus and styloglossus muscles) propels the bolus backward into the pharynx. This part of the act of swallowing is under voluntary control.

● While the thyrohyoid muscle draws the larynx toward the hyoid bone, the pre-epiglottic adipose body presses the epiglottis on to the inlet to the larynx, thus closing it.

● Through contraction of the levator and tensor veli palatini muscles, the soft palate is elevated and brought into a horizontal position. Contraction of the superior constrictor muscle of the pharynx also causes Passavant's cushion to approximate to the soft palate. This results in closure of the nasal part of the pharynx.

● During the act of swallowing there is serial contraction of the constrictor muscles of the pharynx downward from the superior to the inferior.

● During the esophageal phase the bolus is propelled to the stomach in a peristaltic wave.

The swallow reflex

Once the bolus comes into contact with the wall of the pharynx, the further act of swallowing takes place involuntarily. The swallow center is located in the medulla oblongata above the respiratory center. Afferent fibers travel in the glossopharyngeal and vagus nerves to the swallow center. In addition to the named nerves, efferent fibers also travel in the trigeminal nerve (muscles of the floor of the mouth), the hypoglossal nerve (muscles of the tongue), and the cervical nerves (infrahyoid muscles).

In early childhood the act of swallowing occurs as a purely reflex process and is intimately linked to the suckling process.

Note: During the act of swallowing the tongue delivers a flexion impulse to the SBS.

During suckling, too, the tongue exerts pressure on the anterior part of the palate and thus stimulates the SBS.

Waldeyer's lymphoid (tonsillar) ring (Fig. 12.36)

Waldeyer's lymphoid (tonsillar) ring is located at the points where the oral and nasal cavities open into the pharynx. Its principal function is to identify pathogens and, where appropriate, to activate the immune defense mechanism. It also protects the entry portals in the pharynx from pathogens.

The ring consists of the palatine tonsils, the pharyngeal tonsils, the lingual tonsils, the tubal tonsils and, in addition, the lymphatic organs in the wall of the salpingopharyngeal folds, and lymphoepithelial organs with no specific name.

They are lymphoepithelial organs, consisting of primary and, in particular, secondary follicles containing abundant B-lymphocytes and plasma cells.

Figure 12.36 Waldeyer's lymphoid (tonsillar) ring (From: Drenckhahn D, Zenker W (eds). Benninghof, Anatomie, Vol. 1. 15th edn. Munich: Urban & Schwarzenberg)

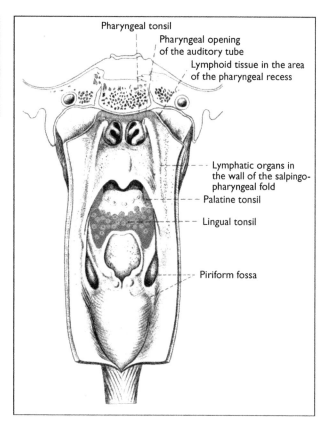

Pharyngeal tonsil

Pharyngeal opening of the auditory tube

Lymphoid tissue in the area of the pharyngeal recess

Lymphatic organs in the wall of the salpingo-pharyngeal fold

Palatine tonsil

Lingual tonsil

Piriform fossa

The palatine tonsils, paired

Each tonsil is placed in the tonsillar fossa between the diverging palatoglossal and palatopharyngeal arches. The tonsil is extremely variable in size. When inflamed, especially in childhood, it may become enlarged to such an extent that swallowing is impaired. It is situated on the superior constrictor muscle of the pharynx, from which it is separated by connective tissue. The surface of the tonsil presents some 10 to 20 orifices that lead into the tonsillar crypts.

Each tonsil is supplied by the facial, maxillary and ascending pharyngeal arteries. Its regional lymph node is the jugulodigastric node. This is located beneath the angle of the mandible, at the intersection of the internal jugular vein and the digastric muscle.

It is a clinically important finding that this lymph node becomes swollen when the palatine tonsils are inflamed.

The palatine tonsils receive sensory innervation from the glossopharyngeal nerve.

The lingual tonsils, paired

These are located at the root of the tongue and present as a collection of lymphoid follicles. Following extraction of the palatine tonsils, the lingual tonsils may exhibit marked compensatory enlargement and produce symptoms similar to those associated with the palatine tonsils.

The pharyngeal tonsil, non-paired

This is located at the roof of the nasal part of the pharynx, behind the choanae. In childhood the pharyngeal tonsil can grow to such a size that nasal breathing is hampered. This may lead to mouth breathing, with development of a raised palate, increased susceptibility to infection due to bypassing the nasal filter, and sleep disturbances with resultant disturbed concentration.

The tubal tonsils, paired *(Fig. 12.37)*

These aggregations of lymphoid tissue are located around the pharyngeal opening of the auditory tube, on a level with the inferior nasal meatus.

TREATMENT OF THE PHARYNX

Chapman reflex points

Pharyngitis:

- Anterior: On the first rib, 2 cm medial to the point of intersection with the clavicle.
- Posterior: Mid-way between the spinous process and transverse process of the axis.

Tonsillitis:

- Anterior: First intercostal space, next to sternum
- Posterior: Mid-way between the spinous process and transverse process of the atlas.

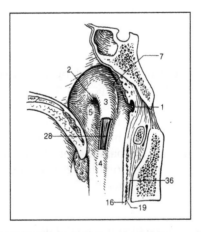

Figure 12.37 The tubal tonsils and the opening of the auditory tube 1, Pharyngeal bursa; 2, Pharyngeal opening of the auditory tube; 3, Tubal elevation; 4, Salpingopharyngeal fold; 5, Torus levatorius; 7, Pharyngeal recess; 16, Submucosal layer; 19, Muscular tunic of the pharynx; 28, Salpingopharyngeus muscle; 36, Retropharyngeal space (From: Feneis H. Anatomisches Bildwörterbuch. 6th edn. Stuttgart: Thieme; 1988)

Laryngitis:

- Anterior: Superiorly, on the first rib, 5–6 cm lateral to sternum.
- Posterior: Mid-way between the spinous process and transverse process of the atlas.

Treatment methods for the pharyngeal structures and sore throat

When treating sore throat, it is important first to exclude a diagnosis of group A β-hemolytic streptococcal infection or diphtheria. Antibiotics are indicated for these diseases because of the risk of dangerous complications.

Therapy is directed primarily at stimulating the immune system, at removing toxic waste products, and at improving venous return. In this context, too, treatment must of course be preceded by a global examination.

- Treatment of the craniocervical fascia.
- Treatment of the cervicothoracic diaphragms: superior costal articulations, sternoclavicular and acromioclavicular joints, sternum (thymus), release of scalene muscles.
- Lymph techniques: (a) Release of diaphragmatic tension (= primary lymphatic pump). (b) Lymphatic pump technique for the feet. (c) CV-4. (d) Recoil technique for the upper thoracic region and the upper cervicothoracic junction.
- Harmonization and stimulation of immune defense organs: spleen, liver, thymus, and appendix.
- Treatment of the muscles of the floor of the mouth, tongue, other hyoid muscles and the hyoid bone.[10]
- Treatment of the upper cervical vertebrae and the occipito-atlantal joint (superior cervical ganglion) and pre-ganglionic treatment on a level with the 7th cervical vertebra to 2nd thoracic vertebra and 1st rib.
- Treatment of the 11th and 12th ribs and thoracic vertebrae (adrenals).
- Local treatment of the tonsils and auditory tube technique (see Temporal bone and Organ of hearing).
- Treatment of the palatines, maxilla, vomer and SBS.
- Possible treatment of the lateral pterygoid muscle (pharyngeal pain) and the digastric muscle (disturbed swallowing).[11]
- Resolution of psychosocial stress factors.
- Regulation of diet: cutting down on or avoiding dairy products, cutting down on refined sugar, bread, flour-based foods, and fried foods. More fruit and vegetables instead.
- Self-help techniques: (a) Palatine tonsil drainage, (b) 'Roaring lion'.

Local treatment for the tonsils

In addition to holistic treatment, local tonsillar drainage using Röder's technique has proved very useful in practice. Although this is not an osteopathic technique *per se*, it may nevertheless be used from an osteopathic perspective. It is therefore described below.

Equipment required: Four glass aspirator tubes, two curved cotton applicators, two straight cotton applicators.

Method: *a)* Aspiration of the palatine tonsils (Fig. 12.38)

Place cotton wool soaked in hydrogen superoxide into the aperture of the aspirator tube. Position the tip of the tube over the palatine tonsil and 'milk' the tonsil by pressing the rubber bulb. The pressure on the rubber bulb must not be so great that you have to forcibly detach the tip of the aspirator tube from the tonsil. Afterwards the drainage products from the tonsil can be inspected on the cotton wool (greasy, possibly yellowish, or granular).

b) Massage of the palatine tonsils (Fig. 12.39)

With the tip of your index finger wrapped in cotton wool, gently massage both palatine tonsils. Soak the cotton wool with tap water and then with a few drops of arnica tincture. Patients may also perform this procedure at home themselves. A gag or cough reflex may be produced when performing the technique.

c) Massage of the pharyngeal tonsil (Fig. 12.40)

Place the curved cotton applicator (with cotton wool soaked in hydrogen superoxide) flat on the tongue. Then position the curved part of the applicator so that it is vertical and wipe it a few times over the nasal part of the pharynx, including the pharyngeal tonsil. Perform this maneuver swiftly because it will provoke a gag reflex.

d) Endonasal massage (see also Fig. 13.24b)

Take a cotton bud moistened with nasal oil and insert it carefully into the inferior nasal meatus (in the direction of the 7th cervical vertebra) until it touches the posterior wall of the pharynx. Gently massage there a few times and withdraw the bud again.

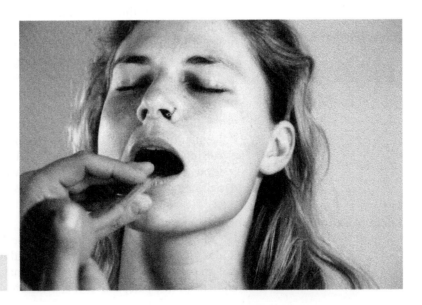

Figure 12.38 Aspiration of the palatine tonsils

Figure 12.39 Massage of the palatine tonsils

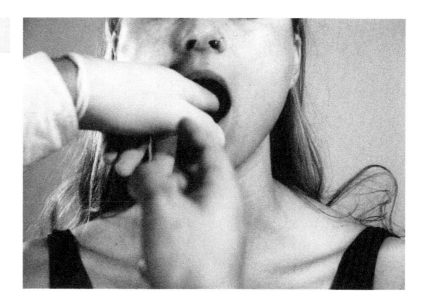

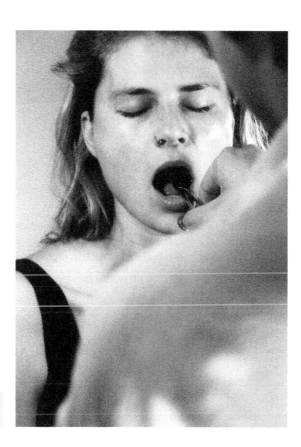

Figure 12.40 Massage of the pharyngeal tonsil

Figure 12.41 Drainage of the palatine tonsils.

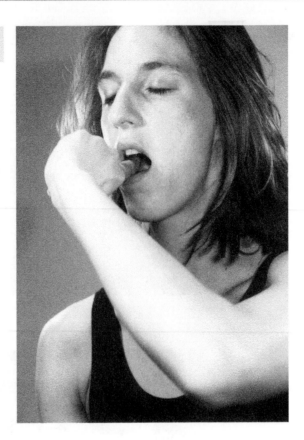

Note: Endonasal massage generally provokes an increasingly runny nose.

Self-help techniques

a) Drainage of the palatine tonsils (Fig. 12.41)
➤ Use your own index finger to demonstrate to the patient how to reach the palatine tonsils that are located bilaterally behind the palatoglossal arch.
➤ The patient may then finger-massage and drain the palatine tonsils once daily.

b) The 'roaring lion' (Fig. 12.42)
This exercise represents another way to improve the milieu in the pharynx, including the tongue and tonsils. It also has a positive effect in people with halitosis.

Method
(instruct the patient as follows): ➤ Squat on your heels, with your hands on your knees, arms straight, and fingers spread.
➤ Shift your bodyweight on to your knees.
➤ Push your stomach and chest forward. Stretch your back so that it is in slight extension. Relax your shoulders.

Figure 12.42 The 'roaring lion'

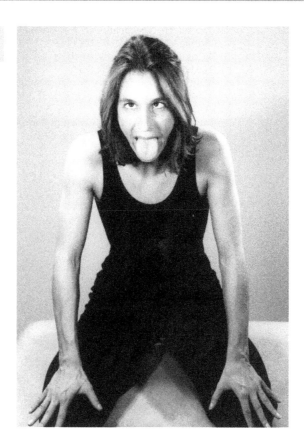

➤ Open your mouth wide and stick your tongue out as far as possible toward your chin. You may also adopt a cross-eyed look.
➤ Start to breathe in; then, while breathing out, roar like a lion.

Over a period of about 3 weeks perform this exercise at least once a day for a 1–2 min.

References

1 Upledger JE. Craniosacral Therapy II. Beyond the Dura. Seattle: Eastland Press; 1987:191.
2 Bahnemann F, ed. Der Bionator in der Kieferorthopädie. Grundlagen und Praxis. Heidelberg: Haug; 1993:28, 30–44.
3 Magoun HI. Osteopathy in the Cranial Field. 3rd edn. Kirksville: Journal Printing Company; 1976:213.
4 Amiguez JP. L'A.T.M. Une Articulation entre l'Ostéopathe et le Dentiste. Aix en Provence: Verlaque; 1991:142.
5 Knapp C. Succion du pouce et charnière cervico-occipitale. Annales de Médécine Ostéopathique 1985; 1.
6 Seider R. Der Einfluss von kraniosakraler Therapie auf den Bewegungsumfang entfernt liegender großer Gelenke, bei Zustand nach kieferorthopädischer Zahnstellungskorrektur mittels Zahnspange. Hamm: Diploma thesis; 1999.
7 Travell JG, Simons DG. Myofascial Pain and Dysfunction. Vol. 1. Baltimore: Williams and Wilkins; 1983:219, 236, 273.

8 Magoun HI. Osteopathy in the Cranial Field. 3rd edn. Kirksville: Journal Printing Company; 1976:214.

9 Magoun HI. Osteopathy in the Cranial Field. 3rd edn. Kirksville: Journal Printing Company; 1976:215.

10 Allain A. Le complexe musculo-aponevrotique sous-hyoidien et la circulation veineuse de retour cranien à propos de 10 études échotomographiques. Dijon: Mémoire; 1992.

11 Travell JG, Simons DG. Myofascial Pain and Dysfunction. Vol. 1. Baltimore: Williams and Wilkins; 1983:249, 276.

13 The nasal cavity and paranasal sinuses

THE NASAL CAVITY *(Figs 13.1, 13.2)*

Together with the pharynx, the nasal cavity forms part of the upper respiratory tract. It is located in the mid-region of the face between the orbits and the oral cavity. The nasal septum divides the nasal cavity into a right and a left half. The nasal cavity has a single anterior opening known as the piriform aperture. Posteriorly, the two halves of the nasal cavity communicate with the nasal part of the pharynx via the paired posterior nasal apertures (or choanae).

The morphology of the nose, paranasal sinuses and ethmoid bone[1]

The ethmoid bone occupies a key position, as important for the adjacent bones of the viscerocranium as the thorax is for the function of the pectoral girdle and upper limbs and for pulmonary respiration. It is the central point for the organization of the viscerocranium: the maxilla, frontal bone, palatine bone and lacrimal bone. It is through the ethmoid that breath is drawn into the olfactory region and respiratory tract, by way of the nasal conchae.

The structural changes occurring during the major phases of fetal growth are also reflected in the development of the paranasal sinuses.

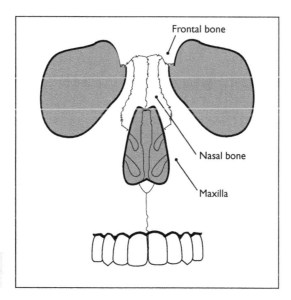

Figure 13.1 The nasal cavity, anterior view

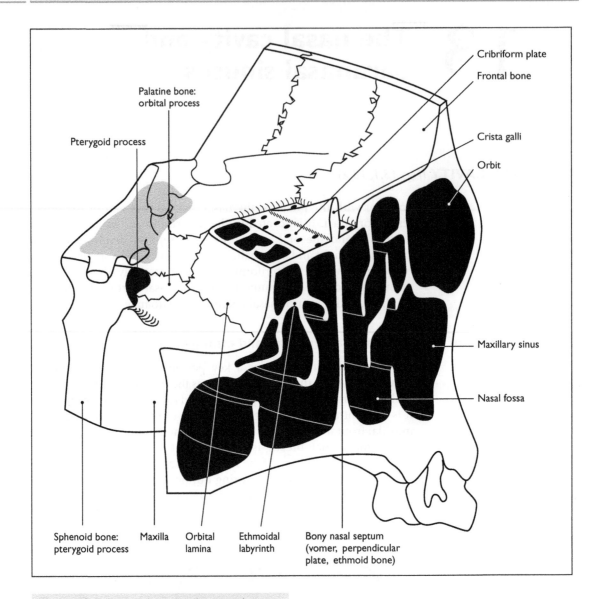

Palatine bone:
orbital process

Pterygoid process

Cribriform plate

Frontal bone

Crista galli

Orbit

Maxillary sinus

Nasal fossa

Sphenoid bone:
pterygoid process

Maxilla

Orbital
lamina

Ethmoidal
labyrinth

Bony nasal septum
(vomer, perpendicular
plate, ethmoid bone)

Figure 13.2 The nasal cavity and paranasal sinuses

These are present in rudimentary form in the embryo but only develop to full size between the ages of 3 and 21 years.

For Rohen, downward-directed pulmonary breathing is involved in the material development of physical substance: by contrast, the upward-directed breathing system evidences itself in a reduction in substance, as shown by the pneumatization of the cranial bones.

In addition, it is probable that respiratory rhythm acts on the CSF system of the brain via the cribriform plate. Olfaction is intimately related to the limbic system.

Development of the nasal cavity

The nasal capsule becomes cartilaginous during the 2nd month of intrauterine life and forms a cavity that is bounded laterally, medially, and above by walls of cartilage. The lateral mass of the ethmoid bone and the inferior nasal concha arise from this lateral wall. The medial wall develops into the cartilaginous nasal septum, except for its postero-inferior portion, which ossifies and forms the anlage for the vomer. The wings of the vomer extend as far as the sphenoid bone and are involved in forming the roof of the nasal part of the pharynx.

During the fetal period the cartilaginous nasal septum develops between the cranial base and the subjacent premaxilla, the palatine process of the maxilla, and the vomer. Its growth exerts a force downward and forward on maxillary growth and it is assisted in this by the appositional growth of the posterior superior border of the vomer.

The structural elements of the external nose *(Fig. 13.3)*

- Above, at the upper angle or root: the nasal bone and the frontal process of the maxilla. The remainder of the external nose is formed by cartilage that has its origin in the nasal capsule.
- On the dorsum of the nose: lateral nasal cartilage.
- At the wings or alae of the nose, in the area around the nostrils: major alar cartilage.
- The cartilaginous framework of the nose also includes other smaller components.
- The piriform (pear-shaped) anterior aperture of the nose is formed by the maxillae and the inferior border of the nasal bones.

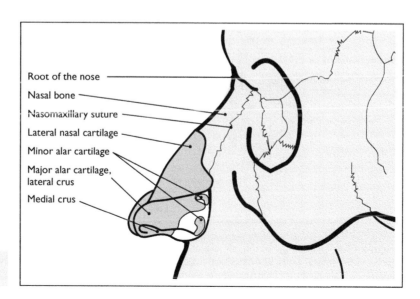

Root of the nose

Nasal bone

Nasomaxillary suture

Lateral nasal cartilage

Minor alar cartilage

Major alar cartilage, lateral crus

Medial crus

Figure 13.3 The external nose

The structure of the nasal cavity *(Fig. 13.4)*

The nostrils and the nasal vestibule

Air inhaled through the nostrils first arrives in the nasal vestibule. The vestibule is lined with stratified keratinized squamous epithelium and contains sebaceous and sweat glands. Short coarse hairs (vibrissae) prevent the passage of insects and particulate foreign matter carried with the current of inhaled air. In the nasal vestibule the nasal septum presents an area of slight thickening, which is the source of most nosebleeds.

The nasal conchae: The nasal conchae are relatively thin curved plates of bone projecting from the lateral wall of the nose. They serve to increase its surface area and are lined with mucous membrane that is permeated by abundant venous networks. In general, humans have three nasal conchae in each half of the nose. While the inferior nasal concha is an independent bone, the other two nasal conchae have their origin in the ethmoid bone. The inferior nasal concha commences posterior to the nasal vestibule and communicates with the nasopharyngeal meatus. It is the largest of the three nasal conchae.

The middle and superior nasal conchae each commence about 1.5 cm behind the anterior border of the immediately subjacent nasal

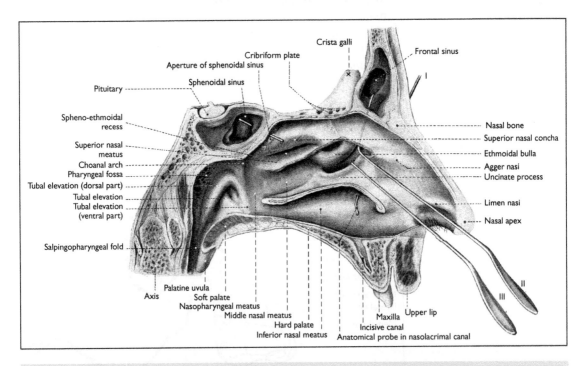

Figure 13.4 Medial view of the left lateral nasal wall. I, Anatomical probe in the nasolacrimal duct; II, Anatomical probe in the frontal sinus; III, Anatomical probe in the ethmoid infundibulum (From: Tillmann B. Farbatlas der Anatomie. Zahnmedizin – Humanmedizin. Stuttgart: Thieme; 1997)

concha. Above the superior nasal concha the spheno-ethmoidal recess communicates with the sphenoidal sinus.

The nasal meatuses

These are passages between the nasal conchae. The inferior nasal meatus lies between the palate and the inferior nasal concha. The middle nasal meatus is located between the inferior and middle nasal conchae, and the superior nasal meatus runs between the middle and superior nasal conchae.

The pharyngeal meatus

The three nasal meatuses unite to form the pharyngeal meatus. From that point the nasal cavity communicates posteriorly with the nasal part of the pharynx via the choanae. The choanae are bounded by the vomer, the ethmoid processes, the palatine bone, and the body of the sphenoid bone.

The functions of the nasal cavity

- To warm the inhaled air: The incoming air flows through the nasal conchae and in so doing it is warmed by the blood in the highly vascular mucous membrane permeated with venous plexuses.
- To moisten the inhaled air: The mucous membrane in the nasal conchae is continuously moistened by nasal glands.
- To filter out dust and bacteria: Dust particles adhere to the nasal mucosa. They are then transported by the mucosal ciliated epithelium into the pharynx, an area that in turn is rich in lymphoid tissue.
- To allow for testing by the sense of smell: e.g. food, harmful foul-smelling gases etc.
- To play a role in phonation (the paranasal sinuses provide resonance spaces for the voice).

The walls of the nasal cavity

Nasal septum (Fig. 13.5)

This comprises a bony, a cartilaginous and a connective tissue component:

- Bone: The perpendicular plate of the ethmoid bone and the vomer. (According to Magoun, rhythmic motion of the vomer stimulates drainage and circulation in the sphenoidal sinus and in the nasal cavity.)
- Cartilage: The septal cartilage of the nose extends to the tip (or apex) of the nose and also sends a process backward between the vomer and the perpendicular plate of the ethmoid bone.
- Connective tissue: This is the membranous part of the nasal septum, a small area behind the tip of the nose.

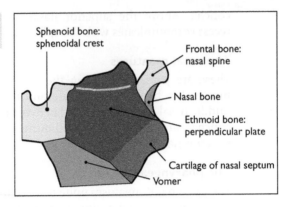

Figure 13.5 The nasal septum

Sphenoid bone: sphenoidal crest
Frontal bone: nasal spine
Nasal bone
Ethmoid bone: perpendicular plate
Cartilage of nasal septum
Vomer

The nasal septum is commonly deflected from the median plane. Breathing may be hindered in cases of marked asymmetry.

Roof (from the front backward)

Nasal bone, nasal part of the frontal bone, the cribriform plate of the ethmoid bone, and the anterior surface of the body of the sphenoid bone.

Floor (from the front backward)

Palatine process of the maxilla with the incisive bone and the horizontal plate of the palatine bone.

Lateral wall (from the front backward) *(see Fig. 13.2)*

- Nasal bone, frontal process and body of the maxilla, uncinate process and nasal conchae of the ethmoid bone, inferior nasal concha, and the perpendicular plate of the palatine bone.
- In addition, the embryological development of the vomer downward and forward plays a key role in the formation of the nasal cavity.
- The lateral wall accommodates the three nasal conchae: the superior and middle nasal conchae of the ethmoid bone, and an independent bone, the inferior nasal concha. The three nasal meatuses (superior, middle and inferior) pass between the nasal conchae.

Anterior sloping part

The nasal bone.

Structures communicating with the nasal cavity

At the lateral wall of the nose (Fig. 13.6):

- Above the superior nasal concha, via the spheno-ethmoidal recess: the sphenoidal sinus.
- Via the superior nasal meatus: the posterior ethmoidal air cells.

Figure 13.6 The nasal cavity: lateral nasal wall

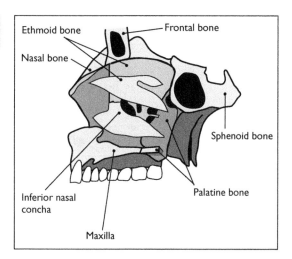

Ethmoid bone

Frontal bone

Nasal bone

Sphenoid bone

Inferior nasal concha

Palatine bone

Maxilla

- Via the middle nasal meatus, above the semilunar hiatus: the maxillary and frontal sinuses and the anterior ethmoidal air cells.
- Via the inferior nasal meatus: the nasolacrimal duct. This carries the superior posterior nasal branches (from CN V2) and the sphenopalatine artery (a branch of the maxillary artery) from the pterygopalatine fossa to the mucous membrane of the nose.

Neighboring structures (Fig. 13.7)

The anterior cranial fossa with the frontal lobe is separated from the spheno-ethmoidal recess of the nasal cavity only by the cribriform plate of the ethmoid bone.

On each side the cribriform plate presents about 20 foramina for the passage of the olfactory nerves. The olfactory bulb lies superior to the cribriform plate. The tubular sheaths of the olfactory nerves form a continuous tissue connection between the intracranial cerebrospinal fluid space and the lymph vessels of the nose.

The nasal mucous membrane

- Respiratory mucous membrane in the respiratory region: lines the major part of the nasal cavity.
- Olfactory mucous membrane in the olfactory region: lines the superior nasal concha (in the spheno-ethmoidal recess) and a small part of the nasal septum.

Respiratory mucous membrane

- This is composed of columnar ciliated epithelium interspersed with goblet cells. It is characterized by a particularly thick basement membrane, seromucous nasal glands, and cavernous venous plexuses over the nasal conchae, and is firmly attached to the bone without a submucosal layer.

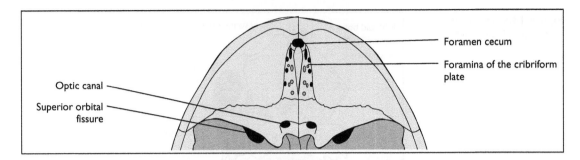

Figure 13.7 Neighboring structures of the nasal cavity: anterior cranial fossa

Olfactory mucous membrane

- This consists of olfactory, supporting (sustentacular) and basal cells.
- The olfactory cells are chemoreceptors. As primary sensory neurons (bipolar ganglion cells), their dendrite terminates at the free surface of the epithelium where it expands slightly to form a bulbous olfactory ending. Scattered over the surface of this bulbous ending, some 10 to 20 olfactory cilia project into a film of mucous secretion, which diffuses odors to the olfactory receptors.
- A non-myelinated axon from each receptor cell body runs in small bundles with other axons; these bundles join with others to form the fasciculi of the olfactory nerve. They pass through the cribriform plate of the ethmoid bone where they synapse with second-order sensory neurons.

THE PARANASAL SINUSES *(Fig. 13.8)*

The air-filled sinuses are excursions from the nasal cavity extending into adjacent bones. They communicate with the nasal cavity and are lined with the same mucous membrane. In the paranasal sinuses, however, this membrane has fewer glands and goblet cells and no venous plexuses. Nasal infections may spread to the paranasal sinuses relatively easily. Since the paired paranasal sinuses develop independently of each other, their shape is often asymmetrical.

Development of the paranasal sinuses

The nasal cavity epithelium grows into the surrounding mesenchyme. The paranasal sinuses increase in size as a result of bone resorption and mucosal growth. The point where they open into the nasal cavity is the site for the development of the sinus in question. The anlage for the paranasal sinuses is already established during the fetal period.

- The embryonic structures for the paranasal sinuses of the middle nasal meatus are the first to develop. Epithelial budding from the

Figure 13.8 The paranasal sinuses

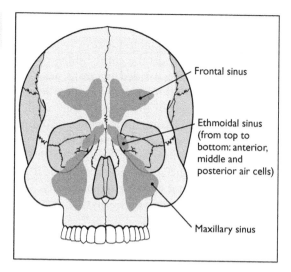

Frontal sinus

Ethmoidal sinus (from top to bottom: anterior, middle and posterior air cells)

Maxillary sinus

infundibular groove gives rise to the anlage for the maxillary and frontal sinuses and for the anterior ethmoidal air cells. The middle and sometimes the anterior ethmoidal air cells develop directly from the middle nasal meatus.

- Epithelial budding from the superior nasal meatus gives rise to the posterior ethmoidal air cells.
- The sphenoidal sinus develops from the posterior region of the nasal cavity.

While the first pneumatization of the sphenoidal and ethmoidal sinuses commences from the 3rd month of fetal life, the paranasal sinuses are still hardly detectable in neonates. They attain half their full size by the age of 10 years, and are fully sized following eruption of the permanent teeth. The development of the paranasal sinuses is therefore closely related to facial growth and dentition.

Factors influencing the development of the sphenoidal sinus:

- The replacement of red by yellow marrow at the level of the presphenoid immediately precedes the further pneumatization and development of the sphenoidal sinus from about the age of 3 years onward.
- A further factor influencing the development of the sphenoidal sinus appears to be the closure of the synchondroses in the sphenoid bone and of the synchondroses with the adjacent ethmoid and occipital bones. Residual synchondroses represent mechanical obstacles to the further development of the sinuses.

The function of the paranasal sinuses

- To provide resonance spaces for the voice.
- To enlarge the surface area of the nasal mucous membrane.
- To save weight: this aspect is trivial because they account for only about 1% of the total cranial weight.

The maxillary sinuses (paired) *(Fig. 13.9)*

These are the largest accessory air sinuses of the nose and, in adults, they fill almost the entire bodies of the maxillae. Each maxillary sinus resembles a 4-sided pyramid, with its base facing medially and its apex extending into the zygomatic process of the maxilla. The nerves and vessels in the walls of the maxillary sinus also become involved relatively easily in the event of inflammation.

Anterior wall: Anterior surface of the maxilla.

Posterior wall: Maxillary tuberosity, behind which lies the pterygopalatine fossa.

Roof: Orbital surface of the maxilla; the infraorbital nerve (CN V2) and the infraorbital vessels pass anteriorly.

Floor: Alveolar process of the maxilla; in intimate contact with the upper teeth.

Several subsidiary recesses may be encountered

The alveolar recess (intimate contact with the teeth), infraorbital recess (close to the nasolacrimal canal and the infraorbital canal), palatine recess (at the roof of the oral cavity), and zygomatic recess (at the lateral wall of the orbit).

Communication with the nasal cavity

The maxillary sinuses communicate with the middle nasal meatus through the semilunar hiatus via the ethmoidal infundibulum. The aperture is clearly above the level of the maxillary sinus floor.

The frontal sinuses (paired) *(Fig. 13.10)*

These are located in the frontal bone. Their size and shape are highly variable. Generally they grow into the squama of the frontal bone.

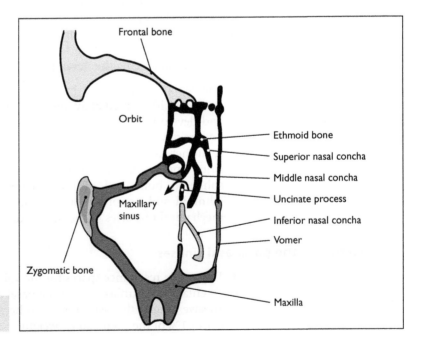

Figure 13.9 The maxillary sinus

Figure 13.10 The frontal sinus

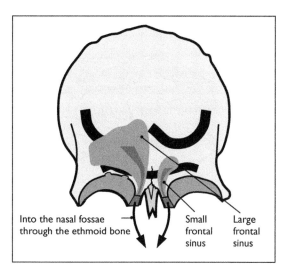

Into the nasal fossae through the ethmoid bone

Small frontal sinus

Large frontal sinus

Sometimes they also extend into the roof of the orbit, and laterally into the zygomatic process and to the lesser wings of the sphenoid bone. In rare cases the frontal sinuses may be absent altogether. The left and right frontal sinuses are separated by a thin bony septum. In most cases the frontal sinuses are asymmetric. Frontal sinus growth is completed by the age of 25 years.

The frontal sinuses are bordered by the anterior cranial fossa, the orbit and the anterior ethmoidal air cells.

Communication with the nasal cavity

The frontal sinuses communicate with the anterior part of the middle meatus of the corresponding half of the nasal cavity, sometimes directly by the frontonasal canal, and sometimes indirectly by the ethmoidal infundibulum. This communicating passage is directed inferiorly, which is advantageous in principle for the drainage of secretions. However, it may be blocked in the event of mucosal congestion, with the result that suppurative infections of the frontal sinuses, like those involving the maxillary sinuses, may be highly resistant to therapy.

The ethmoidal air cells (ethmoidal sinuses) (Fig. 13.11)

The ethmoidal cells are air-filled, thin-walled cavities in the ethmoid bone between the orbit and the nasal cavity. The cavities vary considerably in terms of size and number. Large cavities may encroach upon or subdivide surrounding paranasal sinuses. The ethmoidal air cells are known collectively as the ethmoidal labyrinth. One especially large rounded projection beneath the middle nasal concha is termed the ethmoidal bulla. This is thought to be a rudimentary nasal concha.

Figure 13.11 The ethmoidal air cells (lateral view of the ethmoid bone)

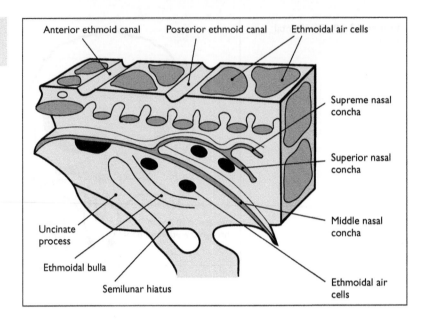

Anterior ethmoid canal   Posterior ethmoid canal   Ethmoidal air cells

Supreme nasal concha

Superior nasal concha

Middle nasal concha

Uncinate process

Ethmoidal bulla

Semilunar hiatus

Ethmoidal air cells

Communication with the nasal cavity

The anterior and middle ethmoidal air cells communicate with the middle nasal meatus, and the posterior ethmoidal air cells communicate with the superior nasal meatus.

The ethmoidal air cells are bordered by the orbit, the anterior cranial fossa, the frontal sinus and the sphenoidal sinus.

The sphenoidal sinuses (paired) *(Fig. 13.12)*

The sphenoidal sinuses are contained within the body of the sphenoid bone beneath the sella turcica. The intervening septum is asymmetric in most cases. The sphenoidal sinuses are situated behind the ethmoidal air cells. They may show considerable extensions, as follows:

- Posteriorly as far as the basal portion of the occipital bone.
- Laterally into the roots of the greater and lesser wings of the sphenoid bone.
- Inferiorly into the root of the pterygoid process of the sphenoid bone.
- Inferiorly and laterally to the foramen rotundum.
- Superiorly and anteriorly to the wall of the optic canal.

Each sphenoidal sinus communicates with the corresponding spheno-ethmoidal recess.

Neighboring structures

- Cranial: The pituitary, optic canal, prechiasmatic sulcus, anterior and middle cranial fossa. A band of tissue (the hypophyseal or craniopharyngeal duct) running obliquely to the pituitary provides

Figure 13.12 The sphenoidal sinus

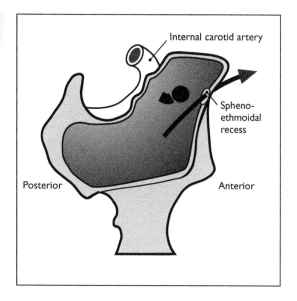

Internal carotid artery

Spheno-ethmoidal recess

Posterior

Anterior

a clue to the developmental pathway of the adenohypophysis from the roof of the pharynx to the sella turcica.

- Lateral: The cavernous sinus, internal carotid artery, CN III, IV, V1, V2, VI and the superior ophthalmic vein, sometimes the foramen rotundum.

Neighboring structures *(see Fig. 13.4)*

- Orbit: Below is the maxillary sinus, medially are the ethmoidal air cells, and above is the frontal sinus.
- Anterior cranial fossa and frontal lobe: The frontal sinus and ethmoidal air cells form a major part of the floor of the anterior cranial fossa.
- Middle cranial fossa: The sphenoidal sinus immediately beneath the sella turcica communicates with the pituitary gland and the cavernous sinus.
- Pterygopalatine fossa: The posterior wall of the sphenoidal sinus forms the anterior wall of the pterygopalatine fossa.
- Pharynx: The floor of the sphenoidal sinus forms the roof of the nasopharynx.
- Teeth: The roots of the upper row of teeth protrude more or less freely into the maxillary sinus.

Innervation of the nasal mucous membrane and external nose *(Figs 13.13a–c)*

1) Sensory innervation (Figs 13.14, 13.15)
- Branches of the ophthalmic nerve (CN V1): anterior and superior parts of the nasal cavity.

Figure 13.13 (a) Innervation of the nasal mucous membrane (From: Feneis H. Anatomisches Bildwörterbuch. 6th edition. Stuttgart: Thieme; 1988) (b) Nerve supply to the lateral nasal wall via branches of the maxillary nerve and ophthalmic nerve (c) Nerve supply to the nasal septum via branches of the maxillary nerve and nasociliary nerve (b and c from: Tillmann B. Farbatlas der Anatomie. Zahnmedizin – Humanmedizin. Stuttgart: Thieme; 1997)

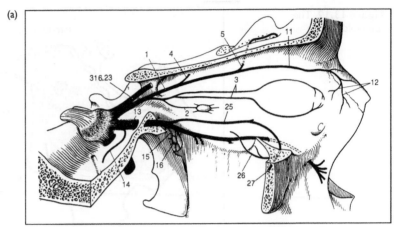

(a)

1	Nasociliary nerve	14	Meningeal branch
2	Communicating branch	15	Ganglionic branches
3	Long ciliary nerves	16	Pterygopalatine ganglion
4	Posterior ethmoidal nerve	25	Zygomatic nerve
5	Anterior ethmoidal nerve	26	Zygomaticotemporal branch
11	Infratrochlear nerve	27	Zygomaticofacial branch
12	Palpebral branches	316.23	Frontal nerve
13	Maxillary nerve		

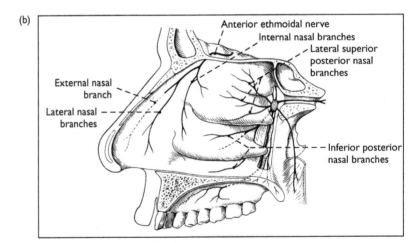

(b)

Anterior ethmoidal nerve
Internal nasal branches
Lateral superior posterior nasal branches
External nasal branch
Lateral nasal branches
Inferior posterior nasal branches

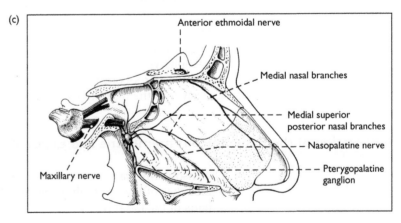

(c)

Anterior ethmoidal nerve
Medial nasal branches
Medial superior posterior nasal branches
Nasopalatine nerve
Pterygopalatine ganglion
Maxillary nerve

Figure 13.14 Schematic diagram of the ophthalmic nerve

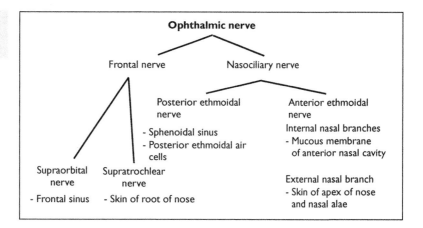

Figure 13.15 Schematic diagram of the maxillary nerve

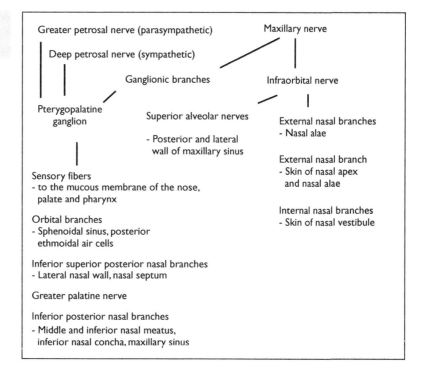

- Branches of the maxillary nerve (CN V2): middle, posterior and inferior parts of the nasal cavity via the pterygopalatine ganglion. The sensory nerve branches generally travel together with the arteries of the same name. The sensory nerves afford protection for the respiratory tract, e.g. by triggering the sneeze reflex. The external nose is also supplied by the trigeminal nerve. Branches of CN V1 supply the root of the nose, and branches of CN V2 the nasal alae.

2) Sympathetic innervation: The cell bodies of the preganglionic neurons are located in the spinal cord segment C8–Th2 between the

7th cervical and 2nd thoracic vertebrae. The postganglionic sympathetic fibers have their origin in the superior cervical ganglion. From the internal carotid plexus these run via the deep petrosal nerve to the pterygopalatine ganglion where they travel with the sensory nerves to the nasal cavity.

3) Parasympathetic innervation: The parasympathetic nerves are derived from the intermedius nerve (CN VII). They travel through the geniculate ganglion and pass via the greater petrosal nerve to the pterygopalatine ganglion. There they are relayed to postganglionic fibers and arrive at the mucous membrane of the nasal cavity.

4) Special sensory innervation: Olfactory nerves (CN I), see Olfactory mucous membrane.

Blood vessels

- Anterior ethmoidal artery (branch of the ophthalmic artery from the internal carotid artery): This passes through the anterior ethmoidal foramen of the ethmoid into the anterior cranial fossa and through the cribriform plate into the nasal cavity. It supplies the anterior part of the nasal cavity, the frontal sinus and the anterior ethmoidal air cells.
- Sphenopalatine artery (terminal branch of the maxillary artery from the external carotid artery): This passes from the pterygopalatine fossa through the sphenopalatine foramen and supplies the posterior part of the nasal cavity.
- Pterygoid venous plexus: This runs to the maxillary veins and further, via the retromandibular vein, into the facial vein to reach the internal jugular vein. A branch of the retromandibular vein also passes to the external jugular vein.
- Superior ophthalmic vein: A small supply of venous blood flows via this vein to the cavernous sinus.
- Facial vein: From the anterior nasal cavity.
- Pharyngeal veins: From the choanae.
- Superior sagittal sinus: In children a vein travels through the foramen cecum to the sinus (possible pathway for the spread of infection).
- External nose: Angular artery from the facial artery, dorsal nasal artery from the ophthalmic artery, facial vein.

Lymph drainage

- Most of the lymph from the posterior nasal cavity and the paranasal sinuses is transported to the cervical lymph nodes located behind the pharyngeal wall at the level of the second cervical vertebra.
- A smaller quantity is transported from the anterior nasal cavity to the submandibular lymph nodes.
- Lymph from the external nose is transported to the facial lymph nodes, the submandibular lymph nodes and, from the root of the nose, to the parotid lymph nodes.

LOCATION, CAUSES AND CLINICAL PRESENTATION OF DYSFUNCTIONS OF THE NASAL CAVITY AND PARANASAL SINUSES

Osseous dysfunction

Disturbances of the nasal cavity/paranasal sinuses may be caused not only by dysfunction of the bones forming the nasal cavity/paranasal sinuses, but also by dysfunction of virtually any cranial bone.

a) Frontal bone, frontal sinus
This may compromise the cribriform plate and the ethmoidal foramina in the ethmoidal notch. As a result, either the olfactory nerve or the anterior ethmoidal artery or vein may be impaired.

Clinical presentation: Functional disturbance of the frontal lobe and the orbits, olfactory disturbances etc.

b) Sphenoid bone, sphenoidal sinus
● The middle cranial fossa and the cavernous sinus are located above the sphenoidal sinus. Under certain circumstances, therefore, paranasal sinus inflammation may spread to involve the entire brain.

Clinical presentation: Functional disturbance of the pituitary, cavernous sinus, internal carotid artery, CN II, III, IV, V1, V2, and VI.

c) Maxilla, maxillary sinus
Causes: ● Because its aperture is clearly higher than the floor of the maxillary sinus, pus and secretions may accumulate there if ciliated epithelium movement is damaged (bacterial toxins etc.). Because of the position of the aperture, maxillary sinus inflammation is quite prolonged in most cases.

Clinical presentation: Sinusitis

● The anterior wall of the pterygopalatine fossa is in immediate proximity to the maxillary sinus.

Clinical presentation: Functional disturbance of the pterygopalatine ganglion.

● Other closely adjacent structures: anterior cranial fossa, orbit.
● Motion restriction of the frontal process is capable of limiting the expansion and retraction of the nasal cavity.

d) Ethmoid bone, ethmoidal sinuses
● A paper-thin layer of bone (the lamina papyracea) separates the ethmoidal air cells from the orbit, with the result that suppurating infections may spread to involve the orbit. However, they may also spread into the anterior cranial fossa or the frontal sinus.
● Dysfunction of the cribriform plate with subsequent disturbance of olfactory nerve function.
● In the course of its further growth during childhood, the perpendicular plate may be exposed to forces resulting in deviation of the nasal septum. This is the case, for example, if

insufficient space is available between the roof of the nose and the hard palate.

e) Orbit: Inflammation of the paranasal sinuses may spread relatively quickly to involve the orbit.

f) Teeth: Inflammatory, suppurating infections of the teeth may affect the maxillary sinuses, and vice versa.
Position of the dental roots:

- Incisor: at the floor of the nasal cavity.
- Canines: in the bone between the nasal cavity and maxillary sinus.
- Second premolars: anterior maxillary sinus.
- First and second molars: beneath the floor of the maxillary sinus (in rare cases they even protrude directly into the sinus).
- The first premolars and third molars generally have no contact with the maxillary sinus.

g) Nasal cavity: The anterior cranial fossa is separated from the spheno-ethmoidal recess of the nasal cavity only by the cribriform plate of the ethmoid bone.

Clinical presentation: Functional disturbance of the frontal lobe.

h) Nasal septum: According to Magoun, septal scoliosis is usually the consequence of dietary deficiencies in the 'civilized' world, which lead to developmental disorders of the perpendicular plate of the ethmoid bone, the vomer and the cartilage of the nasal septum.[2] Later dysfunctions of the ethmoid bone, vomer or maxilla may also develop.

Sequelae and clinical presentation: Impairment of nasal perfusion or innervation, disordered nasal breathing (with consequent mouth breathing), leading to sleep disturbances, concentration and learning difficulties, and changes in the shape of the palate.

i) Temporal bone: Disturbance of the intermedius nerve (CN VII) and at the trigeminal impression, disturbance of the ophthalmic nerve (CN V1) and maxillary nerve (CN V2).

Clinical presentation: Innervation disturbance to the mucous membrane and skin of the nose and disturbed glandular function (parasympathetic system).

j) Cervical spine and C8 to Th2: Disturbance of sympathetic nerve function.

k) Sternoclavicular joint and upper costal dysfunctions may result in venolymphatic stasis.

Muscle dysfunction

a) Abnormal tension on the myofascial masticatory system (masseter muscle etc.) and neck muscles (digastric, sternocleidomastoid, omohyoid muscles etc.) may cause venolymphatic stasis.

b) Muscle spasms may have a minute yet direct adverse influence on the position and motion of the bones of the paranasal sinuses. Such spasms may be secondary to tension on the neck muscles or more rarely be a direct response to injury.

Thus, increased neck muscle tone may move the occiput into PRM flexion. This abnormal tension may be transmitted forward via the falx cerebri to the frontal and ethmoid bones, resulting in minute positional changes to these.

Masseter muscle spasm may draw the maxilla backward, while unilateral spasm of the anterior part of the temporal muscle may move the frontal bone laterally.

c) Orbicularis oculi muscle[3]

Causes: Strabismus, frequent frowning, as a secondary phenomenon following sternocleidomastoid muscle dysfunction.

Clinical presentation: Pain in the nose and tip of the nose.

d) Masseter muscle

Clinical presentation: Pain as in maxillary sinusitis.[4]

e) Lateral pterygoid muscle and sternocleidomastoid muscle (sternal part)

Clinical presentation: Maxillary sinus pain.

Nerve disturbances

a) Olfactory nerves (CN I)

Causes: Ethmoid bone dysfunction: On each side the cribriform plate presents about 20 foramina for the passage of the olfactory nerves. The olfactory bulb lies superior to the cribriform plate. The tubular sheaths of the olfactory nerves form a continuous tissue connection between the intracranial cerebrospinal fluid space and the lymph vessels of the nose.

Clinical presentation: Olfactory disturbances.

b) Ophthalmic nerve (CN V1) and maxillary nerve (CN V2) and their branches

Causes: Dysfunction involving the temporal bone (trigeminal impression), sphenoid bone (superior orbital fissure, foramen rotundum), cavernous sinus, pterygopalatine foramen (CN V2), orbital surface of the maxilla (CN V2).

Clinical presentation: CN V1:

- Disturbed innervation to the mucous membrane of the anterior and superior nasal cavity and of the root of the nose.

CN V2:

- Disturbed innervation to the mucous membrane of the medial, posterior and inferior nasal cavity and of the skin at the nasal alae.

c) Sympathetic system

Causes: Temporal bone dysfunction:

- Foramen lacerum and carotid canal (internal carotid plexus), from the 1st to 4th cervical vertebrae (superior cervical ganglion), from the 7th cervical to 2nd thoracic vertebrae (preganglionic neurons in spinal cord segment C8–Th2).

Sphenoid bone dysfunction:

- Pterygoid canal.

d) Parasympathetic system, via the intermedius nerve (CN VII), greater petrosal nerve, nerve of the pterygoid canal.

Causes: Temporal bone dysfunction:

- Facial canal, sulcus of the greater petrosal nerve.

Sphenoid bone dysfunction:

- Pterygoid canal.

The parasympathetic fibers regulate the mucosal glands and hence the production of secretion in the nose. Parasympathetic and sympathetic fibers jointly innervate the vessels of the mucous membrane. By supplying the arteriovenous communications and the prominent venous plexuses, these nerves are able to regulate their level of filling. As a result, internal nerve stimuli may also be involved in the causation of rhinitis or sinusitis (swelling of the nasal mucosa). Sympathetic stimulation constricts the venous plexuses in the nose and enlarges the nasal spaces. Parasympathetic stimulation produces nasal vasodilatation and contracts the nasal spaces.

e) Pterygopalatine ganglion:

Clinical presentation: see above.

Vascular disturbances

a) Maxillary veins

Cause: Congestion of the internal jugular vein.

b) Superior ophthalmic vein

Cause: Congestion of the cavernous sinus or internal jugular vein.

c) Superior sagittal sinus: Spread of infection in children through the foramen cecum.

d) The facial vein communicates with the superior ophthalmic vein via the angular vein, with the result that suppurating inflammation of the external nose may spread to involve the cavernous sinus.

e) Anterior ethmoidal artery

Cause: Dysfunction of the ethmoid and frontal bones, or of the frontoethmoidal suture.

f) Sphenopalatine artery

Cause: Dysfunction of the sphenoid bone, palatine bone and maxilla, e.g. following a fall on to the face.

g) Lymphatic stasis

Causes of dysfunction in the nasal cavities and paranasal sinuses

- Intraosseous trauma: pre-, peri- and postnatal.
- Falls and blows may result in restricted motion of the bones of the nasal cavity.
- Sphenoid bone dysfunction due to SBS dysfunctions (most likely, extension/IR dysfunctions) may result in restricted motion of the nasal cavity bones or in nasal septum deviation. Also, developmental disorders of the cranial base in the embryo lead to developmental disorders of the nasal cavities.
- Dental inflammation, bacteria, bacterial toxins.
- Excessive stress (psychological and physical).
- Incorrect diet.
- Neurovegetative dysregulation (sympathetic and parasympathetic innervation).
- Allergic disposition.
- Enlarged tonsils or polyps.
- Mouth breathing

Causes: Mechanical obstructions (polyps), septal deviation, sinusitis, recurrent rhinitis,[5] spinal column dysfunction/deformity, especially of the cervical spine, bottle-feeding of infants (absence of the necessary formative stimulus and movement stimulus to develop oral, including lingual, function: e.g. there is no powerful increase in orbicularis oris muscle tone necessary for mouth closure in nasal breathing),[6] tight-fitting clothing,[7] nutritional deficiencies,[8,9] thumbsucking.[10]

Sequelae: Altered palate shape, altered lip position, possibly altered tongue position, jaw anomalies (e.g. a lowered mandible), spinal column changes (extension position, scoliosis etc.) and sometimes altered growth of the lower and middle thirds of the face, lymphatic and venous congestion with hyperplasia of the respiratory mucous membrane, dryness of the lips, oral cavity, and pharyngeal and bronchial mucosa, infections of the pharynx and respiratory tract, tonsillar changes, polyps, neurohormonal dysregulation (e.g. via a neurovascular reflex arc from the nasal mucosa to the anterior lobe of the pituitary), sleep disturbances, problems with concentration and learning.[5,6]

DIAGNOSIS AND ASSESSMENT *(Table 13.1)*

History-taking

- Nasal secretion: for how long, what color (clear, yellowish), what consistency (watery, mucous, crusted)?
- Nasal breathing: impaired, unilaterally or bilaterally (unilateral: possible nasal septum deviation, foreign body, tumor)?

Table 13.1 Differential diagnosis of sinusitis

	Pain (on pressure/percussion)	Secretion discharged into
Maxillary sinusitis	Maxilla (possibly at the parietal bone initially)	Pharynx
Frontal sinusitis	Frontal bone (above the eyes)	Nose
Ethmoidal sinusitis	Behind the nose, medial to the orbit; raised intraocular pressure, possibly lacrimation, conjunctivitis	Pharynx
Sphenoidal sinusitis	Behind the frontal bone, in the whole cranium/mid-cranium in the area of the calvaria	Pharynx

- Is the patient breathing increasingly through the mouth?
- Is there evidence of toothache or dental disease?
- Is the sense of smell reduced or lost?
- Are other symptoms present (fever, sore throat, nervous disorders, general state of health, etc.)?
- Has the patient been taking medication (nasal drops, oral contraceptives, reserpine, alcohol, etc.), and over what time period?
- Are the symptoms seasonal or are they dependent on exposure to certain substances (allergic rhinitis)?
- Local headache, feeling of tension, dull sensation, face/head sensitive to cold, facial pain, possibly fever (sinusitis)?
- Bleeding from the nose (trauma, nose picking, inflammation, dry mucosa, tumor, foreign body, bleeding disorders, leukemia etc.)?
- What is the patient 'fed up with'?

Inspection

- Widened or narrowed nostrils may be the result of maxillary injury or disturbance.
- Acute rhinitis: nostrils reddened, formation of secretion, nasal mucosa swollen, nasal breathing impaired.
- Allergic rhinitis: swollen blue-reddish nasal mucosa, itchy nose, eyes etc., clear, watery secretion.
- Hyper-reflectory/vasomotor rhinitis: symptoms as for allergic rhinitis, but no allergen detected, rhinitis triggered by psychological, emotional stress.
- Furuncle: painful and usually swollen and reddened site at the nasal vestibule; caution, do not burst by squeezing.
- Septal deviation to the left or right.
- Accompanying symptoms in chronic nasal obstruction: Unilateral or bilateral crossbite. Narrow maxillary arch. Enlarged tonsils or polyps. Altered position of tongue and lips. Extension of cervical spine. Disturbance of the TMJ and maxilla. Slightly lowered

mandible. Altered growth of lower and middle thirds of face. Possible upward and forward displacement of hyoid bone.

Motion testing of the nasal cavity and paranasal sinuses

Palpation of primary respiration *(Fig. 13.16)*

Therapist: Take up a position at the head of the patient.

Hand position: ➤ Place the index fingers of both hands on either side of the nose, with the middle fingers on the frontal processes of the maxillae.

Biomechanical approach
Inspiration phase of PR, normal finding (Fig. 13.17):

- Increase in horizontal and decrease in vertical diameter of the nasal cavity.
- The posterior part of the inferior border of the vomer is lowered, and its anterior part is raised.

Expiration phase of PR, normal finding:

- Decrease in horizontal and increase in vertical diameter of the nasal cavity.
- The posterior part of the inferior border of the vomer is raised, and its anterior part is lowered.

Biodynamic/embryological approach
Inspiration phase of PR, normal finding (Fig. 13.18):

- Lateral, anterior and inferior widening of the nasal cavity.
- Lowering of the nasal cavity.
- The nasal septum moves downward and forward.

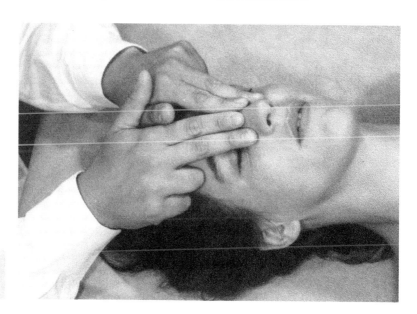

Figure 13.16 Palpation of primary respiration of the nasal cavity

Figure 13.17 The inspiration phase of PR/ biomechanical approach

Figure 13.17 The inspiration phase of PR/ biomechanical approach

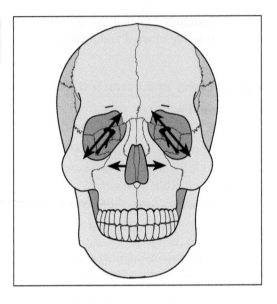

Figure 13.18 The inspiration phase of PR/biodynamic approach

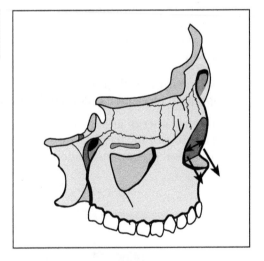

- Compare the amplitude, force, ease and symmetry of nasal cavity motion.
- Other types of motion of the nasal cavity may also sometimes occur during external and internal rotation. These provide an indication as to further dysfunctions of the respective bones of the nasal cavity.
- Unilateral or bilateral dysfunctions of the nasal cavity may be encountered.

In addition, palpate the entire face by placing your thumbs next to the metopic suture and on either side of the nasal bone, your index fingers bilaterally on the maxilla, and your ring fingers on the zygomatic bone.

Motion testing

This differs from palpation of primary respiration only in as much as the external and internal rotation motion of the nasal cavity is now actively induced by the therapist in harmony with primary respiration.

Testing the nasal septum (Fig. 13.19).

Patient: Supine.

Therapist: Take up a position to one side of the patient's head.

Hand position: Cranial hand:

> ➤ Place your index finger below the nasion on the internasal suture. Locate your middle finger on the glabella.

Caudal hand:

> ➤ Place your index finger directly behind the incisor teeth on the median palatine suture. Position your middle finger further back on the median palatine suture.

Method: During the inspiration phase of PR:

> ➤ At the beginning of the inspiration phase, deliver a slight impulse cephalad with the index finger that is on the median palatine suture.
> ➤ With the index finger that is on the internasal suture, you will sense a minute anterior motion (flexion of the ethmoid bone) in response to this pressure. *Remember:* The lower part of the anterior surface of the ethmoid moves anteriorly during the inspiration phase of PR.

During the expiration phase of PR:

> ➤ At the beginning of the expiration phase, deliver a slight impulse cephalad with the middle finger that is on the median palatine suture.

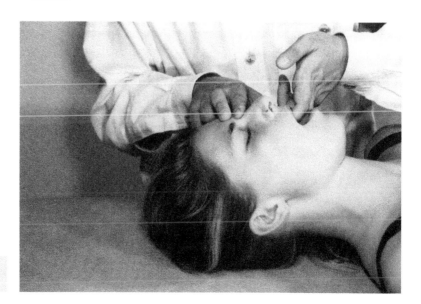

Figure 13.19 Testing the nasal septum

➤ With the middle finger that is on the glabella, you will sense a minute anterior motion (extension of the ethmoid bone) in response to this pressure.

➤ To check this, administer pressure on the nasion (extension) and the glabella (flexion) and palpate the pressure response at the vomer using the fingers that are on the median palatine suture. Compare the amplitude of motion, ease of motion, and the force required to elicit motion.

Note: This method can, of course, also be used as therapy for motion restrictions.

Palpation: Specific palpation of the SBS and of each individual bone of the nasal cavity/paranasal sinuses and their sutural junctions (see the respective chapters in each case):

● Nasal bone: frontonasal, internasal, ethmoidonasal, nasomaxillary, nasoseptal sutures.
● Vomer: sphenovomeral, vomeroethmoidal, vomeromaxillary, vomeropalatine, vomeroseptal sutures.
● Frontal bone: sphenofrontal, frontoethmoidal, coronal, frontomaxillary, frontozygomatic, frontonasal, frontolacrimal sutures.
● Ethmoid bone: sphenoethmoidal, vomeroethmoidal, fronto-ethmoidal, ethmoidonasal, ethmoidomaxillary, palatoethmoidal, lacrimoethmoidal sutures.
● Maxilla: frontomaxillary, ethmoidomaxillary, zygomaticomaxillary, lacrimomaxillary, transverse palatine, palatomaxillary, naso-maxillary, vomeromaxillary, conchomaxillary, median palatine sutures.

Chapman reflex points in sinusitis:

Anterior: At the 2nd costal cartilage and first intercostal space, 8 cm lateral to the sternum.

Posterior: Mid-way between the spinous process and transverse process of the axis.

TREATMENT OF THE NASAL CAVITY

Treatment methods

1. Global examination and, where appropriate, treatment.
2. Treatment of the anterior and posterior cervical fasciae and possibly of the other diaphragms.
3. Examination and treatment of the cranium, especially of the SBS and vomer, in particular using the vomer pump technique.
4. Special examination and treatment of the cervical spine, especially the upper cervical spine (superior cervical ganglion) and C7 to Th2 (preganglionic neurons in spinal cord segment C8 to Th2), and of the sacrum. (According to McIntyre, 31% of patients with

paranasal sinus problems also have upper cervical spine symptoms).[11]

5. Treatment of the nerve supply system: (a) Inhibition of the superior cervical ganglion.[12] (b) Technique for the pterygopalatine ganglion (see Pterygopalatine fossa and Maxilla: decompression of the maxillary complex at the pterygopalatine suture).[13] (c) Technique for the trigeminal ganglion.

6. Improvement of venolymphatic drainage: (a) General: thoracocervical diaphragm (including upper costal joints, sternoclavicular joint), AO release, venous sinus technique, 4th ventricle compression (CV-4), release of diaphragmatic tensions (= primary lymphatic pump). (b) Local: drainage of the pterygoid venous plexus, fascial venolymphatic techniques.

7. Stimulation of the arterial system: treatment of the common carotid artery and external carotid artery.

8. Specific examination and treatment (including V-spread technique) of the individual bones and sutures of the nasal cavity and paranasal sinuses, in particular of the nasal bone, maxilla, frontal, ethmoid, sphenoid, and zygomatic bones.[14] Sutural manipulations that are indicated particularly commonly: widening of the ethmoidal notch of the frontal bone (see Ethmoid bone), ethmoidomaxillary suture (see Maxilla lift and spread technique), frontozygomatic suture, metopic suture.

9. Endonasal massage (Röder's technique).

10. Local treatment of the paranasal sinuses: vomer pump technique (see Sphenoid bone), ethmoid pump technique (see Ethmoid bone), drainage of the frontal and maxillary sinuses, unilateral drainage of the ethmoidal air cells, self-help technique for ethmoidal air cell drainage, drainage of the nasal alae, endonasal massage.

11. Treatment of the floor of the mouth, the masseter muscle and the sternocleidomastoid muscle.

12. Harmonization and stimulation of the immune defense organs: spleen, liver, thymus, appendix, general lymph techniques, lymphatic pump technique for the feet etc.

13. Resolution of underlying causal factors of an emotional nature.

14. Regulation of diet: cutting down on or avoiding dairy products and refined sugar.

Of course, treatment should always be implemented in cooperation with a medical specialist. Sometimes surgical intervention may be required to correct severe nasal septum deviation or other structural pathologies. Häfner and Stadler (2002)[15] investigated the efficacy of osteopathic treatment in refractory chronic sinusitis. Forty-three patients were subdivided into three groups that were assigned to different treatment modalities: Group 1: weekly osteopathic treatment; Group 2: daily nasal lavage with isotonic saline solution; Group 3: a combination of weekly osteopathic treatment and daily nasal lavage. The treatment period for each study participant was 4 weeks and the total assessment period lasted for 10 weeks. The treatments were administered by two osteopaths.

Result: Marked improvements in symptoms (nasal breathing, headache, tension in head, flow of secretion, quality of life) were recorded in participants in both osteopathy groups ($n = 28$); in particular, these improvements were further confirmed in most cases after the 6-week break from treatment. The positive symptom changes recorded in Group 2 ($n = 15$) were frequently not sustained during the 6-week break from treatment.

Inhibition of the superior cervical ganglion *(Figs 13.20a,b)*

Therapist: Take up a position at the head of the patient.

(a)

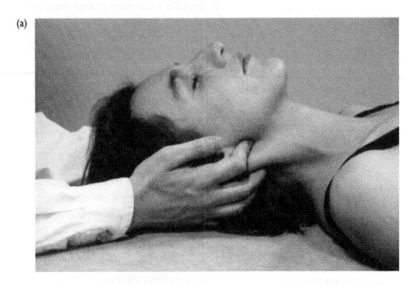

(b)

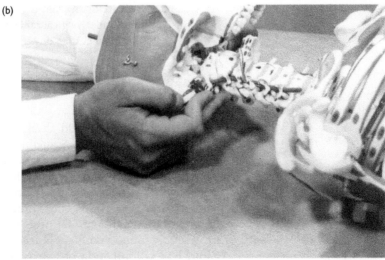

Figure 13.20 (a,b)
Inhibition of the superior cervical ganglion

Hand position: ➤ On each side of the patient's head, place your index fingers on the lateral masses of the first cervical vertebra in front of the sternocleidomastoid muscles.

➤ On each side of the patient's head, place your middle fingers on the posterior margin of the transverse processes of the second cervical vertebra.

Method: ➤ Place the patient's head in slight extension.

➤ With your index and middle fingers, apply gentle pressure in an anterior direction on to the vertebrae. Hold this pressure for 90 s.

Venous pump technique for the clavicle *(Fig. 13.21)*

Therapist: Take up a position beside the patient's head on the side being treated.

Hand position: Cranial hand:

➤ Span the mandible.

Caudal hand:

➤ Place the thenar eminence of your thumb at the medial end of the clavicle, and hold your arm at a slightly oblique angle.

Method: ➤ With your caudal hand, deliver a rhythmic pumping movement at the medial end of the clavicle.

➤ With your cranial hand, fix the patient's head in slight extension and contralateral rotation to ensure traction on the anterior myofascial structure.

➤ Always perform the technique bilaterally. When using this technique, always take care also to release the anterior and lateral myofascial structures.

Note: When used on the right-hand side, this technique not only promotes venous return but also stimulates the right common carotid artery. To stimulate the left common carotid artery, perform the technique on the sternum.

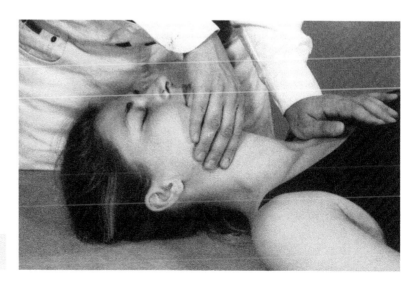

Figure 13.21 Venous pump technique for the clavicle

Pterygoid plexus *(Fig. 13.22)*

Therapist: Take up a position to one side of the patient's head.

Hand position: Place the thumbs of both hands outside on the patient's cheek. Locate the index fingers of both hands on the inner surface of the cheek, on a level with the ascending ramus of the mandible. Position your thumbs and index fingers below the zygomatic arch and take hold of the cheek tissue at the point where the pterygoid venous plexus surrounds the lateral pterygoid muscle.

Method:
➤ Squeeze the tissues and draw them apart between your fingers.
➤ The force employed should never exceed the pain threshold; on the contrary, it should feel pleasant to the patient.
➤ It is also necessary to treat the other venolymphatic structures in the middle and lower face (facial vein, deep facial vein etc.) in a similar way.

Treatment of the external carotid artery *(Fig. 13.23)*

Treat the point where the maxillary artery branches off from the external carotid artery.

Aim: To improve the arterial blood supply to the nasal cavity.

Patient: Head turned away from the side being treated.

Therapist: Take up a position at the head of the patient.

Hand position:
➤ Span the mandible with the cranial hand, positioning your thumb on the angle of the mandible.
➤ Cradle the occiput with the caudal hand, positioning your thumb directly below the angle of the mandible.

Method: ➤ Apply slight pressure to the tissue with your thumbs, moving them in concert toward each other and then apart again.

Endonasal massage (Röder's technique) *(Figs 13.24a,b)*

While your little finger may also be used to treat the individual nasal conchae, this is not really possible without a mild local anesthetic.

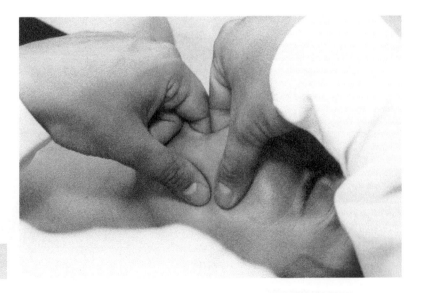

Figure 13.22 The pterygoid venous plexus

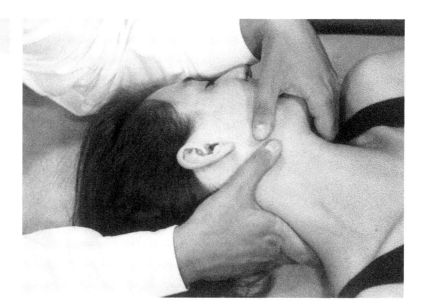

Figure 13.23 Treatment of the external carotid artery

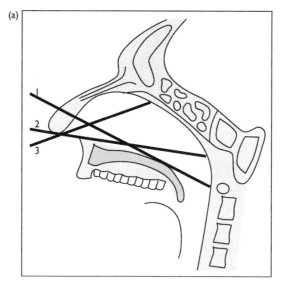

(a)

(b)

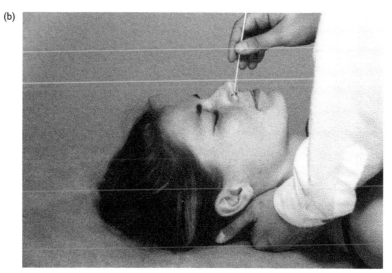

Figure 13.24 (a) Endonasal massage. 1. Inferior nasal meatus: approximately in the direction of the 7th cervical vertebra. 2. Middle nasal meatus: approximately in the direction of the cranial base or 1st cervical vertebra. 3. Superior nasal meatus: approximately parallel to the dorsum of the nose.
(b) Endonasal massage: inferior nasal meatus.
(c) Endonasal massage: middle nasal meatus.
(d) Endonasal massage: superior nasal meatus

(c)

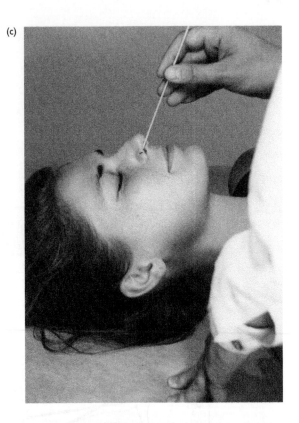

(d)

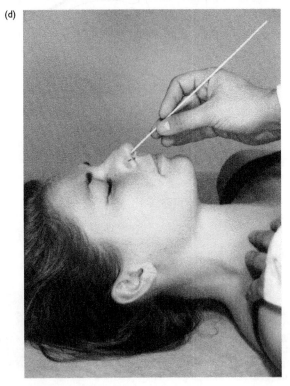

Figure 13.24 *(continued)*

Röder's technique is more appropriate and can be used with similar success.

Indication: Chronic sinusitis, anosmia, and to improve drainage.

Method:
1. Inferior nasal meatus (see Fig. 13.24b): Take a cotton bud moistened with nasal oil and insert it carefully into the inferior nasal meatus (in the direction of the 7th cervical vertebra) until it touches the posterior wall of the pharynx. Gently massage there a few times and withdraw the bud again.
2. Middle nasal meatus (Fig. 13.24c): Take a cotton bud moistened with nasal oil and insert it into the nose in the direction of the cranial base.
3. Superior nasal meatus (Fig. 13.24d): Take a cotton bud moistened with nasal oil and insert it into the nose in a direction parallel to the dorsum.

Note: Endonasal massage generally provokes an increasingly runny nose.

Drainage of the frontal sinuses *(Fig. 13.25)*

Therapist: Take up a position at the head of the patient.

Hand position:
➤ Place your thumbs on the frontal bone bilaterally, above the eyes at the level of the frontal sinuses.
➤ Position your other fingers along the side of the cranium. They are passive.

Method:
➤ With your thumbs, apply gentle circular pressure at the level of the sinuses.
➤ Start directly above the eyes and work gradually in a lateral direction.

Drainage of the maxillary sinuses *(Fig. 13.26)*

Therapist: Take up a position at the head of the patient.

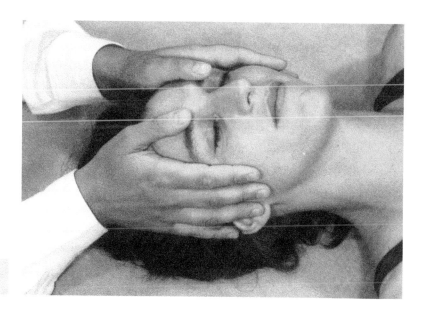

Figure 13.25 Drainage of the frontal sinus

Figure 13.26 Drainage of the maxillary sinus

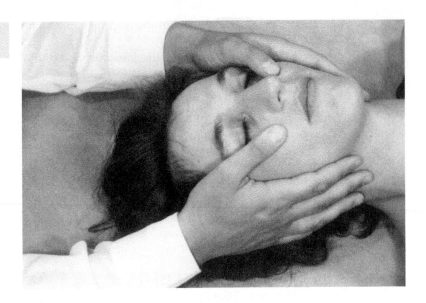

Hand position:	➤ Place your thumbs on the maxillae bilaterally, below the eyes at the level of the maxillary sinuses.
	➤ Position your other fingers along the mandibular angle. They are passive.
Method:	➤ With your thumbs, apply gentle circular pressure at the level of the sinuses.
	➤ Start directly below the eyes and work downward along the nasolabial sulcus.

Unilateral drainage of the ethmoidal air cells (example shown: right side) *(Fig. 13.27)*

Therapist:	Take up a position to the (left) side of the patient's head on the opposite side to that being treated.
Hand position:	Cranial hand:

➤ Place your thumb on the (left) side of the frontal bone, i.e. on the side opposite the dysfunction. Place your index finger on the frontal process of the (right) maxilla. Place your middle finger on the anterior surface of the (right) maxilla. Rest your ring finger and little finger on the (right) zygomatic bone.

Caudal hand:

➤ Place your index finger inside the patient's mouth on the median palatine suture, anterior to the transverse palatine suture. Place your middle finger inside the patient's mouth on the median palatine suture, posterior to the transverse palatine suture.

Alternative hand position:	➤ Place your index finger only on the median palatine suture, both anterior and posterior to the transverse palatine suture. Only use this alternative if you are able to sense and induce the flexion and extension of the vomer using this finger position.

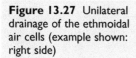

Figure 13.27 Unilateral drainage of the ethmoidal air cells (example shown: right side)

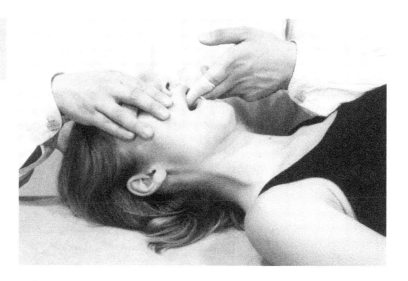

Method: During the inspiration phase of PR:

> ➤ Encourage motion of the frontal bone, maxilla and zygomatic bone into external rotation.
> ➤ At the same time, administer pressure in a superior direction with the index finger of your caudal hand (superiorly directed impulse in front of the transverse palatine suture: flexion). This encourages motion of the ethmoid bone into flexion, via the vomer.

During the expiration phase of PR:

> ➤ Encourage motion of the frontal bone, maxilla and zygomatic bone into internal rotation.
> ➤ At the same time, administer pressure in a superior direction with the middle finger of your caudal hand (superiorly directed impulse behind the transverse palatine suture: extension). This encourages motion of the ethmoid bone into extension, via the vomer.
> ➤ Repeat for several cycles of primary respiration.

Self-help technique for drainage of the ethmoidal sinus *(Fig. 13.28)*

Patient: Seated.

Hand position:
> ➤ Place the thumb of one hand at the intersection of the median and transverse palatine sutures.
> ➤ Support both elbows on a table.

Method:
> ➤ Slowly and gently bend the head forward to increase the pressure on the thumbs.
> ➤ Breathe deeply in this position for several cycles.

Drainage of the nasal alae *(Fig. 13.29)*

Indication: To improve nasal breathing and to regenerate the nasal mucous membrane.

Figure 13.28 Self-help technique for ethmoidal sinus drainage

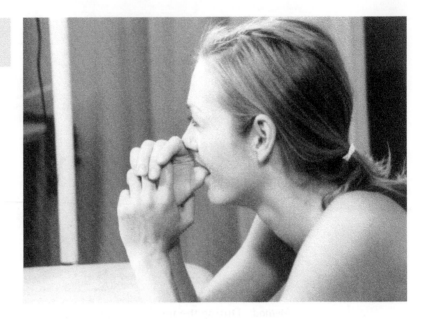

Figure 13.29 Drainage of the nasal alae

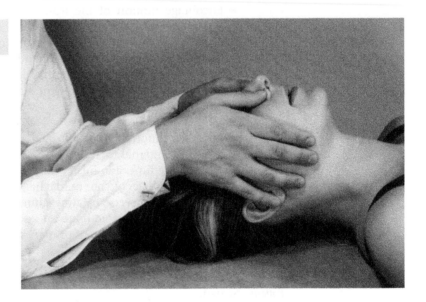

Therapist: Take up a position at the head of the patient.

Hand position: ➤ Position your thumbs on the nasal alae on both sides.

Method: ➤ Use your thumbs to exert medial pressure on the nasal alae.
➤ Start cranially where the soft tissues begin and work in a caudal direction as far as the nostrils.

Note: Discontinue the technique if it feels uncomfortable for the patient. Inform the patient that lacrimation may be induced after the technique has been completed.

Figure 13.30 F. Buset's technique for the sternocleidomastoid muscle

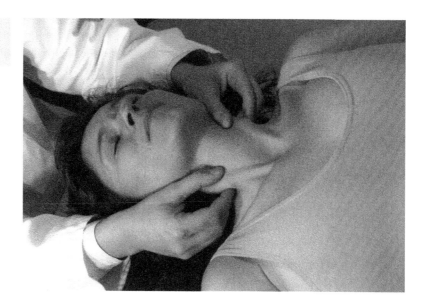

F. Buset's technique for the sternocleidomastoid muscle *(Fig. 13.30)*

Therapist: Take up a position at the head of the patient.

Hand position: ➤ Take hold of both sternocleidomastoid muscles, as shown.

Method: ➤ Move the sternocleidomastoid muscle together with the superficial fascial layer laterally and medially, and mobilize in relation to the pretracheal fascial layer and the hyoid muscles.

References

1 Rohen JW. Morphologie des Menschlichen Organismus. 2nd edn. Stuttgart: Verlag Freies Geistesleben; 2002:391.

2 Magoun HI. Osteopathy in the Cranial Field. 3rd edn. Kirksville: Journal Printing Company; 1976:211.

3 Travell JG, Simons DG. Myofascial Pain and Dysfunction. Vol. 1. Baltimore: Williams and Wilkins; 1983:282, 285.

4 Travell JG, Simons DG. Myofascial Pain and Dysfunction. Vol. 1. Baltimore: Williams and Wilkins; 1983:219.

5 Travell JG, Simons DG. Myofascial Pain and Dysfunction. Vol. 1. Baltimore: Williams and Wilkins; 1983:276.

6 Bahnemann F. Anthropologische Grundlagen einer Ganzheitsmedizin aus kieferorthopädischer Sicht. Heidelberg: Haug; 1992:84.

7 Bahnemann F., ed. Der Bionator in der Kieferorthopädie. Grundlagen und Praxis. Heidelberg: Haug; 1993:28, 30–44.

8 Magoun HI. Osteopathy in the Cranial Field. 3rd edn. Kirksville: Journal Printing Company; 1976:98.

9 Bahnemann F. Anthropologische Grundlagen einer Ganzheitsmedizin aus kieferorthopädischer Sicht. Heidelberg: Haug; 1992:111–119.

10 Magoun HI. Osteopathy in the Cranial Field. 3rd edn. Kirksville: Journal Printing Company; 1976:213.

11 McIntire LD, Hoyt WH III. The ethmoid sinus as an etiology of cephalgia. National Osteopathic Foundation Clinical Presentation, Colorado Springs, COLO, 1984/3.

12 Hoyt WH III. Current concepts in management of sinus disease. J Am Osteopath Assoc 1990; 90(10):913–919.

13 Hoyt WH III. Current concepts in management of sinus disease. J Am Osteopath Assoc 1990; 90(10):183.

14 Magoun HI. Osteopathy in the Cranial Field. 3rd edn. Kirksville: Journal Printing Company; 1976:290.

15 Häfner S, Stadler M. Osteopathie und chronische Sinusitis. Pilotstudie. Diploma thesis, COE, AOD: Schlangenbad; 2002.

The eye

THE MORPHOLOGY OF THE EYE ACCORDING TO ROHEN[1]

In adults the eye displays a three-layered structure that, according to Rohen, reflects the tripartite global organization of the body: the inner layer comprising the retina and retinal pigment epithelium constitutes the information system of the eye; the middle layer comprising the choroid, ciliary body, iris and blood vessels constitutes the circulatory system of the eye, which (with the pigment epithelium) is also responsible for metabolic processes; and the outer layer comprising the sclera, ocular muscles and eyelid apparatus constitutes the limb-locomotor system of the eye.

A certain polarity exists between the anterior and posterior regions of the eye. While the neural processes (the sclera, choroid, pigment epithelium and retina) are concentrated in the posterior region of the eye, the other systems essential to vision (the cornea, iris, ciliary body etc.) are located in the anterior region, with the lens as the centerpiece.

Five functional systems can be distinguished: (1) the neural system (retina, visual pathway and brain centers); (2) the accommodation apparatus; (3) the diaphragm system (iris); (4) the motor apparatus (extraocular muscles and sclera); (5) and protective devices (cornea, eyelid apparatus).

In contrast with hearing, vision is characterized more by antipathy between the internal and the external. The optic cup receives light from an external source, but responds to it with a contrary action. The image is 'dismantled' into its constituent parts (color, shape, movement or position in space) and distributed by the occipital lobe to entirely different areas of the brain. Although the image is dismantled, it is not reassembled. The body's 'powers of thought' are necessary to reconstruct or produce perceived images.

THE METAMORPHOSIS OF THE KIDNEY INTO THE EYE ACCORDING TO ROHEN[2]

The eye (embryonic optic cup) and the kidney (cup-shaped glomeruli) are similar in terms of their structural principle.

However, while each kidney has some 1.2 million glomeruli, each eye has only one optic cup.

In the glomerulus there is invagination of the inner wall of this cup-like structure, carrying with it the vascular loops of the glomerulus. At the same time, the renal tubules communicate with the outside world.

In the eye, in contrast, the blood vessels are displaced outward, and instead of vascular loops, a continuous sheet (the choroid) is formed around the optic cup. At the corresponding site where the tubules emerge in the kidney, the eye is penetrated by the lens, establishing communication between the eye and the outside world.

At the embryonic stage the eye also contains a vascular layer (the hyaloid vascular system), which regresses before birth.

Rohen sees the kidney as a type of sensory organ that 'views' liquids/solids in the body's interior. Blood enters the cup-like structure. During reabsorption in the renal tubules, body water and salt content are viewed and monitored.

The eye, in contrast, is completely outward-directed in order for light from the external world to enter it. Unlike the glomerulus, the choroid, which has an external location and is of the greatest importance for the eye, contains polygonal fields with central arterioles. The outer layer in the eye develops into the pigment epithelium, assumes a mediator role between the retina and blood, and is involved in almost all exchange processes. Whereas in the kidney, therefore, ultrafiltration in the glomeruli and reabsorption in the renal tubules occur separately in space and time, the corresponding processes in the eye both unfold in the cup-like structure.

Striking similarities are also seen in terms of the embryonic developmental dynamics of the two organs. In the kidney, spoon-shaped structures become invaginated to form the glomerular cups. In the eye a cup is formed as the primary anlage from a vesicle. This grows outward from the inner wall of the optic cup. As a result of its eversion, the lens vesicle is drawn into the cup region. For Rohen, therefore, the inner retinal layer plays the active role in this organizational process, drawing the lens inward and the blood vessels into the interior of the cup space, to provide nutrition for the lens and retina. Finally, in comparison with the kidney, embryonic development in the eye is completed as a primary phenomenon and thus, according to Rohen, it possesses higher organizational integrity.

According to Rohen, the eye and kidney are organs of sense and perception in which, unlike the ear, opposing processes come together. These correspond to antipathic gestures of 'soul'. In this context, the kidney is anchored in the metabolic system and the eye is part of the information system.

THE ORBIT *(Fig. 14.1)*

The orbit is shaped like a four-sided pyramid. Its base is directed anteriorly as the orbital opening. Its apex is located in the optic canal. Its longitudinal diameter measures 4 to 5 cm.

Figure 14.1 Anterior view of the right orbit

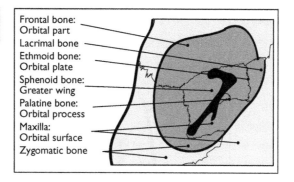

Frontal bone:
Orbital part
Lacrimal bone
Ethmoid bone:
Orbital plate
Sphenoid bone:
Greater wing
Palatine bone:
Orbital process
Maxilla:
Orbital surface
Zygomatic bone

The walls of the orbit

The walls of the orbit are formed by seven bones: the frontal bone, sphenoid bone, maxilla, lacrimal bone, ethmoid bone, zygomatic bone, and palatine bone. Some of these bones originate in the cranial base, while others originate in the cranial vault and the viscerocranium. Because of the large number of cranial sutures present, the walls of the orbit are characterized by a relatively high degree of mobility and capacity for adjustment.

- Roof: the orbital plate of the frontal bone and the lesser wing of the sphenoid bone.
- Floor: the orbital surface of the maxilla, the zygomatic bone, and the orbital process of the palatine bone.
- Lateral wall: the orbital surface of the zygomatic bone, and the greater wing of the sphenoid bone.
- Medial wall: the orbital plate of the ethmoid bone, and the lacrimal bone (frontal process of the maxilla).

Openings into the orbit *(Fig. 14.2)*

- The optic canal: located at the apex of the orbital pyramid in the lesser wing of the sphenoid, this establishes communication between the orbit and the middle cranial fossa and contains the optic nerve (CN II) and the ophthalmic artery.
- Superior orbital fissure: this passes between the greater and lesser wings of the sphenoid and leads to the middle cranial fossa (outside the common tendinous ring):

Laterally: Trochlear nerve (CN IV), lacrimal and frontal branches of the ophthalmic nerve (CN V1), superior ophthalmic vein.

Medially: Oculomotor nerve (CN III), abducent nerve (CN VI), nasociliary branch of the ophthalmic nerve (CN V1) (within the common tendinous ring).

- Inferior orbital fissure: this passes between the maxilla and the greater wing of the sphenoid and leads to the pterygopalatine fossa and the infratemporal fossa. It transmits the inferior ophthalmic vein from the pterygoid venous plexus, and the zygomatic and

Figure 14.2 The openings into the orbit

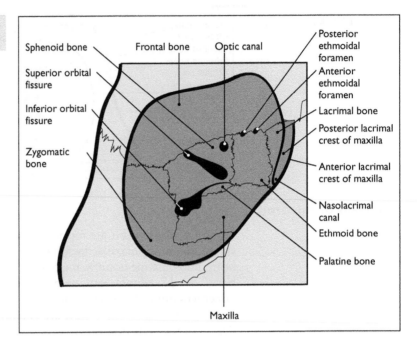

infraorbital branches of the maxillary nerve (CN V2) (from the foramen rotundum).

- Lacrimal groove: located anteriorly inside the orbital cavity, this passes between the lacrimal bone and the maxilla, and leads to the nasal cavity via the nasolacrimal duct.
- Anterior ethmoidal foramen: this leads to the anterior cranial fossa and transmits the anterior ethmoidal nerve and artery.
- Posterior ethmoidal foramen: this leads to the ethmoidal air cells and transmits the posterior ethmoidal nerve and artery.
- Infraorbital canal: this runs anteriorly at the floor of the orbit and transmits the infraorbital nerve (CN V2) and infraorbital artery (maxillary artery), both from the pterygopalatine fossa.
- Zygomatico-orbital foramen: located on the orbital surface of the zygomatic bone, this leads to the face and transmits the zygomatic nerve (CN V2).

Neighboring structures

- Above the roof of the orbit is located the anterior cranial fossa with the frontal cortical lobe.
- Above and anteromedially, the orbit is separated from the frontal sinus only by the orbital part of the frontal bone. Medially it is separated from the ethmoidal air cells by the paper-thin orbital plate of the ethmoid, while below and medially it is separated from the maxillary sinus by the orbital surface of the maxilla. Because the orbit at some points is separated from the paranasal sinuses only by thin layers of bone, paranasal sinus infections may spread to involve the orbit.

- Below and posterolaterally, the orbit communicates via the inferior orbital fissure with the infratemporal fossa.
- Lateral to the orbit is located the temporal fossa with the temporalis muscle.
- Posteriorly, the orbit communicates via the superior orbital fissure and the optic canal with the middle cranial fossa, and via the sphenoid bone with the sphenoidal sinus.

VISCERAL STRUCTURES

The development of the eye *(Fig. 14.3)*

According to Rohen, the auditory system reflects sympathy as a gesture of 'soul' whereas the visual system exhibits more antipathic tendencies. This antipathy of functional processes is already evident here in the embryological organizational dynamics. For example, the eye arises directly from the diencephalon and develops outward toward the skin (inside-to-outside development), whereas the organ of hearing and balance arises from the ectoderm and becomes detached from this during the course of its embryonic development (outside-to-inside development).

The optic vesicle induces the development of the lens anlage in the adjacent ectoderm. Both structures become invaginated. Finally, the rudimentary lens moves to a location completely inside the optic cup. While the anterior cells of the lens vesicle exhibit marked mitotic activity, in the optic cup it is principally the cells of the inner layer that move inward and form the retina. This growth dynamic corresponds to that of the cells of the cerebral cortex.

The lens is therefore formed as a result of cup-like evagination from the outside and 'sucks in' the light from outside, whereas the optic cup grows from inside to outside and, like an open hand, encircles the lens vesicle that is incorporated into it.

- The retina (the inner membrane of the eye), pigment epithelium, optic nerve, and the muscles of the iris develop from the neuroectoderm (neural tube).
- The lens and the anterior corneal epithelium develop from the surface ectoderm.
- The middle and outer eye membranes and the vitreous body develop from the mesenchyme.

Figure 14.3 The development of the optic cup (From: Drews U. Taschenatlas der Embryologie. Stuttgart: Thieme; 1993)

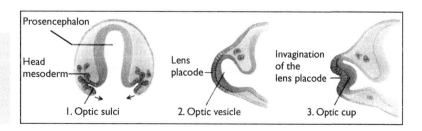

On day 22, at the cranial end of the neural tube, optic sulci develop bilaterally at the inner surface of the neural folds. These grooves deepen to form the two optic vesicles that project laterally from the cranial region by the end of the 4th week of fetal life. The optic vesicle is a kind of evagination from the diencephalon. The development of the optic vesicles appears to be induced by the directly adjacent mesenchyme. Following closure of the anterior neuropore, the CSF in the cerebral ventricles exerts pressure on the wall and influences the further growth of the spherical optic vesicles toward the sides of the head. The proximal part of the optic vesicle becomes the optic stalk, the precursor of the optic nerve. Contact with the diencephalon is maintained via the optic stalk. The lumen of the optic vesicle also communicates with the 3rd cerebral ventricle. The optic vesicles become evaginated proximally in the direction of the epidermis, which becomes thicker and develops into the lens placode. The development of the lens placode is stimulated by the optic vesicles. The central area of the lens placode undergoes invagination to form the lens pit. The margins of the lens pit grow toward each other, causing the lens pit to close and the lens vesicle to form. Simultaneously, the optic vesicle invaginates to form the two cell layers of the optic cup.

The outer cell layer of the optic cup develops into the pigmented layer of the retina, and the inner cell layer becomes the neural stratum of the retina. The outer layer is covered by the dura mater. At the edges of the optic cup the two layers fuse together.

A longitudinal groove (the fetal eye fissure) develops at the caudal end of the optic cup and the optic stalk: through this groove the blood vessels (hyaloid artery and vein) enter the interior of the optic cup. Finally, the edges of the fetal optic fissure become approximated with each other again, causing the vessels to be included within the optic nerve. The vessels in the optic cup close and only the proximal vessels persist to become the central retinal artery and vein.

The development of the retina *(Figs 14.4, 14.5)*

The retina develops from the optic cup. The optic vesicle originated as an evagination from the diencephalon and, even after birth, a neuronal contact persists between the retina, the optic nerve and the diencephalon. The pigment epithelium develops from the outer cell layer of the optic cup, and the neural stratum of the retina from the inner cell layer. During the embryonic period a space (the optic cup lumen) is still present between the two cell layers, but this disappears with increasing development of the retina. After the lens vesicle has formed, the neural stratum begins to develop into light-sensitive rods and cones and into bipolar and multipolar ganglia. The rods and cones accumulate in the pigment epithelium. Behind, the neural stratum continues as the optic nerve stalk. Because of the proliferation of fibers in the embryonic optic nerve, the lumen of the optic nerve stalk (which originally communicated with the 3rd ventricle) finally disappears.

Figure 14.4 The optic cup in an embryo at about 32 days

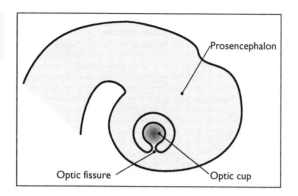

Figure 14.5 (a) Cross-section through the optic stalk, optic fissure and vessels. (b) Formation of the optic cup and lens vesicle

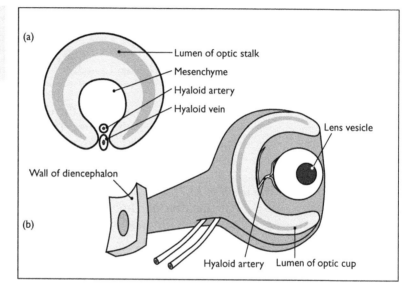

The retina is fully functional at birth, except for the fovea centralis region in the macula. Development of photoreceptors in the central fovea requires a further 4 months. Also, myelination of the optic nerve fibers is not completed until about 10 weeks after contact with light.

The anterior part of the inner cell layer of the optic cup develops to become the cecal part of the retina (see below).

The development of the lens (see Figs 14.4, 14.5)

The lens has its origin in the ectoderm. It develops from the lens vesicle. The cells forming the posterior wall of the lens vesicle lose their nuclei, become elongated and, as transparent lens fibers, gradually fill the lumen of the lens vesicle completely. Secondary lens fibers are formed into adulthood. The lens epithelium at the anterior wall of the lens vesicle forms the highly elastic lens capsule.

The development of the ciliary body (Fig. 14.6)

The outer part of the ciliary body, corresponding to the retinal pigment epithelium, differentiates from the outer cell layer of the

Figure 14.6 The development of (a) the ciliary body and (b) the iris (From: Langmann J. Medizinische Embryologie: die Normale Menschliche Entwicklung und ihre Fehlbildungen. 8th edn. Stuttgart: Thieme; 1989)

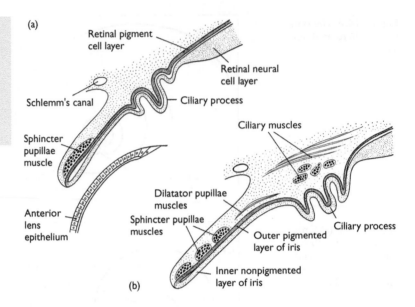

(a)

Retinal pigment cell layer

Retinal neural cell layer

Schlemm's canal

Ciliary process

Sphincter pupillae muscle

Ciliary muscles

Anterior lens epithelium

Dilatator pupillae muscles

Sphincter pupillae muscles

Ciliary process

Outer pigmented layer of iris

Inner nonpigmented layer of iris

(b)

optic cup. The inner part of the ciliary body is a continuation of the neural stratum of the retina. The ciliary muscle and the stroma of the ciliary body develop from the mesenchyme clustered around the anterior part of the optic cup.

The development of the iris *(Fig. 14.7)*

The iris develops from the two cell layers at the anterior rim of the optic cup. The pigment epithelium of the iris is formed from the inner cell layer. The sphincter and dilatator pupillae muscles (neuroectodermal origin) are formed from the outer cell layer. The connective tissue and vessels of the iris have their origin in the mesenchyme. The iris is continuous behind with the ciliary body.

The development of the cornea and sclera *(see Fig. 14.7)*

The formation of the cornea and conjunctiva is induced by the anlage of the lens. The outer surface of the cornea arises from the surface ectoderm. The substantia propria and the internal corneal epithelium are formed from the mesenchyme.

The outer sclera, rich in fibers but poorly vascularized, develops from the surrounding mesenchyme of the optic cup. Anteriorly, the sclera is continuous with the cornea.

The substantia propria of the cornea as well as the sclera develop from a tissue that is continuous with the dura mater.

The development of the choroid

Like the sclera, the choroid derives from the mesenchyme surrounding the optic cup. However, it arises from tissues continuous with the pia mater and becomes differentiated into the highly vascularized middle tunic of the eyeball. The ciliary processes (see below) develop from the choroidal anlage at the rim of the optic cup.

Figure 14.7 Sagittal section through the eye of an embryo at 16 weeks (From: Langmann J. Medizinische Embryologie: die Normale Menschliche Entwicklung und ihre Fehlbildungen. 8th edn. Stuttgart: Thieme; 1989)

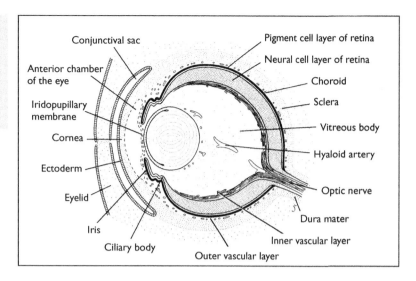

The development of the vitreous body

The outer mesenchyme of the optic anlage enters the optic cup through the aperture of the latter. It also contributes to the origin of the hyaloid artery (branch of the ophthalmic artery, embryonic arterial supply to the lens). Between the lens and retina a fibrous network develops: this is later filled with a gelatinous fluid and so becomes the vitreous body.

The development of the eyelids

The eyelids arise from two skin folds consisting of ectoderm and mesoderm. Initially, the embryonic eye is still wide open. The skin folds grow toward each other and become fused, thus closing the eyes from week 10 onward. The eyelids only start to open again at week 26.

THE EYEBALL *(Fig. 14.8)*

The spherical eyeball comprises three layers (see Fig. 14.8):

● The outer fibrous tunic.
● The middle vascular tunic.
● The inner sensory (or neural) tunic. The outer fibrous tunic corresponds to the inelastic dura mater of the brain, the middle vascular tunic to the vascularized arachnoid and pia maters, and the innermost sensory tunic to the nervous tissue of the cerebral cortex.

The outer fibrous tunic of the eyeball

The outer fibrous tunic of the eyeball consists of the opaque, white sclera and the avascular transparent cornea.

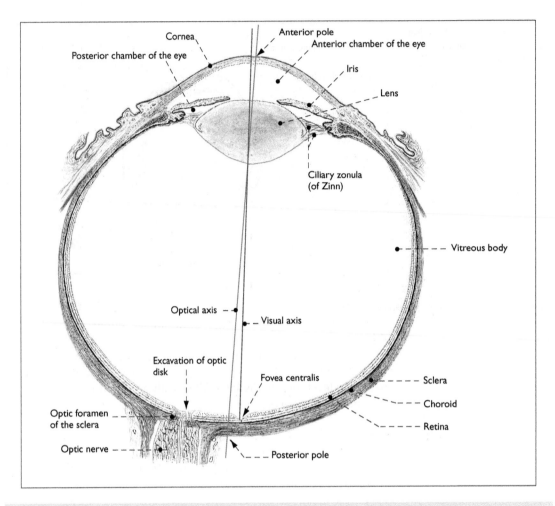

Figure 14.8 Horizontal section through a right eyeball at the level of the optic nerve (From: Tillmann B. Farbatlas der Anatomie. Zahnmedizin – Humanmedizin. Stuttgart: Thieme; 1997)

- The sclera covers the major part of the surface of the eyeball. It consists of a great many collagenous fibers intermixed with a few elastic fibers and, as a stable connective tissue capsule, it is responsible for maintaining the constant shape of the eyeball. The external surface of the sclera serves as an attachment for muscles and is continuous with the outer sheath (dura mater and arachnoid) of the optic nerve. Its inner layer is pierced like a sieve by the fibers of the optic nerve. The sinus venosus sclerae (or Schlemm's canal), which is responsible for the drainage of aqueous humor, is located near to the sclerocorneal junction.
- The avascular cornea forms the front lens of the eye. Because of the special composition of its ground substance (the refractive index of which is identical to that of the aqueous humor and fibers), the cornea is transparent. The cornea is kept moist anteriorly by lacrimal fluid and posteriorly by aqueous humor. Its degree of

curvature is greater than that of the sclera, with the result that it is slightly convex anteriorly (like the glass face of a watch). The cornea consists of five layers: anterior stratified epithelium, anterior limiting lamina (Bowman's membrane consisting of basement membrane, adhesive substance, and fibrils), the collagen-rich substantia propria (corneal stroma), posterior limiting lamina (Descemet's membrane), and posterior monolayer epithelium (=corneal endothelium). Clouding of the cornea occurs when the eyeball dries out, e.g. due to absence of blinking or to swelling (failure of the pump function of the corneal endothelium).

The middle vascular tunic of the eyeball

The middle vascular tunic consists of the iris and the ciliary body in the anterior part of the eyeball, and of the choroid in the posterior part. The inner surface of the sclera is covered by the choroid and to a lesser extent by the ciliary body.

The choroid

The highly vascular choroid is located between the retina and the sclera. From outside to inside it comprises four layers:

1. A pigmented, non-vascular transitional zone (the suprachoroid) that connects it with the sclera. The suprachoroid is characterized by interstices, which contain lymph and accommodate the ciliary nerves, the long and short posterior ciliary arteries, and the vorticose veins.
2. The stroma with large vessels (the vascular lamina), in which run the small twigs of the ciliary arteries and veins that feed into the vorticose veins.
3. The choriocapillaris (the capillary lamina), which provides nutrition to the retinal photoreceptors by diffusion.
4. A limiting membrane in contact with the retinal pigment epithelium (basal lamina (complex) or Bruch's membrane) and containing elastic and collagenous fibers.

The ciliary body (Fig. 14.9)

The ciliary body is an annular thickening located at the lens between the ora serrata and the roots of the iris. The ciliary body contains the ciliary muscles and the ciliary processes. The ciliary body can be divided into two zones – the annular corona ciliaris and the orbiculus ciliaris. The corona ciliaris is ridged by 70 to 80 radiating capillary-rich folds (the ciliary processes). Its outer, very heavily pigmented epithelium is continuous with the retinal pigment epithelium. Its inner nonpigmented layer produces the aqueous humor, which flows into the anterior chamber of the eye. The lens is suspended on the ciliary body by the zonule fibers. These serve to transmit traction forces to the lens. The ciliary muscle with its meridional, radial and circular fibers is specifically concerned with the accommodation of

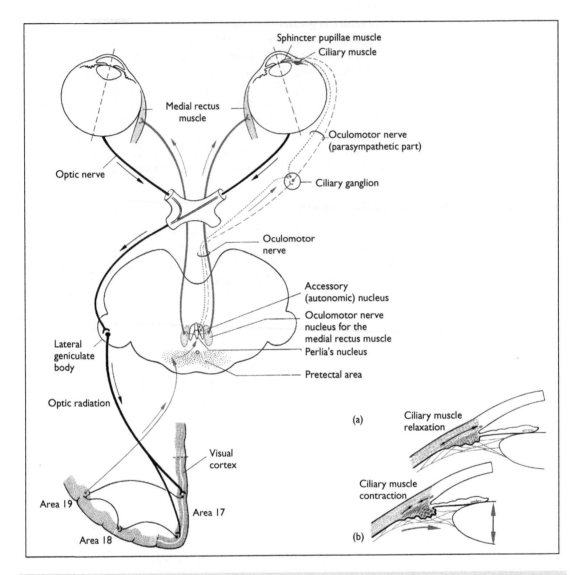

Figure 14.9 The ciliary body and its relations to the CNS for accommodation and convergence. (a) The ciliary muscle relaxes (distance vision); (b) The ciliary muscle contracts (near vision) (From: Tillmann B. Farbatlas der Anatomie. Zahnmedizin – Humanmedizin. Stuttgart: Thieme; 1997)

the lens. Contraction of the ciliary muscle slackens the zonule fibers and the lens assumes its inherent domed shape for close vision. The ciliary muscle is supplied by parasympathetic fibers of the oculomotor nerve (CN III).

The iris

The iris is a rounded disc of individually varying color: it surrounds the pupil and regulates the amount of light entering the eye by constricting the pupil (sphincter pupillae muscle) or dilating it (dilatator pupillae muscle). Both muscles arise from the ectoderm. The sphincter pupillae muscle is under parasympathetic control (via the oculomotor nerve), and the dilatator pupillae muscle is under sympathetic control (ciliospinal center C8-Th1, superior cervical ganglion, ciliary ganglion). The iris consists of loose, highly vascular connective tissue (Fig. 14.10). The posterior aspect of the iris is covered with heavily pigmented epithelium that is impermeable to light. This epithelium, which is of retinal origin, gives the iris its color. The pupillary reflex can be used to test whether the iris is functioning correctly. Covering the eye causes the pupil to dilate. Removal of the covering causes immediate constriction of the pupil in response to light. (Reflex arc: afferent, optic nerve, CN II; efferent, parasympathetic fibers of the oculomotor nerve, CN III).

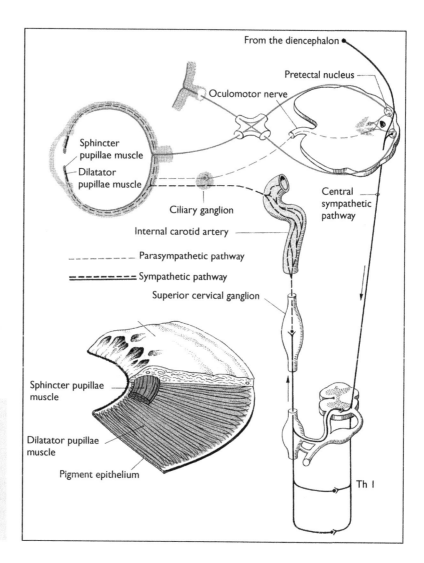

Figure 14.10
Parasympathetic innervation of the sphincter pupillae muscle and sympathetic innervation of the dilatator pupillae muscle (From: Tillmann B. Farbatlas der Anatomie. Zahnmedizin – Humanmedizin. Stuttgart: Thieme; 1997)

The inner sensory tunic of the eyeball

The inner tunic of the eyeball is the retina. It is located between the choroidocapillaris and the vitreous body. Its outer layer consists of pigment epithelium, while the neural retina is in the interior.

The neural retina consists of three sections:

- The optic part of the retina, a light-sensitive area comprising primary sensory cells.
- The ciliary part of the retina, which coats the inner surface of the ciliary body in the anterior half of the eyeball.
- The iridial part of the retina, which covers the posterior aspect of the iris. The ciliary and iridial parts are known collectively as the cecal part of the retina. The majority of the retina (the optic part of the retina) is light-sensitive; only at the ciliary body and on the reverse surface of the iris is the retina insensitive to light (the cecal part of the retina). The optic part is separated from the cecal part by a crenated margin (the ora serrata). The retina can be examined with an ophthalmoscope.

The neural retina contains three orders of neurons linked in series, which are responsible for the reception and onward transmission of light stimuli. These are anchored in a glial framework. From outside to inside, the following orders of neurons can be distinguished (Fig. 14.11):

1. The photosensory layer: rod and cone cells.
2. The ganglionic layer of the retina: bipolar ganglion cells.
3. The ganglionic layer of the optic nerve: multipolar ganglion cells.

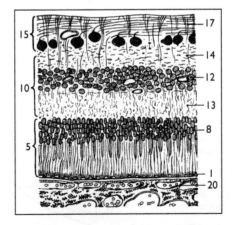

Figure 14.11 The layers of the retina. 1, Pigment epithelium; 5, Photosensory layer; 8, Outer nuclear layer; 10, Ganglionic layer of the retina; 12, Inner nuclear layer; 13, Outer plexiform layer; 14, Inner plexiform layer; 15, Ganglionic layer of the optic nerve; 17, Nerve fiber layer; 20, Choroidocapillaris (From: Kahle W. Taschenatlas der Anatomie: für Studium und Praxis. Vol. 3. Nervensystem und Sinnesorgane. 5th edn. Stuttgart: Thieme; 1986.)

Rod and cone cells (first-order neurons)

These are primary sensory cells. The rods are sensitive for light-dark perception in dim lighting conditions. The cones are receptors for color and their function is for vision in bright daylight. Each person has ~75 to 175 million rod cells and 4 to 7 million cone cells.

Bipolar ganglion cells (second-order neurons)

Their dendrites travel to the rods and cones, while their axons pass to the neurons in the ganglionic layer of the optic nerve.

Multipolar ganglion cells (third-order neurons)

Their short dendrites connect to the bipolar cells. Their axons pass to the optic disk (unmyelinated fibers), where they form the optic nerve (myelinated fibers) and travel to the lateral geniculate body.

In the neural retina two sites stand out in particular (Fig. 14.12).

All the retinal nerve fibers collect at the optic disk where they leave the eye. There are no photoreceptors at the optic disk, giving rise to a blind spot at this location in the visual field. However, this visual field defect is not normally intrusive because it is compensated for by the contralateral eye and the cerebrum. The central part of the optic disk presents a slight depression where the central retinal artery enters the interior of the eye and sends out several branches, and the veins unite to form the central retinal vein.

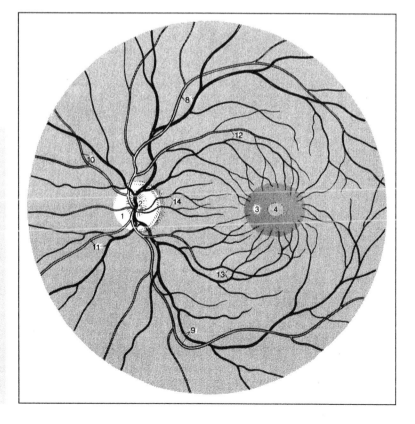

Figure 14.12 The fundus of the eye. 1, Optic disk; 2, Excavation of optic disk; 3, Macula; 4, Fovea centralis; 8, Superior temporal arteriole/venule of the retina; 9, Inferior temporal arteriole/venule of the retina; 10, Superior nasal arteriole/venule of the retina; 11, Inferior nasal arteriole/venule of the retina; 12, Superior macular arteriole/venule; 13, Inferior macular arteriole/venule; 14, Medial arteriole/venule of the retina (From: Feneis H. Anatomisches Bildwörterbuch. 6th edn. Stuttgart: Thieme; 1988)

The avascular macula lutea is located 3–4 mm lateral to the optic disk. It is the area of highest visual acuity. At its center there is a small depression, the fovea centralis. Because the macula contains almost only cones (daylight/color receptors) and no rods (light/dark receptors), it is not possible to see clearly in the dark.

The inner retinal layers are supplied by the central retinal artery, whereas the outer retinal layers are supplied by diffusion, particularly from the choroid.

The pigment epithelium

The pigment epithelium sits on Bruch's membrane of the choroidocapillaris. Its projecting apical regions are in direct contact with the photoreceptor cells. They are responsible for substance exchange between the choroidocapillaris and the photoreceptor cells and for the phagocytosis of fragments shed from the outer surface, especially of rods. Their pigment granules take up scattered light so that the photoreceptors are not impaired by diffused light. The photoreceptors are unable to function without contact with the pigment epithelium.

The lens

The lens is located in the posterior chamber between the iris and pupil (in front) and the vitreous body (behind). Its anterior surface is bathed by aqueous humor, thus maintaining the transparency and hydration status of the lens. The lens has a biconvex shape and is about 9 mm in diameter and 4 mm thick. The convexity of its posterior surface is greater than that of its anterior surface. The marginal circumference of the lens is termed the equator.

The suspensory apparatus of the lens consists of fine fibers (zonule fibers) that are attached to the ciliary body.

The lens is divided into a relatively better-hydrated outer zone (or cortex) and a less well-hydrated nucleus.

It contains no nerves or blood vessels.

The water content and elasticity of the lens decline with age, and accommodation and distance vision are reduced in the elderly. Ageing-related or in rare cases congenital clouding of the lens is known as cataract.

Accommodation (distance adjustment) *(see Fig. 14.9)*

The accommodative apparatus consists of the lens and the suspensory ciliary zonule as passive components, and of the ciliary muscle as the active component.

Distance vision: The eye is adjusted for distance vision. The ciliary muscle slackens, causing the tension of the choroidal membranes to be transferred to the zonule fibers. The lens becomes flattened.

Near vision: The ciliary muscle contracts, causing the zonule fibers to relax. As a result, the inherent elasticity of the lens produces an increase in lens curvature.

The chambers of the eye

- The anterior chamber of the eye is bounded in front by the cornea, and behind by the iris and the lens.
- The posterior chamber of the eye surrounds the lens as a ring bounded by the iris, ciliary body and lens. The two chambers of the eye communicate with each other via the pupil and are filled with a CSF-like, acellular clear fluid (the aqueous humor).

The vitreous body

- The vitreous body is an acellular, gel-like substance consisting largely of water and filling the space between the lens and retina.

The oculomotor apparatus (Figs 14.13, 14.14)

The oculomotor apparatus consists of the four rectus muscles (superior, inferior, lateral, and medial) and the two oblique muscles (superior and inferior) (Fig. 14.15, Table 14.1).

Origin: All the extraocular muscles apart from the inferior oblique originate from a common tendinous ring (the annulus of Zinn). This tendinous ring surrounds the anterior end of the optic canal and the middle third of the superior orbital fissure. The inferior oblique muscle originates from the nasal corner of the orbital floor, next to the nasolacrimal canal (see Figs 14.14, 14.15).

Insertion: The rectus muscles penetrate Tenon's capsule and insert into the sclera anterior to the equator of the eye. True to their names, their insertions are superior, inferior, lateral or medial.

The two oblique muscles have their insertions posterior to the equator of the eye, the superior oblique above on the temporal side, and the inferior oblique below on the temporal side of the eyeball.

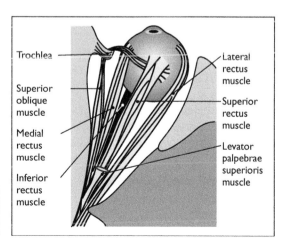

Figure 14.13 The extraocular muscles (viewed from above)

Figure 14.14 The muscles of the eye (right lateral view)

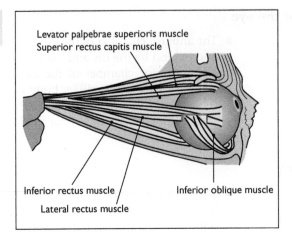

Levator palpebrae superioris muscle
Superior rectus capitis muscle
Inferior rectus muscle
Lateral rectus muscle
Inferior oblique muscle

Figure 14.15 The origins of the extraocular muscles

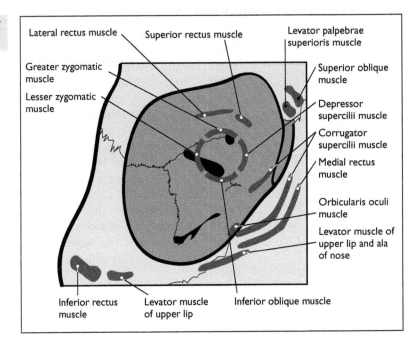

Lateral rectus muscle
Superior rectus muscle
Levator palpebrae superioris muscle
Greater zygomatic muscle
Lesser zygomatic muscle
Superior oblique muscle
Depressor supercilii muscle
Corrugator supercilii muscle
Medial rectus muscle
Orbicularis oculi muscle
Levator muscle of upper lip and ala of nose
Inferior rectus muscle
Levator muscle of upper lip
Inferior oblique muscle

The superior oblique muscle passes from the common tendinous ring to the upper medial corner of the orbit. There its tendon further traverses a fibro-cartilaginous pulley (the trochlea) on the frontal bone and then curves downward and posterolaterally to reach its insertion point on the eyeball.

Innervation:
- Cranial nerves III, IV and VI.
- Oculomotor nerve (CN III): the superior rectus, inferior rectus, medial rectus, inferior oblique and levator palpebrae muscles.
- Trochlear nerve (CN IV): the superior oblique muscle.
- Abducent nerve (CN VI): the lateral rectus muscle.

Table 14.1 The functions of the oculomotor muscles

Muscle	Function
Superior rectus	Elevation and intorsion of the eyeball
Inferior rectus	Downward movement and extorsion of the eyeball
Lateral rectus	Abduction of the eyeball
Medial rectus	Adduction of the eyeball
Superior oblique	Intorsion, downward movement and abduction of the eyeball
Inferior oblique	Extorsion, elevation and abduction of the eyeball
Function	**Muscles**
Elevation	Superior rectus, inferior oblique
Downward movement	Inferior rectus, superior oblique
Abduction	Lateral rectus, inferior/superior oblique
Adduction	Medial/superior/inferior rectus
Intorsion	Superior oblique, superior rectus
Extorsion	Inferior oblique, inferior rectus

Paresis:
- Where there is weakness or failure of specific extraocular muscles, the healthy eye muscles become dominant.

Abducent nerve (CN VI) palsy: limited abduction; the commonest form of extraocular muscle paresis.
- In most cases the oblique muscles can hold the eyeball straight, but it can no longer be rotated laterally beyond the midline. In failure of the left lateral rectus, therefore, when the patient gazes to the left, the left eyeball rotates to the left less than the right eyeball, resulting in diplopia.

Oculomotor nerve (CN III) palsy: due to total paralysis.
- The eye deviates laterally and downward (failure of the superior/inferior/medial rectus muscles and the inferior oblique muscle). Diplopia occurs in almost all gaze directions.
- The upper eyelid can no longer be raised (failure of the levator palpebrae).
- This results in a dilated pupil (failure of the intraocular muscles).

Note: Encountered commonly in cerebral aneurysm.

Trochlear nerve (CN IV) palsy: The eyeball deviates upward and medially or downward and lateral gaze is no longer possible. In paresis of the left superior oblique muscle, diplopia results when the patient gazes down to the right or turns the head to the right.

The levator palpebrae superioris should also be categorized as an extraocular muscle. It arises above and anterior to the optic canal and on the dural sheath of the optic nerve (CN II). Its tendon broadens anteriorly and divides into a superior and an inferior lamella, which attach to the upper eyelid. The levator palpebrae superioris is supplied by the oculomotor nerve (CN III).

Concluding remark: One explanation for the extremely complex innervation of the extraocular muscles lies in the high functional importance of the eyes.

The orbital fascia *(Fig. 14.16, see also Fig. 14.18)*

The periosteal covering of the bones forming the orbit (the periorbita) The periorbita is the periosteum that covers the bones of the orbit. Where the orbit communicates with the cranial interior, the periorbita is continuous with the dura mater. In the optic canal it unites with the dural sheath of the optic nerve. Like the dura mater, it can be detached easily from the bone, but not at those sites where it communicates with the cranial interior. Because of the continuity between the dura and the periorbita, tension may be transmitted from the cranial interior to the orbit or from the orbit to the cranial interior.

In front, the periorbita is continuous with the orbital septum. This forms the anterior boundary of the orbit and serves to attach the eyelids.

Smooth muscle fibers are inserted into the periorbita at the inferior orbital fissure. Their tension influences the position of the eyeball. When these sympathetically innervated muscles relax, the eyeball retracts slightly.

The orbital septum

This layer of connective tissue forms the anterior boundary of the orbit.

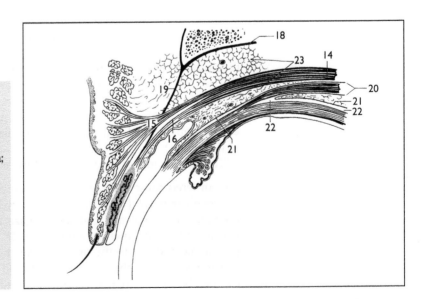

Figure 14.16 Sagittal view of the orbit: orbital fascia. 14, Levator palpebrae superioris muscle; 15, Superficial layer; 16, Deep layer; 18, Periorbita; 19, Orbital septum; 20, Muscular fascia; 21, Tenon's capsule; 22, Episcleral space; 23, Adipose body of the orbit (From: Feneis H. Anatomisches Bildwörterbuch. 6th edn. Stuttgart: Thieme; 1988)

Tenon's capsule

This sliding sheath separates the eyeball from the fatty tissue of the orbit. Posteriorly, where the optic nerve enters, Tenon's capsule is fused with the sclera. Anteriorly, it terminates beneath the conjunctiva.

Muscular fascia

This is the fascia surrounding the four rectus and the two oblique extraocular muscles. The muscular fascia has its origin in Tenon's capsule.

The protective structures of the eye *(Fig. 14.17)*

The lacrimal apparatus

This comprises the lacrimal gland and its excretory tear ducts.

The serous lacrimal gland is located in the lateral corner of the roof of the orbit, in the lacrimal gland fossa of the maxilla. Its outlet ducts feed into the conjunctiva (superior conjunctival fornix).

At the medial angle of the orbit is the lacus lacrimalis, from which the lacrimal fluid drains into the lacrimal sac via the superior and inferior canaliculi. These canaliculi are surrounded by longitudinal and annular muscles of the orbicularis oculi, which act like a type of pressure-suction pump.

The lacrimal sac is located anteriorly in the medial wall of the orbit in the lacrimal groove. This is bounded in front by the anterior lacrimal crest of the maxilla and behind by the posterior lacrimal crest of the lacrimal bone.

The lacrimal fluid drains from the lacrimal sac through the ca. 2.5 cm long nasolacrimal duct anteriorly into the inferior nasal meatus.

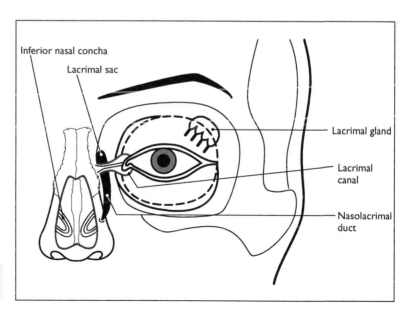

Figure 14.17 Eyelid and lacrimal apparatus

The eyelids

The eyelids cover the anterior surface of the eyeball. They are reinforced by the tarsal plate of the eyelid. The upper eyelid can be raised by the levator palpebrae superioris muscle. The upper and lower eyelids possess smooth muscle fibers to regulate the width of the palpebral fissure. Active eyelid closure is effected by the orbicularis oculi muscle (CN VII).

The conjunctiva

The conjunctiva covers the inner surface of the eyelids: it is reflected at the fornix and covers the eyeball with stratified, non-keratinized squamous epithelium as far as the corneal margin.

Vascular supply

Arterial: Two different vascular systems are present in the eye: the ciliary arteries and the central retinal artery, both of which arise from the ophthalmic artery (uveal and retinal circulation).

The ciliary arteries run to the vascular membrane of the eye. The central retinal artery travels in the optic nerve to the optic disk where it subdivides further. Its branches are terminal arteries. They travel on the inner surface of the retina. The venous blood collects in the central retinal vein, which follows the same course as the artery of the same name.

The photoreceptor cells are supplied internally by the capillaries of the central retinal artery and externally by the capillaries of the short posterior ciliary arteries.

Venous: The venous blood of the orbit, the periorbita and the eyeball is transported to the cavernous sinus via the superior and inferior ophthalmic veins. Additionally, connections run from the superior ophthalmic vein via the nasofrontal vein to the angular vein and further to the veins of the superficial and deep facial region, and from the inferior ophthalmic vein to the pterygoid plexus (Fig. 14.18).

The course of the superior ophthalmic vein corresponds largely to that of the superior ophthalmic artery. It passes behind the upper eyelid at the roof of the orbit, crosses laterally between the superior rectus muscle and the optic nerve, and passes through the superior orbital fissure outside the common tendinous ring to the cavernous sinus.

The smaller-caliber inferior ophthalmic vein passes behind the lower eyelid at the floor of the orbit, between the lateral rectus and inferior rectus muscles, and feeds into the superior ophthalmic vein or directly into the cavernous sinus.

Lymph drainage: The facial and parotid lymph nodes receive lymph from the eyelids and the conjunctiva.

Other structures

The ciliary ganglion *(Fig. 14.19)*

This parasympathetic ganglion is situated approximately 2 cm behind the eyeball, lateral and adjacent to the optic nerve. It contains

Figure 14.18 The orbital veins (lateral view) and their relations with the cavernous sinus and the facial veins

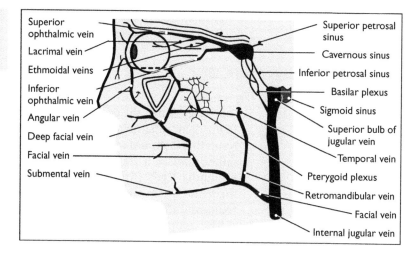

Figure 14.19 The ciliary ganglion

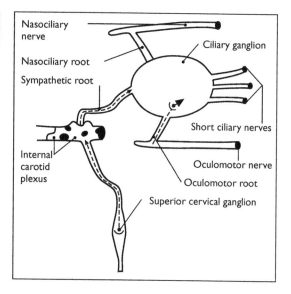

the perikarya of the postganglionic parasympathetic nerve fibers and innervates the ciliary muscle and the sphincter pupillae muscle.

It has connections to the:

● Oculomotor nerve (CN III): the preganglionic fibers of CN III pass via the oculomotor root to the ganglion where they are relayed.
● Sympathetic nervous system: the sympathetic root from the internal carotid plexus (arriving from the superior cervical ganglion) bypasses the ganglion without being relayed and innervates the dilatator pupillae muscle and the tarsal muscle.
● Ophthalmic nerve (CN V1): via the nasociliary root, sensory fibers travel from the eye to the nasociliary nerve (without being relayed).
● Eyeball: via the short ciliary nerves; they contain postganglionic parasympathetic fibers from the ganglion, postganglionic

sympathetic fibers from the sympathetic root, and sensory fibers from the nasociliary root.

The visual pathways *(Fig. 14.20)*

The optic nerve (CN II) *(Fig. 14.21)*

Strictly speaking, the optic nerve is not a cranial nerve. It has its origin in the diencephalon and is directly part of the cerebral tissue, with the result that it should more accurately be described as a cranial pathway rather than as a cranial nerve. It is composed of the axons of the multipolar cells (third-order neurons) from the ganglionic layer of the retina. There are no synapses between the sensory receptors in the retina and the point where the nerve enters the brain.

The optic nerve emerges from the eyeball about 3 mm medial to and 1 mm above the posterior pole of the eye. In total, it is about 4.5 to 5 cm long.

The optic nerve sheaths *(see Fig. 14.21)*

The optic nerve is enclosed by the dura mater, the arachnoid mater and the pia mater.

- The outer sheath of the optic nerve is formed by the dura mater, which blends with the sclera at the posterior surface of the eyeball. The outer sheath is continuous with the periosteum of the orbit. The dura mater protects the optic nerve and offers the eyeball support against the traction exerted by the extraocular muscles.
- The inner sheaths of the optic nerve are formed by the arachnoid mater and the pia mater. The pia mater directly invests the optic

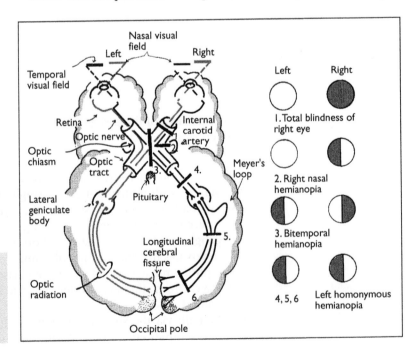

Figure 14.20 Horizontal section through the brain: the visual pathways (From: Liebmann M. Basiswissen Neuroanatomie. Stuttgart: Thieme; 1993)

Figure 14.21 The optic nerve

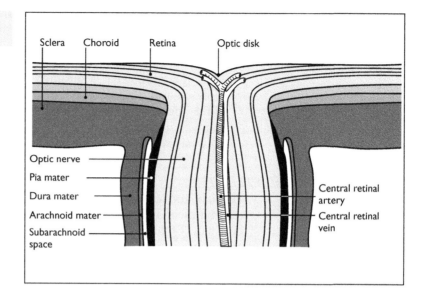

Sclera   Choroid   Retina   Optic disk

Optic nerve
Pia mater
Dura mater
Arachnoid mater
Subarachnoid space

Central retinal artery
Central retinal vein

nerve and passes septa into the nerve; these septa incompletely surround the bundles of nerve fibers. The pia mater is continuous with the choroid of the eyeball. The arachnoid mater is interposed between the dura mater and the pia mater and enables the optic nerve to shift minimally in its dural sheath. The fluid-filled intervaginal space corresponds to the CSF-filled subarachnoid space and very probably communicates with the latter. The intervaginal space terminates blindly at the eyeball. In the eye the arachnoid mater is a lamellar space between the choroid and the sclera.

The path of the optic nerve may be subdivided into four sections:

1. The intraocular part (2 mm). The intraocular part consists of unmyelinated fibers located in the wall of the eyeball. Immediately after passing through the sclera the fibers acquire a myelin sheath.
2. The intraorbital part (2.5 to 3 cm). This extends from where the nerve exits the eyeball as far as the optic canal. The optic nerve is surrounded by the four rectus muscles of the eye. The ophthalmic artery, the ciliary ganglion, the ciliary nerves and the ciliary vessels are located close to the optic nerve. A short distance behind the eyeball the central retinal vessels enter the optic nerve. At the entrance to the optic canal the optic nerve is surrounded by the funnel-shaped common tendinous ring. The nasociliary nerve, the abducent nerve as well as orthosympathetic fibers for the ciliary ganglion also pass through the common tendinous ring.
3. The intracanalicular part (5 mm). Together with the ophthalmic artery, the optic nerve passes through the optic canal. It runs superiorly and medial to the artery. The optic canal is formed from the two original roots of the lesser wing of the sphenoid

bone. In the optic canal the optic nerve travels in close proximity to the sphenoidal sinus and the ethmoidal air cells.

4. The intracranial part (13 mm). This runs in the chiasmatic cistern in a posterior and medial direction to reach the optic chiasm. Here the optic nerve is sheathed only by the pia mater. Via the optic chiasm it is influenced by the pressure of the cerebrospinal fluid. The optic nerve also runs in close proximity to the internal carotid artery and its branches, the cavernous sinus, and the pituitary stalk.

The optic chiasm *(Figs 14.22, 14.23)*

The right and left optic nerves merge to form the optic chiasm, which rests on the diaphragma sellae. The internal carotid artery passes on both sides of the optic chiasm, which is also in close proximity to the cavernous sinus, the 3rd ventricle, the pituitary stalk, the pituitary and the tuber cinereum. In the optic chiasm the fibers from the nasal half of each retina cross the median plane and enter the optic tract of the opposite side. The fibers from the temporal half of each retina do not cross over.

The optic tracts *(see Fig. 14.20)*

The optic chiasm continues posterolaterally on each side into the 3 cm long optic tracts. These contain the uncrossed fibers from the temporal half of the retina as well as the crossed fibers from the nasal half of the retina. The optic tracts pass between the anterior perforated substance and the tuber cinereum and wind themselves around the anterior parts of the cerebral peduncles. At this point each optic tract divides into a lateral and a medial root. The majority of the optic tract fibers run in the lateral root and terminate in an eminence

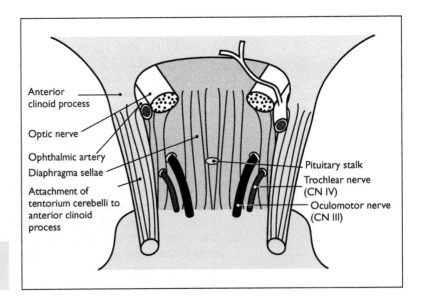

Figure 14.22 The optic chiasm (inferior view): anatomical relations

Anterior clinoid process

Optic nerve

Ophthalmic artery

Diaphragma sellae

Attachment of tentorium cerebelli to anterior clinoid process

Pituitary stalk

Trochlear nerve (CN IV)

Oculomotor nerve (CN III)

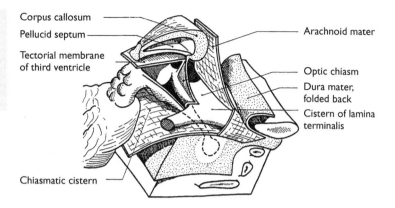

Figure 14.23 The optic chiasm (superior view): anatomical relations (From: Perlemuter L, Waligora J. Cahiers d'Anatomie 1, Système Nerveux Central. Paris: Masson; 1980)

known as the lateral geniculate body, the primary visual center in the thalamus.

The fibers carried in the medial root pass via the medial geniculate body to gain the superior colliculus and the pretectal nucleus.

The optic radiation *(see Fig. 14.20)*

Relay to the fourth-order neurons of the visual pathway occurs in the lateral geniculate body. The majority of the axons are carried in the optic radiation. They curve around the lateral ventricle to reach the visual center in the cortex of the occipital lobe, which is situated above the sulcus of the transverse sinus. There they arrive at area 17 (the striate area). In area 17 the image projected from the retina is not proportional to the retinal surface area. The fovea centralis at the point of highest visual acuity occupies a large projection area whereas the peripheral retinal areas are assigned only a small part of area 17. Some axons also lead to areas 18 and 19.

In each case, the opposite half of the visual field is imaged in each visual center, i.e. the left visual field is imaged in the right visual center, and vice versa.

LOCATION, CAUSES AND CLINICAL PRESENTATION OF DYSFUNCTIONS INVOLVING THE ORBIT

Osseous dysfunction

Dysfunctions of any of the bones forming the orbit may result in disturbances of visual function (Fig. 14.24).

a) Narrowing of the superior and inferior orbital fissures (Fig. 14.25)

- Right torsion of the SBS: narrowing of the fissures on the left side, widening on the right side.
- Right side-bending rotation of the SBS: narrowing of the fissures on the right side, widening on the left side.

Clinical presentation: Congestion of the superior ophthalmic vein. Functional disturbance (due to pressure or traction) of the trochlear nerve (CN IV),

Figure 14.24 The axes of the orbit and petrous portion of the temporal bone (according to V.M. Frymann) (a) Axes of the orbital pyramids and petrosal pyramids. (b) Symmetrical axes of the orbital pyramids. (c) Shifting of the orbital pyramid axis due to right lateral strain dysfunction of the SBS. (d) Symmetrical axes of the petrosal pyramids. (e) Shifting of the petrosal pyramid axis due to right lateral strain dysfunction of the SBS

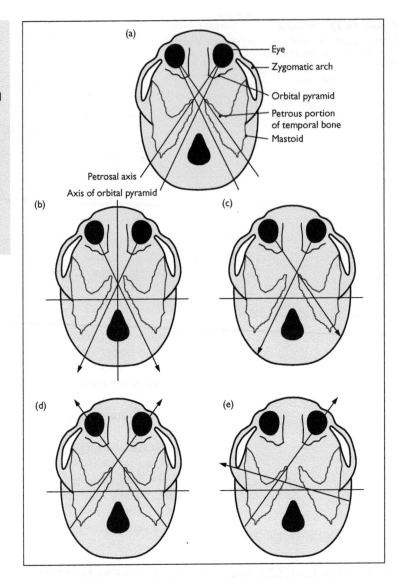

ophthalmic nerve (CN V1), oculomotor nerve (CN III), and abducent nerve (CN VI).

b) Sphenoid bone

Clinical presentation:
- Disturbance of eyeball muscle movements due to changes affecting the attachment of the extraocular muscles to the sphenoid bone.
- Functional disturbance of the oculomotor nerve (CN III), trochlear nerve (CN IV), ophthalmic nerve (CN V1), and abducent nerve (CN VI), and reduced venous drainage from the eyes via the superior and inferior orbital fissures (extension of the SBS: narrowing of the fissures; right torsion of the SBS: narrowing of the fissures on the left side, enlargement on the right side; right side-bending rotation of the SBS: narrowing of the fissures on the right side, enlargement on the left side).

Figure 14.25 The superior orbital fissure

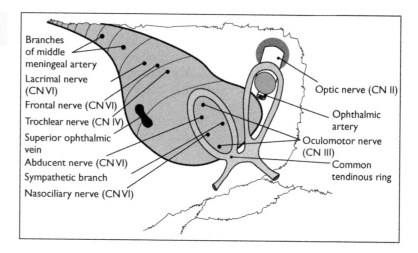

Branches of middle meningeal artery
Lacrimal nerve (CN VI)
Frontal nerve (CN VI)
Trochlear nerve (CN IV)
Superior ophthalmic vein
Abducent nerve (CN VI)
Sympathetic branch
Nasociliary nerve (CN VI)

Optic nerve (CN II)
Ophthalmic artery
Oculomotor nerve (CN III)
Common tendinous ring

- Functional disturbance of the optic nerve (CN II) via the optic canal.
- Functional disturbance of CN III via dural attachments to the sphenoid bone, of CN IV via the petrosphenoidal suture, of CN VI via dural attachments to the dorsum sellae and via the petrosphenoidal ligament.
- In fixed flexion position: reduced longitudinal diameter of the orbit with possible long-sightedness.
- In fixed extension position: increased longitudinal diameter of the orbit with possible short-sightedness.

c) Frontal bone, maxilla: For example, due to birth trauma (obstetric forceps etc.)

Clinical presentation: Functional disturbance of the inferior oblique muscle (disturbed elevation, abduction and extorsion of the eyeball). Functional disturbance of the ophthalmic nerve (CN V1) and maxillary nerve (V2).

d) Occipital bone, temporal bone: compression of the jugular foramen

Clinical presentation: Venous congestion from the internal jugular vein via the cavernous sinus into the ophthalmic vein.

Dysfunction of the occipital condyles may interfere with the nucleus of the abducent nerve (CN VI) in the 4th ventricle. Dysfunction of the petrosal portion of the temporal bone may cause abnormal tension in the petrosphenoidal ligament with impairment of abducent nerve function.

e) Paranasal sinusitis spreading to involve the orbit

f) Palatine bone (orbital process)
This small process acts as a tension regulator for the maxillary nerve. According to Sutherland,[3] it is very important in the treatment of ocular disorders.

g) Ethmoid, lacrimal, and zygomatic bones

Muscle dysfunction

The central nervous system synthesizes proprioceptive information with information in the organ of balance and integrates this with information from the organ of sight. The body seeks to ensure the best possible balance of the horizontal axes in relation to the vertical midline.

Consequently, the extraocular muscles are closely related to body posture, and in particular to neck muscle tone and to the organ of balance.

a) Imbalance of extraocular muscle tone

Causes: Compensated or decompensated postural imbalance, dysfunction of the sphenoid bone, maxilla (inferior oblique muscle), frontal bone (superior oblique muscle), and extraocular muscle nerves, and following stroke etc.

b) Altered eye position

Results in a compensatory change in head position, which in turn leads to a change in the axes of the semicircular ducts. This produces a change in the postural integrity of the body, e.g. increased tone in the extensor muscles of the contralateral lower extremity.

Referred pain of muscular origin

c) In particular, involving the sternocleidomastoid muscle (sternal part)

Clinical presentation: Homolateral pain above and over the eye, excessive lacrimation, reddening (vascular engorgement) of the conjunctiva, drooping eyelid (ptosis).[4]

d) Temporalis muscle

Clinical presentation: Pain along the eyebrows and behind the eye.[5]

e) Splenius cervicis muscle

Causes: Postural imbalance, excessive head extension or rotation, sleeping with cervical spine curved, exposure to cold air on the neck, impulse techniques involving the neck.[6]

Clinical presentation: Homolateral pain of the orbit, near vision blurred.[7]

f) Masseter muscle (superficial part)

Clinical presentation: Pain along the eyebrows.[8]

g) Occipital muscle

Causes: Impaired vision, glaucoma.

Clinical presentation: Pain behind the eye.[9]

h) Orbicularis oculi muscle

Clinical presentation: Pain in the eye, especially toward the nose.[10]

i) Trapezius muscle
Clinical presentation: Retro-orbital pain.[11]

j) Suboccipital muscles[12]

k) Tendinous ring
If this tendinous ring is shortened, the eyeball is drawn backward and fixed in internal rotation.

Dysfunction of the intracranial dural membranes

- Pain referred from the dura to the eye: from the anterior cranial fossa and the tentorium cerebelli.
- Dural tension may be transmitted to the orbit (via the continuity of the dura with the optic nerve and sclera).
- Traction or pressure exerted by the dura on the extraocular muscle nerves and the optic nerve (see below).

Nerve disturbances

a) Optic nerve (CN II)
Causes: Change in position of the sphenoid body, congestion of the intracranial venous return system, abnormal tension exerted by the dura mater in the optic canal, venous congestion in the cavernous sinus, e.g. due to occipitotemporal dysfunction, CSF pressure changes, internal carotid artery aneurysms, cavernous sinus aneurysms, pituitary adenoma.

b) Oculomotor nerve (CN III)
Causes: Dysfunction at the superior orbital fissure; commonly encountered in vertical strain, dysfunction of the greater and lesser sphenoid wings and of the temporal bone, intraosseous dysfunction of the occipital bone, abnormal tension on the tentorium cerebelli and other dural structures, venous congestion in the cavernous sinus, e.g. due to occipitotemporal dysfunction, paranasal sinusitis involving the sphenoid bone, increased CSF pressure, tumor affecting a cranial nerve nucleus, diabetes mellitus, arterial pathologies (see below). Vegetative part of the oculomotor nerve: venous congestion in the pterygoid venous plexus.
Clinical presentation: Lateral deviation of the eyeball, horizontal diplopia, divergent strabismus, impairment of upward, downward and medial gaze.
      CN III, vegetative: dilated pupil (mydriasis), drooping eyelid (ptosis), and impairment of photomotor reflex.

c) Trochlear nerve (CN IV)
Causes: See Oculomotor nerve (CN III)
      The nerve pierces the dura approximately where the free border and the attached periphery of the tentorium cerebelli cross

over and it is especially sensitive to abnormal dural tension in that location.

Clinical presentation: Deviation of the eyeball upward and medially, reduced downward and lateral movement, vertical or oblique diplopia, convergent strabismus.

d) Abducent nerve (CN VI)

Causes: See Oculomotor nerve (CN III), plus: Petrosal apex fracture, carotid artery aneurysm in the cavernous sinus, calcification or tension involving the petrosphenoidal ligament, dural tension on the dorsum sellae and dysfunction involving the occipital condyles, other arterial pathologies (see below).

Clinical presentation: Horizontal diplopia, convergent strabismus, medial deviation of the eyeball, lateral gaze impairment, the patient's head tends to turn laterally to compensate for the dysfunction.

e) Ophthalmic nerve (CN V1)

Causes: Dysfunction of the maxilla (infraorbital canal), palatine bone (orbital process), and sphenoid bone (superior orbital fissure).

Clinical presentation: Disturbed sensibility and pain involving the skin of the forehead and upper eyelid, and the mucous membrane of the frontal sinus and conjunctiva, impaired corneal (blinking) reflex (CN V1), ocular pain and lacrimation (some parasympathetic fibers run in the trigeminal nerve).

Note: The ophthalmic nerve is of major importance for the integration of eye and neck muscle movements. The nerve sends proprioceptive information from the extraocular muscles to the trigeminal ganglion and from there to the mesencephalic nucleus of the trigeminal nerve in the rhombencephalon. Postsynaptic fibers travel to the vestibular nuclei. After further synapsing, fibers reach the vestibulospinal tract where they synapse with alpha and beta neurons before traveling to the major and minor rectus capitis muscles.

f) Anterior and posterior ethmoidal nerve

Causes: Dysfunction of the corresponding foramina between the frontal bone and the ethmoid bone and the cribriform plate of the ethmoid.

Clinical presentation: Disturbed innervation to the mucous membrane of the nasal cavity and paranasal sinuses.

g) Superior cervical ganglion (C1 to C4) and the preganglionic neurons (spinal cord segment C8-Th2) at the level of the 7th cervical to the 2nd thoracic vertebrae. Orthosympathetic stimulation leads to vasoconstriction, reduced secretion, reduced venolymphatic drainage, and metabolic tissue disturbances.

Clinical presentation: Dry eyes, mydriasis. Chronic sympathicotonia may result in lens turbidity.[13]

h) Pterygopalatine ganglion

Causes: Falls on or blows to the maxilla, frontal bone or zygomatic bone, extension dysfunction of the SBS.

(→ zygomatic nerve → communicating branch → lacrimal nerve → lacrimal gland.)

Clinical presentation: Disturbed lacrimation.

Note: Increased parasympathetic activity may result in increased lacrimation and in disturbances of accommodation.

Vascular disturbances

a) Superior ophthalmic artery

Causes: Narrowing of the superior orbital fissure, intracranial venous congestion (cavernous sinus etc.), e.g. due to abnormal dural tensions (diaphragma sellae, tentorium cerebelli) or osseous dysfunction of the cranial bones, especially at the jugular foramen, and increased tension at the craniocervical and thoracocervical junction.

b) Cavernous sinus

Clinical presentation: Possible functional disturbance of CN III, IV, V1, V2, and VI as well as congestion of the superior ophthalmic vein.

c) Inferior ophthalmic vein

Cause: Congestion in the pterygoid plexus.

d) Pain referred from the superior sagittal sinus, transverse sinus, sinus confluence and cavernous sinus into the ocular region

e) Schlemm's canal (or sinus venosus sclerae)
Outflow obstructions may occur at the level of the iridocorneal angle, resulting in increased intraocular pressure and development of glaucoma.[14]

f) Posterior cerebral artery and superior cerebellar arteries
CN IV passes between these arteries and may be adversely affected by vascular pathologies.

g) Posterior cerebral artery, superior cerebellar artery, basilar artery
CN III passes between these arteries and may be adversely affected by vascular pathologies.

h) Supraorbital artery: Pain radiating into the orbit

Psychological factors

What does the patient not wish to see? Is the patient afraid of seeing objects clearly or of seeing them as they are?

Causes of orbital dysfunctions

Primary/traumatic:

- Prenatal dysfunction between pre- and postsphenoid (according to Sutherland's observation, possibly leading to Down syndrome).
- Flickering in front of the eyes may be indicative of disorders of the mesencephalon and of cranial nerve nuclei of CN III, IV and VI. Nystagmus points to involvement of the vestibular organ, central brainstem disturbances, cerebral processes, and involvement of optical and vestibular pathways (vestibular nuclei, quadrigeminal plate, cerebellar nuclei).
- Falls, blows or maxillofacial surgery associated with dysfunction of the orbital bones and the temporal bone.
- Whiplash trauma with trigger points in the sternocleidomastoid (sternal part), temporalis and splenius cervicis muscles.[15]

Secondary:

- SBS disturbances: side-bending rotation, torsion etc.
- Global organization of the body, fascial tension etc.
- Emotional trauma and specific eye movement patterns, e.g. in neurolinguistic programming (NLP) the patient's eye movements are observed to obtain clues as to the use of specific sensory channels (visual, auditory, kinesthetic etc.). Thus it has been found that the eyes generally glance transversely to the left during auditory recall, but upward and to the left during visual recall etc.[16]

DIAGNOSIS

Testing the movements of the eyeball

Ask the patient to look at and track the movements of a pencil or your finger.

Where ocular deviation is present, you should distinguish between non-paralytic and paralytic strabismus.

Non-paralytic strabismus is usually the result of an imbalance in the tension of the extraocular muscles. This may have multiple causes (see above) and usually has its onset in childhood.

A further distinction is made between convergent strabismus (the eyeball deviates medially) and divergent strabismus (the eyeball deviates laterally).

Let us take convergent strabismus of the right eye as an example (weakness of the right lateral rectus muscle or excessively powerful right medial rectus muscle):

- Cover test (cover/uncover test):

Objective: to differentiate unilateral and alternating strabismus.

➤ Ask the patient to focus on a light source. When the straight eye is covered, the deviating eye has to make a corrective movement to focus on the target. In this case, after covering the left eye and leaving the right eye uncovered, you will notice a corrective adjustment of the right eye from medial to lateral as it now takes up fixation. Where definite paralysis of the lateral rectus muscle is present, there is impaired abduction of the affected eye associated with diplopia and a characteristic anomalous head posture.

Testing the extraocular muscle nerves

Abducent nerve (CN VI) palsy *(Fig. 14.26)*

In straight-ahead gaze, the affected eye deviates medially. The patient is unable to gaze laterally with the affected eye. Medial gaze is possible.

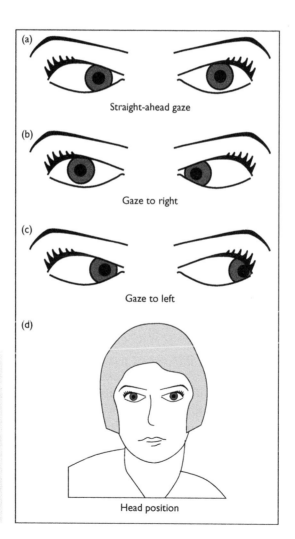

Figure 14.26 Testing the extraocular muscle nerves in right abducent nerve palsy (a) In straight-ahead gaze the affected eye is directed medially. (b) The affected eye is incapable of lateral gaze. (c) The affected eye is capable of medial gaze. (d) Compensatory head position: turned towards the affected (right) side

Figure 14.27 Testing the extraocular muscle nerves in left trochlear nerve palsy. (a) The affected eye is directed minimally upwards and medially (b) The affected eye is incapable of lateral downgaze. (c) Compensatory head position: turned and tilted towards the healthy (right) side

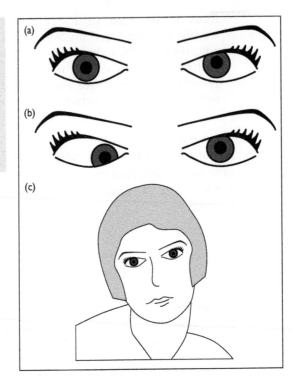

Trochlear nerve (CN IV) palsy *(Fig. 14.27)*

The affected eye deviates slightly upward and medially. The affected eye cannot gaze laterally downward.

Oculomotor nerve (CN III) palsy *(Fig. 14.28)*

The affected eye is unable to gaze downward, upward and medially (or can do so only to a limited extent). Because of the relatively stronger lateral rectus muscle, the eye deviates laterally. Eyelid droop (ptosis) and pupillary dilatation (mydriasis) may also be present, as may impairment of the photomotor reflex (sympathetic fibers of the oculomotor nerve).

Testing the pupils

Direct light response: ➤ Ask the patient to look at a distant object. Then cover both eyes. After several seconds, remove the cover from the test eye and pupillary constriction (miosis) will occur after about 0.1 s in normal circumstances. Then test the other eye.

Consensual pupil response: ➤ Begin as above. Obliquely cover one of the patient's eyes so that it can be observed without being exposed to light. Then shine a light into the other eye. Normally, the pupil of the non-illuminated eye should constrict.

Accommodation response: ➤ Ask the patient to look at a distant point. Then move an object from further away and hold it about 30 cm away from the patient's face. The patient should focus on the object. Normally,

Figure 14.28 Testing the extraocular muscle nerves in left oculomotor nerve palsy (a) Ptosis (left eye). (b) The affected eye is directed laterally (lateral rectus muscle, CN VI). (c) The affected eye is incapable of medial gaze (to the right). (d) The affected eye is incapable of upgaze

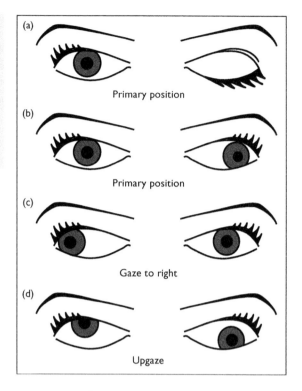

(a)

Primary position

(b)

Primary position

(c)

Gaze to right

(d)

Upgaze

accommodation is accompanied by pupillary constriction that is more pronounced than in the direct and consensual light response.

Assessment of amaurotic (sightless) pupillary rigidity

Both pupils are equally dilated in diffuse light. In the affected eye there is no direct light response and the consensual light response cannot be elicited in the healthy eye.

● Absolute pupillary rigidity:

The direct light response, consensual light response and accommodation are absent in certain diseases of the brain and iris.

● Reflex pupillary rigidity:

The direct light response, consensual light response and accommodation are preserved in certain CNS diseases.

● Tonic pupil:

Mostly unilateral, the pupil is oval and somewhat dilated on moderate illumination, with delayed light response and accommodation and delayed pupillary dilatation.

● Slightly dilated pupil:

Possible sympathicotonic type.

● Slightly constricted pupil:

Possible vagotonic type.

Swinging flashlight test: ➤ After an efferent pupillary disorder, a relative afferent pupillary defect can be detected using this test. Shine a light from below several times into each eye alternately for about 1 s on each occasion. If an afferent pupillary defect is present, pupillary dilatation occurs on direct illumination, and this should be assessed as an objective sign of a unilateral or asymmetric optic nerve or retinal lesion.

Testing intraocular pressure

While the patient looks downward with eyes kept shut, place the tips of both your index fingers on the upper eyelid being tested. Apply light pressure to test the tension of the eyeball. As a guide, first perform the test on your own eyes.

- Raised intraocular pressure: primary and secondary glaucoma.
- Reduced intraocular pressure: dehydration (e.g. due to diabetes mellitus), iritis, eye injury.

Palpation

Palpation of position: orbital diameter *(Fig. 14.29)*

Therapist: Take up a position at the head of the patient.

Hand position: Place your index fingers at the superior medial angles, and your middle fingers at the inferior lateral angles of the orbits.

Method: ➤ Compare the diameter of both eyes.
➤ Superomedial inferolateral diameter: increased (ER) or reduced (IR) in size.
➤ Zygomatic arch: increased (ER) or reduced (IR) in size.
➤ Eyeball: protruding (ER) or retracted (IR).

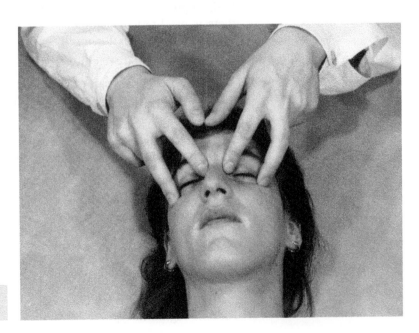

Figure 14.29 Palpation of the diameter of the orbit

Palpation of primary respiration at the orbit *(Fig. 14.30)*

Therapist: Take up a position at the head of the patient.

Hand position: ➤ Place the digits of both your hands on the orbits bilaterally (with your thumb at the superior medial angle of the orbit, index and middle fingers on the maxilla, ring finger on the zygomatic bone, and little finger on the frontal bone).

Biomechanical approach
Inspiration phase of PR, normal finding (Fig. 14.31): ER

● Widening of the orbital opening.

Expiration phase of PR, normal finding: IR.

● Narrowing of the orbital opening.

Note: In right torsion of the SBS, the right orbital diameter is large and the left is small. In right lateral flexion/rotation, the right orbital diameter is small and the left is large.

Biodynamic/embryological approach
Inspiration phase of PR, normal finding (Fig. 14.32):

● Widening of the orbital opening.
● Downward motion of the orbit.

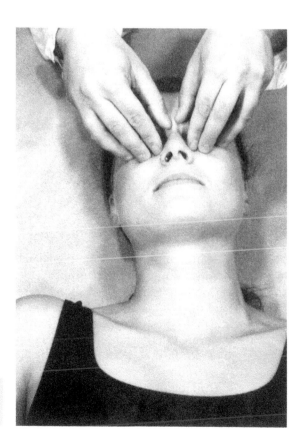

Figure 14.30 Palpation of primary respiration at the orbit

Figure 14.31 The inspiration phase of PR/biomechanical approach

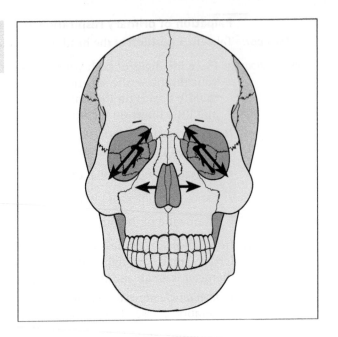

Figure 14.32 The inspiration phase of PR/biodynamic approach

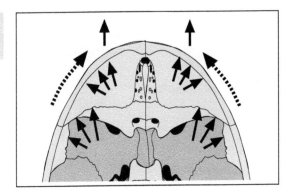

- Motion of the orbit from the lateral toward the midline.
- Forward motion of the orbit.
- Compare the amplitude, force, ease and symmetry of the motion of the orbits.
- Other types of motion of the orbits may also sometimes occur during external and internal rotation. These provide an indication as to further dysfunctions of the particular orbital bone in question.
- Unilateral or bilateral dysfunctions of the orbit may be encountered.

Motion testing

This differs from palpation of primary respiration only in as much as the external and internal rotation motion of the orbit is now actively induced by the therapist in harmony with primary respiration.

Specific palpation

Specific palpation of each individual orbital bone and of the sutures involved (see the respective individual chapters): sphenofrontal, frontozygomatic, sphenozygomatic, ethmoidomaxillary, palato-maxillary, palatoethmoidal, frontoethmoidal, ethmoidolacrimal, frontolacrimal and frontonasal sutures.

Palpation of primary respiration at the eyeball *(Fig. 14.33)*

Patient: Supine with eyes closed.

Therapist: Take up a position at the head of the patient.

Hand position:
- ➤ Place three or four digits of each hand around each eyeball.
- ➤ You may sometimes sense a minimal protrusion of the eyeball in the inspiration phase of PR, and a retraction of the eyeball in the expiration phase of PR.

Note: Patients wearing contact lenses must remove them first.

Palpation of extraocular muscle tone *(see Fig. 14.33)*

Same starting position as for the palpation of primary respiration at the eyeball.

Method: Test the motion of the eyeball and compare the ease and amplitude of motion.

Note: Patients wearing contact lenses must remove them first.

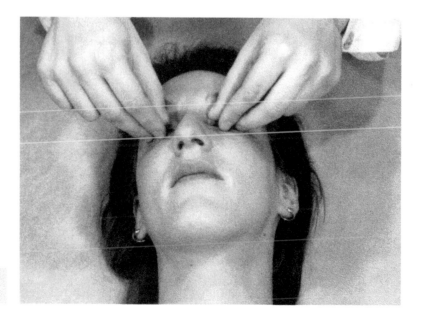

Figure 14.33 Palpation of the eyeball

TREATMENT

Treatment of the orbit

Treatment methods

1. Global examination with special attention to body posture and, where appropriate, treatment.
2. Special examination of the cranium and cervical spine and, where appropriate, treatment, especially of the upper cervical vertebrae and the 7th cervical to 2nd thoracic vertebrae (superior cervical ganglion and its preganglionic neurons in the spinal cord segment C8 to Th2).[17,18]
3. Improvement of venous return:
   a. Thoracocervical diaphragm (including upper costal joints, sternoclavicular joints).
   b. Treatment of the atlanto-occipital joint.
   c. Venous sinus technique.[19]
   d. 4th ventricle compression (CV-4); Magoun recommends starting with this technique.[20]
   e. Drainage of the pterygoid venous plexus.
4. General treatment of the orbit (widening or narrowing of the orbit).
5. Where required, treatment of the dura and craniosacral integration.
6. Specific treatment of the individual bones of the orbit.
7. Treatment of the eyeball and Ruddy's techniques for eye manipulation.[21]
8. Neurovegetative integration of the eye:
   a. CV-4 (stimulation of the parasympathetic system).
   b. Inhibition of the superior cervical ganglion.
   c. Pterygopalatine ganglion in disturbances of lacrimation.
9. Where vision is disturbed, it is generally beneficial for patients themselves to perform regular eye exercises.[22,23] In children, in particular, it is not uncommon for this to obviate the need for aids to vision. Specialist medical advice should be sought on this.

General treatment of the orbit I *(Fig. 14.34)*

Indication: To correct restrictions involving the orbit and to improve the circulation in the orbit.

Therapist: Take up a position at the head of the patient.

Hand position: Position the fingers of both hands bilaterally over the homolateral orbit, with your:

➤ Thumbs on the frontal bone.
➤ Index fingers on the lacrimal bones and the maxillae (frontal processes).

Figure 14.34 General treatment of the orbit I

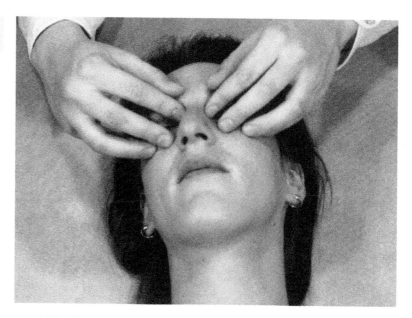

> Middle fingers on the maxillae.
> Ring and little fingers on the zygomatic bones.

Method: For example, where the orbit is in ER.
Indirect technique:

> At the beginning of the inspiration phase of PRM, deliver an impulse into external rotation.
> Hold the orbit in ER until you sense no further release or until you sense a still point at the orbit and the orbit then wishes to move back into IR.

Direct technique:

> At the beginning of the expiration phase of PRM, deliver an impulse into internal rotation.

PBMT, PBFT:

> During the inspiration phase of PRM, allow your digits to go with the affected orbit into external rotation until the best possible balance is achieved in the tension between IR and ER.

General treatment of the orbit II (example shown: right side)
Direct technique *(Fig. 14.35)*

Therapist: Take up a position at the head of the patient.
Hand position: Place your right hand on the patient's right orbit with your:

> Thumb on the frontal bone.
> Index finger on the lacrimal bone and maxilla (frontal process).
> Middle finger on the maxilla.
> Ring finger and little finger on the zygomatic bone.
> With your left hand, cradle the occiput on the opposite side.

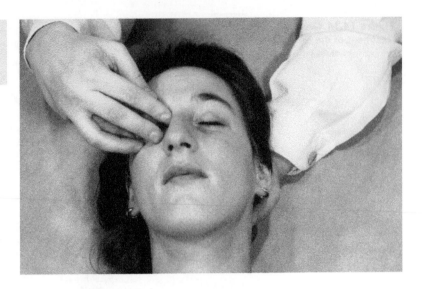

Figure 14.35 General treatment of the orbit II (example shown: right side, direct technique)

Method: Testing for motion restriction:

➤ With your right hand go with the orbit into ER and into IR or deliver a clockwise and a counterclockwise impulse and compare the amplitude and ease of motion.

➤ With your right hand go with the orbit in the direction of the restriction as far as the limit of motion.

➤ Simultaneously, use your left hand at the occiput to deliver a fluid drive impulse to the orbit.

➤ With your right hand take up the slack each time until you sense a release at the orbit.

➤ Establish the PBMT and PBFT.

General treatment of the orbit III

Direct technique *(Fig. 14.36)*

Therapist: Take up a position at the head of the patient.

Hand position: ➤ Place your index finger at the superior medial angle of the orbit.

➤ Place your middle finger at the inferior lateral angle of the orbit.

Method: ➤ Compare the diameter of both eyes.

➤ Where there is fixation in internal rotation, increase the orbital diameter by moving your index and middle fingers further apart.

➤ Where there is fixation in external rotation, reduce the orbital diameter by drawing your index and middle fingers closer together.

Treatment of the eyeball *(Fig. 14.37)*

Indication: To correct abnormal tension of the extraocular muscles, to improve the circulation in the eye, and to treat glaucoma.

Therapist: Take up a position at the head of the patient.

Hand position: ➤ Encircle the patient's eyeballs with your thumbs, index, middle and ring fingers.

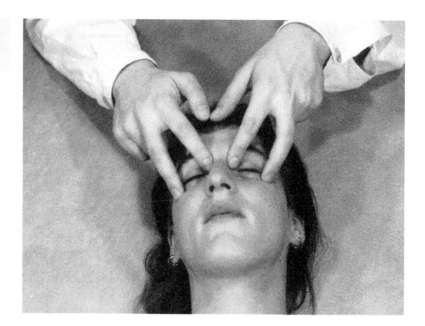

Figure 14.36 General treatment of the orbit III (direct technique)

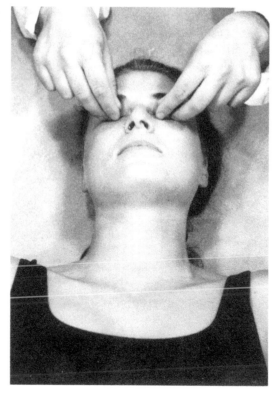

Figure 14.37 Treatment of the eyeball

Method: Unilateral or bilateral.

➤ With your digits, follow the eyeball to the position where the best possible balance is achieved in the tension of the extraocular muscles.

Unwinding:

> ➤ With your digits follow the tensions of the extraocular muscles.

Note: Patients wearing contact lenses must remove them first.

Ruddy's technique for glaucoma *(Fig. 14.38)*

Indication and desired effect: For use in mild forms of glaucoma. The technique improves the drainage of aqueous humor in the eye.

Note: Patients wearing contact lenses must remove these first.

Patient: Supine with eyes closed.

Therapist: Take up a position at the head of the patient.

Hand position: ➤ Point one finger in a lateral to medial direction resting on the patient's closed eye.

Method: ➤ Use the index finger of your other hand to perform gentle tapotement on the finger placed over the closed eye.

Contraindication: Acute glaucoma with obstruction of aqueous humor flow. Results from several research teams have independently confirmed a marked improvement in intraocular pressure from 6 min to 1 h after treatment.

Ruddy's technique for the lacrimal apparatus *(Fig. 14.39)*

Indication and desired effect: Disturbed drainage of lacrimal fluid. Also for use in neonates during the first 6 months of life. The technique improves the drainage of aqueous humor in the eye.

Note: Patients wearing contact lenses must remove these first.

Patient: Supine with eyes closed.

Therapist: Take up a position at the head of the patient.

Hand position: ➤ Place the little finger of one hand on the lacrimal sac of the patient's closed eye.

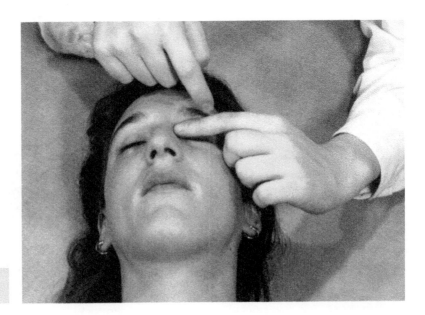

Figure 14.38 Ruddy's technique for glaucoma

Figure 14.39 Ruddy's technique for the lacrimal apparatus

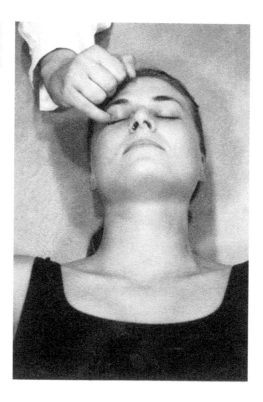

Method: ➤ With your little finger exert a gentle rhythmic pressure on the lacrimal sac (compression and decompression).

Warning: This treatment must always be performed with the prior agreement of a medical specialist. If the condition does not improve, further medical treatment must be given in every case.

Ruddy's technique for the lacrimal gland *(Fig. 14.40)*

Indication and desired effect: To improve drainage in cases of minor inflammation of the lacrimal gland.

Note: Patients wearing contact lenses must remove these first.

Patient: Supine with eyes closed.

Therapist: Take up a position at the head of the patient.

Hand position: ➤ Place one finger under the lower third of the upper eyelid of the patient's closed eye.

Method: ➤ Apply traction with this finger.
➤ Simultaneously, use the tip of the index finger of your other hand to exert a gentle rhythmic pressure on the lacrimal sac (compression and decompression).

Ruddy's technique for the cornea *(Fig. 14.41)*

Indication and desired effect: To treat mild forms of acute keratitis or iritis. To improve arterial blood supply and venous and lymphatic return and exudate drainage.

Note: Patients wearing contact lenses must remove these first.

Patient: Supine with eyes closed.

Figure 14.40 Ruddy's technique for the lacrimal gland

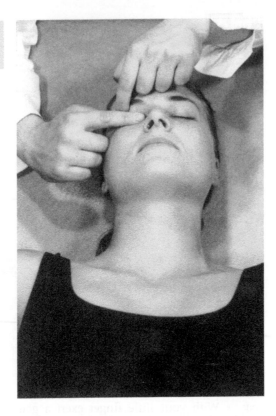

Therapist:	Take up a position at the head of the patient.
Hand position:	➤ With the patient's eyes closed, place one index finger on the eyelid.
Method:	➤ Use your index finger to exert a gentle continuous pressure on the cornea. (With practice it is also possible to place the finger directly on the cornea.)

Ruddy's technique for the eyeball *(see Fig. 14.41)*

Indication and desired effect:	To treat episcleritis, scleritis, iritis, uveitis, retinitis etc. To resolve circulatory stasis in the sclera, episclera, and uvea. Indirectly, the technique also influences the lens and vitreous body. It is a type of lymphatic pump for the eyeball.
Note:	Patients wearing contact lenses must remove these first.
Patient:	Supine with eyes closed.
Therapist:	Take up a position at the head of the patient.
Hand position:	➤ With the patient's eyes closed, place one index finger on the eyelid.
Method:	➤ Use your index finger to exert a gentle rhythmic pressure on the eyeball (compression and decompression).
	➤ According to Ruddy, if used in the early stage, this technique can be used for an evolving cataract and, if performed regularly over a period of weeks and months, can heal this condition.

Ruddy's modified technique for the extraocular muscles

Indication and desired effect:	To treat imbalance of the extraocular muscles, latent strabismus, and signs of paresis.

Figure 14.41 Ruddy's technique for the cornea

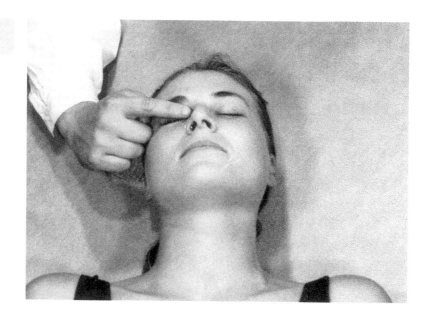

Caution: Any therapeutic measure involving the eye should always be preceded by a precise specialist medical diagnosis. It is essential that strokes etc. should immediately receive further medical care. Nevertheless, ocular dysfunctions, e.g. those due to strokes, may be treated at a later date. Latent strabismus secondary to sinusitis or periodontal inflammation and caused by a subsequent peripheral neuritis generally responds well to treatment (6–8 weeks).

Note: Patients wearing contact lenses must remove these first.

Patient: Supine with eyes closed.

Therapist: Take up a position at the head of the patient.

1. Stretching the extraocular muscles (relaxing the muscles in question)

Lateral rectus muscle *(Fig. 14.42)*

Hand position: ➤ With the patient's eyes closed, place your index finger on the eyelid lateral and posterior to the equator of the eye.

Method: ➤ Ask the patient to gaze medially (toward the contralateral muscle) for about 10 s. This will relax the lateral rectus muscle.

➤ Then mobilize the eyeball in all directions.

Note: ➤ Follow the same procedure for the other rectus muscles.

Superior oblique muscle *(Fig. 14.43)*

Hand position: ➤ With the patient's eyes closed, place your index finger on the eyelid inferiorly at the lateral posterior equator of the eye.

Method: ➤ Ask the patient to gaze upward and medially (to stretch the superior oblique muscle) for about 10 s.

➤ Then mobilize the eyeball in all directions.

Figure 14.42 Stretching the lateral rectus muscle

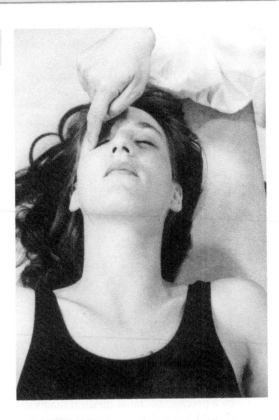

Figure 14.43 Stretching the superior oblique muscle

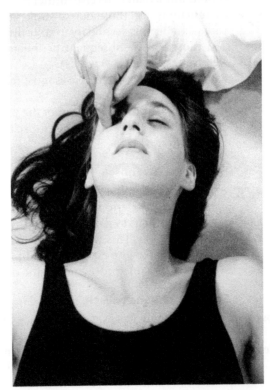

Figure 14.44 Stretching the inferior oblique muscle

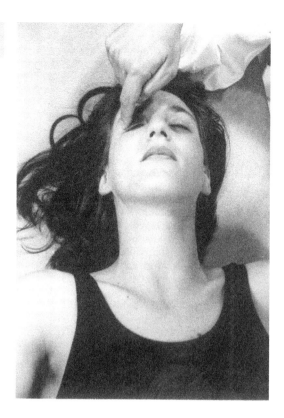

Inferior oblique muscle *(Fig. 14.44)*

Hand position: ➤ With the patient's eyes closed, place your index finger on the eyelid superiorly at the lateral posterior equator of the eye.

Method: ➤ Ask the patient to gaze downward and medially for about 10 s.
➤ Then mobilize the eyeball in all directions.

Muscle energy technique for the extraocular muscles (example: lateral rectus muscle): stretching and increasing tone *(see Figs 14.42–14.44)*

Indication: To treat atonic or paretic extraocular muscles and latent strabismus.

Hand position: ➤ With the patient's eyes closed, place your index finger on the eyelid lateral and posterior to the equator of the eye.

Method: ➤ Ask the patient to gaze laterally for about 10 s while your index finger resists this motion.
➤ During the relaxation phase, encourage the eyeball to move medially as far as the next limit of motion.
➤ Then ask the patient again to gaze laterally for about 10 s and gently resist this motion with your index finger.
➤ Repeat this procedure three times for about three cycles.
➤ According to Ruddy, in patients with latent strabismus, treatment should be administered initially three times a week for 10 min; this regimen can then be reduced to twice weekly and finally to once weekly until healing occurs.

Note: Follow the same procedure for the other extraocular muscles.

References

1 Rohen JW. Morphologie des Menschlichen Organismus. 2nd edn. Stuttgart: Verlag Freies Geistesleben; 2002:278–292, 380–383.

2 Rohen JW. Morphologie des Menschlichen Organismus. 2nd edn. Stuttgart: Verlag Freies Geistesleben; 2002:380–383.

3 Sutherland WG. Teachings in the Science of Osteopathy. Fort Worth: Sutherland Cranial Teaching Foundation; 1991:90.

4 Travell JG, Simons DG. Myofascial Pain and Dysfunction. Vol. 1. Baltimore: Williams and Wilkins; 1983:203.

5 Travell JG, Simons DG. Myofascial Pain and Dysfunction. Vol. 1. Baltimore: Williams and Wilkins; 1983:236.

6 Travell JG, Simons DG. Myofascial Pain and Dysfunction. Vol. 1. Baltimore: Williams and Wilkins; 1983:299.

7 Travell JG, Simons DG. Myofascial Pain and Dysfunction. Vol. 1. Baltimore: Williams and Wilkins; 1983:296.

8 Travell JG, Simons DG. Myofascial Pain and Dysfunction. Vol. 1. Baltimore: Williams and Wilkins; 1983:220.

9 Travell JG, Simons DG. Myofascial Pain and Dysfunction. Vol. 1. Baltimore: Williams and Wilkins; 1983:293, 290.

10 Travell JG, Simons DG. Myofascial Pain and Dysfunction. Vol. 1. Baltimore: Williams and Wilkins; 1983:282.

11 Travell JG, Simons DG. Myofascial Pain and Dysfunction. Vol. 1. Baltimore: Williams and Wilkins; 1983:183.

12 Travell JG, Simons DG. Myofascial Pain and Dysfunction. Vol. 1. Baltimore: Williams and Wilkins; 1983:321.

13 Cole WV. Experimental evidence. In: Hoag JM. Osteopathic Medicine. New York: McGraw-Hill; 1969:119, 385.

14 Schumacher G-H. Anatomie für Zahnmediziner. Heidelberg: Hüthig; 1997:452.

15 Travell JG, Simons DG. Myofascial Pain and Dysfunction. Vol. 1. Baltimore: Williams and Wilkins; 1983:207, 299, 240.

16 Besser-Sigmund C, Siegmund H. Denk dich nach Vorn. Düsseldorf: Econ; 1993:61–62.

17 Misisischia PJ. The evaluation of intraocular tension following osteopathic manipulation. J Am Osteopath Assoc 1981; 80(7):750.

18 Feely RA, Castillo TA, Greiner JV. Osteopathic manipulative treatment and intraocular pressure. J Am Osteopath Assoc 1982; 82(9):60.

19 Masduraud, C. Pression intra-oculaire et sinus veineux. Etude des Variations de la Tension Oculaire Suite à la Technique de Liberation des Sinus Veineux Selon Viola Frymann, Emerinville: Mémoire 1994.

20 Magoun HI. Osteopathy in the Cranial Field. 3rd edn. Kirksville: Journal Printing Company; 1976:208.

21 Ruddy TJ. Osteopathic manipulation in eye, ear, nose and throat disease. Academy of Applied Osteopathy Yearbook 1962:133–140.

22 Scholl L. Das Augenübungsbuch. Berlin: Gillessen-Orlopp; 1981.

23 Goodrich J. Natürlich besser sehen. 2nd edn. Freiburg im Breisgau: Verlag für angewandte Kinesiologie; 1989.

15 The viscerocranium

The viscerocranium forms the bony structure of the face, including the jaw skeleton and the teeth. It comprises the oral cavity, the nasal cavity with the paranasal sinuses, and the orbits.

The face comprises the following bones:

- Ethmoid bone (unpaired)
- Vomer (unpaired)
- Nasal bone (paired)
- Lacrimal bone (paired)
- Inferior nasal concha (paired)
- Mandible (unpaired)
- Maxilla (paired)
- Palatine bone (paired)
- Zygomatic bone (paired)

The anatomical structures and their functional and patho-physiological interactions have already been covered in detail in the sections dealing with the individual bones of the face.

In addition, separate chapters have been devoted to the treatment of specific facial regions (TMJ, oral cavity, orbit, nasal cavity and paranasal sinuses).

This chapter will describe the system of treatment and a few general techniques for the viscerocranium.

THE TRIPARTITE STRUCTURE AND METAMORPHOSIS OF THE VISCEROCRANIUM ACCORDING TO ROHEN[1]

Ossifying endochondrally from inside and standing in relationship to physical substance and the vascular system, the spongiosa system of the extremities, which is adapted to static stresses by its trajectories, is thought to metamorphose into the viscerocranium.

The shape of the facial bones is determined by forces that stand in relationship to the individual expression of personality. Consequently, the forces of the will (which express themselves through the movements of the extremities and which – in contact with resistance from the material world – determine the experiences of the individual) are said to find expression in the viscerocranium.

The lower extremity metamorphoses into the mandible, which is involved in the development of the oral cavity and the TMJ. The lower third of the face is thus associated more with physical substance and with the metabolic sphere and is rather an expression of the natural will of the human individual. The lower third of the face is associated via the sense of taste with the cerebral part of the head. Individuality is expressed in the lower third of the face through the capacity for speech.

The upper extremity, which stands in relationship to the rhythmic system and the world of the emotions, metamorphoses into the middle third of the face and into the maxilla in particular. The arm gains its freedom of movement in that it is able to establish autonomy from the thorax via the clavicle and to glide over the thorax via muscle loops at the scapula. Similarly, the maxilla achieves its expression in the face in that it is supported posteriorly on the cranial base via the zygomatic bone and cranially on the frontal bone and hence on the cranial vault. Polar dynamics come together in the maxilla: the frontal process with its upward, skyward orientation is directed toward the nasal root, the concentration point for the awareness of self. These dynamics are simultaneously involved in the nasal cavity and thus in the respiratory rhythm system of the body.

The alveolar process is involved in mastication and hence in the confrontation with physical substance. Finally, the zygomatic process and the palatine process occupy an intermediate position between the two polarities.

The clavicle is said to metamorphose into the zygomatic bone, which functions as a mediator between the cranium (cranial base, cranial vault) and the viscerocranium and connects the maxilla, temporal bone and frontal bone to each other.

By contrast, the upper third of the face with the frontal bone is fully integrated into the cranium and tends to represent the thought world. Like the scapula, it is a sheet of bone and consisted originally of two bones. Just as the mobility of the scapula enables the arm to move above and beyond the horizontal, the frontal bone is expressive of contact with the heavens and with the world of the intellect.

The palate, as the 'diaphragm of the head', separates the oral cavity from the nasal cavity. The ear is situated at the border between the mandible and the cranium, and has 'detached itself' from physical substance.

The eye is located between the middle third of the face and the cranium and so forms part of the world of the sensations and imagination.

The tripartite structure of the face is also reflected in its innervation by the trigeminal nerve. In a certain sense the trigeminal nerve has combined in itself the function of all spinal nerves because the segmental organization found in the spinal cord is no longer present in the head region. Similarly, the trigeminal ganglion also integrates within itself the function of all spinal ganglia in that, unlike the dorsal root of the spinal nerves, it no longer supplies sensory innervation to just one segment but to the major part of the head.

The ophthalmic nerve supplies the upper third, the maxillary nerve the middle third, and the mandibular nerve the lower third of the face. Each of these divisions sends one branch inwardly to the mucous membrane, one branch outwardly to the skin, and one branch to the respective organ structure.

The trigeminal nerve also shows relationships corresponding to those between spinal nerves and the sympathetic trunk. Thus, each of the three divisions of the trigeminal nerve has a parasympathetic ganglion: the ciliary ganglion for the ophthalmic nerve, the pterygopalatine ganglion for the maxillary nerve, and the otic ganglion for the mandibular nerve.

DIAGNOSIS

Palpation of primary respiration *(Fig. 15.1)*

Therapist: Take up a position at the head of the patient.

Hand position: Position the fingers of both hands over both sides of the patient's face with your:

> Thenar eminences on the frontal bone.
> Thumbs bilaterally on the frontal bone, next to the metopic suture and over the nasal bones.
> Index fingers on the frontal processes of the maxillae.
> Middle fingers on the bodies of the maxillae.
> Ring fingers on the zygomatic bones and the rami of the mandible.
> Little fingers on the TMJs.

Biomechanical approach

Inspiration phase of PR, normal finding:

● Widening of the face and orbital opening.

Expiration phase of PR, normal finding:

● Narrowing of the face and orbital opening.

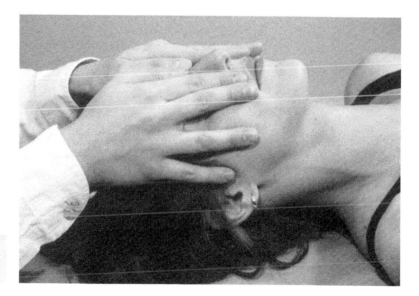

Figure 15.1 Palpation of primary respiration of the face

Biodynamic/embryological approach
Inspiration phase of PR, normal finding:

- The facial parts develop medially. Cranio-caudal lengthening also occurs.
- Compare the amplitude, force, ease and symmetry of facial bone motion.
- Other types of facial bone motion may also sometimes occur during external and internal rotation. These provide an indication as to further dysfunctions of the particular facial bone in question.

Unilateral or bilateral, symmetrical or asymmetrical dysfunctions of the facial bones may be encountered.

Motion testing

This differs from palpation of primary respiration only in as much as the flexion/extension motion and external/internal rotation motion of the viscerocranium are now actively induced by the therapist in harmony with primary respiration.

Specific palpation of individual facial bones (see the respective individual chapters).

TREATMENT OF THE VISCEROCRANIUM

Treatment methods

1. Treatment of SBS dysfunctions, and of the atlanto-occipital joint and sacrum. During the embryonic period and in childhood the growth processes of the cranial base play a very major role in the development of the face. In later life, too, SBS dysfunctions may adversely influence the function of the viscerocranium in a wide variety of ways.
2. (a) Treatment of specific dysfunctions of the individual facial bones and their sutures: frontal bone, zygomatic bone, maxilla and pre-maxilla, palatine bone, nasal bone, lacrimal bone, ethmoid bone, mandible. (b) Treatment of specific facial structures: the orbits, nasal cavity, oral cavity.
3. General harmonization of the face.
4. Treatment of the venous, arterial, lymphatic and nerve supply of the face: e.g. the trigeminal nerve pathway and the nuclei at its origin (cervical spine, atlanto-occipital joint, temporal bone, sphenoid bone, pterygopalatine ganglion).
5. Treatment of the cervical fascia, the thoracocervical transition and the hyoid bone, thus influencing the internal jugular vein, the common carotid artery and the vagus nerve in the cervical fascia.
6. Treatment of the structures in the body as a whole that are linked with the pattern of dysfunction.

General treatment of the face

General harmonization of the face (Fig. 15.2)

Therapist: Take up a position at the head of the patient.

Hand position: Position the fingers of both hands over both sides of the patient's face with your:

> ➤ Thenar eminences on the frontal bone.
> ➤ Thumbs bilaterally on the frontal bone, next to the metopic suture and over the nasal bones.
> ➤ Index fingers on the frontal processes of the maxillae.
> ➤ Middle fingers on the bodies of the maxillae.
> ➤ Ring fingers on the zygomatic bones and the rami of the mandible.
> ➤ Little fingers on the TMJs.

Method:
> ➤ In harmony with the rhythm of the primary respiratory mechanism, gently encourage the motion of the viscerocranial bones with each inspiration and/or expiration phase.

Harmonization of the upper third of the face (Fig. 15.3)

Indication: Falls on or blows to the frontal bone, frontal, ethmoidal or sphenoidal sinusitis, orbital dysfunction, behavioral anomalies, disturbance involving the prefrontal cortex (inappropriate emotional expression).

Therapist: Take up a position at the head of the patient.

Hand position:
> ➤ Place your ring fingers laterally on the zygomatic processes of the frontal bone.
> ➤ Place your little fingers next to the ring fingers.
> ➤ Place your middle and index fingers lateral to the midline of the frontal bone.
> ➤ Allow your thumbs to touch or cross posteriorly.

Method:
> ➤ In harmony with the rhythm of the primary respiratory mechanism, gently encourage the motion of the frontal bone with each inspiration and/or expiration phase.

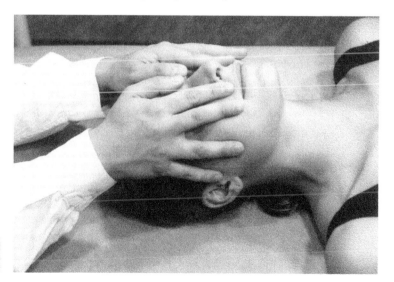

Figure 15.2 General harmonization of the face

Figure 15.3 Harmonization of the upper third of the face

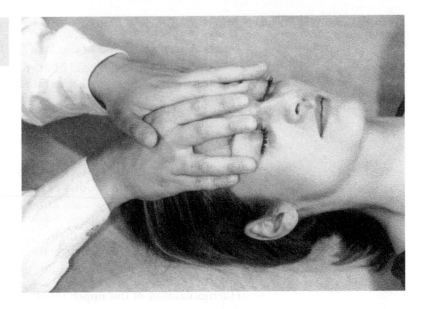

Figure 15.4 Harmonization of the middle third of the face

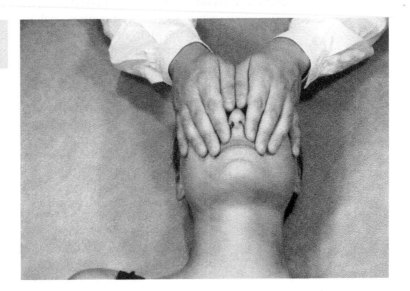

Harmonization of the middle third of the face *(Fig. 15.4)*

Therapist: Take up a position at the head of the patient.

Hand position:
- ➤ Place your thenar eminences on the frontal bone.
- ➤ Place your thumbs either side of the midline of the frontal bone.
- ➤ Place your index, middle and ring fingers on the alveolar arches of the maxillae.
- ➤ Place your little fingers on the zygomatic bones.

Method:
- ➤ In harmony with the rhythm of the primary respiratory mechanism, gently encourage the motion of the maxillae and zygomatic bones with each inspiration and/or expiration phase.

Harmonization of the lower third of the face (Fig. 15.5)

Therapist: Take up a position at the head of the patient.

Hand position:
➤ Position the heels of your hands on the temporal bones bilaterally.
➤ Place your fingers on the mandible.

Method:
➤ In harmony with the rhythm of the primary respiratory mechanism, gently encourage the motion of the temporal bones and the mandible with each inspiration and/or expiration phase.

Harmonization of the frontal bone, maxilla and zygomatic bone (Fig. 15.6)

Therapist: Take up a position beside the patient's head on the opposite side to the one being treated.

Hand position:
➤ Span the frontal bone with your cranial hand, with your thumb on one side and your index and middle fingers on the other.
Caudal hand:
➤ Place your index finger on the frontal process of the maxilla. Place your middle and ring fingers on the zygomatic bone. Place your little finger inside the patient's mouth on the alveolar arch of the maxilla.

Method:
➤ In harmony with the rhythm of the primary respiratory mechanism, gently encourage the motion of the frontal bone, maxilla and zygomatic bone with each inspiration and/or expiration phase. Then treat the other side.

Harmonization of the frontal, sphenoid and zygomatic bones (Fig. 15.7)

Therapist: Take up a position beside the patient's head on the opposite side to the one being treated.

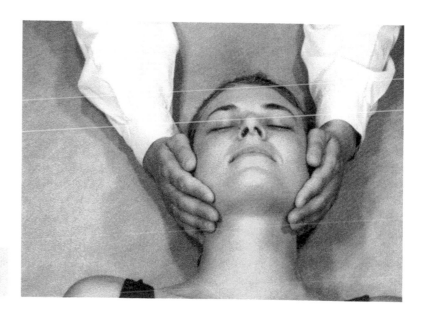

Figure 15.5 Harmonization of the lower third of the face

Figure 15.6 Harmonization of the frontal bone, maxilla and zygomatic bone

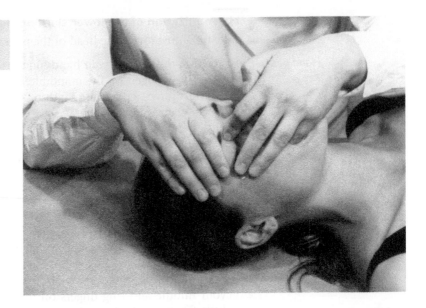

Figure 15.7 Harmonization of the frontal, sphenoid and zygomatic bones

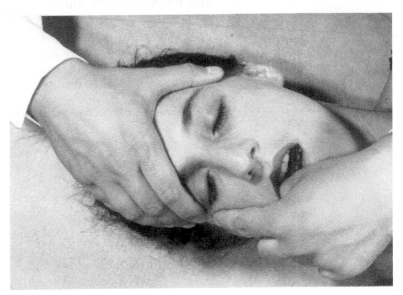

Hand position: Cranial hand:

> With your thumb and middle finger, span the sphenoid bone at the greater wings. Position your index finger with its metacarpophalangeal joint on the frontal bone.

Caudal hand:

> Take hold of the zygomatic bone between your thumb (inside the patient's mouth) and index finger (outside).

Method: > In harmony with the rhythm of the primary respiratory mechanism, gently encourage the motion of the frontal bone, sphenoid bone and zygomatic bone with each inspiration and/or expiration phase. Then treat the other side.

Harmonization of the zygomatic, temporal, sphenoid and frontal bones, and the maxilla *(Fig. 15.8)*

The zygomatic bone is the integration point for influences acting on the occipital bone (via the temporal bone), sphenoid bone, and viscerocranium.

Therapist: Take up a position beside the patient's head on the opposite side from the dysfunction.

Hand position: Cranial hand:

➤ Take hold of the zygomatic bone between your thumb and index finger.
➤ Insert your middle finger into the patient's external acoustic meatus.
➤ Place your ring finger on the mastoid process of the temporal bone.
➤ Place your little finger on the mastoid part of the temporal bone.

Caudal hand:

➤ Place your index finger on the frontal bone.
➤ Place your middle finger on the sphenoid bone.
➤ Place your ring finger on the zygomatic bone.
➤ Place your little finger on the maxilla.

Method: ➤ In harmony with the rhythm of the primary respiratory mechanism, gently encourage the motion of these bones with each inspiration and/or expiration phase. Then treat the other side.

Harmonization of the viscerocranium and cranial vault *(Fig. 15.9)*

Therapist: Take up a position to one side of the patient's head.

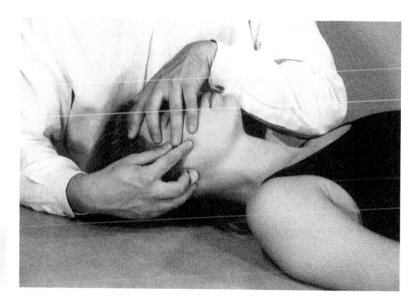

Figure 15.8 Harmonization of the zygomatic, temporal, sphenoid and frontal bones and the maxilla

Figure 15.9 Harmonization of the viscerocranium and cranial vault

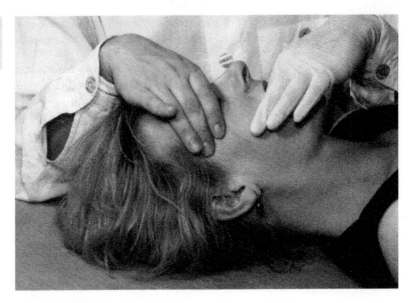

Hand position: Cranial hand:

➤ With your thumb on one side and your index/middle fingers on the other, span the zygomatic processes of the frontal bone and greater wings of the sphenoid.

Caudal hand:

➤ Inside the patient's mouth, position your thumb and index finger laterally on the alveolar arches at the level of the premolars and molars.

Method: Indirect technique
Caudal hand:

➤ Follow the tensions/motions of the maxillae and the other viscerocranial bones (indirect technique), while your cranial hand gently immobilizes the frontal and sphenoid bones.

Cranial hand:

➤ Then with your cranial hand, follow the tensions/movements of the frontal and sphenoid bones (indirect technique) while your caudal hand gently immobilizes the maxillary bones and other viscerocranial bones.
➤ Establish the PBMT and PBFT between the viscerocranium and cranial vault.
➤ In harmony with the rhythm of the primary respiratory mechanism, gently encourage the motion of the viscerocranium via the contact at the maxillae with each inspiration and/or expiration phase.

Viscerocranium (van den Heede's method I)

Testing (Fig. 15.10)

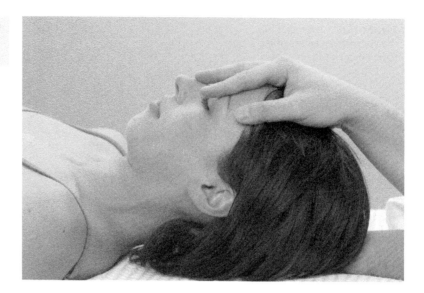

Figure 15.10 Testing of the viscerocranium according to van den Heede

Therapist: Take up a position at the head of the patient.

Hand position: ➤ With one hand, span the cerebellum, pons and occipital lobe. Place your hand on the occipital bone, with the heel of your palm at the lambda point, your thumb and little finger at the asterion, and your middle finger as close as possible to the basion.
➤ With your other hand, span the front of the cerebrum. Position the heel of your palm at the bregma, your thumb and little finger as close as possible to the greater wing, and your middle finger on the nasion and ophryon.

Findings: ● Has it been possible for the brain to develop posteriorly? Is a midline formed between the nasion and basion?
● Where is the electrophysiological point?
● Can you sense a cephalad dynamic of the occipital bone and the interparietal occiput, and a caudad dynamic of the frontal bone and frontoparietal region?

Technique *(Fig. 15.11)*

Therapist: Take up a position to one side of the patient.

Hand position: ➤ With your cranial hand, span the cerebellum, pons, occipital lobe and medulla oblongata. Position your hand on the occipital bone, with the fingers directed caudally. Place the heel of your palm at the lambda point, your thumb and little finger at the asterion, and your middle finger as close as possible to the basion.
➤ Place your caudal hand on the thorax, with the fingers directed cranially. Position the palm of your hand on the sternum, with the fingertips touching the clavicles.

Method: ➤ Move the cranial base and the cardiac region toward each other and compress gently so as to produce a resonance with the embryonic

Figure 15.11 Treatment of the viscerocranium according to van den Heede

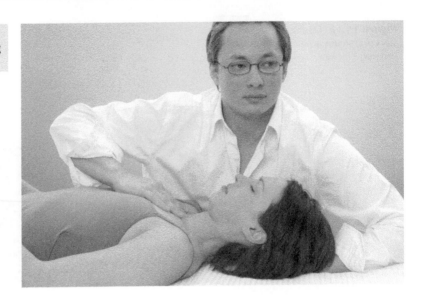

growth dynamics. While applying gentle compression, sense all the tissue dynamics but do not actively intervene.

➤ As a rule you will sense the formation of a fulcrum between the two regions. Once the fulcrum has been established, you will sense the two structures moving apart.

➤ Maintain gentle compression between the cranial base and the heart and go with the decompression of the two structures – in a caudal direction in the cardiac region and in a cranial direction in the cranial base.

Viscerocranium (according to van den Heede's method II)
(Fig. 15.12)

Therapist: Stand beside the head of the patient.

Hand position: ➤ Take hold of the patient's chin in the palm of your caudal hand. Position your index and middle fingers on the frontal processes, and your ring finger and thumb on the zygomatic bones.

➤ Position the palm of your cranial hand over the bregma, with your middle finger on the midline. Place your index and ring fingers on the superciliary arches, and your thumb and little finger as close as possible to the greater wings.

Method: ➤ Gently move both hands toward each other and, in so doing, gently compress the ectomesenchymal facial tissue.

➤ As a rule, you will sense the development of a fulcrum and, as this happens, craniocaudal distraction or disengagement of the two structures. Encourage this process by maintaining gentle compression and going with the disengagement.

Figure 15.12 Treatment of the viscerocranium II according to van den Heede

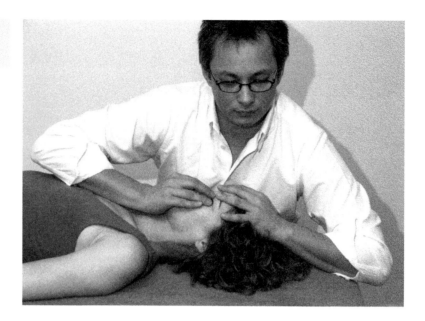

Reference

1 Rohen JW. Morphologie des Menschlichen Organismus. 2nd edn. Stuttgart: Verlag Freies Geistesleben; 2002:367, 377–379, 389.

16 Head, face and neck pain

Note: Any therapy should be associated with a global assessment and examination of the body and should also take account of far-reaching structural, functional interactions as well as of energy-related, psychological and external factors. Given the limitless variables and the huge variety of possible interactions, only close structural physiological connections will be considered in the discussion of suggested treatments.

TRIGEMINAL NEURALGIA

Trigeminal neuralgia is almost always unilateral, and is usually characterized by excruciating, paroxysmal episodes of pain in the territory innervated by the divisions of the trigeminal nerve, generally the maxillary nerve (CN V2) and the mandibular nerve (CN V3). The condition is commonly associated with contraction of the muscles of facial expression (tic douloureux). While its cause is unknown, trigeminal neuralgia is commonly elicited by trigger point stimulation, temperature changes, cold beverages, chewing, brushing the teeth, sneezing or talking. In true (essential) trigeminal neuralgia there are no pathological findings.

Diagnosis

The diagnosis is usually established by a typical history and by trigger point testing:

1. Pain history:
   - Mandibular nerve: in the region of the mandible, lower lip, and lower gingiva, anteriorly on one side of the tongue.
   - Maxillary nerve: in the region of the maxilla, the nasal alae, palate, upper lip, and upper gingiva. Ophthalmic nerve: unilateral, involving the forehead and eye.
2. Trigger points: Regions located within the territory innervated by the respective division of the trigeminal nerve.
3. Pressure points: Mental foramen (CN V3), infraorbital foramen (CN V2), and supraorbital foramen (CN V1).

Differential diagnosis

'Symptomatic' trigeminal neuralgia:

1. Tumors and vascular malformations at the cranial base: pontine lesions (sensory and motor deficit), medullary damage (loss of pain and temperature sensation, loss of corneal reflex).
2. Sinusitis.
3. Dental problems, dental root inflammation, dental extractions.
4. Herpes infection: preceded by typical skin eruption, usually in the territory innervated by CN V1.
5. Migraine and atypical facial nerve pain: longer episodes of throbbing or burning pain.
6. Rheumatic disorders: Sjögren's syndrome, rheumatoid arthritis (associated with a sensory nasal or perioral deficit).
7. Chronic meningitis, rare: possible trigeminal nerve defect.

Osteopathic treatment

Treatment of the structures in the pathway of the trigeminal nerve and its divisions

1. Upper cervical spine and atlanto-occipital joint (region of the trigeminal nerve nucleus).
2. Temporal bone, e.g. with an internal rotation dysfunction: the trigeminal ganglion occupies the trigeminal cave (Meckel's cavity) at the apex of the petrous part of the temporal bone. A recess in the dura surrounds the ganglion at that point.
3. Sphenopetrosal synchondrosis (Gruber's sphenopetrosal ligament): dental extraction in the upper jaw may produce a homolateral dysfunction, whereas dental extraction in the mandible may produce a contralateral dysfunction of the ligament.
4. Dural membrane techniques: intracranial and extracranial.
5. Sphenobasilar synchondrosis/synostosis (SBS).
6. Sacrum.
7. Possibly, the temporomandibular joint (TMJ).
8. Sphenofrontal suture.
9. In infraorbital pain in the territory supplied by CN V2: possibly, the palatine bone, maxilla, pterygopalatine suture, pterygopalatine ganglion.

GLOSSOPHARYNGEAL NEURALGIA

Glossopharyngeal neuralgia is characterized by recurrent attacks of severe pain involving the back of the pharynx, tonsils, tongue base and middle ear, the retro-auricular region and possibly extending into the neck. It is encountered very rarely and its cause is unknown. Usually there are no pathological findings.

The episodes of pain may be of spontaneous onset or may be triggered in the same ways as trigeminal neuralgia. In most cases, pain begins at the base of the tongue and extends to involve the neck and throat region. It is possible that increased vagus activity impairs cardiac impulse formation, thus resulting in disturbed cerebral blood flow with transient syncope.

Glossopharyngeal neuralgia can be diagnosed by obtaining a specific history with regard to pain location and on the basis of the exacerbation of pain during swallowing or when the tonsils are touched.

Differential diagnosis: tumors of the cerebellopontine angle, tonsils and pharynx, as well as neck metastases.

Osteopathic treatment

1. Atlanto-occipital joint.
2. Jugular foramen: temporal bone and occipital bone (occipitomastoid suture, petrojugular suture).
3. Temporomandibular joint.

OCCIPITAL NEURALGIA

Occipital neuralgia is characterized by recurrent attacks of severe pain along the distribution of the greater occipital nerve (a branch of the 2nd cervical dorsal ramus). This emerges from between the 2nd cervical vertebra and the obliquus capitis inferior muscle and passes through the trapezius and semispinalis capitis muscles. It supplies the muscles of the neck and the skin of the occiput. An increase in the tone of the trapezius or semispinalis capitis muscles, e.g. as a result of trauma or following exposure to cold etc., may lead to headache with or without other trigger factors.

Osteopathic treatment

1. Upper cervical spine and atlanto-occipital joint.
2. Cervical fascia and release of the trapezius and semispinalis capitis muscles.
3. Intraspinal and intracranial dural membranes, including the sacrum.
4. The occiput and its sutures.
5. Compression or expansion of the 4th ventricle (CV-4, EV-4).

HEADACHE (CEPHALGIA) *(Tables 16.1–16.5)*

Headache is an accompanying or hallmark symptom of numerous general, systemic or organic diseases. However, no organic disturbance can be detected in the vast majority of patients with headache.

Table 16.1 Pain sensitivity of the dural membranes and their patterns of pain referral

Dura	Pain referral pattern
Anterior cranial fossa	Homolateral eye, retro-orbital, frontal region
Middle cranial fossa	Facial region, temporal region
(a) Trigeminal cavity	Facial region
(b) Sella turcica	Crown of head
(c) Diaphragma sellae	Retro-orbital
Posterior cranial fossa	Occiput, behind the ear, neck, shoulder
(a) Transverse and sigmoid sinus	Behind the ear
(b) Area around the foramen magnum	Occiput and nuchal region
(c) Falx cerebelli	Nuchal region
Falx cerebri	Along the superior sagittal sinus, ocular region and frontoparietal region
Tentorium cerebelli	
(a) Pressure from above	Eye, lateral anterior region of head
(b) Pressure from below	Behind the ear, anterior region of head, eye

Table 16.2 Pain sensitivity of the dural sinuses and their patterns of pain referral

Dural sinuses	Pain referral pattern
Superior sagittal sinus and supplying veins	Frontoparietal region and ocular region
Transverse sinus, confluence of the sinuses	Homolateral anterior region of head, eye
Superior petrosal sinus, transverse sinus	Temporal region
Cavernous sinus	Homolateral eye, maxillary region (via the maxillary nerve)

The majority of intracranial structures are insensitive to pain. Those structures that are pain-sensitive are the dura membranes as well as the venous sinuses and adjacent veins, the arteries of the dura and cranial base, and the cranial nerves with sensory components (CN V, CN IX and CN X).

The dura membranes are sensitive to pain particularly in the region of the cranial base, tentorium cerebelli, and in the territory surrounding the branches of the middle meningeal artery. Other areas of the dura though appear to be virtually insensitive to pain. Compression and stretching of the blood vessels, choroid plexus, pia mater and the dura mater sinuses may cause pain in just the same way as compression or traction of the trigeminal nerve (CN V), intermedius nerve (CN VII) or the first three cervical nerves.

Table 16.3 Nerve structures involved in pain conduction

	Innervation	Structures involved
Anterior cranial fossa	Ophthalmic nerve (CN VI) Sympathetic: superior cervical ganglion, nerve fibers in the arterial adventitia	Superior orbital fissure, trigeminal cavity, occipital bone to C3 Foramen lacerum, pterygoid canal, pterygopalatine ganglion, pain conducted via CN V, CN IX, CN X
Lateral cranial wall	Maxillary nerve (CN V2), mandibular nerve (CN V3)	Supra- and infra-orbital foramina, trigeminal cavity, occipital bone to C3
Middle cranial fossa	Maxillary nerve (CN V2), mandibular nerve (CN V3), filaments of the trigeminal ganglion	Supra- and infra-orbital foramina, trigeminal cavity, occipital bone to C3
Posterior cranial fossa	Vagus nerve (CN X), Glossopharyngeal nerve (CN IX)	Jugular foramen
Foramen magnum region	Meningeal branches from C1, C2 and C3 via branches of the hypoglossal nerve (CN XII)	Occipital bone to C3, canal of hypoglossal nerve
Occipital skin	Greater occipital nerve from C2, lesser occipital nerve, great auricular nerve from C2, C3	Occipito-atlanto-axial joint, obliquus capitis inferior, semispinalis capitis, trapezius, and sternocleidomastoid muscles
Skin of the neck	Third occipital nerve from C3 and the cervical plexus	
Facial skin	Trigeminal nerve	Frontal bone, maxilla, palatine bone, mandible, temporal bone, sphenoid bone, occipital bone to C3

The parasympathetic intermedius nerve (CN VII) is not involved in pain conduction.

Outer components of the cranial vault are also sensitive to pain. The brain itself and the cranium, however, are not sensitive to pain.

Extracranial structures possibly involved in the causation of pain in the head include the nuchal and masticatory muscles in particular, as well as their arteries and veins.

Other pain-sensitive structures include the skin (see Trigeminal neuralgia), the mucous membrane of the oral and nasal cavities and paranasal sinuses, the TMJ (especially the joint capsule and the retrodiskal tissue), as well as the orbital contents, the tongue and the teeth.

Diagnosis

The diagnosis of headache is based primarily on history-taking, on the clinical findings (location, frequency, duration and severity of

Table 16.4 Arteries and headache

Arteries	Pain referral pattern
1. Intracranial arteries, e.g. middle meningeal artery*	Pain is referred via nerve fibers in the adventitial coat of the blood vessels

2. Extracranial location:
   Superficial temporal artery
   Occipital artery
   Supraorbital artery
	
	Parietal region
	Nuchal region and area behind the ear
	Pain in the orbit and forehead

*According to Magoun,[1] hypertensive headache and congestive headache develop due to compression in the vertical course of the sphenosquamous suture, at the point where the middle meningeal artery crosses the suture.

Table 16.5 Referred pain of muscular origin, according to Travell

Region	Muscles
Nuchal region	Trapezius, multifidi (levator scapulae, splenius cervicis, infraspinatus)
Occipital region	Trapezius, sternocleidomastoid (semispinalis capitis and cervicis, splenius cervicis, deep neck muscles, occipital belly of occipitofrontalis, digastric, temporalis)
Vertex	Sternocleidomastoid (sternal part), splenius capitis
Temporal region	Trapezius, sternocleidomastoid (sternal part), temporalis, semispinalis (splenius cervicis, suboccipital muscles)
Frontal region	Sternocleidomastoid, frontal belly of occipitofrontalis, zygomaticus major (semispinalis capitis)

pain, as well as pain type), and on the results of a neurological examination (Table 16.6).

A pulsating pain is generally encountered in hypertension, fever or migraine. A 'one-off' headache may occur in response to alcohol abuse, over-tiredness, fever or going without food. A generalized, ill-defined headache suggests a process with a hemodynamic etiology. The diagnosis in chronic headache is more problematic.

Further investigations (sight testing, blood tests, lumbar puncture, X-rays, and computed tomography) are indicated in ill-defined and atypical headache with specific warning symptoms.

Warning symptoms:
- Headache occurring for the first time or taking a particularly severe course.
- Headache with fever and chills: infectious etiology.
- Additionally, with nuchal rigidity, neck and back pain: blood or pus in the subarachnoid space.
- Headache associated with exhaustion, increasing fatigue, loss of concentration, dizziness, and ataxia: raised intracranial pressure.
- Headache associated with chronic muscle and joint pain and fatigue: temporal arteritis.

Table 16.6 Differential diagnosis of headache

	Symptoms
1. Raised intracranial pressure	Local or generalized, mild to severe pain Papilledema
(a) Brain tumor	Brief antecedent history Responds to changes in head posture Pain initially may be local to the area of the tumor Pain later becomes increasingly generalized due to raised intracranial pressure Vomiting, papilledema Increasing neurological deficits and unilateral weakness, epileptiform seizures Personality changes Visual disturbances
(b) Brain abscess: due to otitis media, petrous bone caries, sinusitis, bronchiectases, pulmonary abscess, peripheral suppuration, cardiac damage	Symptoms as for brain tumor
(c) Subdural hematoma: following cranial trauma, more rarely due to chronic alcoholism, rarely due to chronic oozing hemorrhage	Increasing headache, possibly over weeks and months Dizziness, vomiting Seizures, signs of paralysis, sensory disturbances Dilated pupil on the focal side
(d) Meningitis	Severe generalized headache radiating into the nuchal region Febrile illness of sudden onset Nuchal rigidity, opisthotonos (hyperextension of the neck) Kernig's sign (patient unable to extend leg while seated), Brudzinski's sign (passive flexion of the neck results in spontaneous flexion of the knee)
(e) Subarachnoid hemorrhage: danger of massive hemorrhage	Severe headache of sudden onset Unremitting pain Prodromal sign: pain over or in the eye
(f) Chronic meningitis, syphilis, tuberculosis	Headache and moderately high fever Occasionally, cranial nerve palsy and confusional states More or less definite signs of meningeal irritation
2. Cranial changes due to Paget's disease, metastases	Paget's disease: increased head circumference; cranial nerve signs Metastases: localized headache, cranial nerve signs, primary tumor symptoms
3. Sensory nerve disturbances of the skin of the head in herpes zoster	Pain along the distribution of the nerve, tenderness Herpes vesicles on the skin
4. Vascular disturbances: (a) Migraine (see below) (b) Hypertensive headache: possibly due to renal disease (c) Hypotensive headache (d) Toxemia (uremia, alcoholism, CO_2 poisoning, chronic constipation etc.) (e) Cluster headache	Throbbing headache of sudden onset in occipital region or at crown of head Edema, retinal changes, cardiac symptoms Steady, moderately severe throbbing headache, generalized occurrence Further signs of toxicity Mostly in men between the ages of 35 and 50 years Sudden onset, usually at night or after an afternoon nap Duration: usually 20–60 min Daily for 4–12 weeks Unilateral retro- or periorbital pain May change to other side in following episode

Table continued

Table continued

	Symptoms
	Unilateral reddening and unilateral flush
	Lacrimation and nasal secretion
	Redness of the eyes and occasionally Horner's syndrome
5. Extracranial causes:	
(a) Middle ear infections: otitis media, mastoiditis	Headache in temporal region
	Other ear symptoms
	Fever and malaise, possibly meningeal irritation
	Tenderness over the mastoid
	Tympanic involvement
(b) Eye disorders: glaucoma, iritis, eye strain	Frontal and supraorbital headache
	Usually intensified by certain sight tests
	Pain in the eye
	Possibly, raised intraocular pressure
	Possibly, visible eye changes
(c) Paranasal sinusitis: e.g. due to dental (root) lesions	Location dependent on sinus affected: forehead, maxilla
	Dull to severe pain, especially in the mornings
	Worse in damp cold weather
	Tender/painful on percussion
	Purulent nasal discharge
(d) Muscle tension headache: e.g. triggered by psychological stress, depression, overexertion Causes: whiplash injury, degenerative spinal cord changes, chronic incorrect neck posture, muscle strain, excessive PC monitor work, visual disturbance	Bilateral continuous non-pulsating pain
	Usually morning onset and increasing through to evening, occurring over a period of days to months
	Usually occurs in adults
	Location: nuchal, occipital and frontal region
	Dull sensation of pressure, like a vise around the head
	Unlike migraine, headache is improved by alcohol and physical activity
– Increased tone of longissimus capitis muscle (see above)	Often accompanied by dizziness
	Location: initially in temporal bone region or entire head
	Made worse by heat (increases vasodilatation)
	Improved by cooling
– Increased tone of occipitofrontalis muscle, especially the frontal belly	Location: frontal region
	Made worse by cold and stress
(e) Barré-Liéou syndrome: arthrotic changes in cervical spine with irritation of the vertebral artery and sympathetic nervous system	
(f) TMJ arthropathy, bruxism	
6. Psycho-emotional states due to anxiety, conversion hysteria	Pain usually bilateral in the temporal region or generalized
	Vise-like around the crown of the head
	Unremitting pain, lasting all day
	Occurs daily
	Headache intensified by emotional stress
	Neurovegetative signs
	Usually no organic findings
	Emotional headache usually starts in the neck or forehead, spreading to involve the entire cranium as a sensation of pressure or contraction in the head
7. Post-traumatic following whiplash injury, a blow to or fall on the head	Headache locally at the site of injury or generalized
	Dizziness, made worse by changing position
	Irritability, disturbed sleep or concentration

MIGRAINE

The term migraine describes periodic attacks of headache that are not infrequently accompanied by visual and gastrointestinal symptoms. Migraine has a genetic basis and, in conjunction with altered internal physiological (e.g. hormonal) cycles, this results in an inherent propensity to respond to external triggers with a migraine headache. In this process there is an alteration in perfusion and cortical brain activity, a change in neurotransmitter levels, and very probably, aseptic perivascular inflammation of the dura arteries.

Migraine is the most commonly encountered cause of headache. It usually first appears in childhood or by the third decade of life. Women are affected more often than men. Familial clustering has been reported in 50% of cases.

Despite scientific research on a wide range of fronts, the cause of migraine has still not been completely elucidated. It is probable that the cause is to be found in the interplay between a genetic disposition and alterations in internal physiological cycles, in hormone levels (menstruation, ovulation), or in sympathetic responsiveness (due to physical or psychological stress factors). These ultimately create an inherent propensity to react to external stimuli (alcohol, chocolate etc.) with a migraine attack.

Prodrome causation: It is unclear whether the prodromal symptoms (paresthesia etc.) are caused by the inhibition of cortical activity in the brain, which in turn leads to reduced cerebral blood flow, or whether intracranial vaso-constriction causes inhibition of cortical activity.

Headache causation: It has been established that altered activity in the locus ceruleus and in the trigeminal nerve nuclei produces a change in cerebrovascular tone and causes the release of vasoactive substances (serotonin, substance P). In a final step, as a result of prostaglandin activation and mast cell degranulation, aseptic perivascular inflammation develops in the dura arteries, leading to the clinical symptom of headache.

It was once thought that vasodilatation of the cutaneous arteries of the head was responsible for causing headache. However, it has been demonstrated that vasodilatation of the cutaneous arteries of the head can also be produced by stimulation of the trigeminal nerve nuclei.

The characteristic accompanying symptoms such as nausea and vomiting etc. arise when further vegetative centers in the brainstem are affected.

Trigger factors: Food (alcohol, chocolate, cheese etc.), hunger, medication (reserpine), psychological and physical stress factors, apprehensive anxiety, post-stress phase, time changes, changes in the sleep/waking cycle, menstruation, ovulation, noise, cold, smoke etc.

Clinical presentation:
- Migraine attacks may occur daily or even monthly, and usually have their onset early in the morning.
- Initially, specific prodromal features may be evident (migraine with aura): flashing lights, visual field losses and paresthesia.

In some circumstances, the prodromal features may take the form of depression, confusional states, irritability, aphasia, dizziness, nystagmus and even paresis affecting one or both sides of the body. These neurological symptoms generally subside again after about 1 h at most.

- The headache then starts immediately afterward or within 1 h of the prodromal phase.
- Generally, the headache begins in the temporal and frontal region or in the nuchal region and then spreads to involve other areas.
- It is usually unilateral, but often changes from one side to the other. Generalized headache may also be experienced.
- The headache is throbbing, pulsating or hammering. In rare instances it is described as continuous and persistent. It is exacerbated by physical activity.
- Accompanying vegetative symptoms include nausea, retching, vomiting, photophobia and phonophobia.
- The patient's extremities are cold.
- The cutaneous arteries of the head generally stand out prominently.
- Polyuria and diarrhea may follow the migraine attack.

Special forms:
- Ophthalmologic migraine is associated with paresis of the lateral extraocular muscles.
- Basilar migraine is characterized by diplopia, dizziness, ataxia and dysarthria, in addition to headache.

Interactions with the digestive system have also been detected in routine practice. 'Digestive' migraine occurs preferentially during the digestive phase. Further accompanying symptoms include anorexia, bitter taste in the mouth, sensitivity to odors, physical and psychological asthenia, and (possibly) achylia.

STRUCTURES INVOLVED IN THE CAUSATION OF HEADACHE

Osseous factors

- Cranial pain may be caused by bone tumors and bone diseases, such as Paget's disease.
- Pain involving the head may also result from trauma, cranial bone restrictions, TMJ dysfunctions, and restrictions of the sacrum or coccyx due to continuity with the dura.
- Further causes of headache include vertebral dysfunctions, e.g. of the upper cervical vertebrae (superior cervical ganglion, jugular vein, cervical nerves, region of the trigeminal nerve nucleus etc.), C8 to Th2 (preganglionic neurons of the superior cervical ganglion) etc.
- Dysfunctions of the upper ribs, sternoclavicular joints and jugular foramen may impair venous return.

Muscular factors

The nuchal and masticatory muscles may be involved in the causation of pain involving the head, face and neck. The tone of these muscles may be increased by a wide range of factors, for example, by whiplash injury, falls, blows, structural problems, incorrect posture, unbalanced working postures, jaw disturbances, visual disturbances, and psychological problems.

a) Nuchal muscles: trapezius, rectus capitis posterior minor (continuity with the dura mater),[2] splenius capitis etc.

Cause: Commonly, trauma etc. Increased tone in these muscles may exert compression on the cervical nerves. For example, spasm of the trapezius or semispinalis capitis can bring pressure to bear on the greater occipital nerve.

In particular, spasm of the longissimus capitis at its attachment to the mastoid process may exert traction inferiorly and medially. By drawing the temporal bone toward the occiput, it produces compression at the occipitomastoid suture and narrowing at the jugular foramen.

In most cases this condition remains unrecognized and asymptomatic. It is only in response to trigger factors such as physical or psychological overexertion, stress, fatigue, cold etc. that there may be a further increase in muscle tension, with consequently reduced venous drainage in the cranium. The premenstrual phase in women may also act as a trigger factor. Thus, an increase in intracranial CSF volume, intensifying intracranial congestion, has been recorded during the premenstrual phase.

Reduced perfusion in the cerebral arteries may result from venous congestion and this is responsible in the final analysis for minimal yet significant cerebral hypoxia. Headaches may ultimately be triggered by additional factors (alcohol, phenylalanine in chocolate, sodium glutamate, wine or cheese etc.) that do not increase muscle tone but cause vasodilatation. The increased supply of blood leads to raised intracranial pressure with subsequent headache.

b) Sternocleidomastoid muscle: (this passes obliquely across the occipitomastoid suture): increased tone in the sternocleidomastoid or trapezius muscles may adversely affect venous return and the nerve structures at the jugular foramen.

c) Muscles at the cranial base: longus capitis, rectus capitis anterior, superior constrictor muscle of the pharynx.

d) Increased muscle tone in the occipitofrontalis muscle, especially its frontal belly, may give rise to headache.

e) Masticatory muscles: masseter, temporalis, lateral pterygoid muscles etc. Increased muscle tone in the temporalis muscle may compress the squamous suture or, in the event of unilateral spasm, fix the frontal bone to one side.

The dura mater and extracranial fascia

a) Tension, due to unilateral traction on the dural membrane system of the cranium may provoke severe and sometimes dull pain, e.g. due to fibrosis, meningitis etc.

The dural structures may cause traction on the sinuses, arteries or sensory nerves. In this context, the innervation of the dural structures is of importance.

b) There exist a large number of fascial connections with the cranium and dural system:

- The dural membranes of the cranium are continuous with the cranial nerve sheaths and vascular sheaths that penetrate into or emerge from the cranial interior. Abnormal tensions on these structures may not only be perpetuated into the cranial interior but may also directly affect the nerves and vessels concerned.
- The cervical fascia are adherent to the cranial base, and externally at the occiput, temporal bone, sphenoid bone and mandible.
- Multiple fascial connections exist between the cranium and the diaphragm; via these connections, abdominal or thoracic dysfunctions may have repercussions in the cranium.
- A myofascial connection exists between the pelvis and the cranium, and the temporal bone in particular (locomotor apparatus dysfunction).

Because of these relationships, extracranial fascial tensions may be transmitted to the cranium, and consequently, even remote dysfunctions in the body may be involved in the causation of headache.

For example, abnormal tensions on the cervicothoracic and craniocervical fascia may reduce venous return from the cranium and cause impairment of nerve structures (see also Muscles).

Arteries

Over-distension, traction or compression of the arteries produces pain. These impulses are transmitted onward via the nerve fibers in the vascular adventitia. Paroxysmal, pulsating headache may arise as a result of over-distension of the branches of the external carotid artery, as in migraine and cluster headache. Over-distension of the cerebral arteries due to hypertension, and arterial vasodilatation due to fever, allergic shock states, hypoglycemia, or carbon monoxide poisoning, for example, may elicit continuous persistent generalized headache.

Arterial compression or traction due to brain tumors causes severe fluctuating headaches, usually lasting for hours, without any prior history.

In addition, arteriovenous perfusion disorders modify the intracranial biochemical and bioelectric environment (altered pH, increased metabolic breakdown products).

1. Intracranial arteries.
2. Superficial temporal artery (pain in the parietal region).
3. Occipital artery (pain in the nuchal region and behind the ear).
4. Supraorbital artery (pain in the orbit and forehead).

Veins

Headaches may result from venous congestion in the following structures:

a) Internal jugular vein: due to narrowing of the jugular foramen, e.g. as a result of cranial trauma, edema in this region, increased sternocleidomastoid or trapezius muscle tone, fascial and dural tensions.

b) Intracranial sinuses: dural tensions and brain tumors, as well as the causes listed above.

c) Veins at the cervicothoracic junction: due to dysfunction of the skeleto-myofascial structures in this region.

d) Lymphatic stasis: at the cervicothoracic diaphragm appears to aggravate the symptoms.

e) Right heart failure, with congestion in the superior vena cava.

f) Pressure in the head when bending is caused by congestion in the vertebral valveless veins.

Nerves

Neuralgic pain may occur episodically or be continuous and persistent. Episodic headache is generally caused by stimulation of specific trigger points (see Trigeminal neuralgia). Continuous and persistent headache is not infrequently the result of compression or traction due to tumors, aneurysms, inflammatory disease, increased CSF pressure, and disturbed venous return at the jugular foramen, or due to fibrosis, for example, after an episode of meningitis. Tumors of the cranial bones or scarring and inflammation of the skin of the head may also be causally involved. Abnormal muscle tensions in the neck as well as suture compression may exert traction or pressure on nerves. Reduced axonal conductivity and synaptic transmission may be consequences of venous congestion.

a) The sensory cranial nerves may be affected, especially the trigeminal nerve with its divisions, and more rarely the glossopharyngeal nerve (CN IX) and vagus nerve (CN X) (innervation of the posterior dura mater), and the greater occipital nerve arising from the 2nd cervical nerve.

Clinical presentation: Pain impulses emanating from the nose, paranasal sinuses, teeth and ears may produce pain in the occipital, frontal or temporal region via the trigeminal nerve.

b) The trigeminal nerve nucleus in the spinal column extends to the level of the 1st and 2nd cervical vertebrae.

c) The superior cervical ganglion (C1–C4) and its preganglionic neurons (C8 to Th2) may also be involved in the pain process.

d) Cervical nerves: irritation of the 1st cervical nerve causes pain at the vertex. Irritation of the 2nd and 3rd cervical nerve roots elicits pain in the nuchal and occipital regions.

Biochemical factors

Toxic metabolites or allergenic substances may also cause pain in the head and face.

Psychological factors

In particular, pain originating in the neck and spreading over the cranium in a localized or generalized manner may be of psycho-emotional origin. Such pain may be vise-like or merely be experienced as paresthesia of the head or face. In most cases it is difficult to identify a specific structure affected.

DIAGNOSIS

The treatment of head, face and neck pain is complicated by the fact that multiple mechanisms are frequently involved simultaneously in the causation of pain in this region. Meticulous history-taking with specific reference to pain, together with carefully implemented examination and palpation techniques, are prerequisites for successful treatment.

History-taking

- Where does the pain start, where does it continue, does the pain radiate, and does it change from one side of the body to the other?
- What type of pain is involved – continuous and persistent, throbbing, dull etc.?
- How long has the pain been present, what is its course, and does it occur at regular intervals?
- Is it responsive to intervention, what makes it worse or better?
- What triggers the headache?
- Are there any traumatic events in the patient's history?
- Are there any accompanying symptoms?

Location and intensity of headache *(see Tables 16.1–16.5)*

Very severe headache:

- Subarachnoid hemorrhage: diffuse at the occiput.
- Cluster headache: frontal region, above the eyes.

- Trigeminal neuralgia: territories innervated by the divisions of the trigeminal nerve.

Severe headache:

- Migraine: frontal and temporal region.
- Meningitis: diffuse at the occiput.
- Hemorrhage: usually diffuse.
- Temporal arteritis: temporal artery palpably hardened and tender.

Mild to moderate pain:

- Hypertension: diffuse.
- Muscle tension headache: nuchal, occipital and frontal region.
- Sinusitis: frontal and facial region.

Palpation

Palpate the cranium, sacrum and coccyx for PRM rhythm and motion.

TREATMENT

Treatment methods

Atypical headaches of uncertain etiology must always be elucidated by an appropriate medical specialist and malignant disease must be excluded.

Note: At the initial treatment, especially for headaches caused by congestion, do not use direct techniques for the cranium (or use only with extreme caution).

Treatment should not be instigated where there is a risk of cerebral hemorrhage (aneurysms, stroke), after whiplash injury or cranial base fracture. Treatment of the cranium and atlanto-occipital joint may be started about 2 months after stroke or whiplash injury.

1. Global examination, focusing particularly on the diaphragms and body posture, with treatment as appropriate.
2. Examination and treatment of fascial relationships: (a) Craniocervical, including muscle release. (b) Craniodiaphragmatic connections. (c) Fascial connections between the temporal bone and pelvis. (d) Diaphragm harmonization using Frymann's method.
3. Abdominal tension release.
4. Improvement of venous return at the thoracocervical diaphragm: (a) Upper costal joints. (b) Sternoclavicular and acromioclavicular joints. (c) Scalene muscle release. (d) Lymphatic pump technique for the thorax.
5. Improvement of venous return at the craniocervical diaphragm: (a) Treatment of the atlanto-occipital joint. (b) Occipitomastoid suture.

6. Improvement of intracranial venous return: (a) Venous sinus technique. (b) 4th ventricle compression or expansion (CV-4 or EV-4).
7. Special examination of the spinal column, with treatment as appropriate, especially of the upper cervical vertebrae (superior cervical ganglion, region of the trigeminal nerve nucleus and upper cervical nerves) and of C8 to Th2 (preganglionic neurons of the superior cervical ganglion in the spinal cord), 2nd to 6th thoracic vertebrae (zona ingrata).
8. Dural treatment and integration of the cranium, sacrum and coccyx.
9. General treatment of the cranium.
10. Specific treatment of the cranial bones: (a) SBS. (b) Occipitomastoid, petrojugular and petrobasilar sutures (petro-occipital synchondrosis) (jugular foramen). (c) Sphenosquamous suture (middle meningeal artery). (d) Sphenopetrosal synchondrosis (foramen lacerum) etc.
11. Treatment of the nerves involved: (a) Trigeminal nerve, see Trigeminal neuralgia. (b) Vagus nerve (CN X), glossopharyngeal nerve (CN IX), AO release, sutures between the occipital and temporal bones. (c) First three cervical nerves, upper cervical vertebrae and the atlanto-occipital joint.
12. Neurovegetative integration: CV-4 (stimulation of the parasympathetic system), inhibition of the superior cervical ganglion.
13. Temporalis muscle release (squamous suture).
14. Cerebral integration: Jealous' CV-3 technique, PBT of the CNS.
15. Depending on the individual case: dietary regulation, psychoemotional integration, eye treatment, detoxification etc.

References

1 Magoun HI. Osteopathy in the Cranial Field. 3rd edn. Kirksville: Journal Printing Company; 1976:76, 176, 282.
2 Hack GD, Koritzer RT, Robinson WL, Hallgren RC, Greenman PE. Anatomic relation between the rectus capitis posterior minor muscle and the dura mater. Spine 1995; 20:2484–2486.

17 The organ of hearing and balance

The ear, which accommodates the organ of hearing and balance, is divided anatomically into the external ear, the middle ear, and the internal ear.

The external ear consists of the auricle and the external acoustic meatus; the tympanic membrane is a partition separating the external ear at its medial limit from the middle ear.

The middle ear consists of the tympanic cavity, the auditory ossicles, the auditory (Eustachian) tube and the mastoid antrum (an air sinus in the mastoid process), and (as an inconsistent finding) the pneumatic system of the temporal bone.

The internal ear, located within the petrous part of the temporal bone, consists of two structures – an outer bony labyrinth that encloses an inner membranous labyrinth. The bony labyrinth is divided into the cochlea (containing receptors for hearing), and the vestibule and semicircular canals (containing receptors for balance). The membranous labyrinth is filled with a fluid called endolymph and is surrounded by a fluid called perilymph.

Relations with other structures: The external ear (external acoustic meatus and auricle) projects from the side of the head. The middle ear communicates with the nasal part of the pharynx via the auditory tube. The internal ear communicates with the posterior cranial fossa via the internal acoustic meatus.

The external acoustic meatus, the tympanic membrane as well as the organ of hearing and balance are of ectodermal origin. The mucous membrane of the middle ear arises from endodermal tissue.

The following pages will describe only those structures that are of practical relevance for the osteopath.

THE MORPHOLOGY OF THE ORGAN OF HEARING AND BALANCE ACCORDING TO ROHEN [1]

The organ of hearing

The internal ear, which has the capacity to create awareness of the inner nature of the spatial world, is located in the petrous part of the temporal bone.

Just as the pelvis in women provides space for the growth of a new living being – for the transition from the non-dimensional to the physical – the petrous part of the temporal bone provides space for the organ of hearing and balance where the spatial world of different frequencies and three-dimensionality can be experienced. As a result, however, the petrous part is required to forsake all life of its own: it loses its hematopoietic bone marrow at a very early stage and becomes the hardest bone in the body.

The organ of hearing can be differentiated into three regions: the sound-receiving external ear, the sound-conducting middle ear, and the internal ear with its lining of sensory cells. The malleus registers the vibrations of the tympanic membrane. Via the stapes, waves are generated that move onward at varying velocity in the perilymph of the scala of the cochlea and in turn produce vibrations in the endolymph and thus on the basilar membrane of the organ of Corti. A sound is 'dismantled' into a large number of waves traveling at differing velocities: they address different basilar membrane regions, which in turn produce receptor potential changes in the nerves involved. The afferent information is thus transmitted not only to one brain region for processing, but is distributed over different brain regions.

While spiral winding is already recognizable in the external acoustic meatus, Rohen likens the definitely spiral configuration of the cochlea in the internal ear to a spiral coil of intestine. The processes of nutrient breakdown and assembly of endogenous substances in the intestinal tract also have their counterparts in the organ of hearing. The double spiral structure of the cochlea reflects a process that begins with a dismantling from the outside inward and, at the transition from the scala vestibuli to the scala tympani, is transformed into a reassembly process from the inside outward. However, this dismantling and reassembly also occurs in another sense: words heard are first dismantled into individual sounds, vibrations, and potential differences and then reassembled in different regions of the brain to form meaningful words.

According to Rohen, the physical events in the auditory process reach a null point as a result of the transition from air to fluid and ultimately to solid through bending of the sensory cells. This null point marks the beginning of the inner neural and mental process. He likens it to a passive, spiraled 'wrapping' of information from an external source and an active, listening 'unwrapping' of information from an internal source.

The organ of balance

The endolymph in the semicircular ducts is the only body fluid that does not follow the fluid movements of the body, but is set in motion by the external world. This mechanism registers body position in response to sudden movement (dynamic equilibrium). In contrast, the otoliths of the macular region are organs of gravitation, registering body position with respect to gravity (static equilibrium). Through the organ of balance, therefore, body position in space is experienced in both dynamic and static terms.

The spatially-oriented organ of balance is the diametric opposite of the organ of hearing in its ontogenetic and phylogenetic development as well as in its structure. For example, the sensory cells are stimulated directly by fluid movement. In phylogenetic terms, the organ of balance is already present in the earliest vertebrates, whereas the organ of hearing is only properly developed in mammals.

Spatial perception definitely occurs at a less conscious level than auditory perception. For Rohen, the hearing of sounds and tones opens up the inner (mental) aspect of the material world, of space and the interior world of other people. These are examined from outside by the organ of hearing.

The organ of balance, in contrast, examines the external (physical) world, so to speak, and provides sensory information on the position of the body in space.

THE METAMORPHOSIS OF THE UPPER ABDOMINAL ORGANS INTO THE ORGAN OF HEARING AND BALANCE ACCORDING TO ROHEN[2]

For Rohen, the spatial problem is the focal point of these metamorphoses. Organs that accommodate spiraled structural forces and that fulfill similar functional processes, only in the material world in this case, are the liver, biliary system and spleen. In functional terms the liver also embodies a spiraled process working in opposite directions. The liver receives nutrients from the intestine and assembles them into the substance of the body, thus enabling entrance into the spatial realm. Waste substances and breakdown products are excreted with the bile. For Rohen, the monitoring process that takes place in the liver (e.g. of protein breakdown and assembly) symbolizes an auditory process unfolding in the material world. In the spleen, substances from the outside are screened and tested immunologically, highlighting the importance of the question of the endogenous versus the exogenous. To a certain degree this process corresponds to the spatial perception provided by the organ of balance. The iron-blood-biliary system is more closely related to the static spatial perception controlled by the macular organs.

THE DEVELOPMENT OF THE INTERNAL EAR

During the course of its development the internal ear becomes detached from the ectoderm, in structural terms resulting in an internalization process from the outside inward. An upper and a lower part, which are connected via the utricle and the saccule, develop already at an early stage.

A wound spiral plate is formed in the upper part. While the central areas of the plate coalesce and ultimately disappear, the three semicircular ducts of the organ of balance are formed from the peripheral tubes. These communicate with the utricle.

The cochlea of the organ of hearing originates in an entirely contrasting manner. Arising from the saccule, it develops as a tubular anlage and ultimately becomes elongated to form the spiral cochlea.

THE EXTERNAL EAR

The auricle

With the exception of the ear lobe, the auricle consists of elastic cartilage. It is covered with facial skin.

The external acoustic meatus

- It extends from the auricular concha to the tympanic membrane (a distance of about 30 mm).
- The lateral third of the meatus consists of a cartilaginous canal that is deficient posterosuperiorly. A connective tissue plate closes the canal to form a tube.
- The medial two-thirds are osseous. The squama of the temporal bone forms the roof, while the tympanic element of the temporal bone forms the remainder of the osseous meatus. It is of interest to note that the greatest part of the osseous wall is not formed until after birth.
- The external acoustic meatus is slightly curved and angled to protect the tympanic membrane from direct trauma.
- The external acoustic meatus is about 5 to 10 mm in diameter. The narrowest point is the isthmus at the cartilage-bone junction.
- Course: The external acoustic meatus follows a relatively transverse path, with the cartilaginous and osseous parts being at a slight angle to each other.
- The skin of the external acoustic meatus consists of stratified keratinized squamous epithelium furnished with sebaceous glands and apocrine glands. The entrance is protected by coarse hairs. The subcutis is absent. Even minor swelling here produces severe tension in the skin and is extremely painful.
- Glandular secretions together with epidermal flakes produce ear wax (also known as cerumen).

Relations of the external acoustic meatus

- In front: the TMJ.
- Behind: the mastoid process.
- Below: the parotid salivary gland; inflammation may migrate from this gland through the bone into the external acoustic meatus, and vice versa. The facial nerve (CN VII) (passes beneath the external acoustic meatus)
- Above the osseous part: the middle cranial fossa.

The tympanic membrane

- The tympanic membrane is thin (~0.1 mm thick), oval, and funnel-shaped.

- It marks the transition from ectoderm to endoderm and separates the tympanic cavity from the external acoustic meatus and thus from the external regions of the head. It is covered by an outer cuticular layer and an inner mucous layer.
- The tympanic membrane is attached to the bone by a fibro-cartilaginous ring. For most of its circumference the membrane is attached in the tympanic sulcus to the tympanic element of the petrous part of the temporal bone. The tympanic membrane attached here is taut. The upper part is attached to the squama of the temporal bone. The small area of tympanic membrane attached here above the malleolar folds is flaccid and composed of loose connective tissue.
- The handle of the malleus draws the tympanic membrane slightly inward, producing a funnel shape.
- The tympanic membrane is placed obliquely, from lateral superoposterior to medial inferoanterior, forming an angle of about 45°. In neonates, in contrast, the tympanic membrane is virtually horizontal.

Innervation of the skin of the external ear *(see also Fig. 17.5)*

- Auriculotemporal nerve (from CN V3): the anterior surface of the auricle, the anterior wall and roof of the external acoustic meatus.
- Great auricular nerve (from the cervical plexus): the posterior and anterior surfaces of the auricle.
- Auricular branch of the vagus nerve: the floor and posterior wall of the external acoustic meatus.

Innervation of the tympanic membrane

- Outer surface: auriculotemporal nerve (from CN V3); a small area is also supplied by the auricular branch of the vagus nerve (CN X) and a communicating branch from the facial nerve (CN VII). According to Tomatis,[3] the branch of the vagus nerve also provides sensory innervation to the outer surface of the tympanic membrane. Even the stapedius muscle seems to receive sensory innervation from this branch (motor innervation is provided by CN VII).
- Inner surface: the tympanic plexus via the glossopharyngeal nerve (CN IX).

Vessels

- The arteries have their origin in the external carotid artery.

Lymph vessels

- These feed into the superficial and deep parotid lymph nodes as well as the mastoid lymph nodes. The mastoid lymph nodes also receive lymph from the mastoid air cells.

THE MIDDLE EAR *(Fig. 17.1)*

The tympanic cavity

- The tympanic cavity is located between the external ear and the internal ear. This narrow, irregular space has a vertical diameter of about 18 mm, an anteroposterior diameter of about 10 mm, and a transverse diameter of 3 (5) mm.
- The chorda tympani, a branch of the facial nerve, traverses the tympanic cavity.
- The tympanic cavity consists of three parts: the epitympanic recess, which is an upper area above the level of the membrane; the mesotympanum, a middle area on a level with the membrane; and the hypotympanic recess, a lower area situated beneath the promontory and the membrane.
- Its epithelium is single-layered, flattened to cuboid.

The tympanic cavity has six boundaries

The lateral (or membranous) wall

This consists mainly of the tympanic membrane and, to a lesser extent, of bone (the squama above, and the tympanic element below).

The medial (or labyrinthine) wall

This also constitutes the lateral wall of the internal ear. In the center there is an identifiable rounded eminence (known as the

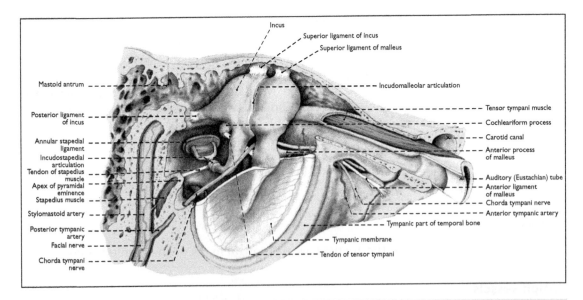

Figure 17.1 The lateral wall of the tympanic cavity; lateral view (From: Tillmann B. Farbatlas der Anatomie Zahnmedizin – Humanmedizin. Stuttgart: Thieme; 1997)

promontory) formed by the basal turn of the cochlea. Posterior to this is the round window (fenestra cochleae). Situated superior to the promontory is a reniform opening known as the oval window (fenestra vestibuli), which is occupied by the base of the stapes.

Inflammation may spread through these windows to the labyrinth. In front of the promontory, at the end of the bony canal of the tensor tympani muscle, there is a process around which bends the tendon of tensor tympani. The tympanic plexus containing fibers for the parotid salivary gland lies beneath the mucous membrane of the promontory.

The roof (or tegmental wall)

The tegmen tympani, a thin plate of the petrous part of the temporal bone, forms the upper boundary of the tympanic cavity and its upper surface is at the floor of the middle cranial fossa. In some circumstances there may be contact between the mucous membrane and the dura mater at this point.

The posterior (or mastoid) wall

This is directed toward the mastoid process. In its superior part is the entrance (aditus) to the mastoid antrum leading further to the mastoid air cells. On the medial wall of the aditus to the antrum is the rounded eminence of the lateral semicircular canal and the facial nerve canal. Below it lies the bony pyramidal eminence, which contains the stapedius muscle.

The floor (or jugular wall)

This thin plate of bone lies immediately above the superior bulb of the internal jugular vein.

The anterior (or carotid) wall

Its inferior part is formed by the wall of the internal carotid artery canal. The fine caroticotympanic canaliculi for nerves and vessels afford communication with the tympanic cavity. In the superior part of the anterior wall lies the tympanic orifice of the auditory tube.

Innervation of the tympanic cavity mucosa

- The tympanic plexus containing fibers from the facial nerve (CN VII), the glossopharyngeal nerve (CN IX), and the internal carotid plexus.

Vessels

- The anterior tympanic artery (branch of the maxillary artery): enters the tympanic cavity via the petrotympanic fissure.
- The superior tympanic artery (branch of the middle meningeal artery): enters via the sulcus of the lesser petrosal nerve; this forms a vascular anastomosis between the dura and the middle ear.
- The posterior tympanic artery (branch of the stylomastoid artery): travels with the chorda tympani.

- The inferior tympanic artery (branch of the pharyngeal artery): enters via the tympanic canaliculus.
- Tympanic veins travel to the pterygoid plexus and pharyngeal plexus.

Lymph vessels

Regional lymph nodes embedded in the parotid salivary gland.

The three auditory ossicles: malleus, incus and stapes

The auditory ossicles articulate together, are clothed with mucous membrane, and have ligamentous attachments. The tensor tympani and stapedius muscles are attached to the auditory ossicles.

The malleus (hammer) consists of a head, neck and handle, and of superior, anterior and lateral ligaments. The malleus is attached to the tympanic membrane and articulates with the incus.

The incus (anvil) consists of a body, short and long processes or limbs, and superior and posterior ligaments. The incus articulates with the malleus and the stapes.

The stapes (stirrup) consists of a head, an anterior and a posterior limb, and the stapedial membrane. The annular ligament of the base of the stapes fixes the stapes to the margin of the oval window, enabling it to move.

The tensor tympani muscle: This is contained in the canal of tensor tympani; its tendon bends laterally round the cochleariform process and is attached to the handle of the malleus, near its root.

Innervation: Mandibular nerve (CN V3).

The stapedius muscle: This is contained in the cavity of the pyramidal eminence and its tendon is inserted into the neck or posterior surface of the head of the stapes.

Function: To dampen the movement of the stapes in the oval window.

Innervation: Facial nerve (CN VII).

The auditory tube *(Fig. 17.2)*

The auditory tube is about 4 cm long and is the channel through which the nasal part of the pharynx communicates with the tympanic cavity. Medially to laterally, it leads upward and backward at an angle of about 45°.

The walls of the auditory tube are formed partly of cartilage and partly of bone.

In its medial section close to the pharynx, the cartilaginous part of the auditory tube (~2.5 cm long) consists of elastic cartilage. On transverse section, the hook-shaped auditory tube cartilage becomes progressively narrower laterally, and it is completed laterally by a membranous connective tissue wall to form a tube.

The bony part of the auditory tube, together with the tensor tympani muscle, is located in the musculotubal canal of the petrous part of the temporal bone. Medially, it is bounded by the carotid canal and it communicates with the tympanic cavity.

Figure 17.2 The auditory tube. 2, Tensor tympani muscle; 14, Tympanic orifice of the auditory tube; 15, Bony part of the auditory tube; 16, Isthmus of the auditory tube; 17, Air cells; 18, Cartilaginous part of the auditory tube; 19, Auditory tube cartilage; 22, Membranous lamina; 25, Pharyngeal orifice of the auditory tube (From: Feneis H. Anatomisches Bildwörterbuch. 6th edn. Stuttgart: Thieme; 1988)

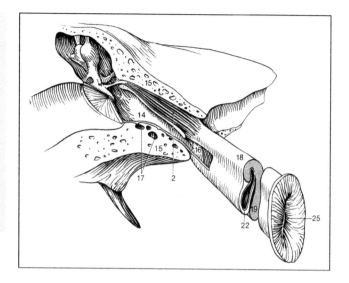

The mucous membrane of the bony part is continuous with that of the tympanic cavity, whereas the mucous membrane of the cartilaginous part increasingly resembles that found in the pharynx.

The function of the auditory tube is to equalize air pressure on the medial and lateral surfaces of the tympanic membrane. During swallowing, contraction of the levator veli palatini and tensor veli palatini muscles causes dilatation of the pharyngeal orifice of the auditory tube.

The air-filled sinuses

The mastoid air cells communicate with the tympanic cavity via the mastoid antrum. The air cells themselves do not form until after birth with the development of the mastoid process. They may vary greatly in size and number.

Relations: in front, the facial nerve (CN VII), and behind, the sigmoid sinus.

In rare cases, the pneumatic system of the temporal bone may extend as far as the zygomatic process.

Sound conduction

The function of the tympanic membrane and the auditory ossicles is to transmit and amplify sound and to convert sound waves into pressure waves in the perilymph and endolymph. This function is achieved thanks to the larger diameter of the tympanic membrane compared with the oval window, and the articulated suspension of the auditory ossicles (the longer lever is at the tympanic membrane, the shorter lever is near to the oval window). However, hearing is still possible without the auditory ossicles, with the result that a middle ear defect is not necessarily synonymous with complete deafness.

The internal ear

The membranous cavity system of the internal ear (the labyrinth) is located in the petrous part of the temporal bone between the tympanic cavity and the internal acoustic meatus. It accommodates the receptors of the organ of hearing and balance.

The bony labyrinth

The outer bony labyrinth has the same general shape as the inner membranous labyrinth and it surrounds the latter as an osseous capsule. The bony labyrinth can be divided into four areas: the vestibule, the semicircular canals, the cochlea, and the internal acoustic meatus.

- The vestibule is ~0.5 cm in diameter. It contains the two sacs of the membranous labyrinth (the saccule and the utricle).
- The semicircular canals: Both ends of the three C-shaped semicircular canals open into the vestibule. The lateral, anterior and posterior semicircular canals are perpendicular to each other.
- The cochlea: The bony spiral canal of the cochlea takes about two and a half turns around its hollowed conical central axis, known as the modiolus. The cochlear nerve and the spiral ganglion are lodged in the bony canal. The osseous spiral lamina projects from the cochlear axis into the interior of the canal. It is a bilamellar spiral of bone which winds round like the thread of a screw. The basilar membrane of the organ of hearing is attached to the osseous spiral lamina.
- The internal acoustic meatus: Its orifice is on the posterior surface of the petrous part of the temporal bone, above the jugular foramen. The internal acoustic meatus communicates with the bony labyrinth. It is approximately 1 cm long. The internal acoustic meatus is divided by the transverse crest into a superior and an inferior area.

The following pass through the internal acoustic meatus:

- The vestibulocochlear nerve (CN VIII) with the vestibular ganglion.
- The intermedius branch of the facial nerve (CN VII).
- The labyrinthine artery (branch of the basilar artery).
- The labyrinthine veins, which are received by the inferior petrosal sinus.

The membranous labyrinth (Fig. 17.3)

The receptors for the organ of hearing are contained in the cochlear duct, while those for the organ of balance are contained in the utricle, saccule, and the three semicircular ducts.

The cochlear duct (organ of hearing) communicates with the saccule (organ of balance) via the ductus reuniens. The utricle and saccule communicate with each other via the utriculosaccular duct. The endolymphatic duct passes from the saccule in a thin bony canal

Figure 17.3 The membranous labyrinth

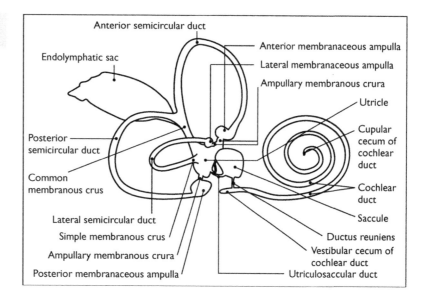

Anterior semicircular duct

Endolymphatic sac

Anterior membranaceous ampulla

Lateral membranaceous ampulla

Ampullary membranous crura

Utricle

Cupular cecum of cochlear duct

Posterior semicircular duct

Common membranous crus

Cochlear duct

Lateral semicircular duct

Saccule

Simple membranous crus

Ductus reuniens

Ampullary membranous crura

Vestibular cecum of cochlear duct

Posterior membranaceous ampulla

Utriculosaccular duct

(known as the aqueduct of the vestibule) to the posterior surface of the petrous part of the temporal bone and ends in a blind dural pouch, the endolymphatic sac.

The perilymphatic and endolymphatic spaces

The perilymphatic space is located between the bony labyrinth and the membranous labyrinth.

The endolymphatic space is located inside the membranous labyrinth. In terms of volume, the perilymphatic space is clearly larger than the endolymphatic space.

Relations between the middle ear and internal ear (labyrinth)

- The lateral labyrinthine wall is simultaneously the medial wall of the tympanic cavity.
- The inferior turn of the cochlea produces an eminence (the promontory) in the medial wall of the tympanic cavity.
- The semicircular canals are bounded by the mastoid antrum and the upper area of the tympanic cavity (epitympanic recess).

The facial nerve (CN VII) *(Fig. 17.4)*

The facial nerve enters the internal acoustic meatus in company with the vestibulocochlear nerve (CN VIII). It passes further into the facial nerve canal and then bends sharply backwards at the geniculum of the facial nerve. It runs to the medial wall of the tympanic cavity, arches downwards at the aditus to the tympanic antrum, and finally descends to the stylomastoid foramen.

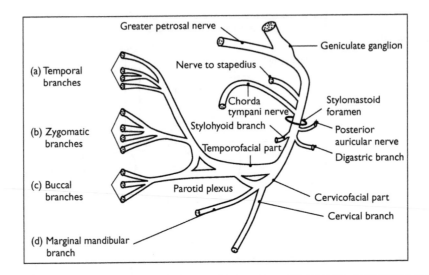

Figure 17.4 Schematic diagram of the territory innervated by the facial nerve (CN VII). Motor innervation. (a) Occipitofrontalis (frontal belly), temporoparietal, orbicularis (upper eyelid), procerus, corrugator supercilii, superior auricular (anterior part), anterior auricular muscles. (b) Orbicularis oculi (upper eyelid), nasalis, levator labii superioris alaeque nasi, levator labii superioris, levator anguli oris, greater and lesser zygomatic, orbicularis oris (upper lip), depressor septi muscles. (c) Buccinator, orbicularis oris (angle of mouth), depressor anguli oris, risorius muscles. (d) Orbicularis oris (lower lip), depressor labii inferioris, mentalis muscles

The branches of the facial nerve:

- The nerve to stapedius innervates the stapedius muscle.
- The communicating branch with the tympanic plexus runs in the mucous membrane of the tympanic cavity and ramifies in the tympanic plexus of the glossopharyngeal nerve.
- The communicating branch with the vagus nerve unites with the vagus nerve after leaving the chorda tympani, directly below the stylomastoid foramen.
- The posterior auricular nerve branches off below the stylomastoid foramen and passes upward between the mastoid process and the external acoustic meatus, sending branches to the muscles behind the auricle and to the occipital belly of the occipitofrontalis muscle.
- The digastric branch divides immediately after the stylomastoid foramen and supplies the posterior belly of the digastric and the stylohyoid muscle. It joins the glossopharyngeal nerve (communicating branch with the glossopharyngeal nerve).
- The parotid plexus forms a network between the two parotid lobes, and has the following branches: The temporal branches pass over the zygomatic arch to the muscles of facial expression above the palpebral fissure and at the ear. The zygomatic branches supply the lateral parts of the orbicularis oculi muscle and the muscles of facial expression between the palpebral and oral fissures. The buccal branches supply the buccinator and the muscles of facial expression at the mouth. The lingual branch (inconstant) provides

sensory innervation to part of the tongue. The marginal mandibular branch runs to the chin and innervates the muscles of facial expression below the oral fissure. The cervical branch descends steeply, behind the mandibular angle to the platysma and innervates this, together with the transverse nerve of the neck from the cervical plexus.

The following branches arise from the intermedius nerve (CN VII):

- The greater petrosal nerve: This leaves the facial nerve canal at the geniculum of the facial nerve. In the hiatus of the canal of the greater petrosal nerve it arrives at the anterior surface of the petrous part of the temporal bone and travels through the foramen lacerum. Together with the deep petrosal nerve it passes forward through the pterygoid canal of the sphenoid bone to reach the pterygopalatine ganglion.

Function: To supply secretory fibers to the lacrimal gland, the nasal glands, and glands of the palate.

- The chorda tympani nerve: This leaves the vertical section of the facial nerve canal and enters the tympanic cavity in a bony canal of its own. Having passed between the malleus and incus close to the tympanic membrane, it leaves the tympanic cavity together with the anterior ligament of the malleus in a groove (the petrotympanic fissure) between the petrous and the tympanic parts of the temporal bone. In the infratemporal fossa it unites with the lingual nerve (CN V3).

Function: To supply sensory fibers for taste perception to the anterior two-thirds of the tongue, and secretomotor fibers to the submandibular ganglion.

The auditory pathways

Afferent:
- First-order neuron: in the spiral ganglion of the cochlea (neurites from the cochlear duct).
- The central processes travel with the cochlear nerve to the internal acoustic meatus. This then unites with the vestibular nerve to form the vestibulocochlear nerve (CN VIII), which enters the rhombencephalon on a level with the cerebellopontine angle.
- Second-order neuron: in the cochlear nuclei in the medulla oblongata. Ventral cochlear nucleus: most fibers cross over to the opposite side (trapezoid body); some fibers remain on the same side and ascend to the inferior colliculus of the midbrain. Dorsal cochlear nucleus: fibers cross over at the floor of the rhomboid fossa and then travel to the trapezoid body nuclei and the olivary nuclei. Other fibers ascend to the inferior colliculus of the midbrain.
- Third-order neuron: in the trapezoid body nuclei of the olivary nucleus, the lateral lemniscus nuclei, and the inferior colliculus.

- Fifth-order neuron: in the medial geniculate body. Here connections exist with the optic-acoustic reflex center in the superior colliculus of the midbrain.
- The auditory projection passes through the posterior limb of the internal capsule to the auditory cortex in the temporal lobe (transverse temporal gyri of Heschl).
- Auditory cortex: tonotopic projection according to cochlear areas; fibers also cross to the contralateral temporal lobe.
- Further connections exist with the reticular formation and from there onwards to motor nuclei in the midbrain and rhombencephalon and in the spinal cord (ocular reflex movements, control of innervation of the stapedius and tensor tympani muscles).

Efferent pathway: From the superior olivary nucleus of the rhombencephalon to the sensory cells of the organ of hearing.

Equilibrium pathways

- The sensory receptors are located in the maculae and ampullae of the semicircular ducts of the membranous labyrinth. The sensory receptors (otoliths) of the maculae register head position, while those of the ampullae register the rotatory acceleration of the head.
- The first-order neuron is located in the vestibular ganglion in the internal acoustic meatus. The peripheral processes form three nerves that unite to become the vestibular nerve.
- This combines with the cochlear nerve to form the vestibulocochlear nerve (CN VIII), which enters the rhombencephalon on a level with the cerebellopontine angle.
- The vestibular nerve terminates at the second-order neuron in the medial, lateral, superior and inferior vestibular nuclei in the rhombencephalon.
- These vestibular nuclei have connections with almost all brain areas (the nuclei of origin for the eye muscles, cerebellum, motor neurons of the spinal cord, especially of the neck, reticular formation, hypothalamus, thalamus, cerebral cortex).

Efferent pathway: From the vestibular nuclei to the receptor cells.

LOCATION, CAUSES AND CLINICAL PRESENTATION OF OSTEOPATHIC DYSFUNCTIONS OF THE ORGAN OF HEARING AND BALANCE

Osseous dysfunction

a) Temporal bone

Causes: Pre-, peri and postnatal trauma, e.g. birth trauma, blows and falls, may lead to intraosseous or sutural restriction involving the temporal bone.

- Internal acoustic meatus (communicates with the posterior cranial fossa).

Clinical presentation: Disturbances of the vestibulocochlear nerve (CN VIII), facial nerve (CN VII) and intermedius nerve (CN VII), labyrinthine artery and labyrinthine veins.

- External acoustic meatus (the middle cranial fossa is located above this).
- Petrous part of the temporal bone (contains the organ of hearing and balance, attachment of the tympanic membrane).
- Squamous part of the temporal bone: Attachment of tympanic membrane.
- Mastoid process: Otitis media generally results in (transient) accompanying mastoiditis. Because the aditus to the antrum lies above the mastoid air cells, it is difficult for secretions to drain away. In addition, mucosal swelling may cause the aditus to close. Danger of pus spreading, for example, into the sigmoid sinus (sepsis), the meninges, and the brain (meningitis, cerebral abscess), the skin behind and in front of the ear, the sternocleidomastoid muscle, the external acoustic meatus, the petrous part of the temporal bone (dizziness, vomiting, auditory disturbances etc.), and the facial nerve canal (facial nerve paresis).
- Infections may spread from the middle to the internal ear via the round window and the oval window.

b) Auditory tube and nasal part of pharynx: In the event of pharyngitis, mucosal swelling may close the orifice of the auditory tube and thus impair pressure equalization in the middle ear. Further causes of impaired auditory tube function: sequelae of tonsillectomy, disturbances of the vagus, glossopharyngeal and trigeminal nerves (swallowing and yawning cause the tube to open), and abnormal myofascial tension involving the nasopharynx, the medial pterygoid muscle (trigger point) and suprahyoid muscles may impair tubal opening.

According to Magoun,[4] dysfunction of the temporal bone in internal rotation leads to narrowing of the cartilaginous part of the auditory tube, possibly resulting in a high-pitched noise. Dysfunction of the temporal bone in external rotation causes the tube to be held open, the consequence being a low roar. This sound is probably produced by the blood flow in the internal carotid artery at its bend in the petrous portion of the temporal bone because the artery is separated from the internal ear only by a fine plate of bone (pulse-synchronous tinnitus). Also, according to Magoun, while the auditory tube in children is shorter and has a larger lumen (so that it discharges more easily), it is also more horizontal, and therefore more subject to recurrent infections (e.g. due to food intake).

Clinical presentation: Ear pain in response to altitude changes, recurrent otitis media, unilateral tinnitus, and possible dizziness.

c) Mandible: TMJ

d) Occipital bone: Occipitomastoid, petrojugular and petrotympanic sutures.

e) Sphenoid bone: SBS

f) Atlanto-occipital joint

Muscle dysfunction

a) Sternocleidomastoid muscle (clavicular part)

Clinical presentation: Unilateral auditory impairment, possibly with dizziness in automobiles or on water, ear pain.[5]

b) Masseter muscle (deep part)

Clinical presentation: Ear pain, unilateral tinnitus.[6]

c) Medial pterygoid muscle

Clinical presentation: Possibly dull earache, ear pain or auditory tube dysfunction.[7]

d) Lateral pterygoid muscle

Clinical presentation: Pain anterior to the ear.

e) Occipital belly (occipitofrontalis muscle)

f) Tensor tympani muscle

g) Stapedius muscle

Clinical presentation: Paresis of the stapedius due to facial nerve problems will cause sounds to be heard with excessive loudness.

h) Levator veli palatini and tensor veli palatini muscles

Clinical presentation: Functional disturbance of the auditory tube with ventilation disturbance of the middle ear and sometimes tympanic effusion, otitis media, and cholesteatoma.

Disturbances of the ligaments, fascia and intracranial dura

a) Anterior ligament of malleus: e.g. due to TMJ disturbances

b) Pintus' ligament (irregular; extends from the malleus through the petrotympanic fissure to the head of the mandible), e.g. due to TMJ disturbances

c) Abnormal myofascial tension involving the nasal part of the pharynx, masseter, medial pterygoid and suprahyoid muscles, also involving the temporal fascia, interpterygoidal aponeurosis, tensor veli-styloid fascia, and the superficial and paravertebral layers of the cervical fascia

d) Abnormal intracranial dural tension

Nerve disturbances

a) Vestibulocochlear nerve (CN VIII) and facial nerve (CN VII): e.g. due to dural tension in the internal acoustic meatus

Note: The vestibulocochlear nerve is of major importance for the integration of input with regard to equilibrium and neck muscle movements. The vestibular nerve terminates at the second-order neuron in the vestibular nerve nuclei. Postsynaptic fibers travel in the vestibulospinal tract and, after synapsing with alpha and beta neurons, pass to the major and minor rectus capitis muscles.

b) Facial nerve (CN VII)

Causes: Mastoiditis, also inflammation of the tympanic cavity may adversely affect the facial nerve by crossing the frequently non-intact wall of the prominence of the facial nerve canal.

Clinical presentation: Peripheral facial nerve palsy (buccal asymmetry, frowning and eye closure not possible), taste disturbances to the anterior two-thirds of the tongue, reduced salivary flow, hyperacusis, retroauricular pain and disturbed innervation of the lacrimal gland.

c) Auriculotemporal nerve (from CN V3), great auricular nerve (from the cervical plexus), auricular branch of the vagus nerve (CN X)

Clinical presentation: Possible pain or paresthesia of the skin of the ear.

d) Auricular branch of the vagus nerve (CN X): Stimulation and touching the skin, as well as foreign bodies in the external acoustic meatus, may trigger cough via this nerve (Hitselberger's sign)

Note: This branch is described by Tomatis[8] as the external antenna of the vagus nerve. It may be the source of neurovegetative symptoms and psychosomatic disturbances in other remote organs. In Tomatis' view, the vagus nerve appears to be irritated in particular by low sounds. In an ear that is capable of good high-tone perception, the tympanic membrane is maximally taut and does not tend to vibrate excessively; for Tomatis, this is necessary for good neurovegetative equilibrium.

e) Tympanic plexus containing fibers from the facial nerve (CN VII), the glossopharyngeal nerve (CN IX) and the internal carotid plexus

Clinical presentation: Dysfunctions of these nerves may cause dystrophy of the mucous membrane of the tympanic cavity.

f) Temporal lobe: auditory disturbances

g) Ear pain (see Sensory nerve supply, Fig. 17.5)

Vascular disturbances

a) Internal carotid artery: The canal of the internal carotid artery forms part of the anterior wall of the tympanic cavity. Fine canaliculi permit communication with the tympanic cavity and thus constitute possible transmission pathways for infection; the carotid artery may also be involved in the causation of tinnitus (see above).

b) External carotid artery (branches for the external ear)

c) Labyrinthine artery (branch of the basilar artery): Supplies the internal ear

Figure 17.5 The sensory nerve supply of the auricle and external acoustic meatus

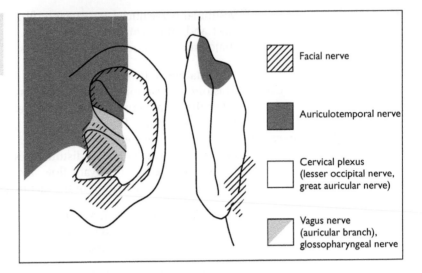

Facial nerve

Auriculotemporal nerve

Cervical plexus (lesser occipital nerve, great auricular nerve)

Vagus nerve (auricular branch), glossopharyngeal nerve

d) Vessels of the tympanic cavity: Anterior, superior, posterior, and inferior tympanic arteries

e) Internal jugular vein: The floor of the tympanic cavity is placed directly above the superior bulb of the internal jugular vein. Because the bone is frequently non-intact, inflammation may spread to involve the internal jugular vein. Conversely, congestion in the internal jugular vein may cause reflux into the sinuses, leading to drainage disturbances of the ear.

f) Sigmoid sinus, inferior petrosal sinus etc.: The labyrinthine veins of the internal ear open into the sinuses

Clinical presentation: Venous congestion in the sinuses may lead to drainage disturbances involving the internal ear.

g) Pterygoid plexus and pharyngeal plexus (drainage territories for the tympanic veins)

Causes of signs of congestion: Disturbances of the pterygoid muscles, the temporalis muscle and the TMJ, signs of congestion in the cervico-thoracic region.

h) Lymph reflux in the cervico-thoracic junction and especially of the lymph nodes in the parotid gland serving the tympanic cavity and the external ear (including reflux to the mastoid lymph nodes).

i) Disturbed endolymph absorption may encourage the development of endolymphatic hydrops and fibrosis of the endolymphatic duct, with the possible consequence of Ménière's disease.[9]

Glandular disturbances

Inflammation of the parotid salivary gland (situated beneath the external acoustic meatus) may spread through the bone into the external acoustic meatus.

Psychological factors, stress

Causes: Psychological and physical overload, psychological illness.

Words and phrases typically used: Listen, fail to hear, have an open ear, give someone a hearing.

DIAGNOSIS

A detailed medical history must always be taken to elucidate causes, accompanying factors, and trigger factors in patients with disturbances of balance and hearing.

For example, familial clustering, excessive stress (psychological and physical), psychological illness, exposure to noise, neurovegetative dysregulation (sympathetic and parasympathetic innervation), venous-lymphatic congestion, inflammation in neighboring regions, alcohol consumption (dizziness), medication (ASA, barbiturates), (cerebral) trauma, previous surgical procedures etc.

Dizziness

Dizziness of vestibular origin may be associated with sensations of swaying, spinning, or up-and-down motion. It may be permanently present or occur episodically and may be caused by certain body positions or when changing position. Patients experience apparent motion either of the environment or of their own body. In most cases, dizziness of vestibular origin is accompanied by symptoms such as nausea, sweating etc. This condition affects the structures of the vestibular apparatus: the vestibule, semicircular canals/ducts, vestibulocochlear nerve (CN VIII), vestibular nerve nuclei in the brainstem, vestibular nerve pathways to the temporal lobe, the eyes.

Otogenic dizziness may occur in association with tinnitus, auditory impairment, pressure sensations in the ear, or peripheral facial nerve palsy.

A disturbance of the organ of balance is associated with nystagmus, even without external irritation of the vestibular organ.

Causes of peripheral vestibular dizziness: Ménière's disease, labyrinthine disease, vestibular neuronitis, benign paroxysmal positional vertigo (BPPV), herpes zoster involving the auditory nerves.

Causes of central vestibular dizziness: Multiple sclerosis, acoustic neuroma, intoxication (alcohol etc.), transient ischemic attacks (TIAs).

Causes of non-vestibular dizziness: Cervical dysfunction, cranial trauma, ocular disturbance, cerebral sclerosis, orthostatic dysregulation, anemia, hypoglycemia, hypovitaminosis, temporal lobe epilepsy, psychological disorders.

Tests

Romberg test:

➤ The patient stands upright with legs together – but not pressed tightly together – and with arms held forward, horizontal to the floor and palms facing upwards. To begin with the patient should stand for 1 min with eyes open, gazing at a fixed point, and then with eyes closed. Patients should remove their shoes for the test, and they should not be able to orient themselves to any light or sound source. A tendency to sway and fall with eyes closed is suggestive of a spinal disorder (e.g. polyneuropathy). A tendency to sway and fall that is already evident with eyes open is suggestive of dizziness of vestibular or cerebellar origin.

Unterberger stepping test:

➤ The patient takes 50 paces on the spot, each time raising the thighs to the horizontal. The patient's arms should be held out in front, horizontal to the floor. If there are muscle tone differences referable to the labyrinthine system (e.g. labyrinthine lesion etc.), the patient gradually rotates towards the side of the lesion. Rotation of more than 60° to the right and more than 40° to the left is pathological (rotation towards the side of the lesion).

Babinsky-Weil test:

➤ The patient takes 2–3 steps alternately forward and then backward. In cases where pathology is present, there is gradual rotation to the side of the lesion.

Orthostatic hypotension: ➤ The patient sits on the treatment table. From the seated position the patient lies down on one side and then sits up again. Dizziness occurring as a result may be of venous origin.

Vertebral artery/organ of balance: ➤ While sitting on the treatment table and without otherwise changing body position, the patient rotates the head or suddenly extends the neck. Dizziness occurring as a result may either be of arterial origin (vertebral artery) or stem from the organ of balance. More rarely, a tumor in the fourth ventricle may be responsible.

Differential diagnosis for the vertebral artery:

➤ The patient sits on the treatment table and rotates the body while the cranium is held firmly in position and not permitted to go with the rotation. Dizziness occurring as a result is more likely to be related to a vertebral artery problem.

Adson's test:

Investigation of subclavian artery status: ➤ While palpating the patient's radial pulse, perform passive abduction, retroversion and external rotation of the arm. Ask the patient to breathe in deeply and to rotate the head to the test side (or contralaterally). Where the artery is compressed there is a reduction in the radial pulse.

Possible causes: Abnormal tension of the anterior/medial scalene muscle, cervical rib.
Note: Abduction of less than 90° leads to compression in the coracopectoral tunnel, and abduction in excess of 90° produces narrowing between the first rib and the clavicle.

Cerebellar test:

> The patient stands on one leg. Dizziness occurring as a result may be of cerebral (cerebellar) origin.

Further causes of dizziness must, of course, be investigated: Lesions to CN VIII or the balance nuclei, and to their cerebral pathways, which travel to the brainstem and cerebellum, as well as hypotension, anemia and alcohol consumption.

Further specialist medical investigations include nystagmus testing with illuminated goggles, thermal testing of the labyrinth, electronystagmography, tests for otolith function, rotation tests etc.

Auditory disturbances

The Weber and Rinne tuning fork tests

> Weber's test (Fig. 17.6) Place the stem of a vibrating tuning fork (frequency: 440 Hz) in the midline at the top of the head or at the upper margin of the forehead.

Note: Where hearing is normal or in cases of symmetrical conductive/sensorineural deafness, there is no lateralization of sound perception, i.e. the patient hears the sound 'in the middle'.

Rinne's test *(Fig. 17.7)*

Rinne's test is based on the principle that air conduction is more efficient than bone conduction. First, hold the vibrating tuning fork near the auricle so that the sound is conducted through the air. Then place the still vibrating tuning fork on the mastoid process for bone conduction (normally less efficient than air conduction). Ask the patient to indicate which stimulus is louder.

Negative Rinne test: in conductive or middle ear deafness (bone conduction is longer than air conduction).

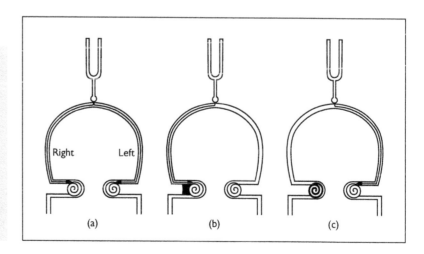

Figure 17.6 Weber's tuning fork test. (a) Normal hearing: the sound is heard in the middle of the head. (b) Conductive deafness (e.g. right side): the sound is heard on the side of the diseased ear (right). (c) Sensorineural deafness (damage to the internal ear or a more central lesion) (e.g. right side): the sound is heard on the side of the healthy ear (left)

Right   Left

(a)   (b)   (c)

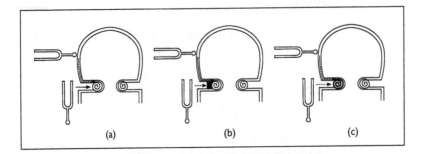

Figure 17.7 Rinne's tuning fork test. (a) Normal hearing: the sound is heard more loudly and for longer by air conduction than by bone conduction. (b) Conductive deafness (pathology affecting the external acoustic meatus or middle ear): the sound is heard more loudly and for longer by bone conduction than by air conduction. (c) Sensorineural deafness (internal ear pathology): the sound is heard for a shorter time by air and bone conduction. However, the duration and loudness relationship between air and bone conduction is as for normal hearing. Where the patient is deaf in one ear, the sound on bone conduction is heard on the opposite side

Positive Rinne test: in patients with normal hearing and in sensorineural or labyrinthine deafness (air conduction is louder and longer than bone conduction, but where pathology is present, air and bone conduction perceptions are reduced.)

Note: In combined conductive and sensorineural hearing loss, tuning fork tests yield only very limited information.

Spoken voice test

This measures the distance at which a spoken voice can be heard:

➤ Hearing is impaired if a conversational voice at a distance greater than 6 m, or whispered monosyllables at a distance of 6 m are inaudible (or only partly audible). During testing the contralateral ear must be muffled. This can be done by inserting a finger in the ear (for whispered monosyllables) and additionally wiggling the finger in the ear (for conversational voice).

Further specialist medical investigations include electroacoustic hearing tests, impedance measurements, retrocochlear tests, and evoked acoustic brainstem and cerebral cortex potentials.

TREATMENT

It is important to identify all pathological conditions that require pharmacological or surgical intervention (bacterial otitis media, carcinoma etc.). It is therefore always essential to have the symptoms assessed by a medical specialist.

After excluding all disease processes of the type referred to above, treatment is indicated for: serous otitis media, tinnitus, auditory impairment, pain in the ear, dizziness, and Ménière's disease.

Treatment methods

1. Global examination, with special attention to body posture and, where appropriate, treatment.
2. Special examination of the cranium and cervical spine and, where appropriate, treatment, especially of the upper cervical vertebrae and of C7 to Th2 (superior cervical ganglion and its preganglionic neurons in the spinal cord, C8 to Th2).
3. Improvement of venous return: (a) Thoracocervical diaphragm (including upper costal joints, sternoclavicular joints). (b) AO release and resolution of suboccipital muscle tension. (c) Venous sinus technique. (d) Fourth ventricle compression (CV-4). (e) Drainage of the pterygoid venous plexus.
4. Improvement of lymph drainage: e.g. recoil technique for the upper thoracic region.
5. Improvement of the arterial blood supply: JP Barral's technique for the vertebral/basilar arteries.
6. Treatment of the cranial bones, especially: (a) Treatment of the SBS.[10] (b) Treatment of the temporal bone, also intraosseous, and possible release of sutural restrictions. (c) Auditory tube technique. (d) Treatment of the TMJ.
7. Tissue technique for the external acoustic meatus and technique for the auditory ossicles.
8. Dural treatment and integration of cranium and sacrum.
9. Harmonization of fluctuation.
10. Neurovegetative integration of the ear: (a) CV-4 (stimulation of parasympathetic system). (b) Inhibition of the superior cervical ganglion. (c) Inhibition of preganglionic neurons in the spinal cord (C8 to Th2): examine and treat C7 to Th2 and the upper ribs.
11. Release of myofascial structures of the nasal part of the pharynx, the suprahyoid muscles and other cervical fascia, as well as of the sternocleidomastoid, masseter, medial and lateral pterygoid, and tensor veli palatini muscles.
12. Reduce psychological stress, and advise dietary change.

- In addition to the points listed above, treatment of the auditory tube, SBS and nasal part of the pharynx is of prime importance in serous otitis media and as concomitant and follow-on treatment for bacterial otitis media.
- Where otitis media or an auditory tube disturbance invariably accompany sinusitis, the latter should be treated as a matter of course. Schiefer and Weis-Ayari[11] performed a pilot study in 62 children (no control group) suffering from chronic tubal ventilation disturbances and showing no improvement despite long-term medical care. The primary efficacy variable (pressure in

the middle ear) and the secondary efficacy variables (nasal breathing, nasal mucous membrane status, nasal secretion and tympanic membrane findings) were assessed by an ENT specialist before and after the 4 osteopathy treatment sessions.

Results: Normalization of middle ear pressure was detected, as were improvements in nasal breathing, nasal mucous membrane status and nasal secretion. The normalization in the middle ear was evident in the reduction in retractions and the smaller number of effusions. Overall, the objective and subjective efficacy variables revealed a definite improvement in findings.

Auditory tube technique *(Fig. 17.8)*

Indications: Chronic inflammation/catarrh of the middle ear, tinnitus, tubal catarrh, ocular swelling (stimulates drainage of the ophthalmic vein, cavernous sinus, petrosal sinus and jugular vein).

Note: Always treat the SBS first.[10]

Patient: Supine.

Therapist: Take up a position at the head of the patient.

Hand position:
➤ Place your thumb at the anterior tip of the mastoid process on both sides, with your thenar eminence on the mastoid part.
➤ Cradle the occiput in your palms.
➤ Interlink the fingers of both hands.
➤ Rest both your elbows on the treatment table.

Method:
➤ During the inspiration phase of the PRM, follow the mastoid tips postero-medially with your thumbs (external rotation). (Stretching of the auditory tube.)
➤ Hold this position and instruct the patient to breathe in and out sharply.
➤ While the patient is breathing in, administer gentle pressure with your shoulder on the glabella and release again while the patient

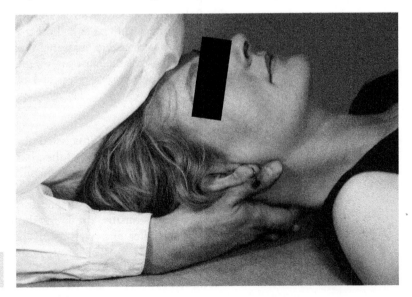

Figure 17.8 Auditory tube technique

breathes out. This pump-like motion is transmitted to the auditory tube and the ethmoid bone.

➤ Continue for several breathing cycles until you sense tissue release.
➤ At the end of the technique, re-synchronize the temporal bones with the rhythm of the PRM.

H. Klessen's alternative position (Fig. 17.9)

Indicated for use especially in children.[12]

Patient: Seated.

Therapist: Take up a position behind the patient and support the patient's head against your stomach.

Hand position: ➤ Place your thumbs on the glabella, with your ring and middle fingers on the mastoid processes on both sides.

Method: As above.[10]

Auditory tube technique II (Magoun and Galbreath) (Fig. 17.10)

Indications and desired effects: To release the TMJ, medial pterygoid muscle and myofascial structures of the nasal part of the pharynx, to drain the pterygoid venous plexus, and to improve auditory tube function. (Release of the medial pterygoid muscle improves the function of the tensor veli palatini muscle, which is responsible for opening the auditory tube.) To release the cranial base.

Patient: Supine, with head slightly raised and turned toward the side opposite the dysfunction.

Therapist: Take up a position beside the patient's head on the side opposite the dysfunction.

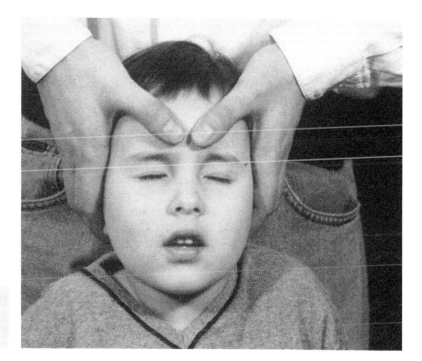

Figure 17.9 H. Klessen's auditory tube technique: alternative position for use in children

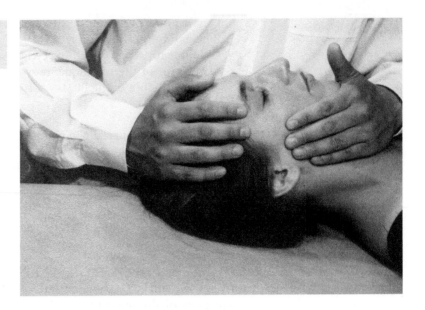

Figure 17.10 Auditory tube technique II (Magoun and Galbreath)

Hand position:	➤ Position your cranial hand frontoparietally to stabilize the head.
	➤ Position your caudal hand pointing cephalad. The heel of your palm should be close to the chin, with your fingers below the zygomatic arch on the TMJ.
Method:	➤ Instruct the patient to relax the jaw as far as possible.
	➤ With your caudal hand administer pressure forward, downward and medially.
	➤ Release the pressure again after a few moments.
	➤ Repeat this process several times. This will exert rhythmic traction on the pterygoid muscles and release the medial pterygoid muscle.
Note:	The osteopathic literature also describes intraoral techniques for treating the auditory tube. However, we have not been able to apply these techniques without making the patient retch.

Treatment of the TMJ (Ruddy's method) *(Fig. 17.11)*

Indication and desired effect:	Abnormal tissue tension around the angle of the jaw and the condylar process adversely affects the region of the external acoustic meatus and tympanic membrane. Aside from the specific techniques described in Chapter 11, a non-specific technique may be used to release this tension.
Patient:	Supine.
Therapist:	Take up a position at the head of the patient.
Hand position:	➤ Place both your hands over the angles and the ascending rami of the mandible on both sides. Do not rest on your elbows.
Method:	➤ Instruct the patient to move the mandible sideways (right and left), while you resist this movement.
	➤ Instruct the patient to tense the muscles for mouth opening and closure while you resist this movement.

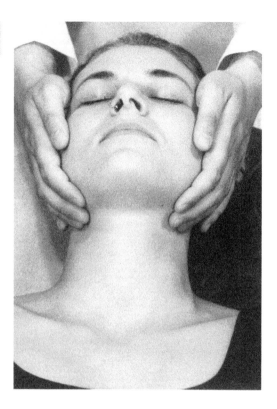

Figure 17.11 Treatment of the TMJ (Ruddy's method)

Tissue technique for the external acoustic meatus *(Fig. 17.12)*

Patient: Supine, with head turned to one side.
Therapist: Take up a position at the head of the patient.

Hand position: ➤ Gently insert your little finger into the external acoustic meatus.
Method: ➤ With your little finger, gently go with the existing tissue tensions, as for fascial release.

JP Barral's technique for the vertebral/basilar artery *(Fig. 17.13)*

Indications: Tinnitus, disturbances of hearing and balance, trauma (with subsequent abnormal dural tension, which may cause narrowing of the vertebral artery), decreased muscle tone (usually unilateral), patient anxiety when reclining into the supine position; generally, symptoms are absent in the prone position. According to ultrasound investigations conducted by Barral, arterial blood flow can be improved by about 30% with this technique.
Therapist: Take up a position at the head of the patient.
Hand contact: Place your left hand under the occiput, as close as possible to the foramen magnum. Position your right hand on a level with the right shoulder and the first rib.
Alternative hand position: With your right hand, fix in position the 6th/7th cervical vertebra.

Method: ➤ With your hand under the occiput, encourage contralateral side-bending and homolateral rotation at the cervical spine and head.
➤ With your right hand, fixate the shoulder/first rib in position by exerting caudad traction on these structures. This will fix the

Figure 17.12 Tissue technique for the external acoustic meatus

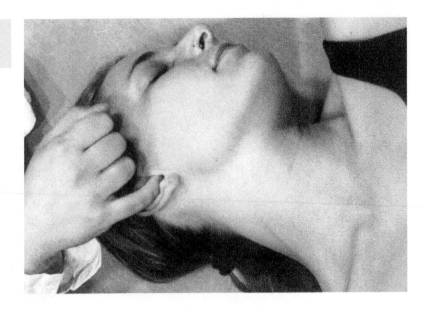

Figure 17.13 JP Barral's technique for the vertebral/basilar artery (example shown: right side)

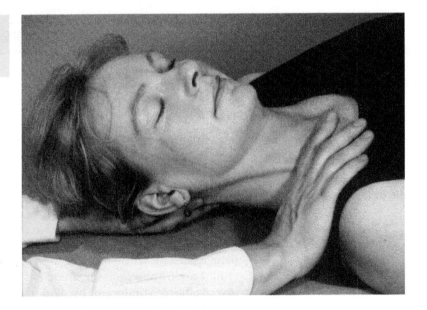

position of the subclavian artery, and hence the vertebral artery.

➤ Now, with your hand at the occiput, exert cephalad traction on the occiput and cervical spine during the inspiration phase of the PRM. Release this traction again during the expiration phase.

➤ Repeat this procedure several times in rhythm with the PRM.

Note: In patients with tinnitus, treatment of the homolateral kidney is also commonly indicated.

References

1 Rohen JW. Morphologie des Menschlichen Organismus. 2nd edn. Stuttgart: Verlag Freies Geistesleben; 2002:263, 270.
2 Rohen JW. Morphologie des Menschlichen Organismus. 2nd edn. Stuttgart: Verlag Freies Geistesleben; 2002:385–386.
3 Tomatis AA. Der Klang des Lebens. Reinbek: Rowohlt; 1987:211.
4 Magoun HI. Osteopathy in the Cranial Field. 3rd edn. Kirksville: Journal Printing Company; 1976:215.
5 Travell JG, Simons DG. Myofascial Pain and Dysfunction. Vol. 1. Baltimore: Williams and Wilkins; 1983:204.
6 Travell JG, Simons DG. Myofascial Pain and Dysfunction. Vol. 1. Baltimore: Williams and Wilkins; 1983:221.
7 Travell JG, Simons DG. Myofascial Pain and Dysfunction. Vol. 1. Baltimore: Williams and Wilkins; 1983:249.
8 Tomatis AA. Der Klang des Lebens. Reinbek: Rowohlt; 1987:22, 212.
9 Gibson WPR. The diagnosis and treatment of Ménière's disease. The Practitioner 1978; 221:718–722.
10 Cozzolino V. Osteopathic treatment of tympanic compliance. 1st International Conference on Advances in Osteopathic Research, London 12/1999.
11 Schiefer M, Weis-Ayari B. Stellt die osteopathische Therapie bei der chronischen Tubenbelüftungsstörung von Kindern eine Alternative zur üblichen chirurgischen Behandlung dar? Pilotstudie. Diploma thesis, COE, AOD: Schlangenbad; 2002.
12 Klessen H. A study about the influence of an osteopathic eustachian-tube technic on the pressure on the middle ear and on the compliance of the tympanic membrane in children from two to six years of age with otitis media with effusion. Dissertation, Hamburg; 1998.

18 Midline

IMPORTANCE OF THE SITE OF SPERM ENTRY INTO THE OVUM

In the absence of information from the outside, unfertilized frogs' eggs do not have the capacity to develop bilateral symmetry. This information is imparted by the site of sperm entry into the ovum. Only then does differentiation occur between meridians or lines of longitude, i.e. one meridian is differentiated from all others. Without this information being imparted from the outside, the ovum cannot know which of the existing lines of longitude will be the future symmetry-determining line of longitude, epigenesis cannot begin, and no embryo will develop. In general, the sperm enters the ovum a little below the level of the equator. The meridian joining the two poles and the entry site becomes the median plane of the ovum. The first cell division follows this meridian and the side on which the sperm enters becomes the ventral aspect of the frog. This information is not transmitted by DNA because even a camel-hair prick can mark the necessary difference to initiate bilateral symmetry development. The ovum would divide and continue to develop into a fully-grown frog, the sole difference being that it would possess only half the normal complement of chromosomes and would not be able to reproduce.

However, frogs' eggs should not be regarded as exemplifying the development of symmetry in higher animals and in humans. The amphibian ovum is already organized before fertilization. The cytoplasm recognizes gradients that are located in the ovum in organized form. In contrast, this type of intracellular cytoplasmic organization in the as yet unfertilized ovum is thought to be virtually absent in higher animals and totally absent in humans.

Nevertheless, in the human ovum too, the site of sperm entry is of some importance because two centrioles originating in the sperm spread out from this site and organize the spindles of the first cell division. These align themselves with the poles at opposite ends and the first cell division plane arises in the equator thus 'formed'. However, as already known, this is thought to be unconnected with the later development of the symmetry plane of the body. In humans, this plane is not laid down until the emergence of the primitive streak and the primitive node.[1]

Cleavage planes

The 1st cleavage plane determines the right–left dimension, the 2nd cleavage plane is perpendicular to the 1st, and the 3rd is perpendicular

635

to the first two, thus differentiating the animal pole from the vegetative pole.

The first three cleavage planes thus result in organization in the three dimensions of space. At this stage of the morula, however, the dimensions are not yet determined in the embryo, but surround it like a sphere.[2]

Gradient between the center and periphery

Even at the 8- or 12-cell stage of the morula, no cellular or intracellular gradients are yet present, and thus no symmetry plane can be identified. The first gradient to appear in human ontogenesis is the gradient between the center (later to form the embryoblast or inner cell mass) and the periphery (later to form the trophoblast or outer cell mass). This first appears as a dynamic phenomenon, i.e. differentiation occurs as a result of metabolic relationships: the metabolic conditions confronting the cells at the periphery are different from those confronting the centrally located cells. Later, this difference also becomes established in genetic-morphological terms and structurally different trophoblasts and embryoblasts are formed.[1]

Dorsal and ventral aspects

The future dorsal and ventral aspects of the embryo are already morphologically identifiable at the start of the 2nd week by the formation of the embryonic disk between the amniotic cavity and the yolk sac.[3]

The axis between the ventral aspect (endoderm: metabolic pole) and the dorsal aspect (neurosensory pole) has also been described by van der Wal as the axis of the will and of motion.[4]

The craniocaudal axis

For Rohen, the craniocaudal dimension already has its beginning with the emergence of the primitive node and the primitive groove.

According to van der Wal, it is the attachment of the connecting stalk in the region of the future rump during the second week that determines the craniocaudal axis of the embryonic disk. While a cranial and a pelvic region have already started to differentiate, a thoracic and an abdominal region have not yet developed. The site of attachment of the connecting stalk determines the position of the rump and of the head at the opposite end. The craniocaudal axis simultaneously represents the axis of polar opposition (of the information and metabolic system) and of its rhythmic balance in the middle. Blechschmidt and Gasser have noted that the craniocaudal ends, the dorsal and ventral aspects, and the lateral margins of the entocyst disk develop once the axial process has identifiably formed.[5] This principal body axis is also the principal axis for molecular orientation in the organism as a whole.

For osteopaths, the formation of the longitudinal axis expresses itself as a potency, which assumes a type of fulcrum function not only for the embryonic development of further structures, but also throughout the whole of life.

Polarity between the connecting stalk and heart

The embryonic disk, the 'earthbound central body', is linked via the connecting stalk at its pelvic pole to the 'skyward-oriented peripheral body'.

Blood vessel formation and hematopoiesis have their beginnings in the periphery. Hemodynamics come into being through osmotic forces and blood starts to flow in the capillaries of the chorionic mesoderm and collects in the connecting stalk. Finally, driven by metabolic forces, it flows from the connecting stalk via the yolk sac, the amniotic cavity, and the flanks to the head region, the cranial end of the embryonic disk. It is there that the primordium of the heart is ultimately formed, due to congestion of the blood. The blood 'comes to rest' at the cranial pole and then finally returns along other capillaries toward the periphery. For van der Wal, this is the moment when a 'presence' is formed in the embryo, a center that stands in opposition to the periphery. Now the embryonic disk becomes the center of attention, and developmental forces orientate themselves in the embryonic disk.[6]

To some extent, the connecting stalk and the heart represent polarities:

- The connecting stalk (later to become the sacral region) symbolizes an opening from the periphery.
- The heart (located cranially) symbolizes a 'coming to rest'.

Embryologically, this polarity is also expressed in the growth dynamics of the arms and legs: the growth direction of the arms is oriented toward the center, and that of the legs toward the periphery.

A further craniosacral polarity exists between the unconscious and the conscious: the more caudal the regions of the body, the more unconscious they are, and the more cranial the regions of the body, the more conscious they are.[6]

Development of left-right symmetry

At the cranial pole, which is closely associated with the heart, there is space for expansion, which is not present in the rump region due to the attachment of the connecting stalk. In the coccygeal region, therefore, the growth dynamic is directed inward and the impulse is created for the development of a new tissue layer, which is inserted between the ectoderm and the endoderm. This impulse ascends from below.[7]

The result is the mesoderm. Starting at the cranial end, a thin strand (the chorda dorsalis or notochord) develops, and this ultimately establishes the median body axis, the axis between left and right. However, the future longitudinal axis of the body is already preformed with the development of the primitive streak.[8] Cell movements to the right and left of the primitive streak characterize the beginning of bilateral symmetry in the embryo.[9]

Differentiation in the sense of left-right symmetry appears at the start of the 3rd week due to a polarity in the direction of movement of the cilia of the primitive node cells. These cilia beat synchronously to the left, causing fluid to flow over the dorsal aspect of the embryo. By this fluid motion, factors inducing left-right determination flow to the left side of the embryonic disk, causing flow-sensitive calcium receptors to be triggered only on the left side. The result is a left-right axis in the embryo in relation to its primordial organs. Blockade of ciliary movement (either experimentally or due to a genetic defect) leads to partial or total lateral transposition. (In contrast, Bateson believes that the information governing asymmetry must already be present in the ovum before fertilization, and he suspects the presence of a spiral of non-quantitative relationships, with the result that each meridian (no matter where it is drawn) must be asymmetric.[10] However, his data were obtained from experiments in frogs' eggs and, as has been noted already, this situation cannot be transposed automatically to that in humans.)

The direction of the flow of intercellular fluid determines the cells in which a specific cascade of chemico-genetic reactions will unfold, which in turn will activate specific genes etc.[11]

The same rule applies in this context: specific metabolic conditions and specific positional relationships come into being first, to be followed later by genetic 'determination'.

Whereas the ectoderm and mesoderm show a tendency to form symmetrical structures, endodermal structures tend to exhibit asymmetry. Thus, asymmetrical structures appear at a very early stage. As early as day 13 to 14, the later asymmetry of the organs, especially of the cardiac primordium, is identifiable by a slight divergence of the principal axes of the anterior and posterior endoblast chambers.[12,13]

Development of three-dimensional structure

Despite this trilaminar form, the embryo still appears flat. It is only with the formation of somatic segments and the resultant onset of mesenchymal development that the body begins to take shape as a three-dimensional structure and the anterior-posterior dimension – already adumbrated in the axis between endoderm and ectoderm – becomes clearly apparent.

Electrical fields

Research with embryos from a wide range of animal species consistently confirms that in all body tissues the anterior-posterior axis is the axis with the greatest polarizing potential. From the axis of the maximum voltage gradient in the electrical field of frogs' eggs, Burr was able to detect the later developmental direction of the nervous system.[14] The fluid membrane matrix of the embryo is thought to be oriented within this median electrical voltage gradient. However, these investigations are limited to work in frogs' eggs.

Liquid-crystalline properties of tissue

According to Ho, antero-posterior or dorso-ventral polarization is based on the liquid-crystalline structure of living organisms. In temporal terms, the antero-posterior axis is established before the dorso-ventral or proximal-distal axis. Ho regards the living organism as a uniaxial liquid-crystalline organism.[15]

Depending on their expression, liquid-crystalline mesophases may range from more liquid structures with only one-dimensional orientation through to very solid structures with three-dimensional orientation. In embryology, large tissue components undergo development from a more liquid to a more solid liquid-crystalline structure. The properties of the liquid-crystalline structures act as a shaping force for the development of a uniform organism because they shape the parts into a unified whole. This therefore constitutes an important morphogenetic organization field. This is substantiated by research demonstrating that non-linear vector fields were responsible for supernumerary or incorrect limb-bud growth.[16]

Dorsal, middle (ventral) and anterior midline

According to van den Heede it is possible to differentiate between a dorsal 'midline' (neural tube), a middle (the former ventral) 'midline' (chorda dorsalis to the sphenoid and the cellulae ethmoidales) and an anterior 'midline'. Nasion and the sacrum are reference points for the development of the middle midline.

The development of the first two midlines induces the formation of a third (anterior) midline, anterior to the former ventral one. This anterior midline draws a line from the nose to the hyoid, the sternum, the xiphoid, linea alba to the pubic symphysis. It develops through the meeting points of the outstretching dorsoventral growth movements. The hyoid is the balance point of the anterior midline (to the dorsal midline). The heart is the balance point for the fluid middle (previously ventral) midline. Sutherland's fulcrum is the balance point for the dorsal midline.

Exchange and memorization occurs in the dorsal 'midline', the middle 'midline' acts as a support for the body, and in the anterior 'midline' the potential body presents itself.[17]

For Jealous, in terms of the bioelectrical potency of the midline, the orientation of structure and function has therapeutic significance.[18]

Orientation to the midline is re-established spontaneously when dysfunctional tension is released following osteopathic treatment. According to Jealous, tidal organization occurs at the midline before the tide spreads to the body functions. All suspended, automatically-shifting fulcrums present should be oriented around this midline. Jealous states that the most important and primary midlines are found in the chorda dorsalis with an anterior orientation, and in the fluid of the ventricular system, which is thought to represent bioelectrical potential in the CNS. A close relationship between the umbilicus and midline is thought to exist, particularly during birth.

Each part of the body has its own midline, around which it is organized and around which it develops; according to Blechschmidt, for example, the vessels represent a type of organizational structure for the development of the limbs. (In this context, a space-time unit exists for each development.) Simultaneously, each structure also orientates itself around a specific primary midline or matrix of fluid potency, for example, around the primitive streak as a fluctuating midline or around one situated in the chorda dorsalis.

However, the body is not absolutely symmetrical. Even the brain or the spinal column is not symmetrical. There are midline structures, however, which represent an integration point for asymmetries and which exert symmetry-stabilizing function.[19]

The term midline may also denote the mean or mesor of rhythmic phenomena. The emotions too are oriented around a specific midline. One important midline in diagnostic and therapeutic terms relates to the dynamics of energy uptake and release, and this also includes sensory stimuli. One of the first and most important diagnostic questions may be to consider whether patients consume more energy than they release or release more energy than they consume, and which tension patterns and etiologies sustain this imbalance.

Traumatic and other factors may disturb the relationship of median and peripheral structures to the primary midline. This is also of major diagnostic importance.

The midline of stillness

- Allow stillness to come and give the stillness space to become full.
- Allow a dynamic stillness to become established between yourself and the patient.
- This stillness may be regarded as a type of midline that is always retained during the techniques described below.

Midline from the vertex to the tip of the coccyx *(Fig. 18.1)*

Patient: Supine.

Therapist: Take up a position to one side of the patient.

Hand position: ➤ Place the index and middle fingers of your caudal hand on either side of the coccyx.

Method: ➤ First sense the midline, the space around this midline, and the potency in the midline.

➤ Then sense the relationship between the vertex and the tip of the coccyx.

Figure 18.1 Midline from the vertex to the tip of the coccyx

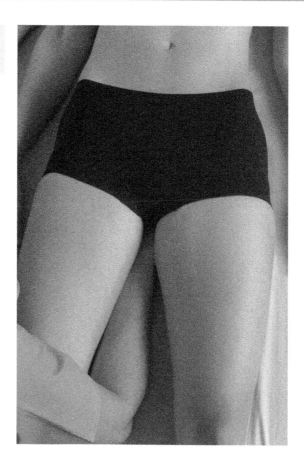

➤ Establish a point of balance between the two.
➤ If there is a lack of potency in the midline, direct attention to the tip of the coccyx.
➤ Ascending from the coccyx, sense the flow of potency and the inherent tissue motions that accompany this flow of potency.
➤ You may also gently amplify motion in the direction of ease (indirect technique).
➤ You will sense an influx of potency between the coccyx and vertex. Direct attention to the rising flow of potency from the coccyx tip in the midline around the region of the former chorda dorsalis as far as the 3rd ventricle of the CNS.
➤ Finally, sense the spread of this potency throughout the entire body.
➤ Re-orientate the vertex and coccyx to the primary midline.

Sacrococcygeal-lumbosacral or thoracolumbar midline
(Fig. 18.2)

Therapist: Take up a position to one side of the patient on a level with the pelvis.
Hand position: ➤ Position the index and middle fingers of one hand on either side of the coccyx. Place the other hand on or span the spinous

Figure 18.2
Sacrococcygeal-lumbosacral
or thoracolumbar midline

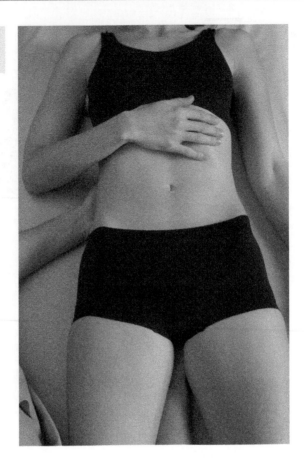

processes at the level of the lumbosacral or thoracolumbar junction.

Method: ➤ First sense the midline, the space around this midline, and the potency in the midline.

➤ Sense the relationship of the structures involved to the primary midline.

➤ Next assess the sacrococcygeal and lumbosacral or thoracolumbar structures in relation to each other. Focus your sensing on the expression of the primary respiration of the membranous-fluid aspects of the structures involved. Assess the synchronous expression of primary respiration in these structures.

➤ While continuing to focus your sensing on the expression of primary respiration, additionally start to go with the tissue tensions and amplify motion in the direction of ease (indirect technique).

➤ Establish a dynamic tension balance.

➤ Establish a fulcrum between the structures involved in order to balance the tensions between the two structures.

➤ Through resonance with the forces contained in the fulcrum, release the bound potency and make it accessible again.

➤ Potency will flow into the structures involved.

➤ You will sense an increase in synchronicity.

Figure 18.3
Sacrococcygeal-sternal
midline

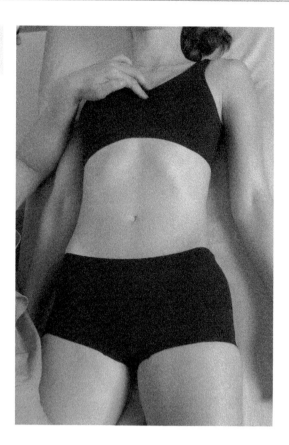

Sacrococcygeal-sternal midline *(Fig. 18.3)*

Hand position: ➤ Place the cranial hand on the sternum. Place the index and middle fingers of your caudal hand on either side of the coccyx.

Method: ➤ Follow the steps described above.

Inion-SBS midline *(Fig. 18.4)*

Therapist: Take up a position at the head of the patient.

Hand position: ➤ Place your thumbs on the greater wings of the sphenoid on both sides. Position the tips of your middle and ring fingers on the inion.

Method: ➤ Follow the steps described above.

Nasion-inion *(Fig. 18.5)*

Therapist: Take up a position at the head of the patient.

Hand position: ➤ Place the tips of your index and middle fingers of one hand on the nasion. Place the tips of the index and middle fingers of your other hand on the inion.

Method: ➤ Follow the steps described above.

Bregma *(Fig. 18.6)*

Therapist: Take up a position at the head of the patient.

Hand position: ➤ Place your thumbs on the bregma, with the tips of your other fingers on the squamous margin of the parietal bone.

Method: ➤ Follow the steps described above.

Figure 18.4 Inion-SBS midline

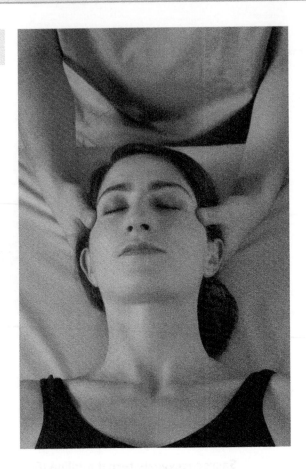

Figure 18.5 Nasion-inion

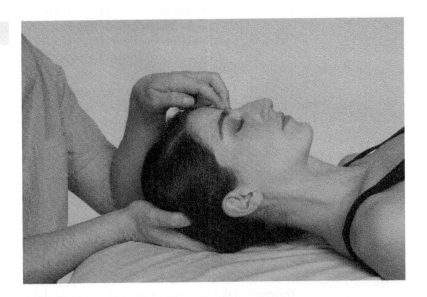

Figure 18.6 Bregma

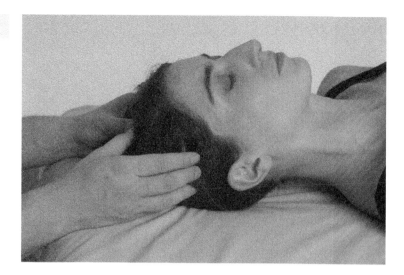

Figure 18.7 Bregma-inion

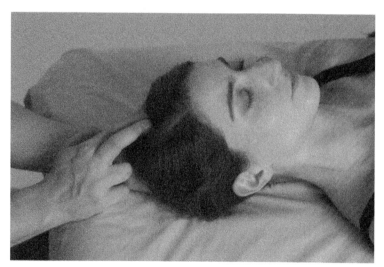

Bregma-inion *(Fig. 18.7)*

Hand position: ➤ Place the tips of your middle and ring fingers of one hand on the bregma. Place the fingertips of your other hand on the inion.

Method: ➤ Follow the steps described above.

Midline from the vertex to C1 *(Fig. 18.8)*

Therapist: Take up a position at the head of the patient.

Hand position: Place your cranial hand on the vertex. The fingers of your caudal hand should be in contact with the posterior tubercle of C1.

Method: ➤ Follow the steps described above.

Atlanto-occipital midline *(Fig. 18.9)*

Therapist: Take up a position at the head of the patient.

Hand position: ➤ Cradle the occipital bone in your hands. Your middle, ring and little fingers should touch at the median line of the occipital

Figure 18.8 Midline from the vertex to C1

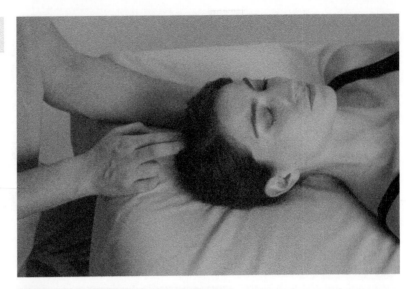

Figure 18.9 Atlanto-occipital midline

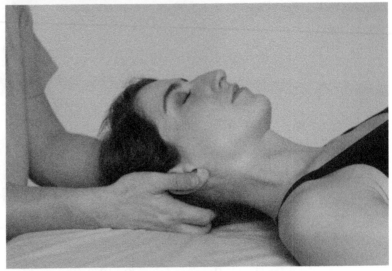

squama, inferior to the inion. Your index fingers should touch at the posterior tubercle of C1.

Method: ➤ Follow the steps described above.

Occipito-sternal midline *(Fig. 18.10)*

Therapist: Take up a position at the head of the patient.

Hand position: ➤ Place your cranial hand on the occipital bone. Place your middle finger on the midline of the squama. Place your caudal hand on the sternum.

Method: ➤ Follow the steps described above.

Navel-occiput (vertex) midline *(Fig. 18.11)*

Indication: Important technique for use in birth trauma and emotional trauma.

Therapist: ➤ Take up a position to one side of the supine patient, on a level with the navel.

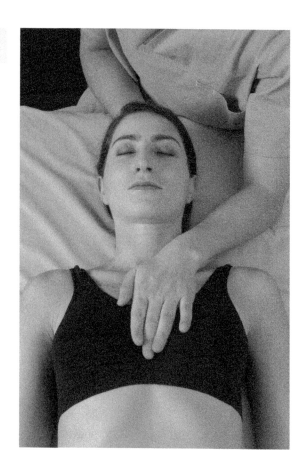

Figure 18.10 Occipito-sternal midline

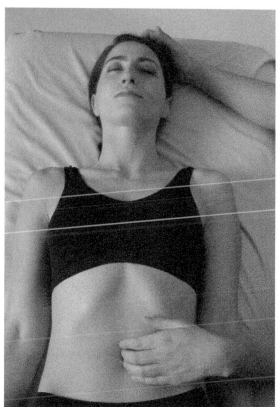

Figure 18.11 Navel-occiput (vertex) midline

Figure 18.12 The chorda dorsalis technique of Jim Jealous

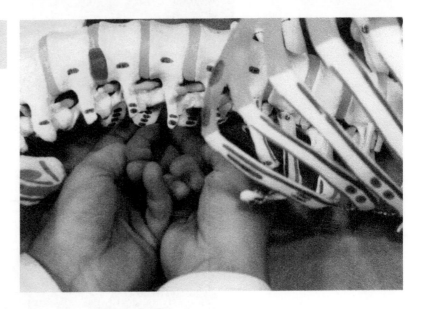

Hand position: ➤ Place one hand on the navel. Rest your other hand on the occiput or the vertex.

Method: ➤ First palpate the tension at the level of the navel and produce a resonance.
➤ Next sense the midline and the space around this midline.
➤ Then connect the navel and the midline to each other.
➤ In individual cases it may be necessary to exert a compressive force to support the inherent forces and bring them into action.
➤ Establish a point of balance between the midline and navel.

The chorda dorsalis technique of Jim Jealous *(Fig. 18.12)*

Indication: For example, to correct vertebral dysfunction.

Therapist: Take up a position to one side of the patient on a level with the vertebrae affected.

Hand position: ➤ Take hold of the two vertebrae involved in the dysfunction. Place your cranial hand on the upper vertebra.
➤ Place your caudal hand on the lower vertebra.

Method: ➤ In line with the embryonic development of the vertebra, gently compress together the lower half of the upper vertebra and the upper half of the lower vertebra.
➤ Then establish a point of balance between the two vertebrae.

A sacrosternal midline, and a midline of the two cerebral hemispheres or only of the frontal lobes may also develop, in addition. CV-3 may also be performed.

References

1 Van der Wal J. Personal correspondence; 2003.
2 Rohen JW. Morphologie des Menschlichen Organismus. 2nd edn. Stuttgart: Verlag Freies Geistesleben; 2002:58.
3 Hinrichsen KV. Humanembryologie: Lehrbuch und Atlas der vorgeburtlichen Entwicklung des Menschen. Berlin: Springer; 1990:112.
4 Van der Wal J, Glöckler M. Dynamische Morphologie und Entwicklung der Menschlichen Gestalt. Dornach: Freie Hochschule für Geisteswissenschaft am Goetheanum; 1999:82.
5 Blechschmidt E, Gasser RF. Biokinetics and Biodynamics of Human Differentiation. Illinois: Charles C. Thomas; 1978:34.
6 Van der Wal J. Course transcript. Hamburg: Osteopathic Schule Deutschland COSD; 9/2003.
7 Van der Wal J, Glöckler M. Dynamische Morphologie und Entwicklung der Menschlichen Gestalt. Dornach: Freie Hochschule für Geisteswissenschaft am Goetheanum; 1999:83.
8 Hinrichsen KV. Humanembryologie: Lehrbuch und Atlas der vorgeburtlichen Entwicklung des Menschen. Berlin: Springer; 1990:113.
9 Rohen JW. Morphologie des Menschlichen Organismus. 2nd edn. Stuttgart: Verlag Freies Geistesleben; 2002:66.
10 Bateson G. Geist und Natur. Frankfurt am Main: Suhrkamp; 1982:204.
11 Poelmann RE. Er bestaat een gen voor links of rechts. Bionieuws 2003;10:3.
12 Blechschmidt E. Die Pränatalen Organsysteme des Menschen. Stuttgart: Hippokrates; 1973:128.
13 Blechschmidt E. Humanembryologie-Prinzipien und Grundbegriffe. Stuttgart: Hippokrates; 1974:21.
14 Burr HS. Blueprint of Immortality. 5th edn. Saffron Walden: CW Daniel; 1991:33.
15 Ho MW. The Rainbow and the Worm. 2nd edn. Singapore: World Scientific; 1998:178.
16 Ho MW. The Rainbow and the Worm. 2nd edn. Singapore: World Scientific; 1998:180.
17 Van den Heede P. Course transcript. Hamburg: Osteopathic Schule Deutschland COSD; 3/2002.
18 Jealous J. Emergence of originality: a biodynamic view of osteopathy in the cranial field. Course transcript: 1997; 112.
19 Van den Heede P. Course transcript. Hamburg: Osteopathic Schule Deutschland COSD; 5/2003.

19 Special technique

THE FULFORD TECHNIQUE *(Fig. 19.1)*

Indication: For the release of tension in the celiac ganglion or solar plexus, therapy blockage, emotional trauma, diaphragm dysfunction, and pulmonary respiratory disturbance.

Therapist: Take up a position to one side of the patient on a level with the solar plexus.

Hand position: ➤ Place one or both your hands on the patient's solar plexus.

Method: ➤ Apply gentle pressure in a posterior direction.
➤ Administer gentle vibrations or go with the tissue tension until you sense marked softening of the tissue.

Note: According to Robert Fulford, the solar plexus is the emotional memory of the body. Emotional traumas are 'stored' in the solar plexus in the autonomic nervous system. For treatment to be successful, it is imperative to release tension at the level of the solar plexus. In so doing, this technique has far-reaching effects similar to those of CV-4.

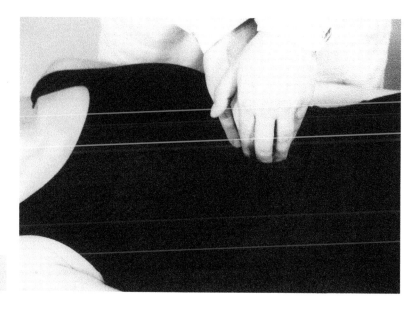

Figure 19.1 The Fulford technique

20

The biodynamic model of osteopathy in the cranial field

'The Tao that can be completely explained is not the Tao itself'
Lao Tzu, *Tao Te Ching*

INTRODUCTION

This chapter concerns the philosophy underlying the Biodynamic model of osteopathy in the cranial field (BOCF). To do this, we employ a Hegelian dialectic, a weave of BOCF principles with BOCF science, presented within an historical context.

We will compare biomechanical OCF with Biodynamic OCF, or 'left-brained versus right-brained cranial' as Fred Mitchell likes to quip. No treatment methods will be described here; BOCF techniques are illustrated in other chapters. Some information presented herein is an amplification of material appearing in other chapters, such as Still's concept of the Health, and Jealous's description of the Midline. Note that certain words in this chapter will be capitalized, indicating the usage of a defined BOCF meaning, not a standard dictionary sense.

BOCF's legacy extends back to Hippocrates, as reflected in the Hippocratic Oath's axiom 'do no harm' and its concern for our triune (body-mind-spirit) integrity. Threads of Paracelsus-style empiricism and Avicennian experimentalism color the BOCF tapestry. The foundation of BOCF, however, is firmly grounded in the philosophy and practice of three osteopathic teacher-physicians, evolving from three lifetimes spent in general medical practice, working alongside the self-balancing, self-healing principles present in their patients.

The first of these teacher-physicians is Andrew Taylor Still (1828–1917), who founded osteopathy in 1874. Dr Still sought 'the Health' in his patients, which was always present no matter how sick his patients presented. This concept was fundamental to Still's hands-on approach to care. 'I love my patients', he declared, 'I see God in their faces and their form'.[1] The physician's task, Still always reminded his students, was to remove with gentleness all perceived mechanical obstructions to the free-flowing rivers of life (blood, lymph, and cerebro-spinal fluid). Nature would then do the rest. Still formulated innovative concepts regarding the cranium, the cranial nerves, and he famously proclaimed, 'the cerebrospinal fluid (CSF) is the highest known element that is contained in the human body'.[2] His treatment techniques included gentle pressure on cranial bones, for example in the treatment of pterygium.[3]

The second of these teacher-physicians is William Garner Sutherland (1873–1954), who founded Osteopathy in the Cranial Field (OCF). Dr Sutherland was a student of Still and became imbued with Still's thinking, methods, and practice. Sutherland formulated his first cranial hypothesis as a student in 1899 while examining a temporal bone from a disarticulated skull. The thought struck him that its edges were bevelled like the gills of a fish, as if part of a respiratory system. Sutherland's 1899 revelation initiated a life-long evolution of thought, described in subsequent sections of this chapter.

The third teacher-physician is James S. Jealous (1943–present) whose Biodynamic Model of OCF (BOCF) has attracted great interest and controversy within the profession. Jealous adapted the term 'Biodynamic' from his study of the German embryologist Erich Blechschmidt and not from the Swiss philosopher Rudolf Steiner, although Steiner's Biodynamic concepts resonate with BOCF principles. For over 30 years Dr Jealous has compiled oral histories from Sutherland's students, and he continues to research Sutherland's writings (both published and unpublished). This 'work with the elders' enabled Jealous to compile an authoritative chronology of Sutherland's journey. Thus BOCF dedicates itself to the perceptual odyssey where Sutherland left off at the end of his life.

METAPHOR AND ARCHETYPE: THE KEEPERS OF THE KEYS

Still[4] wrote, '...that life and matter can be united, and that the union cannot continue with any hindrance to free and absolute motion'. Still's concepts, from the beginning, were already beyond the capabilities of double-blind trials. What Still saw and understood, and Sutherland came to refine in his later writings, was the universal principle that the natural world is constantly changing, and what is fixed (or without motion) becomes out of balance with its environment. Still considered osteopathy a science, but when Still's osteopathy extended beyond known science and rational explanation, he imparted his lessons by using metaphorical language. A metaphor uses familiar information to describe an unfamiliar idea. Metaphor provides a verbal bridge to gap the space between the speaker's intention and the listener's interpretation.[5] This transformational space, metaphorically speaking, characterizes the learning space between teacher and student, the theatre space between actor and audience, and the healing space between the practitioner and patient, where at a certain moment during an exchange something greater than the sum of the parts emerges.

Metaphors, despite being inherently non-rational, have long provided heuristic tools for approaching scientific problems.[6] Western culture, however, has difficulty grasping non-rational thought. The non-rational aspects of osteopathy (and other alternative medical systems) are the most difficult lessons to impart and the most difficult traditions to maintain. The man-as-triune truths that lay behind Still's osteopathy became the victims of medical reductionism, casualties of our Western way of emphasizing the intellectual and eschewing the intuitive and instinctual. Reductionism limits our view of reality and our faculty of awareness (sense of consciousness). Alternative forms of consciousness, as expressed through dreams, poetry, music, painting, or as found in cultures outside the West, such as meditation or trance states, have remained undeveloped in our society. Limiting our knowledge to what can be proven in a reductionist experiment has consistently succeeded in excluding the human spirit from the Western medical model.

This lack of spirit has been a concern of BOCF practitioners, who gained insight and inspiration from Laurens van der Post,[7] 'Man's awareness since the Reformation has been so narrowed that it has become almost entirely a rational process, an intellectual process associated with the outside, the so-called physical, objective world. The invisible realities are no longer real. This narrowed awareness rejects all sorts of things that make up the totality of the human spirit: intuition, instincts and feelings, all the things to which natural man had access'. Van der Post's anthropological concepts have played an important role in our understanding of health and disease in society.

Still no doubt acquired the skill of communicating symbolically-rich language from his father, a Methodist Minister. Sutherland, like Still, was a practiced wordsmith, having worked as a newspaper editor before training as an osteopath. Still's and Sutherland's language reflected the intimacy of their connection with the natural world. Still matured among the Shawnee and other Native American peoples – primal cultures, in anthropological terms. 'In indigenous, oral cultures, nature itself is articulate; it speaks ... There is no element of the landscape that is definitively void of expressive resonance and power...'.[8] Abram quotes a Native American healer, whose words resonate with the writing of Dr Still, 'In the act of perception, I enter into a sympathetic relation with the perceived, which is possible only because neither my body nor the sensible exists outside the flux of time, and so each has its own dynamism, its own pulsation and style. Perception, in this sense, is an attunement or synchronization between my own rhythms and the rhythms of the things themselves, their own tones and textures'.

Still's landscape was peopled by individuals who saw things from a totally different cultural perspective. Highwater[9] wrote, 'Though the dominant societies usually presume that their vision represents the sole truth about the world, each society (and often individuals within the same society) sees reality uniquely'. Still's and Sutherland's unique cultural perspectives have been revived by BOCF practitioners. BOCF initially evolved in New England, a land imbued with the spirit of Ralph Emerson and Henry Thoreau. These 19th century

New England philosophers believed that the study of Nature, or being out-of-doors in the natural world, offered a cleansing of the mind and spirit, and enhanced the journey of self-discovery.

At the time Sutherland[10] first published his insights, osteopathy was undergoing a period of reductionism. Most practitioners focused on the mechanistic aspects of osteopathic principles and practices. Sutherland's OCF represented a Renaissance of Still's osteopathy. But by the time of Sutherland's death in 1954, the OCF Renaissance itself entered a Reformational period, a reclaiming of the rational. Reformational OCF and its basic texts[11,12] has been embraced by many osteopaths as well as massage therapists, physical therapists, and chiropractors. But Sutherland's original Renaissance has carried on, under the aegis of his osteopathic students including Paul Kimberly, Anne Wales, Ruby Day, Rollin Becker, and Robert Fulford.[13]

As OCF has led to BOCF, the use of metaphor has led to the use of archetype. Whereas a metaphor is a figure of speech used to suggest a resemblance, an archetype is a term used to describe a universal symbol that evokes deep and sometimes unconscious responses in a reader or listener. Archetypes symbolically embody basic human experiences and their meaning is instinctually and intuitively understood. Jealous's concept of 'the embryo' as *ever present in the living organism* is a key BOCF archetype. When studying the writings of the embryologist Blechschmidt (described below), Jealous was impressed by Blechschmidt's conclusion that embryonic function (fluid motion) creates form and precedes structure. Jealous[14] intuited from Blechschmidt's reports that the embryologist must have witnessed the organizational forces of primary respiration at work, without the palpatory confirmation, given the reverence with which Blechschmidt and Gasser[15] wrote, 'The originality of embryonic human beings is discernible in many ways; for example, the early human conceptus is master of the whole geometry that it applies to itself. It is never mistaken about any angular sum, and it is never deceived in any surface to volume ratio. It never sets an intersecting point on the wrong site and is master of every physical as well as chemical reaction'.

The embryo, as an archetype of perfect form, serves as a blueprint for our body's ability to heal itself. The formative, resorbative, and regenerative fluid forces that organize embryological development are present throughout our life span, ready for our cooperation in harnessing their therapeutic potency. In other words, the forces of *embryogenesis* become the forces of *healing* after birth.

Among BOCF practitioners, every event within the therapeutic arena has a name. Nothing is referred to vaguely in terms of 'energy'. The importance of naming is shared by primal cultures worldwide, notably the Bushmen of the Kalahari.[16] According to the Bushman, an individual's separation from that part of themselves that is connected to 'everything else' leads to fear and a sense of aloneness, and this facilitates the disease process. Because treatment using the BOCF connects the patient to nature, the patient receives an immediate experience of 'not-aloneness' or 'belonging' in a deep way. Patients gain a physical sense of 'community', possibly for the first time in their life. As Wendell Berry[17] emphasized, 'The community is the smallest unit of health'.

In the next three sections of this chapter, we review OCF's and BOCF's evolution of thought, evolution of perceptual skills, and evolution of treatment approaches – from the *Bones* to the *Dura* to the *CSF* to the *Fluid Body*. See Figure 20.1 for a summary.

EVOLUTION OF THOUGHT

Bones

From his student days until the late 1920s, Sutherland concentrated on cranial bones, their sutures, and foramina. Sutherland proposed that cranial sutures remain mobile throughout a person's life. His hands-on insights predicted what is now known through histological studies – that most cranial sutures never completely ossify.[18] Living sutures contain connective tissue, blood vessels, and nerves. They maintain articular function and serve as crossroads of metabolic motion and somatic information. Sutherland's deductive observations were confirmed by research completed by his osteopathic contemporary, Charlotte Weaver. She conducted fetal dissections that led her to regard the bones of the cranium as modified vertebrae.[19,20] The sphenobasilar symphysis is embryologically homologous to an intervertebral disk – plastic and capable of motion.[21] Thus Weaver proved true the insights Goethe had in 1790, that the bones of the cranium are metamorphized vertebrae.[22]

Dura

In the early 1930s Sutherland shifted his emphasis to the dura and its bilaminar infoldings that form the falx and the tentorium, collectively known as the reciprocal tension membrane, which balances motion within the skull. Sutherland accessed the dura by

1910s–1920s:	Sutherland studies the cranial bones and their sutures and foramina
1930s, early:	Sutherland begins experimenting with the dura and its infoldings (falx, tent)
1930s, late:	Sutherland shifts his focus to the fluctuation of cerebrospinal fluid and elucidates the Primary Respiratory Mechanism
1943:	Sutherland describes the Breath of Life
1948:	Sutherland begins working with Tidal potency
1951:	Sutherland stops motion testing, all fulcra occur in still points
1960s:	Sutherland's writings are published, after editing by Ada Sutherland and Anne Wales
1970s:	Sutherland's students Rollin Becker and Robert Fulford expand his post-1943 work
1980s:	Bar Harbor: at a meeting of osteopaths from England and New England, James Jealous links Sutherland's insights to the works of Blechschmidt and van der Post

Figure 20.1 A chronology of OCF and BOCF evolution

gently gripping the cranium. The external periosteum is contiguous with the internal dura. Sutherland visualized one continuous web of connective tissue, from the cranium down to the sacrum – which he characterized as the tadpole-shaped 'core link'.

CSF

In the middle 1930s Sutherland shifted his focus to the fluctuation of CSF, driven by what he termed the *Primary Respiratory Mechanism* (PRM). He postulated that the PRM consists of five phenomena[11]:

- The inherent motility of the brain and the spinal cord
- Fluctuation of the CSF
- Motility of the intracranial and intraspinal membranes
- Articular mobility of the bones of the cranium
- Involuntary mobility of the sacrum between the ilia

Sutherland described CSF circulating down and around the spinal chord in a rhythmically pulsatile and spiral fashion. Science has again caught up with his hands-on insights, thanks to advances in radionuclide magnetic resonance imaging.[23] Many practitioners call the pulsation the cranial rhythmic impulse (CRI), a term coined by Rachel and John Woods.[24] Clinical studies report a palpable CRI rate of 6–12 cycles/min, independent of cardiac or diaphragmatic rhythms.[11]

The CRI phenomenon is poorly understood and its origin remains unknown (acupuncturists face a similar situation when asked to describe *chi*). Many researchers have made hypotheses regarding its source, as described in this book. Initially, Sutherland[10] proposed that pulsations arise from rhythmical motions of the brain, causing dilatation and contraction of cerebral ventricles, generating a pulse wave of CSF. Magoun[11] elaborated on this proposal and also posed an alternative hypothesis – that the choroid plexus produces CSF in rhythmic cycles, and this oscillation generates brain motility. Upledger and Vredevoogd[12] refined the choroid plexus hypothesis, calling it the 'pressurestat model'. McPartland and Mein[25] called the CRI a palpable *harmonic frequency*, a summation of several pulsations such as CSF oscillations, the cardiac pulse, diaphragmatic respiration, Traube-Hering modulations, rhythmically contractile lymphatic vessels, pulsating glial cells, and other polyrhythms. This 'entrainment hypothesis' has been put forward independently and recently supported by experimental data.[26] Many of these biological oscillators are lesioned by imbalanced autonomic tone[27] making the CRI variable and ephemeral. Thus from a BOCF perspective the CRI is a lesion phenomenon.

Fluid body

Many osteopaths today work within the CRI models proposed by Magoun or Upledger, but Sutherland moved on. In the final ten years of his life, Sutherland described the PRM being generated by *external* forces. He sensed his patients being moved by an external ubiquitous force, which he called the *Breath of Life* (BoL). Sutherland perceived the BoL to be an incarnate process, passing through the patient's body and the practitioner's hands, undiminished. With the BoL concept Sutherland's reverence for a self-correcting system had fully flowered. 'Sutherland arrived at a conceptual transition, leaving those who followed with a bridge to the depth of osteopathic research and practice that places us upon a new and deeply challenging renewal of the ultimate truths of our profession'.[28] Sutherland's bridge linked his students to Still's earlier insights, such as 'Life is the highest known force in the universe' and 'We are the children of a greater mind'.[4]

In the final years of his life, Sutherland's perceptual language drew upon the natural world around his home in Pacific Grove, California. He spoke of his patients as if they were part of a sea, with *waves* that rhythmically move through the water, and a tide that moves deeper, through both water *and* waves.[29] Sutherland was describing a polyrhythmic system (Table 20.1). As the BoL transubstantiates into the PRM, it generates various harmonic rhythms in the body, such as the 'Long Tide', the '300 second cycle', the '2 to 3 cycle', and CRI Becker[30] described the Long Tide as the basal rhythm, its rate directly correlating with that of the BoL, oscillating at a frequency of 6 cycles every 10 min. Around 1988, Jealous described the '2 to 3' (aka the 2.5 CPM cycle) with a mean frequency of 2.5 cycles/min.[28] The 2.5 CPM is a harmonic of the Long Tide. It is not modulated by the central or autonomic nervous systems, making it a stable rhythm. Liem[31] described the 300-s cycle, which has also been described by others. Polyrhythms may explain the poor agreement seen in some OCF inter-examiner reliability studies. For example, the inter-examiner study by Norton,[32] reported low reliability between OCF practitioners. This study was flawed because one practitioner recorded the CRI rate while the other practitioner recorded the 2.5 CPM cycle (Jealous, personal communication, 1997).

Sutherland[33] compared the BoL with the cyclic, sweeping beam of light emitted from a lighthouse, 'lighting up the ocean but not touching it'. The BoL sweeps through the patient, enlightening the healing forces already present in the patient. This allows the 'Fluid Body' to emerge, where the whole body behaves as if it were a single unit of living substance. The Fluid Body represents the BOCF

Table 20.1 Polyrhythmic cycles described in OCF and BOCF

Cycle name	Cycle rate	Cycle source
Cranial rhythmic impulse	6–12 cycles/min	Unknown. Possibly entrained autonomics or pre-neutral CNS activity
2.5 CPM cycle	2.5 cycles/min	Primary respiration
Long Tide	0.6 cycles/min	Breath of Life
300 s cycle	0.2 cycles/min	Unknown. Possibly a third order wave

equivalent of a Bose-Einstein condensate, where individual molecules lose their identity and form a cloud that behaves as a single entity.[34]

EVOLUTION OF PERCEPTUAL SKILLS

Bones

Sutherland's initial osseous approach to OCF requires a sound palpatory comprehension of all surface landmarks of the cranium, at all stages of human development. This includes the contours of the 22 cranial bones, their interlocking articulations, and many fissures and foramina. Normal and abnormal levels of tonus in extracranial muscles must also be appreciated, as well as tissue texture changes in cutaneous tissues.

Dura

The dural model of OCF, like the osseous approach, requires a comprehensive grasp of anatomy. Perceptually, sensing the dura and the reciprocal tension mechanism requires the practitioner to palpate tissues beyond his or her fingertips. This seeming esoteric skill is familiar to anyone who has driven an automobile on wet roads – feeling a slippery road surface through the steering wheel, sensing the road surface indirectly, through a series of linkages from the road through the tires through the wheel axles through the steering wheel.

CSF

For practitioners working with the CSF and fluid fluctuations, anatomical knowledge is not sufficient. Rollin Becker admonished, 'Studying the cadaver is like studying a telephone pole to find out how a tree works'.[35] The requisite education comes from a study of living tissues in one's patients. The practitioner visualizes 'a state of rapport in the fluid continuity between the physician and the patient'[11] by 'melding the hands with the head'.[12] With training and practice the practitioner feels a subtle motion, much like the respiratory excursion of the chest, sensed as a broadening and narrowing of the head between the hands. This type of palpation represents a harmonic signal of several senses, including temperature receptors, mechanoreceptors, and proprioceptors.[25] Other yet-unelucidated sensors may detect piezoelectricity or electrical fields as described by yogic practitioners.[36]

Fluid body

Detecting polyrhythms and the Fluid Body requires practitioners to augment their 'afferent' activity and reduce their 'efferent' activity. In other words, practitioners must emphasize reception rather than transmission – the difference between listening to a radio and conversing on a cell phone. Even 'melding the hands with the head' may be too efferent. Conveying efferent forces into a patient creates a jumbled sense of 'I-thou'. To detect the Long Tide and the 2.5 CPM cycle requires defacilitation of the practitioner's central nervous system.[14] Our consciousness, like our spinal cord, can become facilitated and noisy. According to Jealous, a quiet mind requires the cranial, thoracic, and pelvic diaphragms to function without inhibition. This is accomplished by allowing the breath to become slow and regular, and by softening the muscles above the pubic bone. These actions reportedly serve to 'synchronize the practitioner's attention'. As attention synchronizes and has room to breathe, the practitioner senses deeper rhythms, and the signal shifts from the CRI rate to the 2.5 CPM cycle. With deeper defacilitation, perception of the 2.5 CPM cycle disappears into the Long Tide.[14]

With enhanced perceptual skills, the practitioner eventually perceives a sense of *Neutral*, which is experienced as a homogenization of tissue, fluid, and potency – the Fluid Body, where nothing under the fingertips can be discerned as a separate entity. This lysergic entity lies at the perceptual center of BOCF. The Neutral cannot be conceptualized, it can only be experienced. It is here that 'holism' becomes more than a philosophical concept, it can be appreciated as an actual sensory perception. A summary of some of the differences between OCF and BOCF are presented in the Glossary, Table G.1.

EVOLUTION OF TREATMENT APPROACHES

Bones

Directly adjusting sutures and foramina affects the function of cranial nerves and vessels that traverse these apertures, as well as the function of muscles that originate or insert upon cranial bones. Some of Sutherland's students continue to focus on bones and sutures, such as the American chiropractor Dejarnette, who founded Sacral-Occipital Technique.[37] Treatment of suboccipital muscles directly impacts the dura and may be helpful in patients with dural headaches and chronic pain syndromes.[38]

Dura

Treating the reciprocal tension membrane with balanced membranous tension (BMT) is an indirect technique, performed by gently exaggerating the membrane's strain patterns, balancing the tension in strained fibers with the tension present in normal fibers, effecting a release of the strain.[33] Many osteopaths work with this dural model and get good results. Lawrence Jones used his counterstrain technique to mould the falx and the tent. Beryl Arbuckle was an extraordinarily gifted practitioner of BMT.

CSF

Sutherland initially used direct hydraulic force, such as the CV-4 technique for compressing CSF in the 4th ventricle.[11,12] The CV-4 induces therapeutic changes around the body, possibly via periaqueductal gray (PAG) tissue, which surrounds the 4th ventricle. The PAG is lined with neuroreceptors (opioid and cannabinoid receptors), and it responds to stimuli (such as hydraulic pressure) by activating these neuroreceptors, by releasing endorphins and endocannabinoids, and by propagating pain-inhibitory signals to the dorsal horn. The PAG is homuncular, like the somatosensory cortex, so the topography of the PAG corresponds to different parts of the body (J. Giodarno, personal communication, 2002).

Most practitioners who work with the rhythmic fluctuation of CSF focus upon the CRI rate, as exampled by Magoun's and Updelger's models. The CRI rate is also the focus of the Sutherland Cranial Teaching Foundation (SCTF), although the SCTF now incorporates the 2.5 CPM cycle and the Long Tide into their curriculum (A. Norrie, personal communication, 2002).

CRI-oriented practitioners may bring about therapeutic changes by inducing entrainment.[25] Entrainment was first described in 1665 by Christiaan Huygens.[39] He noted that collections of pendulum clocks began swinging in synchrony with each other. This coupling phenomenon also arises within organisms (e.g. cardiac pacemaker cells) and between organisms (e.g. simultaneously flashing fireflies, harmoniously chirping crickets, and women whose menstrual phases cycle together). Huygens noted that 'strongest' clocks (those with the heaviest pendulums) established the eventual, overall rhythm. McPartland and Mein[25] proposed that practitioners transferred their 'strong clock' rhythms onto their patients, and enhanced this transfer by assuming a meditative state before treating patients. Meditative, centered states are known to produce strong entrainment.[40] Centering to harness entrainment may be a widespread therapeutic technique, albeit unrecognized by practitioners of Feldenkrais, Network Chiropractic, Polarity therapy, Reiki, Therapeutic Touch, and Tragering. Chinese practitioners center on *tan tien*, the 'one point', about 5 cm above the pubic bone, whereas Tibetan practitioners meditate on an image of the Medicine Buddha centered at *sahar chakrã*, the crown of the head.[41] The new 'Freeze-Frame' technique focuses on the heart to achieve entrainment.[40] All these techniques center attention on parts of the body rich in biological oscillators (intestines, brain and heart).

Tiller et al.[40] stated that feelings of empathy and love lead to strong entrainment. Jahn[42] described the *resonant bond* between practitioner and patient as a form of love, transmitting 'beneficial information'. Wirkus[43] emphasized that the healer '… must feel and be the heart chakra … It is not thinking the word "love", it is the real sensation of pure love which brings warmth, delicate vibrations in your heart area'. Fulford[44] was precise: 'You the [practitioner] stand neutral, acting as a conduit for the flow of divine love. As you learn to use love properly in healing work, your body vibrations increase and it becomes easier to handle the potency of the love energy'.

Entrainment has its limitations. It can only be employed by practitioners who work with the CRI. Practitioners working with slower rhythms avoid efferent activity, so no entrainment may be possible, or desired. We limit our therapeutic potential when we focus solely on the CNS – whether we work with the CSF like Sutherland's early years, or the cellular vibrations of entrainment. We may also cause side-effects and iatrogenesis.[45,46]

Fluid body

According to a précis by Jealous (personal communication, 2004), 'Cranial Osteopathy is not about the cranium. It is about Primary Respiration'. Sutherland's move from the CSF to the fluid body began with a technique he called 'automatic shifting'. Paulsen[47] described Sutherland's sensation of a 'motor' starting in the CSF and then carrying on of its own accord, generating a healing force that treated several lesions around the body. 'The core of this work is perceptual', wrote Jealous,[14] 'We learn to sense the Whole. When one meets a patient, one sees the Whole – a very rare event in our modern world'. When a patient achieves a *Neutral* as described previously, the CNS becomes quiet (the person often falls asleep). With the CNS 'out of the way', the whole person – the CNS, CSF, all other fluids, and all other tissues – merges into the fluid body. Within the protoplasmic fluid body, motion is purely metabolic, responding freely to the outside presence of the natural world and the BoL.

To harness the potency present in the BoL as expressed in the Tide requires ever-more subtle techniques. In the final years of his career, Sutherland stopped all motion testing of the head, and applied no forces to osteopathic lesions. He worked with fulcrums in still points, and stated, 'treat not with techniques but gentle contact'.[33] Working with the Health is a BOCF imperative, echoing Still,[2] 'To find health should be the object of the doctor. Anyone can find disease'. Jealous[28] described therapeutic changes requiring an 'aboriginal and instinctual consciousness' on the part of the practitioner, not intellectual or even intuitive, 'The moment is filled with the effort to be present with the Health in the patient and the story as it unfolds into its own answer'.

BOCF SCIENCE: QUANTUM CONSCIOUSNESS

Osteopaths base their science in *physics*, whereas Western medical practitioners practice *chemistry* – their pharmacodynamic tools treat chemical moieties known as genes and gene products. Osteopaths recognize the A-T-C-G chemistry of genes, but focus on the physics of the midline within the double helix itself. To wit, osteopaths focus on the double helix's fourth dimension: Time. DNA converts time into space. Surprisingly, this transmutation can be explained within the mechanistic model of Newtonian physics.[48] Many new ideas proposed by New Age healers operate within a Newtonian paradigm. Pert[49] hypothesized that energy therapists heal their patients by inducing a vibrational tone that shifts neuroreceptors into their constitutively-active state, or the vibrations trigger the release of endorphins that active the neuroreceptors. Oschman[50] described crystalline materials within biological structures (e.g. phospholipids within cell membranes, collagen in connective tissues) that generate electric fields when compressed or stretched (piezoelectricity). These energy fields may be the source of hands-on healing, a radical proposition, but safe within a mechanistic paradigm.

Newtonian physics has undergone a paradigm shift to Quantum physics, thanks to relativistic studies addressing subatomic phenomena and consciousness. Still's writings suggest he had undergone a Quantum paradigm shift. He knew intuitively that the healing events in his patients happened at the subatomic level, but he did not have the words or the concepts of Quantum physics to draw upon, to express the transformation he was experiencing in his treatments. Instead, he ascribed the return to health to God or Divine Nature at work.

Sutherland's BoL exhibits characteristics that can only be explained by Quantum theory (e.g. the theory of implicate order[51]). The BoL transubstantiates into primary respiration, a field force that generates a spatial orientation, so it shares characteristics with the 'morphogenetic fields' described by Sheldrake.[52] Sheldrake's concepts are very Quantum: Morphogenetic fields carry information only (no energy) and are available throughout time and space without any loss of intensity after they have been created. These nonphysical 'blueprints' guide the formation of physical forms through three-dimensional patterns of vibration he called *morphic resonance*. The morphic resonance that generates form in the embryo is the same process that generates healing in the adult.

The role of consciousness in Quantum theory is a radical departure from classical physics. The outcome of any experiment depends upon the consciousness of the observer. Indeed, the term *observer* should be replaced by the term *participator*. We cannot observe the universe, we are participants in it. Our individual consciousness is a small hologram of the universal consciousness shared by all living things. Capra[53] named consciousness ('the process of knowing') as a key feature of life, including life forms such as plants and protozoans that lack a central nervous system. The protoplasmic Fluid Body shares this consciousness, which explains its 'sensitive' and 'decision-making' attributes.[14]

From a BOCF perspective, Jealous[14] acknowledged that the practitioner's consciousness has a primary role in the depth of therapeutic changes arising in the patient. Jealous discovered that his therapeutic results improved in proportion to the extent to which he could free himself from conscious rationalization. He discovered, as did Sutherland, that the practitioner's effort '… is to let the Breath of Life move us, allow us vision … One's effort must be from a 'sense of the possibilities'.[14] The next couple of sections of this chapter review new research 'around the edges' of BOCF science.

BLECHSCHMIDT'S EMBRYOLOGY *VIS À VIS* THE BoL

Jealous[14] characterized traditional osteopathy as a science based on anatomy, whereas BOCF is a science based on embryology. BoL practitioners have followed the work of Erich Blechschmidt (1902–1992), an unabashedly holistic embryologist. According to Blechschmidt,[54] each part of the embryo develops in motion, and each motion impacts the development of each subsequent development. Early embryological development is largely *epigenetic*, guided by fluid dynamics. Blechschmidt's concepts agree with BOCF practitioners, who postulate that the BoL, the external force described by Sutherland, generates a spatial orientation in the embryo. The spatial orientation becomes expressed in the material plane by fluid forces, perhaps by electromagnetic water hydrogen bonds (a concept that resonates with the 'water imprint' theory of homeopathy), generating a matrix that governs the embryo's development. This conceptual agreement between Blechschmidt and BOCF places them on one side of a great debate. For the past 50 years scientists have argued over two theories regarding embryonic development: is it *passive* and '*external*', driven by fluid dynamics, or *active* and '*internal*', driven by the molecular activity of genes?

Neural crest cells (NCCs) are a focus of this debate. Migratory NCCs appear in the 4th week of human embryogenesis. As the lateral edges of the neural plate fold up and fuse at midline to form the neural tube, NCCs surf the crest of the wave generated by this zipper-like action. NCCs follow highly replicated, stereotypical pathways. In our age of molecular medicine, advocates of *active* cell migration uphold the dominant paradigm. According to this view, migrating NCCs are directed by genes that express cell membrane receptors. NCC receptors sense molecular gradients in the extracellular fluid. Thus NCC migration has been described as *chemotaxic*, guided by molecules such as integrins, cadherins, and connexins.[55] This molecular view is challenged, however, by phylogenetic inconsistencies – NCCs only appear in vertebrate embryos. Invertebrate embryos have no NCCs yet they express genes linked with NCC migration, such as *BMP2/4*, *Pax3/7*, *Msx*, *Dll* and *Snail*.[56] Vice versa, genes associated with vertebrate cell migration, such as *CNR1*[57] are absent in invertebrates.[58,59] Plants, which are devoid of a CNS, also express integrin receptors,[60] which aid plant cells in the perception of gravity (a very subtle force in non-ferrous materials). Perhaps integrin receptors are not chemotaxic guides, but in fact respond to subtle electromagnetic forces such as the BoL.

Blechschmidt argued that fluid dynamics permit migrating cells to overcome the inertial, thixotropic (viscous) behavior of embryonic extracellular fluid. The tensile quality of the fluid matrix provides a scaffolding for the migration and movement of NCCs. BOCF practitioners correlate this concept with Sutherland's description of the Tide acting as a fluid within a fluid, expressing a tensile quality, with the ability to direct force. Blechschmidt's theory has been verified by researchers around the world[61] who injected latex beads into living embryos. Latex beads are inert objects incapable of molecular chemotaxis and lack inherent motility. They nevertheless follow the migratory pathways of NCCs. The tensile fluid forces required for this kind of movement were demonstrated by Schwenk,[62] who used micropipettes to inject streams of fluids into water. Boundary surfaces arising between the moving fluid and the still water vortexed into organic forms (Fig. 20.2). Experimental changes in fluid density or injection speed created different forms. In some experiments, the tensile quality of the fluid matrix created shapes that resembled the migratory path of neural crest cells. In other experiments the spatial orientations of fluid-in-a-fluid suggested CNS formation in the embryo, complete with dura and pia, cerebral hemispheres, and a corpus callosum connected the hemispheres (Fig. 20.3). Schwenk's experiments with fluid mechanics suggested that the geometric configuration of the embryo is present *before* the structure develops.

GENETIC CONTRIBUTIONS

After the fluids lay down a matrix or blueprint, genetic expression subsequently organizes the cells, and cell migration does indeed become active. For example, the initial wave of NCCs stops migrating and establishes a reticular lattice. This lattice provides a scaffolding for the active chemotaxic growth of neurons, presaging the mature organization of the autonomic nervous system.[63]

Similar phenomena govern the growth of neurons, via a sensory and motor apparatus in their tip termed the growth cone. Growth

Figure 20.2
Photomicrograph of micropipette injecting a stream of fluid into water, forming a vortex. The boundary surface between the moving fluid and the still water creates organic forms. (Redrawn from Schwenk, 1996).

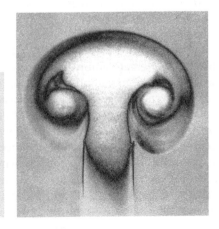

Figure 20.3
Photomicrograph of micropipette injecting a stream of fluid into water, an experimental variation from Fig. 20.2, changing the density of the fluid. The spatial orientation of boundary surfaces suggests that of embryonic CNS formation (Redrawn from Schwenk, 1996)

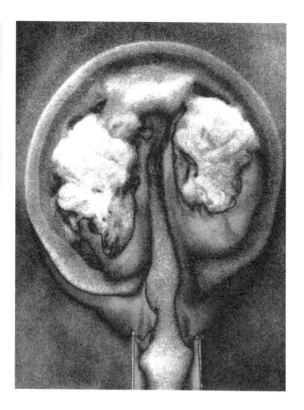

cone pathfinding is partially guided by fluid forces, a passive process again demonstrated by the translocation of inert latex beads.[64] But genes also contribute to growth cone pathfinding, by expressing cell membrane receptors that are activated by extracellular 'attractant' or 'repellent' compounds. For example *UNC-40* and *Eph* receptors are activated by netrins and ephrins, proteins secreted into extracellular fluid. Activated *UNC-40* and *Eph* receptors begin a molecular cascade that directs the cell's actin cytoskeleton, thereby regulating growth cone motility.[65] A veritable molecular soup guides neurons to their destinations. This complexity can be appreciated by the daunting task faced by commissural axons, which must grow towards the midline, cross it, and then continue on their path without turning back.

Nevertheless, Blechschmidt emphasized that genes do not act, they react to external forces. The reaction of genes to hydrostatic pressure during embryogenesis has recently been termed 'the morphogenetic mechanism'.[66] Wal[67] likened genes to the clay that forms a piece of pottery. Clay by itself cannot form into shape, it requires the hands of the artist. And the hands of the artist cannot act without the mind of the artist. From a BOCF perspective, clay represents the genes, the hands represents the fluid forces, and the artist's mind represents the BoL – the 'deific plan' or the 'master mechanic' often alluded to by AT Still. Anecdotally, we (JM and ES) attended a BOCF workshop the week that Venter et al.[68] published the human genome sequence.

While scientists around the world pondered the paradox that an organism of our complexity could operate on only 30,000 genes,[69] our workshop of BOCF practitioners confirmed the obvious necessity for epigenetic forces to make 'decisions' that shape embryogenesis.

METABOLIC MOTION

Blechschmidt[54] elaborated six different mechanisms by which fluids 'behave internally', creating function out of which emerges structure: contusion, distusion, dilatation, retension, detraction, and densation. Later he added corrosion, loosening, and suction mechanisms.[15] These mechanisms are driven by the metabolism of cellular tissues. Cell metabolism potentizes or depletes various fluids, which Blechschmidt termed 'metabolic fields'. For example, the earliest bending of the embryonic disk – flexing into a 'C' shape – is due to a decrease in pressure from the collapse of the yolk sac.[70] Cellular metabolism depletes nutrients in extracellular fluids, and causes a build-up of metabolic wastes. Sheets of cells adjacent to depleted fluids slow their growth, and become the concavity of tissue curvatures. Concentration gradients of nutrients and wastes create fluid movements between sources and sinks. When these fluid movements cannulize tissues they become embryonic blood vessels.

Sheets of cells, tissues, and organs grow at different rates. The epithelial linings of these assemblages become restraining structures, generating form. The embryonic face, for example, arises as folds and furrows between an expanding brain and a beating heart.[71] Growth differentials within the embryonic cranium create fluid patterns that later condense into mechanical tension zones or mesenchymal restraining bands known as the dural girdles. They guide the position, shape, and inner structure of the brain, 'The resistances are not crude mechanical forces but delicate living developmental resistances'.[72] The midline dural girdle between the cerebral hemispheres serve as a strong restrainer against the pull of the descending viscera and the eccentric growth of the cerebrum. This midline dural girdle is retained into adulthood as the falx cerebri. It initially cleaves the frontal bone, which is why the frontal bone, a single midline structure in most adults, functionally behaves like a paired bone. In some individuals this midline function is retained as structure, the metopic suture.[11] Several paired dural girdles arise in the embryo, and one of them is retained into adulthood as the tentorium cerebelli.

FUNCTIONAL MIDLINE

Another aspect of embryology that informs BOCF is the concept of a *functional midline*, around which our bodies and health must organize. The midline is the earliest expression of function within the embryo. A series of structures arises from the midline – first the primitive streak appears in the ectoderm, beginning at the caudal pole of the embryonic disk. Subsequently, the notochord develops within the endoderm, again growing from caudad to craniad. Days later, the neural groove forms along the midline, arising tail to head. During the 4th week of development, the neural tube closes at its two ends, and the movement of fluid is no longer a *circulation*, but a *fluctuation*. The amniotic fluid becomes the CSF. The lamina terminalis marks the closure of the cephalgic end of the tube. This midline structure persists in the adult, at the roof of the 3rd ventricle. It is the pivot point for all neural movement. During the inhalation phase of the PRM (i.e. Liem's 'inspiration' phase), the entire central nervous system spirally converges upon lamina terminalis. During the exhalation phase, all tissues move away from lamina terminalis.

Jealous[28] described the midline arising from the Stillness, generated by the BoL. The functional midline remains present throughout our life, and our structure and physiological motion remain oriented to the midline. The BoL comes into the body at the coccyx and ascends along the midline, cascading like a fountain of life. The conveyance of a midline bioenergetic force from tail to head has been described by numerous workers, perhaps first by the medical polymath Wilhelm Reich. Reich and his students independently described the PRM, '... confirmation of brain movement can be obtained from individuals who are free of armoring ... this movement is relatively slow and unrelated to arterial pulsations'.[73] Interestingly, genetic mechanisms tend to work in the opposite direction, in a cephalad to caudad progression. This is best exemplified by the activation of a dozen *Hox* transcription factor genes (the '*Hox* clock') that direct the formation of embryonic somites from head to tail. The sequence of *Hox* gene expression is collinear with their gene order on the chromosome.[74]

The movement of the Tide can be palpated throughout the body, termed 'Zone A' by BOCF practitioners.[14] Asian practitioners conceptualize this energy moving in channels, such as Chinese *chi* and Ayurvedic *vata* and its subdosha *prana*.[75] The movement of the Tide can also be palpated outside the body, in the 'auric field' of various Eastern and Western energy workers, termed Zone B in BOCF lexicon. Osteopaths such as Randolph Stone and Robert Fulford primarily worked in Zone B, Rollin Becker worked in Zone C, a field diffusing from the midline to the edges of the room (personal communication, J Jealous, 1999). Jealous[14] emphasized that all these zones exist simultaneously, as do other domains, such as Zone D, which extends from the patient's midline to the horizon. The zones are useful diagnostic tools, augmenting the practitioner's perceptual fields.

EMBRYOLOGY LEARNS FROM BOCF

BOCF has learned from embryology, but the relationship is reciprocal – BOCF has informed the science of embryology. Take the anterior dural girdle (ADG) for an example. The ADG arises around the 8th week of pregnancy, as a condensate of strain patterns between the evaginating telencephalic vesicles (Fig. 20.4). According to most embryologists, the ADG regresses before birth. However, one of Jealous's colleagues alerted him to a cranial strain pattern that he detected in several of his adult patients. They started calling it 'the hoop', describing its sensory feel. They organized perinatal dissections with Frank Willard, PhD, and discovered that the anterior dural girdle does not always involute before birth, but sometimes remains as an anterior transverse septum (Fig. 20.5). In other cases, the girdle regresses, although a strain pattern may remain in the fluids.

BOCF palpation also presaged the discovery of a dural bridge in the suboccipital region (J Jealous, personal communication, 1999), and this structure is now known to persist in adults.[76] The dural bridge attaches the dura to the posterior atlanto-occipital membrane (PAOM), a ligament that spans the OA joint.

CARE AND FEEDING OF THE ATTENTION FACULTY

BOCF is taught within a clinically-based program, where each step is designed as a journey to reawaken the intuitive and instinctual aspects of the practitioner's mind. Our intuitive and instinctual faculties were called 'primary perceptions' by Pearce,[77] who described them as 'part of nature's built-in system for communication and rapport with the earth'. These abilities tend to disappear, like muscle atrophy, if they go unused. Thus intuition and instinct are present at

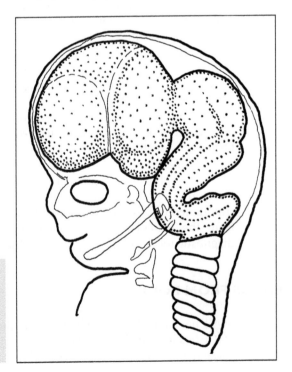

Figure 20.4 The anterior dural girdle forming in an 8-week-old embryo, drawn as a thin double line between anterior and lateral telencephalic vesicles (McPartland)

Figure 20.5 Neonate dissection of the anterior cranial fossa, looking from posterior to anterior, with the pons sliced and brain removed. Bilateral anterior transverse septae angle between the dissected midline falx and paired tentoria (Photograph courtesy of FORT Foundation, www.BioDO.com)

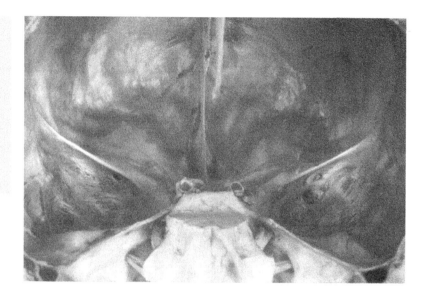

birth, but wither due to lack of use given today's societal and educational burdens. Our intuition, instinct, and perceptual vitality is also dulled by the stress of urban living, and by the pressures of our professional life.

Great care is taken in the choice of where practitioners receive BOCF training. The natural world is a necessary participant and instructor. Through his own experiences in the wildernesses of New England and Canada, Jealous learned how the deeper self, the human spirit, emerges upon encountering the nature world. Nature's 'spell of the sensuous' quiets a person's CNS, allowing boundaries to fall away between the individual and the whole. John Muir, a 19th century American naturalist, spoke like an osteopath, 'In nature, when we try to pick out anything by itself, we find it hitched to everything else in the universe'.[78] The BOCF practitioner transports this natural-world phenomenon to the urban treatment room, incorporating an indigenous state of consciousness into everyday clinical practice.

It is important to recognize that what is observed during the course of treatment is not the result of mesmerism, colored by a vaguely vitalistic theory, but evidence of a precisely organized natural system which requires discipline and dedication in order to develop the practitioner's perceptual faculty. Practitioners at this time in history are in a unique position. Given our training in medical science and hands-on manipulative techniques, combined with the principles of Still and Sutherland, we can consult with the blueprint for health, namely, embryological growth and development recapitulated as the forces of healing. But there is a caveat: without the proper preparation, this approach can be dangerous for the patient and an abuse of the practitioner's commitment to the Hippocratic Oath. This model does not work with 'energy' but with the consciousness of the natural world.

References

1 Still AT. Autobiography of Andrew T. Still, revised edn. Kirksville, MO: Published by the author; 1908.

2 Still AT. Philosophy of Osteopathy. Kirksville, MO: The Journal Printing Company; 1899.

3 Still A. Osteopathy Research and Practice. Kirksville, MO: The Journal Printing Company; 1910.

4 Still A. The Philosophy and Mechanical Principles of Osteopathy. Kirksville, MO: Hudson-Kimberly; 1902.

5 Artaud A. The Theatre and its Double. New York: Grove Press; 1938.

6 Chew MK, Laubichler MD. Natural enemies – metaphor or misconception? Science 2003; 301:52–53.

7 Van der Post L. Patterns of Renewal. Chester, PA: John Spencer, Inc.; 1962.

8 Abram D. The Spell of the Sensuous. New York: Vintage Books; 1996.

9 Highwater J. The Primal Mind. Harper and Row, New York; 1981.

10 Sutherland WG. The Cranial Bowl. Mankato, MN: Free Press Co; 1939.

11 Magoun HI. Osteopathy in the Cranial Field, 3rd edn. Kirksville, MO: Journal Printing Co.; 1976.

12 Upledger JE, Vredevoogd JD. Craniosacral Therapy. Chicago: Eastland Press; 1983.

13 Cardy I. Experience in Stillness: a hermeneutic study of the Breath of Life in the Cranial Field of Osteopathy. Masters dissertation, School of Osteopathy, UNITEC, Auckland, New Zealand; 2004:103.

14 Jealous J. Emergence of Originality, 2nd edn. Farmington ME: Biodynamic/Sargent Publishing; 2001:145.

15 Blechschmidt E, Gasser RF. Biokinetics and Biodynamics of Human Differentiation. Springfield, Illinois: Charles Thomas Publishing; 1978.

16 Van der Post L. The Heart of the Hunter. London: Hogarth Press; 1961.

17 Berry W. The Unsettling of America: Culture and Agriculture. New York: Random House; 1996.

18 Retzlaff EW, Mitchell FL. The Cranium and its Sutures. Berlin: Springer-Verlag; 1987.

19 Weaver C. Cranial Vertebrae. J Am Osteopath Assoc 1936a; 35:328, 35:374–379, 35:421–424 (in three parts).

20 Weaver C. Etiological importance of cranial intervertebral articulations. J Am Osteopath Assoc 1936b; 35:515–525.

21 Weaver C. Symposium on the plastic basicranium. J Am Osteopath Assoc 1938; 37:298–303.

22 Rohen JW. Morphologie des Menschlichen Organismus. Stuttgart: Verlag Freies Geistesleben; 2002.

23 Greitz D, Greitz T, Hindmarsh T. A new view on the CSF-circulation with the potential for pharmacological treatment of childhood hydrocephalus. Acta Paediatri 1997; 86:125–132.

24 Woods RH, Woods JM. A physical finding related to psychiatric disorders. J Am Osteopath Assoc 1961; 60:988–993.

25 McPartland JM, Mein EA. Entrainment and the cranial rhythmic impulse. Alternative Therapies in Health and Medicine 1997; 3(1):40–44.

26 Nelson KE, Sergueef N, Lipinski CL, Chapman A, Glonek T. The cranial rhythmic impulse related to the Traube-Hering-Mayer oscillation: comparing laser-Doppler flowmetry and palpation. J Am Osteopath Assoc 2001; 101:163–173.

27 Schleip R. Neurobiological aspects of the cranial rhythmic impulse. Somatics Web Page, www.somatics.de/cranial.htm; 2002.

28 Jealous J. Healing and the natural world. Alternative Therapies in Health and Medicine. 1997; 3(1):68–76.

29 Sutherland WG, Sutherland AS, Wales A, eds. Contributions of Thought, the Collected Writings of William Garner Sutherland. Kansas City, MO: Sutherland Cranial Teaching Foundation; 1967.

30 Becker RE. Be still and know. Cranial Academy Newsletter, Dec 1965:5–8.

31 Liem T. Praxis der Kraniosakralen Osteopathie. Stuttgart: Hippokrates Verlag GmbH; 2003.

32 Norton JM. A challenge to the concept of craniosacral interactions. J Am Acad Osteopath 1996; 6(4):15–21.

33 Sutherland WG, Wales A, eds. Teachings in the Science of Osteopathy. Portland, OR: Rudra Press; 1990.

34 Cornell EA, Wieman CE. Bose-Einstein condensation: the first 70 years and some recent experiments (Nobel Prize Lecture). Chemphyschem 2002; 3(6):476–493.

35 Speece CA, Crow WT, Simmons SL. Ligamentous Articular Strain. Seattle: Eastland Press; 2001.

36 Green E. 'Foreword'. In Upledger JE, Vredevoogd JD, eds. Craniosacral Therapy. Chicago: Eastland Press; 1983:xi–xiv.

37 Hesse N. Major Betrand DeJarnette: six decades of sacro occipital research, 1924–1984. Chiropractic History 1991; 11(1):13–15.

38 McPartland JM, Brodeur R, Hallgren RH. Chronic neck pain, standing balance, and suboccipital muscle atrophy. J Manip Physiol Ther 1997; 21(1):24–29.

39 Strogatz SH, Stewart I. Coupled oscillators and biological synchronization. Scientific American 1993; 269(12):102–109.

40 Tiller WA, McCraty R, Atkinson M. Cardiac coherence: a new, noninvasive measure of autonomic nervous system order. Alternative Therapies 1996; 2:52–65.

41 McPartland JM. Manual medicine at the Nepali interface. J Manual Med 1989; 4:25–27.

42 Jahn RG. Information, consciousness, and health. Alternative Therapies in Health and Medicine 1996; 2(3):32–38.

43 Wirkus M, Wirkus M. Bioenergy-A Healing Art. Bethesda, MD: Bio-Relax Press; 1992.

44 Fulford RC. Integration of love with the cranial concept. The Cranial Letter 1988; 41(4):2–3.

45 Greenman PE, McPartland JM. Cranial findings and iatrogenesis from craniosacral manipulation in patients with traumatic brain syndrome. J Am Osteopath Assoc 1995; 95:182–192.

46 McPartland JM. Side effects from cranial-sacral treatment: case reports and commentary. J Bodywork Movement Ther 1996; 1(1):2–5.

47 Paulsen AR. Automatic shifting. J Osteopath Cranial Assoc 1953:65–66.

48 Pourquié O. The segmentation clock: converting embryonic time into spatial pattern. Science 2003; 301:328–330.

49 Pert C. 'Foreword'. In: Oschman JL, ed. Energy Medicine. Edinburgh: Churchill Livingstone; 2000:ix–xi.

50 Oschman JL. Energy Medicine. Edinburgh: Harcourt Publishers; 2000.

51 Bohm D. Wholeness and Implicate Order. London: Routledge and Kegan Paul; 1980.

52 Sheldrake R. A New Science of Life. Great Britain: Blond & Briggs, Limited; 1981.

53 Capra F. The Web of Life. London: Harper Collins; 1996.

54 Blechschmidt E. Beginnings of Human Life. Berlin: Springer-Verlag; 1977.

55 Maschhoff KL, Baldwin HS. Molecular determinants of neural crest migration. Am J Med Genet 2000; 97:280–288.

56 Holland LZ, Holland ND. Evolution of neural crest and placodes: amphioxus as a model for the ancestral vertebrate? J Anat 2001; 199:85–98.

57 Song ZH, Zhong M. CB1 cannabinoid receptor-mediated cell migration. J Pharmacol Exp Ther 2000; 294:204–209.

58 McPartland JM, Di Marzo V, De Petrocellis L, Mercer A, Glass M. Cannabinoid receptors are absent in insects. J Comp Neurol 2001; 436:423–429.

59 McPartland JM, Glass M. The nematocidal effects of cannabis may not be mediated by cannabinoid receptors. New Zealand Journal Crop & Horticultural Science 2001; 29:301–307.

60 Lynch TM, Lintilhac PM, Domosych D. Mechanotransduction molecules in the plant gravisensory response. Protoplasma 1998; 201:92–100.

61 Jesuthasan S. Neural crest cell migration in the zebrafish can be mimicked by inert objects: mechanism and implications of latex bead movement in embryos. J Exp Zool 1997; 277:425–434.

62 Schwenk T. Sensitive Chaos: The Creation of Flowing Forms in Water and Air (revised edn). London: Rudolf Steiner Press; 1996.

63 Conner PJ, Focke PJ, Noden DM, Epstein ML. Appearance of neurons and glia with respect to the wavefront during colonization of the avian gut by neural crest cells. Developmental Dynamics 2003; 226:91–98.

64 Newman SA, Frenz DA, Tomasek JJ, Rabuzzi DD. Matrix-driven translocation of cells and nonliving particles. Science 1985; 228:885–889.

65 Dickson BJ. Molecular mechanisms of axon guidance. Science 2002; 298:1959–1964.

66 Van Essen DC. A tension-based theory of morphogenesis and compact wiring in the central nervous system. Nature 1997; 385:313–318.

67 Wal JC van der. De spraak van het embryo. In: Steven De Batselier, ed. Liber Amicorum; 1997. (Accessed from www.home.uni-one.nl/walembryo/esve.htm)

68 Venter JC, Adams MD, Myers EW, et al. The sequence of the human genome. Science 2001; 291:1304–1351.

69 Claverie JM. What if there are only 30,000 human genes? Science 2001; 291:1255–1257.

70 Drews U. Color Atlas of Embryology. New York: Thieme Medical Publishers; 1995.

71 Blechschmidt E, Gasser RF. Biokinetics and Biodynamics of Human Differentiation. Springfield, Illinois: Charles Thomas; 1978.

72 Blechschmidt E. The Stages of Human Development before Birth. Philadelphia: Saunders; 1961.

73 Konia C. Brain pulsations, Part I: Normal functioning. J Orgonomy 1980; 14:103–113.

74 Kmita M, Duboule D. Organizing axes in time and space: 25 years of collinear tinkering. Science 2003; 301:331–333.

75 McPartland JM, Foster F. 'Ayurvedic Bodywork'. In Coughlin P, ed. Principles and Practices of Manual Medicine, Edinburgh: Churchill Livingstone; 2002:155–164.

76 McPartland JM, Brodeur RR. The rectus capitis posterior minor: a small but important suboccipital muscle. J Bodywork Movement Ther 1999; 3(1):30–35.

77 Pearce JC. Magical Child. New York: Penguin Books; 1977.

78 Muir J. My First Summer in the Sierra. Cambridge: The Riverside Press; 1911.

Further reading on BOCF

Jealous J. (2001, with annual updates) The Biodynamics of Osteopathy (interactive audio CD series), Marnee Jealous Long, 6501 Blackfin Way, Apollo Beach, FL 33572 (Available from: mjlong@tampabay.rr.com)

Glossary

'Breath of Life', 'Potency', 'Fulcrum' and other concepts

> I believe in the unlimited possibilities for the development of our spiritual and mental organizations, just as I do the physical…You have this infinity in yourself, and it is only a question of whether you will recognize and cultivate it.
>
> When I study anatomy, I not only develop understanding of the physical but I unfold and enlarge my mental and spiritual qualities.
>
> AT Still[1]

The art of osteopathy finds expression especially in the intelligent and meaningful palpation of living organisms. These act and react as a whole entity, and the parts and organ systems of which they are composed relate both to each other and to the world outside.

The writings of Sutherland and Still were characterized by metaphorical language which appears unscientific, but – however vaguely and unclearly – offer the basis from which to develop the instructional communication of palpatory experience, of making contact with living organisms and the unseen living forces within them. Gaines says that phenomenology as a philosophy and as a discipline, adapted to suit a strict systematic methodology[2] and based on the empiricism of the osteopath's palpatory experience, can help to develop a clear, unified 'osteopathic' language. Some of the following concepts are very important in the practice of osteopathy, but are nevertheless often used differently from one osteopath to another and so need to be further specified and defined. There is certainly a communication problem in the osteopathic community over the concepts described here. What is less clear is whether the solution really does lie in giving a descriptive account, or whether an epistemological insight is also needed to help us understand the knowledge itself. Nor has it yet been shown whether the problem is primarily one of perception, or one related to the overarching paradigm or world view. Klein states the nub of the matter when he writes that we cannot presume that what we perceive corresponds to reality, illustrating the point with reference to optical illusions. He also asks whether the truth content of statements would automatically be greater simply if several persons (osteopaths) believed that they perceived the same thing. In his view it is a mistake to assume that objectivity can be gained by multiplying subjectivity.[3]

The concepts addressed below are viewed and explained with the aid of classical osteopathic literature. The descriptions mainly follow the publications of WG Sutherland and RA Becker, and the first edition of Magoun's *Osteopathy in the Cranial Field* (1951), which Sutherland participated in producing and expressly approved. In certain individual instances we may now see some things as outdated from the point of view of the present day. A considerable number of his chosen concepts seem directed toward the description of palpatory experience, to clarify certain palpatory approaches to his students and lead them toward certain subtle points in palpatory experience. The epistemological problems of these concepts are not dealt with here.

BALANCE/EQUILIBRIUM

The normal state of acting and reacting between different parts within the body.[4]

Sutherland writes that the movements of the tide or fluctuation in their entirety derive from a 'balance' between two points on a given scale, a point where the mechanism is motionless, exactly at the 'neutral point'.[5]

BALANCE POINT (See Point of Balance)

BENT TWIG

An expression frequently used by Sutherland, referring to the saying 'as the twig is bent, so doth the tree incline'. It is intended to show how the slightest tensions in the cranium or spine of a newborn or young child can develop into visible asymmetries as the structures increase in size with the progressive growth of the child.[6]

'BE STILL AND KNOW'

Sutherland often used this biblical quotation (from Psalm 46:10) to make clear the significance of a particular attitude of consciousness during palpation, and also to indicate a particular fulcrum/point of balance between inspiration and expiration in the fluctuation of the fluids.[7]

BIODYNAMICS/BIOMECHANICS

From 1948 Sutherland devoted himself exclusively to the biodynamic approach. In *Tour of the Minnow* for example, he describes the biomechanical and biodynamic principles of the PRM.[8]

Other osteopaths such as Ruby Day, RE Becker and others have taught this model,[9] but it is James Jealous who chose this concept for the title of his courses, and who elaborated and developed the biodynamic approach.[10]

The key distinction is that in the biomechanical model it is necessary to know the limits of the lesion, in the sense of the restriction and the force vectors. The method involves establishing the degree of mobility of the lesion. In the biodynamic approach the wave and the presence of the primary respiration communicate the diagnosis and prescribe the treatment.[9] Whether the biomechanical components should by definition be integrated as part of the biodynamic model, or whether it makes better sense to speak of an integration of the biomechanical and biodynamic models, has not been clarified. Jealous believes that the biodynamic model incorporates all the aspects of the biomechanical model.

Table G.1 A brief comparison of biomechanical and biodynamic models of OCF

Biomechanical approach	Biodynamic approach
Sutherland's first theories date from between 1936 and 1948	Late theories of Sutherland (from 1948 onwards)
The SBS was seen as the primary location of dysfunctions of the cranium	All levels can be affected. A dysfunction is multifaceted; Becker speaks of biodynamic and biokinetic forces
Mechanical approach: bones, sutures, membranes, and axes of motion (sutural; membranous)	Inherent self-regulatory and self-correcting forces come to the fore of consideration. These possess intelligence, the capacity for decision, and goal-direction. See 'breath of life' and 'potency'
Definition of the five structures of the PRM	*Open model:* according to Jealous other factors participate in the creation of the PRM
Examination: mainly by active motion testing, but also by passive sensing	Examination: mainly by passive sensing, harmonization and synchronization
Correction: mechanical; the therapist performs the correction. The therapist approaches motion barriers	*Correction:* the 'Breath of Life' performs and directs the correction. The therapist acts more as a fulcrum through which the forces act; direction of the 'potency' of the CSF
The focus is on dysfunctions, motion barriers/resistances/restrictions	No motion barriers are addressed
Inherent self-regulating forces were hardly mentioned or defined. No use of 'potency' or the 'Breath of Life'	The focus is on the 'potency' of the 'Breath of Life', the inherent homeostatic forces, and 'health'. This approach calls on the personal immediate perception of ordering principles in nature and spiritual experience
Axial motion in bones	Transmutational, Translational motion
CRI is a primary expression of the BoL	CRI is not an expression of the BoL, nor is it a therapeutic force
CRI 8–14 cycles per min. Slower rates not identified	Basic rate is 2-3 cycles per min; slower rates are specifically identified as primary to the system
Perception is automatic. Skills not delineated	Perception is a conscious, skillful act, requiring training and moment-to-moment adjustment, not automatic
SBS is a primary site of orientation for lesion activity. Lesions are diagnosed and reduced by conceptual sequences beginning at SBS	Primary site is variable. Lesions are not automatically corrected, sequences are not conceptual. Priorities are established by the Tide

Source: Liem and McPartland

BIODYNAMIC AND BIOKINETIC FORCES ACCORDING TO BECKER

A 'total rhythmic balanced interchange' takes place in relation to the entirety of the system: between the physiology of the body, life (space-time movement) and environmental processes (genetic factors, trauma, sickness and diseases of all types, physical and psychological stress, and nutritional factors).[11]

Biodynamic energy describes health or the bioenergy of health. This starts at conception and ends at death.[12]

During a traumatic event, vectors of force or biokinetic energy (K) enter the bioenergetic systems (D) of the body. Becker expresses this $D + K = DK$. The concept of 'biokinetic energy' comprises the forces affecting the body and acting to disturb it: physical trauma, psychological trauma, infection, poisoning, errors of nutrition, etc.

The invading environmental energy that led to the development of tissue tensions remains in the tissue, even years later, bringing about a change in the arterial supply and venous drainage of the affected tissue, and so producing the osteopathic dysfunction.[13]

There is an environmental energy field that is part of the tension pattern, and there is also the body's own energy field, the compensatory mechanism of the body that creates the osteopathic dysfunction in its anatomical and physiological aspects.[13]

The osteopathic dysfunction (lesion) could be described as representing a response to these forces. It forms a complex with the environmental energy. To dissipate this, both the osteopathic dysfunction and the environmental energy must be taken into account in diagnosis and treatment.[14]

The 'potency' is continually active to redirect the kinetic energy back out into the environment, by a process that Becker himself sees as mysterious and describes in the words 'something happens', a process aimed at improving the state of health. This is successful to a varying extent according to the strength of the biokinetic forces. This process happens in the hours or weeks following the trauma.

Becker describes the contribution of therapy by saying that biokinetic forces are active in patients in the acute stage or in whom the process was not successfully completed. The osteopath investigates the bioenergetic factors. Treatment assists the 'potency' in its work of dissipating excess biokinetic energy to the world outside.

BREATH OF LIFE

The 'Breath of Life' carries out the correction, not the therapist. It is described as the 'fluid' in the cerebrospinal fluid, as 'liquid light', 'potency', and AT Still's 'highest known element'; as something that disperses the darkness when it is switched on.[15] It represents the fundamental unity in the functioning of the mechanism;[16] the first spark, the release of the involuntary motion, something that releases the motion, something invisible in the cerebrospinal fluid,[17,18] something in the motion of the tides, not the breath of air,[19] comparable with the lightning that shines through the cloud without touching it. Sutherland also sees the breath of life as 'transmutation' (q.v.). He frequently used a quotation from the Bible to show that the breath of life was not to be confused with the air: 'The Lord God ... breathed into his nostrils the breath of life, and man became a living being' (from *Genesis* 2:7).[20]

For Sutherland there was a connection between the fluctuations of the CSF and the Breath of Life.[21]

'A body of fluid that has the Breath of Life. That has 'something' invisible, not only of potency but an Intelligence spelled with a capital 'I'. In that potency of the fluctuation you have an unerring intracranial and intraspinal force, with the tendency toward the normal use as the motive power for the reduction of the lesions'.[5]

Becker says that the fulcrum is the place where the 'tide' changes from one direction to another, the point of exchange between the Breath of Life and the CSF.[22]

The 'Breath of Life' is then transmuted into lesser energies that can be used by the body.

According to Jealous, the Breath of Life is expressed in a rhythm of 100 s per cycle. His fulcrum is a sort of dynamic stillness. This slow rhythm is most easily sensed externally to the body. It suffuses the body; it is a source of motion in the fluids of the body and it is able to transform dysfunctions. The spark of the Breath of Life engenders the form and the function in the form. If this rhythm enters the body it engenders motion in bioelectrical, biomolecular and biomechanical structures with a rhythm of 24 s per cycle.[23]

Sutherland continued until shortly before his death to aid his students in finding the 'liquid light', the 'potency' of this substance, in their lives.[24]

The function of the PRM is absolutely dependent on the 'Breath of Life', the 'still point' and 'potency'. The expression of the 'Breath of Life' in the form of certain outworkings of rhythmic motion are the result of a spark, called the 'Breath of Life', which is transmuted into the PRM.[25]

Becker says that the patterns present are mostly compensatory adaptive ones that reflect the life of the particular individual and in which the PRM, in the healthy state, is able to receive the spark of the 'Breath of Life'. The therapist's task is to recognize any deviation from this compensatory pattern and to lead it back by means of the treatment to the compensatory state of normality for that individual.[25]

Sutherland's hypothesis of the primary respiratory mechanism (PRM) was founded on his recognition of the supreme potency of the Breath of

Life as the spark that initiates the involuntary activity in the PRM:

'It was the recognition of the supreme potency of the 'Breath of Life' as the initiative spark to involuntary activity that interpreted my hypothesis relative to the primary respiratory mechanism'.[26,27]

Jealous emphasizes that the key as regards the Breath of Life is that we cannot experience it when we set out to do so and that we do not choose to approach it; rather, it approaches us. For Jealous, the Breath of Life is a mysterious presence of love itself, which is everywhere present, its first effect everywhere being to create wholeness. It is then that the change takes place.[9]

CANT HOOK

This is a technique that operates by means of leverage.

Hand position:
- A hand position to the side enables one part to act as a fulcrum for the movement of another, like the hinge of a door, e.g. release of the frontosphenoidal suture.
- One hand spans the frontal bone between the thumb and index or middle finger.
- The thumb on one side acts as the fixed point and the fingers lift the frontal bone on the other.[6]

CORE LINK

The structural and functional link of the reciprocal tension membrane (the spinal dura mater as the continuation of the cranial dura mater) that connects the occiput with the sacrum, and thus the cranium with the pelvis. Each pole reciprocally affects the other. According to Sutherland, it is via this link that the involuntary, inherent cranial motion is transmitted to the sacrum.[28]

CRANIO RHYTHMIC IMPULSE

This concept was introduced only after Sutherland's death, and was intended to denote simply the physiological involuntary and rhythmic fluctuation of the cerebrospinal fluid, as a palpable motion of expansion and retraction of the cranium, unassociated with the primary respiratory mechanism. The term was coined by the psychiatrists and osteopaths Woods and Woods to enable other physicians to palpate and evaluate this motion without having to confront the notion of the primary respiratory mechanism. According to both Woods and Woods and Magoun, the CRI is shown by palpation and by electronic measurements to have a frequency of 10–14 cycles per min. Sutherland himself never specified a frequency.

According to Magoun the CRI can still be palpated even after death (for up to about 15 min).[29,30] He states that it influences the physiological centers of the body, including pulmonary breathing.[31]

FLUID DRIVE

The PRM has a 'fluid drive' brought about by the activity of the cerebrospinal fluid.[32] The concept is frequently used in practice to express the hydrodynamic relationship between the CSF, interstitial fluid and lymph.

FLUCTUATION OF THE CEREBROSPINAL FLUID

The cerebrospinal fluid does not circulate but fluctuates. This fluctuation is a motion of the CSF in a natural hollow space, a wave motion with successive rise and fall. This fluctuation can be palpated.[33,34]

The motion of the intracranial dural membranes exerts a pressure on the CSF, causing motion of the fluid.[35]

The inherent motility of the nervous system moves the CSF. There is a fluctuation in volume caused by the increase in size of the ventricles and subarachnoid space.[36]

This can be influenced by compression of the 4th ventricle.[37]

Sutherland emphasizes that it is the fluid fluctuation that leads the structures being treated to a membranous point of balance during therapy.[38]

FREQUENCY OF PRM RHYTHM

Different data exist as to the rhythm of the PRM or craniosacral rhythm. The data derive from findings obtained by palpation, carried out by individual osteopaths, and also from various measurement methods.

The list below gives only a selection of possible rhythms:

- 10–14 cycles per min: 4–6 s cycle (Magoun, Traube-Hering oscillation)[39-45]
- 6–12 cycles per min: 5–10 s cycle (Upledger)[46]
- 8–12 cycles per min: 5–7.5 s cycle (Becker, Upledger)[47,48]
- 2.5 cycles per min: 24 s cycle (Jealous)[49]
- 6–10 cycles per 10 min: 60–100 s cycle (Becker's slow (large) tide, Mayer oscillation)[45,50]
- 1 cycle per 5 min: 300 s cycle (Liem, Lewer-Allen, Bunt et al.)[51,52]
- A rhythm of 1 cycle in around 33 min (2000 s cycle) has also been recorded, by Lewer-Allen, Bunt et al. in the brain. No recorded data based on palpation of this rhythmic pattern presently exist. Personal experience of palpation does also seem to offer some evidence of very slow impulses of expansion and retraction, but these results tend to be inconsistent and irregular.

FULCRUM

A fulcrum is like a point of rest or movable fixed point that can be used, for example, to lift a weight. Its inherent potency acts as an orientational organizing factor for patterns of motion and organization. In nature, the eye of a whirlwind would be a fulcrum.

In the human body there are many fulcrums. The pivot points of cranial sutures (the point at which the bevel of the suture margins changes direction from inward to outward-facing) constitute a fulcrum, a resting or turning point for the motion of the cranial bones (see Ch 6).

The sternal end of the clavicula is a bony fulcrum for the function of the entire upper limb. A bony fulcrum at the SBS, a membranous fulcrum at the straight sinus and a fulcrum of the nervous system at the laminae terminales have also been described. Sutherland also detected a fulcrum in the fluctuations of the CSF.[53]

In addition, fluid fulcrums are stated to exist in the body for a variety of fluid functions.

Sutherland and Becker have also described spiritual fulcrums.[54,55] Examples of this would be regular meditation, a particular religion, a life principle or motto such as 'love your neighbor as yourself'. By directing their lives in accordance with this principle, people can realize its potential power in their lives. Just as regular meditation can represent a point of rest, of taking stock, or a ship on the boundless ocean of life, so a fulcrum can be a regular calling to mind, as Chila emphasizes, so as to empty oneself before and during therapy and to be open to the patient as a whole being.

All inherent motions, motion patterns, tensions and physiological processes in the body, as well as dysfunctions, abnormal tension and motion patterns, are organized from a fulcrum.

A fulcrum acts as an organizational factor for motion. It possesses potency, like the eye of a whirlwind.[56]

A fulcrum is a sort of concentration of potency. Cells and tissues arrange themselves with respect to the potency and the fulcrums.

All natural fulcrums act as an 'automatic shifting suspension fulcrum' and so change their position in synchrony with the respiratory cycles. Dysfunctional fulcrums, which account for the internal organization of a dysfunction, differ in that they represent a barrier or restriction to motion, a densification of energy or matter, and an increase in stagnation.

The eye or still point of the whirlwind carries the potency and pattern of the storm. In the same way, there is a point of rest in the dysfunction that embodies the potency of this dysfunction. This potency in a fulcrum centers the abnormal forces and tensions in the dysfunction. It is like another limb of the body, which organizes itself around that limb.

This eye of the dysfunction, this area of stillness in the tension patterns of the tissues, is the place that represents the specific potency of the particular dysfunction. It is like the soul of the dysfunction, its energy, and the motion that manifests itself and maintains the tension pattern. Any change here, in this place, results in a change in the structural and functional conditions of the tension pattern.

Osteopaths can learn to palpate and locate such places.

Fulcrum: automatic shifting suspension fulcrum

A suspended automatic shifting fulcrum is a point of rest or orientation that is mobile or suspended, such that it can move automatically.

A striking example of this in nature, which gives an idea of the potential power of a fulcrum, is the eye of a whirlwind. Becker describes this as a point of stillness and potential source of power for the force of the whirlwind.

At the same time this type of fulcrum is also 'automatic, shifting, and suspended' in that it moves across land and sea. Another example is the axle of a wheel, where the fulcrum of the wheel's turning is a point of rest. But it is at the same time an 'automatic shifting suspended' fulcrum in that it moves along with the bicycle, while never losing its function as a point of rest for the turning of the wheel. All natural fulcrums in the body act as an automatic shifting suspension fulcrum so that they can react dynamically to internal and external events and to continuous rhythmic impulses.[4]

They are responsible for the organization of states of reciprocal tension balance in the body.

Sutherland chose this term to describe a functional area on the course of the straight sinus, where the falx cerebri, falx cerebelli and tentorium cerebelli unite. It is also called Sutherland's fulcrum. It is a movable point of rest for the reciprocal tension membrane in the cranium and spinal canal. In order to ensure the balance of membranous motion and tension equally in all directions, the membranes need to operate from a fulcrum, a point of rest. If this fulcrum is to shift automatically, it must be in 'suspension' so that any pressure or pull is evenly distributed in the dural membranes.

Sutherland writes that the changing position of the automatic shifting suspension fulcrum can be palpated at the beginning of respiration, and that a sense of warmth arises from the fluctuation of the CSF.[4,57] These fulcrums are important in understanding and diagnosing normal function by examining whether they move with the 'tide' or are static.[10]

Fulcrum: dysfunctional fulcrums

This term describes fulcrums that function as the organizing factor for dysfunctions, in other words, for abnormal tissue tensions and motion restrictions. In contrast to natural fulcrums, these are able to react little if at all to rhythmic events such as pulmonary respiration and the 'Breath of Life' or to the physiological demands of internal and external stimuli by either shifting or moving.

These fulcrums can rather be seen as factors of disturbance that require the body to compensate in a particular way, and to which the natural fulcrums react to create for themselves the best possible subsequent balance of tensions in the body. Consequently, a dysfunctional fulcrum does not just have a local effect; it affects the whole body, depending on the degree of disturbance. Various models can be called upon to explain the effects of these fulcrums, such as the tensegrity model, electromagnetic fields, biophoton fields, the fluid crystalline properties of bodies, or Sheldrake's morphogenetic fields, as well as neurophysiological and endocrine interactions.

Dysfunctional fulcrums result in various acquired states, varying in character and extent from one individual to another: certain patterns of motion and tension, changes in elasticity, densification of energy or matter, or increased stagnation, associated with resistance to motion, motion restriction (partial or complete) in the tissue and fluids. These are as it were the imprint of the individual's history on the tissue. They are the result of events whose intensity or duration made them too strong to be completely resolved by the homeostatic forces of the body. These events include physical injuries, including birth trauma, diseases and psychological trauma. Becker calls these forces 'biokinetic energy'.

According to Becker, biokinetic and biodynamic forces are at work at the heart of every dysfunction. The biokinetic forces are centered by the potency; this describes a homeostatic process that strives to dissipate the biokinetic forces, dispersing them into the biosphere or, if this is not successful, compensating as well as possible.

The therapist uses palpation to sense the interaction between the operation of the life forces/homeostatic forces that are immediately present and the way they have been conditioned, the forces bound and fixed by the habits and conditions of life, physical or psychological trauma, diseases, etc. (biokinetic energy).

A particular pattern comes about when some suffering on the part of the body proves such a hindrance to the system that the body can no longer remember how to heal itself.[58]

HIGHEST KNOWN ELEMENT (See Also 'Breath Of Life')

Still states that this 'highest known element' is found in the cerebrospinal fluid. Sutherland repeatedly refers to it. For him, on the basis of practical experience, it is the constant seat of an intelligent potency with the ability to transcend everything else in the body. He uses this potency for diagnosis and therapy.[59,60]

LIGAMENTOUS ARTICULAR STRAIN (See Membranous articular strain)

'LONG TIDE'

Rollin A. Becker used this term to denote the concept of a very slow rhythm. He states that this rhythm enters the body from outside, originating anywhere and spreading through the body. He palpated a rhythm that took 1.5 min to permeate into the body and the same length of time to ebb away.[61]

MEMBRANOUS ARTICULAR STRAIN

Sutherland terms dysfunctions and abnormal tensions affecting the joints of the vertebral column and their associated ligaments as 'ligamentous articular strain'. Dysfunctions affecting the bones of the craniosacral system and their associated intracranial and intraspinal dural membranes (falx cerebri, tentorium cerebelli, falx cerebelli, spinal dura mater) he called 'membranous articular strain'. These strains can impinge on cerebrospinal fluctuation, cranial arterial and venous perfusion, and the lymphatic drainage of the head and neck. His treatment is therefore above all aimed at a resolution of these imbalances of tension. The treatment principle for the ligamentous and membranous articular types is the same.[62,63]

MIDLINE *(See Ch. 18)*

NEUTRAL, OF THE PATIENT

NEUTRAL POINT, BALANCE POINT

'where the mechanism is idling, neither ebbing out or flowing in', and:

- rhythmic balanced interchange: 'the period where all the fluids of the body have an interchange'.[5]
- during a period when the CSF is 'neutral'.
- all the fluids of the body are influenced: 'an interchange that occurs between all the fluids of the body'.[64]

PIVOT *(See also Fulcrum)*

The pivot points of the cranial sutures (these are the points where the bevel of the cranial sutures changes direction) represent a fulcrum, a point of rest or turning for the motion of the cranial bones. They are the place where the inward-facing border meets the outward-facing border of the articulating bones; where there is a change in the direction of inclination of the suture margins. They serve as fulcrums, points of rest or of turning, and are potential bony axes for the movement of the cranial bones. They are often used in treatment as the place where disengagement techniques can be applied, e.g. Sphenosquamous pivot (SSP); condylosquamosomastoid pivot point (CSMP).[65]

Dynamic pivot points have also been described, for example in the balance of acids and bases or in the blood sugar curve.[66]

POINT OF BALANCE, MEMBRANOUS, LIGAMENTOUS

Magoun defines this as the point in the range of movement of a joint articulation where the membranes are in a state of balance. This is a point between normal tension, which can be seen in the free range of movement, and the increased tension that results from strains and restrictions and appears when the joint is moved beyond its natural physiological range of movement.[67]

The same principle applies to the ligamentous point of balance, e.g. in the joints of the vertebrae.

Sutherland says that the reciprocal membranous tension and the fluctuation of the fluids should be kept at 'balance point' during treatment.[68]

The midpoint between inspiration and expiration is also referred to as 'balance point'.[69]

The concept of the point of balance can also be extended to include the body fluids, electromagnetic fields, etc.

POTENCY

The 'Breath of Life' has 'potency', which operates as 'the thing that makes it move' and is called intelligent potency, more intelligent than the human mentality,[18] or 'an unerring intelligent motive force'.[70]

Becker defines potency as the 'motive power of life from the highest spiritual manifestations down to the simplest physical phenomena'.

It is an 'automatic shifting entity of function in the balanced area of all rhythmic balanced interchange mechanisms'.[71]

Potency is a functional factor in the cycle of action and reaction, found wherever it is met with in nature. Becker calls potency the stillness in the middle of a whirlwind.[72]

The potency in the CSF is also described as an electrical potential, constantly becoming charged and uncharged[73] and producing a specific, selective fluctuating motion or transfer of energy in the cranium.[74]

It has been compared with the potency of the tide. Sutherland not only calls the 'potency' in the CSF a fundamental principle in the functioning of the primary respiratory mechanism (PRM) but also explains that the potency in the fluctuation of the CSF can be used for diagnosis and treatment.[75]

The potency in the fluid can be directed (see under 'fluid drive').[74] According to Becker, a potency is at work in bioenergetic fields (by which he means biomechanical, biochemical, bioelectric, biodynamic and other fields) and forms a focus or fulcrum around which these are organized. He defines potency as a functional point of stillness, a fulcrum in the bioenergetic field of the physiology of the body, through, around and by means of which the patterns of activity of the bioenergetic fields manifest themselves.[12]

The potency operates as an organizing factor in the living body. It refers to a principle of organization, an original force, primary in direction, that can be palpated and used, and that is expressed in the primary respiratory mechanism.[76]

Potency acts as an inherent homeostatic force in the bioenergetic fields, which is continually working to maintain and restore the basic pattern of health.[12]

This means that biokinetic energies and potency are simultaneously present in a dysfunction. The potency can vary in its patterns of activity in order to achieve its purpose, the continuous effort to dissipate excessive biokinetic forces to the environment, and to resolve and normalize abnormal tension patterns. If this proves impossible, it strives to keep the limitations to the functioning of the body to the minimum, or to compensate as well as possible for the dysfunction. The potency does so by centering the biokinetic energies.

'There is something that centers disabilities, traumas, and disease within the human anatomicophysiology, that carries the power, the authority, the potency for the pattern for that particular problem'.[77]

The consequences are reduced vitality in this area, the abnormal tensions, motion restrictions and loss of elasticity of the involved tissues.

Sutherland uses this potency at the point of balanced membranous tension and articular release that is found in direct or indirect techniques, disengagement, or molding. The use of leverage increases the 'potency of the fluid energy'.

Jealous describes potency on the one hand as the presence of the breath of life, which he makes responsible for the shaping of all forms in life, a meaning that places it beyond sensory experience.[78] On the other hand he distinguishes two further types of potency:[79]

- a 'sharp' and 'pointed' force that is sensed when directing the tide, or that is sensed in the fluid, in lateral fluctuation. This potency has a 'vectorial' quality and only acts along geometric lines in relation to the form of the body. To palpate this type of potency, therapists must focus their attention on health. Jealous states that the exact positioning of the therapist's hands is extremely important, so as not to impair this type of potency.[80]
- a soft, sweet potency that acts as a healing force in the body. It has a light, airy quality that permeates everything and acts to transmute, working much more slowly than the first kind.[81]

RECIPROCAL TENSION MEMBRANE

Sutherland chose this term to describe the mechanical function of the inner layer of the dura mater, which is a mechanical functional unity.

The reciprocal tension membrane in the cranium is organized around Sutherland's fulcrum and regulates the motion and integrity of the cranial bones. In the spinal canal the tension membrane links and coordinates the motion of the cranium and sacrum.[82,83]

SPEED REDUCER

Some bones in the cranium have a motion that is greater than that of the bones with which they articulate.[84]

Sutherland quotes the sphenoid as an example of this; its motion is greater than that of the palatine bones. These in turn have greater motion than the maxillae. The palatine bones act as mediators. The zygomatic bones are a further example of speed reducers.[85]

The importance of the speed reducers appears to be to integrate the motion of various structures with one another.

STILLNESS

See also Introduction: 'Principles and methods of palpatory diagnosis' and 'Principles and methods of treatment'.

The art of palpation without preconceived ideas can be developed in stillness. Therapists should act as an 'empty vessel', allowing themselves to be touched by the impressions deriving from the patient. Becker expresses a similar idea when he says that we have to learn not to get in the way of – or go out of the way of – the body's problems in our treatment and in our 'listening'.[86]

For Becker, stillness is the key to understanding Sutherland's teaching and the true factor that brings about a change during treatment.[87]

STILL POINT

- Sutherland's fulcrum is a still point around which the tension membranes operate.[88]
- A fulcrum is a still point that enables a weight to be lifted.[89]
- The fulcrum of the cerebrospinal fluid or the point when the fluctuation of the fluid stops is called the 'still point'.[90,91]
- The craniosacral motion stops.[92]

A still point can occur spontaneously, without any external stimulus, or can be induced therapeutically. It can occur suddenly or may emerge gradually, and may be local, regional, or system-wide. Woods and Woods were able to demonstrate the spontaneous stopping of the rhythm in intense emotional experiences, in 1961.[93]

The occurrence of a still point was also registered using electronic measuring equipment.[94]

During the still point, a general relaxation of the body occurs. This enables the body to recover, re-organize and re-integrate itself. Clear vegetative signs may appear. The still point can last from a few seconds to several minutes.

SUTHERLAND'S FULCRUM *(See Fulcrum)*

TIDE

The 'tide' fluctuates like the tides of the sea; not like the motion of the waves but like the ocean. The tide rises during the inspiration phase and ebbs during the expiration phase. It possesses more 'potency' and 'intelligence' than any force applied from outside. For the later Sutherland it was essential to perform treatment, not by applying external force, but by allowing the 'tide' to work.[95] According to Sutherland, the tide can be directed even from a foot, and even without touching it.[96]

A spiral outward motion and spiral inward motion of the tide has been described.[97]

TRANSMUTATION

The transformation from one form, nature, or substance to another.[98]

References

1 Pickler EC, ed. Early impressions of Dr Still. J Am Osteopath Assoc 1921:244.
2 Gaines E, Chila AG. Communication for osteopathic manipulative treatment (OMT): the language of lived experience in OMT pedagogy. J Am Osteopath Assoc 1998; 98(3):164–168.
3 Klein P. Zum mythos der schädelknochenmobilität. Einige überlegungen eines freien osteopathen. Osteop Med 2002; 2:17–20.
4 Sutherland WG. Teachings in the Science of Osteopathy. Sutherland Cranial Teaching Foundation 1991:285.
5 Sutherland WG. Contributions of Thought. Sutherland Cranial Teaching Foundation 1967:142.
6 Sutherland WG. Teachings in the Science of Osteopathy. Sutherland Cranial Teaching Foundation 1991:286.
7 Sutherland WG. Teachings in the Science of Osteopathy. Sutherland Cranial Teaching Foundation 1991:16, 285.
8 Sutherland WG. Contributions of Thought. Sutherland Cranial Teaching Foundation 1967:33.
9 Doucoux B, Liem T. Interview with Jim Jealous. Osteopath Med 2002; 2:26–31.
10 Jealous J. Emergence of originality. A biodynamic view of osteopathy in the cranial field. Course notes; 1997.
11 Becker RE. In: Brooks, RE, ed. The Stillness of Life. Portland: Stillness Press; 2000:75.
12 Becker RE. Diagnostic touch: Its principles and application, Part IV. AAO Yearbook 1965:165–177.
13 Becker RE. In: Brooks RE, ed. The Stillness of Life. Portland: Stillness Press; 2000:114.

14 Becker RE. In: Brooks RE, ed. The Stillness of Life. Portland: Stillness Press; 2000:115, 118.

15 Sutherland WG. Contributions of Thought. 2nd edn. Sutherland Cranial Teaching Foundation 1998:347.

16 Sutherland WG. Contributions of Thought. Sutherland Cranial Teaching Foundation 1967:207.

17 Sutherland WG. Contributions of Thought. 2nd edn. Sutherland Cranial Teaching Foundation 1998:191.

18 Sutherland WG. Teachings in the Science of Osteopathy. Sutherland Cranial Teaching Foundation 1991:14.

19 Sutherland WG. Teachings in the Science of Osteopathy. Sutherland Cranial Teaching Foundation 1991:5.

20 Sutherland WG. Teachings in the Science of Osteopathy. Sutherland Cranial Teaching Foundation 1991:35, 286.

21 Sutherland WG. Contributions of Thought. 2nd edn. Sutherland Cranial Teaching Foundation 1998;147.

22 Becker RE. In: Brooks RE, ed. The Stillness of Life. Portland: Stillness Press; 2000:6.

23 Jealous J. A biodynamic view of osteopathy in the cranial field. Course notes; 1997.

24 Duval JA. Introduction aux Techniques Ostéopathiques d'Équilibre et d'Échanges Réciproques. Paris: Maloine; 1976:23.

25 Becker RE. In: Brooks RE, ed. The Stillness of Life. Portland: Stillness Press; 2000:124.

26 Sutherland WG. Contributions of Thought. Sutherland Cranial Teaching Foundation 1967;99.

27 Magoun HI. Osteopathy in the Cranial Field. 1st edn. Kirksville: Journal Printing Company; 1951:140.

28 Sutherland WG. Contributions of Thought. 2nd edn. Sutherland Cranial Teaching Foundation 1998:224–226, 344, 350.

29 Frymann V. Course notes; 1995.

30 Magoun HI. Osteopathy in the Cranial Field. 3rd edn. Kirksville: Journal Printing Company; 1976:25, 86, 313–323, 340.

31 Magoun HI. Osteopathy in the Cranial Field. 3rd edn. Kirksville: Journal Printing Company; 1976:40

32 Sutherland WG. Contributions of Thought. 2nd edn. Sutherland Cranial Teaching Foundation 1998:298.

33 Sutherland WG. Contributions of Thought. 2nd edn. Sutherland Cranial Teaching Foundation; 1998:215.

34 Sutherland WG. Teachings in the Science of Osteopathy. Sutherland Cranial Teaching Foundation; 1991:13, 166.

35 Sutherland WG. The Cranial Bowl. Mankato, Minnesota: Free Press Company; 1939:56.

36 Sutherland WG. Teachings in the Science of Osteopathy. Sutherland Cranial Teaching Foundation 1991:34.

37 Magoun HI. Osteopathy in the Cranial Field. 1st edn. Kirksville: Journal Printing Company; 1951:16.

38 Magoun HI. Osteopathy in the Cranial Field. 1st edn. Kirksville: Journal Printing Company; 1951:73.

39 Woods JM, Woods RH. A physical finding related to psychiatric disorders. J Am Osteopath Assoc 1961; 60:988–993.

40 Magoun HI. Osteopathy in the Cranial Field. 3rd edn. Kirksville: Journal Printing Company; 1976:25.

41 Becker RE. Craniosacral trauma in the adult. Osteopath Ann 1976; 4:43–59.

42 Lay E. Cranial field. In: Ward RC, ed. Foundations for Osteopathic Medicine. Baltimore: Williams and Wilkins; 1997:901–913.

43 Lay EM, Cicorda RA, Tettambel M. Recording of the cranial rhythmic impulse. J Am Osteopath Assoc 1978; 78:149.

44 Wirth-Patullo V, Hayes KW. Interrater reliability of craniosacral rate measurements and their relationship with subjects' and examiners' heart and respiratory rate measurements. Phys Ther 1994; 67:1526–1532.

45 Nelson KE, Sergueef N, Lipinski CM, Chapman AR, Glonek T. Cranial rhythmic impulse related to the Traube-Hering-Mayer oscillation: comparing laser Doppler flowmetry and palpation. J Am Osteopath Assoc 2001; 101:163–173.

46 Upledger JE, Vredevoogd JD. Craniosacral Therapy. Seattle: Eastland Press; 1983:6, 243.

47 Brooks RE, ed. Life in Motion: The Osteopathic Vision of Rollin E Becker. Portland: Stillness Press; 1997:120.

48 Upledger JE, Vredevoogd JD. Lehrbuch der Kraniosakral-therapie 2. Auflage. Haug; 1994:292.

49 Jealous J. Emergence of originality. Course manual; 1997:12, 35, 36.

50 Brooks RE, ed. Life in Motion: The Osteopathic Vision of Rollin E Becker. Portland: Stillness Press; 1997:122.

51 Liem T. Lecture OFM in Munich: 1998.

52 Lewer-Allen KL, EA Bunt, Lewer-Allen CM. Hydrodynamic Studies of the Human Craniospinal System. London: Janus Publishing Company; 2000:5.

53 Sutherland WG. Contributions of Thought. Sutherland Cranial Teaching Foundation 1967:153, 208, 244.

54 Sutherland WG. Teachings in the Science of Osteopathy. Sutherland Cranial Teaching Foundation 1991; 14, 46.

55 Sutherland WG. Contributions of Thought. 2nd edn. Sutherland Cranial Teaching Foundation 1998:238.

56 Becker RE. Be still and know. A dedication to William G. Sutherland DO. Cranial Academy Newsletter 1965; 12:6.

57 Sutherland WG. Contributions of Thought. Sutherland Cranial Teaching Foundation 1967:215.

58 Becker RE. In: Brooks RE, ed. The Stillness of Life. Portland: Stillness Press; 2000:8.

59 Magoun HI. Osteopathy in the Cranial Field. 1st edn. Kirksville: Journal Printing Company; 1951:15.

60 Sutherland WG. Teachings in the Science of Osteopathy. Sutherland Cranial Teaching Foundation 1991:32, 55, 166, 176.

61 Cranial Academy. The Cranial Letter. Cranial Academy; 1994:7.

62 Sutherland WG. Teachings in the Science of Osteopathy. Sutherland Cranial Teaching Foundation 1991:119–122.

63 Sutherland WG. Contributions of Thought. 2nd edn. Sutherland Cranial Teaching Foundation 1998:80.

64 Sutherland WG. Contributions of Thought. Sutherland Cranial Teaching Foundation 1967:137.

65 Magoun HI. Osteopathy in the Cranial Field. 1st edn. Kirksville: Journal Printing Company; 1951:70, 118, 123.

66 Becker RE. Force factors with body physiology. AAO-year book; 1959:89–97.

67 Magoun HI. Osteopathy in the Cranial Field. 1st edn. Kirksville: Journal Printing Company; 1951:68.

68 Sutherland WG. Contributions of Thought. 2nd edn. Sutherland Cranial Teaching Foundation 1998:349.

69 Sutherland WG. Teachings in the Science of Osteopathy. Sutherland Cranial Teaching Foundation 1991:14, 16.

70 Sutherland WG. Contributions of Thought. Sutherland Cranial Teaching Foundation 1967:143.

71 Becker RE. In: Brooks RE, ed. The Stillness of Life. Portland: Stillness Press; 2000:80.

72 Becker RE. In: Brooks RE, ed. The Stillness of Life. Portland: Stillness Press; 2000:84.

73 Magoun HI. Osteopathy in the Cranial Field. 1st edn. Kirksville: Journal Printing Company; 1951:72.

74 Magoun HI. Osteopathy in the Cranial Field. 1st edn. Kirksville: Journal Printing Company; 1951:59.

75 Sutherland WG. Contributions of Thought. 2nd edn. Sutherland Cranial Teaching Foundation 1998:220, 239.

76 Duval JA. Introduction aux Techniques Ostéopathiques d'Équilibre et d'Échanges Réciproques. Paris: Maloine; 1976:20.

77 Becker RE. In: Brooks RE, ed. The Stillness of Life. Portland: Stillness Press; 2000:121.

78 Jealous J. A biodynamic view of osteopathy in the cranial field. Course manual; 1997:104.

79 Jealous J. The Biodynamics of Osteopathy. CV-4. no.2 (audio CD series). Marnee Jealous Long, 6501 Blackfin Way, Apollo Beach, FL 33572: USA. mjlong@tampabay.IT.com. 2001.

80 Jealous J. A biodynamic view of osteopathy in the cranial field. Course manual; 1997:104.

81 Jealous J. A biodynamic view of osteopathy in the cranial field. Course manual; 1997:106.

82 Sutherland WG. Teachings in the Science of Osteopathy. Sutherland Cranial Teaching Foundation 1991:289.

83 Magoun HI. Osteopathy in the Cranial Field. 3rd edn. Kirksville: Journal Printing Company; 1976:343.

84 Magoun HI. Osteopathy in the Cranial Field. 3rd edn. Kirksville: Journal Printing Company; 1976:347.

85 Sutherland WG. Teachings in the Science of Osteopathy. Sutherland Cranial Teaching Foundation 1991:78.

86 Becker RE. In: Brooks RE, ed. The Stillness of Life. Portland: Stillness Press; 2000:15, 16.

87 Becker RE. In: Brooks RE, ed. The Stillness of Life. Portland: Stillness Press; 2000:66, 67.

88 Sutherland WG. Teachings in the Science of Osteopathy. Sutherland Cranial Teaching Foundation 1991:18.

89 Sutherland WG. Teachings in the Science of Osteopathy. Sutherland Cranial Teaching Foundation 1991:46.

90 Sutherland WG. Teachings in the Science of Osteopathy. Sutherland Cranial Teaching Foundation 1991:135.

91 Sutherland WG. Contributions of Thought. 2nd edn. Sutherland Cranial Teaching Foundation 1998:342, 348.

92 Upledger JE, Vredevoogd JD. Craniosacral Therapy. Seattle: Eastland Press; 1983:40.

93 Woods JM, Woods RH. A physical finding related to psychiatric disorders. J Am Osteopath Assoc 1961; 60:988.

94 Upledger JE, Karni Z. Mechanical electric patterns during craniosacral osteopathic diagnosis and treatment. J Am Osteopath Assoc 1979; 78:782–791.

95 Sutherland WG. Teachings in the Science of Osteopathy. Sutherland Cranial Teaching Foundation 1991:14, 166.

96 Sutherland WG. Teachings in the Science of Osteopathy. Sutherland Cranial Teaching Foundation 1991:168.

97 Sutherland WG. Teachings in the Science of Osteopathy. Sutherland Cranial Teaching Foundation 1991:16.

98 Sutherland WG. Teachings in the Science of Osteopathy. Sutherland Cranial Teaching Foundation 1991:290.

Index

Printed and bound by CPI Group (UK) Ltd, Croydon, CR0 4YY

03/10/2024

01040345-0016